Safe and Healthy School Environments

Safe and Healthy School Environments

EDITED BY

Howard Frumkin, M.D., Dr.P.H.
Robert J. Geller, M.D.
I. Leslie Rubin, M.D.

WITH

Janice Nodvin

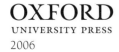

OXFORD
UNIVERSITY PRESS
2006

OXFORD
UNIVERSITY PRESS

Oxford University Press, Inc., publishes works that further
Oxford University's objective of excellence
in research, scholarship, and education.

Oxford   New York
Auckland   Cape Town   Dar es Salaam   Hong Kong   Karachi
Kuala Lumpur   Madrid   Melbourne   Mexico City   Nairobi
New Delhi   Shanghai   Taipei   Toronto

With offices in
Argentina   Austria   Brazil   Chile   Czech Republic   France   Greece
Guatemala   Hungary   Italy   Japan   Poland   Portugal   Singapore
South Korea   Switzerland   Thailand   Turkey   Ukraine   Vietnam

Copyright © 2006 by Oxford University Press, Inc.

Published by Oxford University Press, Inc.
198 Madison Avenue, New York, New York 10016

www.oup.com

Oxford is a registered trademark of Oxford University Press

Library of Congress Cataloging-in-Publication Data
Safe and healthy school environments / Howard Frumkin . . . [et al.].
        p.   cm.
    Includes bibliographical references and index.
    ISBN-13 978-0-19-517947-7
    ISBN 0-19-517947-1
    1. School hygiene—United States.   2. School environment—United States.
3. Schools—United States—Safety measures.   I. Frumkin, Howard.
    [DNLM: 1. Environmental Health—Child—United States.   2. Schools—
organization & administration—United States.   3. Safety Management—
organization & administration—Child—United States.   4. Environmental Pollution—
prevention & control—United States.   5. Food Services—organization &
administration—Child—United States.
WA 30 S128 2006]
LB3409.U5S23 2006
371.7'1—dc22   2005025173

9 8 7 6 5 4 3 2 1

Printed in the United States of America
on acid-free paper

Foreword

Children spend much of their life at school. They are at school to learn the skills they will need for life, to form the foundation that will determine the course of their future, and to develop values and social skills. Schools are building the citizens of the world of tomorrow. Although school districts strive to create environments that are nurturing, safe, and conducive for learning, many school buildings fall far short. They are antiquated, in need of renovation, and sometimes understaffed.

Children are vulnerable. They depend on parents and other adults placed in positions of responsibility for their well-being, their education, their transportation from place to place, their food and shelter, and their health care. These adults need to be advocates for children.

This book is the first to address the school setting utilizing the principles of environmental health. Written by leading experts in topics from noise to crowding, from indoor air quality to safety, from building design to crime prevention, from managing illness at school to accommodating individuals with disabilities, this book explores key topics and applies an evidence-based approach to each. It reviews the evidence we have and points out issues remaining unresolved. The authors present steps that could be taken to address shortcomings that may be present at a school and to help prioritize among them.

This book is important reading for everyone who designs schools, leads them, works at them, or attends them. Parents, teachers, school administrators, and school board members will all find the material presented current yet firmly founded on the best available information. Readers of all types will find this book a valuable reference to have at hand.

Jay Berkelhamer, MD, FAAP
Senior Vice President for Medical Affairs
Children's Healthcare of Atlanta
Atlanta, Georgia

Acknowledgments

Assembling a book like *Safe and Healthy School Environments* is first and foremost an expression of dedication—to the well-being of children at school, and to the well-being of the teachers and other staff members who work in schools. We feel that commitment deeply, and we are keenly aware that many other people, without whose support this book could not have been completed, exemplify the same dedication.

We came together under the auspices of the Pediatric Environmental Health Specialty Unit at Emory University, which serves the southeast region. PEHSUs are responsible for providing technical assistance and information to parents, health care providers, agency officials, and others, regarding children's environmental health. Over the years, we received many inquiries regarding school environments, and it was these inquiries that led us to assemble this book. We thank all the concerned parents, members of Boards of Education, teachers, administrators, and others, who helped us understand the importance of the school environment and who alerted us to their concerns.

We thank the fine professionals at the U.S. Environmental Protection Agency who have championed the field of Children's Environmental Health.

Here in Region 4, we thank Wayne Garfinkel, who coordinates Children's Environmental Health activities, and Dee Rogers-Smith, a long-time supporter of this work. We thank the entire staff of the Office of Children's Health Protection (http://yosemite .epa.gov/ochp/ochpweb.nsf/homepage) in Washington, DC, directed over the last few years successively by Ramona Trovato, Joanne Rodman, and Bill Sanders. We also thank the National Center for Environmental Health and Agency for Toxic Substances and Disease Registry at the Centers for Disease Control and Prevention, which have joined EPA in generously supporting the Pediatric Environmental Health Specialty Units (PEHSUs). And we thank the staff of the Association of Occupational and Environmental Clinics (AOEC), especially Kathy Kirkland and Paula Wilborne-Davis, who work with EPA and NCEH/ATSDR to administer the PEHSUs. In supporting the activities of our PEHSU and others around the nation, including projects such as the completion of this book, these individuals and agencies make enormous contributions to advancing the health and safety of America's children.

We thank our chapter authors, all of them exceedingly busy people, who generously agreed to contribute chapters, accepted our editorial suggestions with grace and professionalism, and tolerated our nagging with good humor.

We thank Janice Nodvin, Project Manager of the Southeast Pediatric Environmental Health Specialty Unit, who has contributed her insight as a former teacher, a mother, and a champion for children with disabilities to every step in the book's preparation. We thank Hope Jackson, who served as editorial assistant on this book during her transition between Emory College and George Washington University medical school (where she will be an asset to our sister PEHSU in Region 3). Hope managed hundreds of files and thousands of tasks big and small with skill and professionalism. On her departure, Hope's responsibilities were assumed by Leslie Greene, who skillfully brought the project to completion with grace, poise, and perseverance. We also thank the dedicated and hardworking staff, past and present, in Emory's Department of Environmental and Occupational Health—especially Robin Thompson, Adrienne Tison, Erica Weaver, Rachel Wilson, and Suzanne Mason—who have directly and indirectly supported the work of the PEHSU. We also recognize with gratitude the contributions of the staff of Emory's Department of Pediatrics, especially Vanessa Walker, Janis Wright, Adam Castellaw, and Renee Dunbar-Scott.

We thank our PEHSU friend and colleague Dr. Gerald Teague, M.D. Clinical responsibilities kept Gerry from collaborating extensively on this book, but his early contributions to the concept were critical, and his return to full PEHSU participation toward the end of the book project delighted us all.

We thank the members of our Editorial Advisory Committee, who provided numerous comments and suggestions, especially during the early stages of the project when we were defining the scope of the book. These individuals are listed on page xvii with institutional affiliations for identification purposes only.

We thank our counterparts at the other PEHSUs across the nation and abroad. In meetings, in telephone consultations, in e-mail exchanges, and in publications, they have shared many of our concerns and have helped build our understanding of the issues discussed in this book.

At many of our editorial work sessions, we were joined by students, residents, and fellows from Emory and Morehouse who were on various clinical rotations. These young people contributed insightful comments and questions, and we thank them for keeping us on our toes. We hope to have inspired them with a lifelong commitment to safe and healthy environments for children.

Finally, we thank our families—Beryl, Gabe, and Amara; Janice and Ken; and Barbara, Justine, Mandy and Tiran, Laila, Xandy, and Mikayla—who put up with early departures for morning meetings, late arrivals from evening meetings, and innumerable other signs that this book was competing with family time. We thank our wives for being wonderful mothers, and we thank our children for teaching us, each and every day, the wonder of the next generation and reminding us of the mandate to bequeath them a safe, healthy world.

Contents

Contributors

Darryl Alexander, M.S.
Director, Occupational Health and Safety
American Federation of Teachers
Washington, DC

Stephen Ashkin
President, The Ashkin Group, LLC—The Green
  Cleaning Experts
Bloomington, IN

Jennifer Audi, M.D.
Assistant Professor of Emergency Medicine
University of Nebraska Medical Center
Omaha, NE

Robert Axelrad
Senior Policy Advisor, Indoor Environments
  Division
U.S. Environmental Protection Agency
Washington, DC

Angelo J. Bellomo, M.S., Q.E.P.
Director, Office of Environmental Health
  and Safety
Los Angeles Unified School District
Los Angeles, CA

Cheryl Bennett, M.S.
Chair, International Ergonomics Association,
  Ergonomics for Children and Educational
  Environments Technical Committee, and Youth
  Ergonomics Strategies Foundation
Livermore, CA

Linda B. Crider, Ph.D.
Program Director, Traffic and Bicycle Safety
  Education Program
University of Florida
Gainesville, FL

Charles Eley, F.A.I.A., P.E.
Vice President, Architectural Energy Corporation
Collaborative for High Performance Schools
San Francisco, CA

Richard Ellis, J.D.
Senior Project Manager, The Ashkin Group,
  LLC—The Green Cleaning Experts
Bloomington, IN

Barbara Erwine
Private Consultant
Seattle, WA

Howard Frumkin, M.D., Dr.P.H.
Professor and Chair, Environmental and
    Occupational Health
Rollins School of Public Health of Emory
    University
(Currently Director, National Center for Environ-
    mental Health and Agency for Toxic Substances
    and Disease Registry, U.S. Centers for Disease
    Control and Prevention, Atlanta, GA)

Robert J. Geller, M.D.
Director, Emory Southeast Pediatric
    Environmental Health Specialty Unit
Medical Director, Georgia Poison Center at Grady
    Health System
Associate Professor of Pediatrics, Emory University
    School of Medicine
Atlanta, GA

Kathy Gips
Director of Training, Adaptive Environments, Inc.
Boston, MA

Amanda Hall, M.H.S.E.
Assistant Program Director, Traffic and Bicycle
    Safety Education Program
University of Florida
Gainesville, FL

Chinonye Harvey, M.P.H., M.T.(A.S.C.P.)
Research Associate and Project Coordinator,
    Mid-Atlantic Center for Children's Health and
    the Environment
The George Washington University School of
    Public Health and Health Services
Washington, DC

Andrea Hricko, M.P.H.
Associate Professor of Preventive Medicine, Keck
    School of Medicine
University of Southern California
Los Angeles, CA

Jouni J.K. Jaakkola, M.D., D.Sc., Ph.D.
Professor and Director, Institute of Occupational
    and Environmental Medicine
University of Birmingham
Birmingham, United Kingdom

Hope T. Jackson
Former Research Assistant, Emory Southeast
    Pediatric Environmental Health Specialty Unit

Former Study Coordinator, Division of Pulmonary
    Medicine
Department of Pediatrics
Emory University School of Medicine
Atlanta, GA

Harry L. Keyserling, M.D.
Professor of Pediatrics, Division of Infectious
    Diseases, Epidemiology and Immunology
Emory University School of Medicine
Atlanta, GA

Nicole Larson, M.P.H., R.D.
Division of Epidemiology and Community Health
University of Minnesota School of Public Health
Minneapolis, MN

Julia Graham Lear, Ph.D.
Research Professor, Department of Prevention and
    Community Health
School of Public Health and Health Services
Director, Center for Health and Health Care in
    Schools
The George Washington University
Washington, DC

David L. Marshall, M.D.
Medical Director, Sports Medicine Program
Children's Healthcare of Atlanta
Clinical Assistant Professor, Department of
    Pediatrics
Emory University School of Medicine
Atlanta, GA

Lorraine E. Maxwell, Ph.D.
Associate Professor and Director of
    Graduate Studies
Department of Design and Environmental Analysis
Cornell University
Ithaca, NY

Robin Moore, M.C.P., Dipl. Arch.
Professor of Landscape Architecture, College of
    Design
Director, The Natural Learning Initiative
North Carolina State University
Raleigh, NC

David Mudarri, Ph.D.
Senior Economist, Indoor Environments Division
U.S. Environmental Protection Agency
Washington, DC

Janice Nodvin
Project Administrator, Emory Southeast Pediatric
    Environmental Health Specialty Unit
Emory University
Atlanta, GA

Jerome Paulson, M.D.
Associate Professor of Pediatrics and Public Health
Co-Director, Mid-Atlantic Center for Children's
    Health and the Environment
The George Washington University
Washington, DC

Troy Pierce, Ph.D.
Pesticides Section, Region 4
U.S. Environmental Protection Agency
Atlanta, GA

H. Douglas Robertson, Ph.D., P.E.
Former Director, Highway Safety Research Center
University of North Carolina
Chapel Hill, NC

I. Leslie Rubin, M.D.
Visiting Scholar, Department of Pediatrics
Morehouse School of Medicine
President, Institute for the Study of Disadvantage
    and Disability
Medical Director, the Team Centers
Participating Physician, Emory Southeast Pediatric
    Environmental Health Specialty Unit
Atlanta, GA

Tod Schneider, M.S.
Crime Prevention Specialist, Eugene Police
    Department
National Consultant, Safe, Healthy and Positive
    Environmental Design for Schools
Eugene, OR

Jeannie Sneed, Ph.D., R.D., C.F.S.P., S.F.N.S.
Professor of Hotel, Restaurant and Institution
    Management

Department of Apparel, Educational Studies, and
    Hospitality Management
Iowa State University
Ames, IA

Mary Story, Ph.D., R.D.
Professor, Division of Epidemiology and
    Community Health
Associate Dean of Academic and Student Affairs
University of Minnesota School of Public Health
Minneapolis, MN

W. Gerald Teague, M.D.
Professor of Pediatrics
Director, Emory Pediatrics Asthma Research
    Center
Emory University School of Medicine
Participating Physician, Emory Southeast Pediatric
    Environmental Health Specialty Unit
Emory University
Atlanta, GA

Diane Tien
Technology Specialist, Family Learning Center
Lake Washington School District
Redmond, WA

Jeffrey C. Tsai, M.S.
Director, School Transportation Group
The Institute for Transportation Research and
    Education
North Carolina State University
Raleigh, NC

Sandra S. West, Ph.D.
Associate Professor of Biology
Texas State University
San Marcos, TX

Andree Woodcock, Ph.D.
Senior Research Fellow, Coventry School of Art
    and Design
Coventry University
Coventry, UK

Editorial Advisory Committee

Darryl Alexander, M.S.
Director, Occupational Health and Safety
American Federation of Teachers

Robert Axelrad
Senior Policy Advisor, Indoor Environments
  Division
U.S. Environmental Protection Agency

Sophie Balk, M.D.
Attending Pediatrician, Children's Hospital at
  Montefiore
Professor of Clinical Pediatrics, Albert Einstein
  College of Medicine

Angelo Bellomo, M.S., Q.E.P.
Director, Office of Environmental Health and Safety
Los Angeles Unified School District

Jim Bogden
Project Director, Safe and Healthy Schools Project
National Association of State Boards of Education

William A. Brenner, A.I.A.
Vice President, National Institute of Building
  Sciences

Director, National Clearinghouse for Educational
  Facilities

Leslie C. Campbell, M.S.
Environmental Health Scientist
Agency for Toxic Substances and Disease Registry

Daniel L. Duke, Ed.D.
Professor of Educational Leadership and Research
  Director for the Darden-Curry Partnership for
  Leaders in Education
University of Virginia

Lloyd J. Kolbe, Ph.D.
Professor of Applied Health Science, Indiana
  University
Former founding Director, Division of Adolescent
  and School Health
U.S. Centers for Disease Control and Prevention

Julia Graham Lear, Ph.D.
Director, Center for Health and Health Care in
  Schools
The George Washington University

David K. Lohrmann, Ph.D., C.H.E.S.
Past-President, American School Health Association
Associate Professor of Applied Health Science
Indiana University

William Modzeleski
Associate Assistant Deputy Secretary, Office of
    Safe and Drug Free Schools
U.S. Department of Education

Rabbi Daniel J. Swartz
Former Executive Director, Children's Environ-
    mental Health Network

Coordinator, Greater Washington Interfaith Power
    and Light

Elizabeth Sword
Former Executive Director, Children's Health En-
    vironmental Coalition

Howard Taras, M.D.
Professor of Pediatrics, University of California,
    San Diego
American Academy of Pediatrics; Council on
    School Health

Safe and Healthy School Environments

Howard Frumkin

Introduction

In the United States, more than 48 million students attend 94,000 public elementary, middle, and secondary schools each day (Hoffman 2003; Wirt et al. 2004), and an additional 5.3 million students attend 30,000 private schools (Broughman and Pugh 2005). Children spend more time in schools than in any other environment except their home. In addition, more than 4.7 million teachers and hundreds of thousands of administrators, janitors, food service workers, security guards, and other personnel staff these schools.

Schools are unique environments in many ways. No other category of building can claim to house one in five Americans every day. In virtually no other settings do people spend extended periods of time in such close quarters; the average school has an occupant density somewhere between those of prisons and commercial airplanes and several times that of the average workplace. Few other buildings house such a wide variety of functions, from education to athletics to health care to food preparation and even to automobile repair and chemical processes.

But the most important feature of schools is that we send our children there to learn—to learn reading and writing and mathematics and sciences, to learn values and social skills, to prepare for their

futures, to become all that they can be. It is no exaggeration to say that schools harbor our collective dreams for the future: they are the places where values are passed on, technical solutions originate, and the world of tomorrow is shaped. These high expectations stand in sharp contrast to the realities of many school environments. In a nation of gleaming office buildings, sumptuous gated communities, and luxurious shopping malls, many of our schools do not measure up.

Research by the U.S. General Accounting Office in the mid-1990s (GAO 1995, 1996a, 1996b) described the conditions of U.S. schools in detail. The GAO found that one in three schools had buildings in need of extensive repair or replacement, and almost 60 percent reported one major building feature that needed extensive repairs, an overhaul, or replacement. In addition, about half of the schools reported at least one unsatisfactory environmental condition such as poor ventilation, heating or lighting problems, or poor physical security. There were schools in warm climates without functioning air-conditioning, schools in cold climates without adequate heating systems, and schools across the country without good lighting. The report documented overcrowded schools, noisy schools, and schools with blatant safety hazards. One example provided was a school ceiling that had been weakened by leaking water and that collapsed just 40 minutes after students left the building. Media reports have continued to reveal such incidents: an elementary school in Cleveland discovered hidden structural problems in the roof after a ceiling leak was noted (Okoben, 2006); a ceiling collapsed in an elementary school in Mechanicville, New York, injuring a fourth-grade teacher (NY Teacher, 1999); and a 30-foot by 30-foot section of the roof of an elementary school in Christina, Delaware, collapsed after accumulation of snow and ice (Christina School District, 2003). In the GAO reports, most problems were not isolated; a school with one problem often had multiple problems.

Later research by the U.S. Department of Education (2000) found similar results. Nearly half the schools in this study also reported at least one environmental factor in unsatisfactory condition: ventilation in 26%, acoustics or noise control in 18%, indoor air quality in 18%, heating in 17%, and lighting in 12%. Ongoing research has continued to corroborate these findings. For example, a recent review of air quality in schools revealed that inadequate ventilation, excessive levels of carbon dioxide, volatile organic compounds, bioaerosols, bacteria, dust mites, and animal allergens are common (Daisey et al. 2003). Conditions such as these pose both short-term and long-term threats to children's health and productivity and may translate into health-care costs as well.

Courts and the U.S. Congress have recognized that high-quality learning environments are crucial to educating children well. One court defined "decent facilities" as those that are "structurally safe, contain fire safety measures, sufficient exits, an adequate and safe water supply, an adequate sewage disposal system, sufficient and sanitary toilet facilities and plumbing fixtures, adequate storage, adequate light, [are] in good repair and attractively painted as well as contain acoustics for noise control" (*Pauley v. Kelly,* 1982; *Edgewood Independent School District v. Kirby,* 1987). In passing the Education Infrastructure Act of 1994 (an act that was never implemented), Congress recognized that "improving the quality of public elementary and secondary schools will help our Nation meet the National Education Goals."

The public health field has also long recognized that wholesome environments are necessary for people's health, safety, and well-being. Indeed, historic efforts by public health officials have helped rescue Americans from many hazards: Fresh water systems have been constructed, sewage treatment facilities built, safer roads engineered, air pollution emissions controlled, and toxic exposures ended, all in order to protect health. Traditional sanitarian functions, still performed in most health departments, include oversight of sewage systems and food establishments, as well as conditions in facilities such as nursing homes and control of vector-borne diseases. However, environmental health does not stop there. Modern environmental health professionals are also concerned with exposures to indoor and ambient air pollutants, toxic substances such as lead and pesticides, and safety hazards. Environmental health, broadly defined, addresses the health and safety of air, water, food, waste materials, transportation, building design, and many other aspects of the places people live, work, play, and learn (Frumkin 2005).

This book applies the perspectives of environmental health to a critically important environment: our schools. We take a broad approach. The school environment, in our view, is the totality of what surrounds students not only in the classroom but also on the playing fields, in the cafeteria, and on their way to and from school. It includes obvious factors such as noise, light, and air quality, as well as less obvious factors such as the "food environment" (e.g., what food choices confront students at school), environmental factors that affect crime, and the walkability of the neighborhood between home and school.

We begin in chapters 2 through 9 by addressing the physical environment—factors such as crowding, lighting, noise, temperature, the biomechanical challenges of backpacks and furniture, animals in schools, playground design, and other safety hazards. Next, in chapters 10 through 12, we deal with indoor and ambient air quality, with special attention to mold, a topic of recent concern. In chapters 13 through 15 we move to toxic hazards such as pesticides and cleaning materials. Subsequent chapters address other aspects of school environments: food selection and preparation (chapters 16 and 17); sports facilities (chapter 18); environmental factors relevant to crime prevention (chapter 19); emergency management (chapter 20); and school travel (chapters 21 and

22). In chapter 23 we introduce the concept of high-performance schools, which blend health, performance, environmental, and economic considerations. Finally, chapters 24 through 30 provide guidance on practical approaches to achieving safe and healthy school environments through programs such as school environment audits and health services.

The vision that motivates this book is simple: it is a vision of safe, healthy schools in which children can feel well, learn and play safely, thrive, and reach their full potential and in which teachers and staff can perform effectively without fear of work-related injury or illness. Accordingly, the mission of this book is to provide a practical tool to help make that vision a reality.

Themes of This Book

Throughout the book, several themes recur—ideas that we believe are central to achieving safe and healthful school environments. We describe them in the following pages.

Children Are Not Just Little Adults

In recent years scientists have increasingly realized that children are especially vulnerable to the effects of hazardous environmental exposures (Gitterman and Bearer 2001; Landrigan et al. 2004). Their organ systems are developing, especially during the younger years, making them susceptible to developmental toxins such as lead (Weiss 2000). Children breathe more air, eat more food, and drink more water per pound of body weight than do adults. Certain behaviors, such as tactile exploration and hand-to-mouth contact, increase the probability of some exposures. As a result, environmental health scientists and regulators have recognized the need to exercise special caution in protecting children from potentially hazardous exposures—setting margins of safety to minimize children's exposures, avoiding the use of potentially toxic chemicals near children, and so on (National Research Council 1993; Lanphear et al. 2005). Because the school is a child's environment for much of the day, this same sense of vigilance and care is clearly appropriate.

School Is an Opportunity to Promote Health

In the same way that schools merit special concern because of children's vulnerability, schools present an unparalleled opportunity to promote children's health. Healthy school environments reduce risks of respiratory illness, injury, musculoskeletal pain, and other ailments. In a more positive sense, wholesome school environments promote health and well-being in many ways. For example, environmental cues at school can result in healthier eating habits (Perry et al. 2004; chapter 17). Similarly, when schools are small, sited in relatively dense residential neighborhoods, and located close to children's homes and when the route to school is relatively free of heavy traffic, children are more likely to walk or bike to class (Dellinger and Staunton 2002; Braza, et al. 2004; chapter 22). The school environment (together with curriculum content and programming) sends important signals to students, providing rich opportunities to promote their health.

A Team Approach Is Critical

Throughout this book, the importance of a team approach to safe and healthy school environments is emphasized. Schools are complex social systems with many stakeholders. Safe and wholesome school environments are not accomplished by a few school administrators alone, even if they are energetic, popular, and visionary. Nor can a few parents or students do it by themselves. Administrators, parents, staff, neighbors, students, health-care providers, and others need to work together. In particular, people need to collaborate across different professions, disciplines, and administrative boundaries—cafeteria personnel and custodians, science teachers, coaches, principals, and bus drivers. Even for problems whose solutions seem purely technical—say, an improved heating/ventilating/air-conditioning (HVAC) system—planning, funding, installation, maintenance, and monitoring work best with a team approach. One example of this tactic is the Monroe Method for implementing integrated pest management in schools, which is described in chapter 13.

Adult Involvement and Presence Are Also Critical

Again and again the chapters of this book offer examples of the positive influence of involved adults. During the transportation of children to school, the most hazardous modes of travel are those in which the children are in control (especially when they are driving), and the safest are those in which adults are in control (chapter 21). In designing school environments for crime prevention, an adult presence is a strong deterrent to improper behavior by students (chapter 19). Comedian Woody Allen is said to have observed that "Eighty percent of success is just showing up." If parents, teachers, administrators, and other adults "just show up," they help by their presence to achieve safe and healthy school environments.

Teachers have a special role: They not only teach but they also model attitudes and behaviors for students. Teachers can take the lead in promoting safe and healthy school environments by learning about them, taking steps to prevent or control hazards, and demonstrating to students the importance of these initiatives.

Resources Are Limited

No school has all the resources it needs to pay its teachers and staff, educate its children, and improve its physical plant. If a school cannot afford a deluxe approach, optimizing every aspect of the school environment, then a more selective method may be necessary. Schools can set priorities by systematically addressing needs and opportunities. What are the major safety and health hazards present in the school? (Chapter 25 provides a structured approach to answering this question.) For each danger, what are the options for addressing it, what are the associated costs, and how much benefit can be expected? (Chapter 24 discusses cost-benefit analysis of school environmental interventions.) It is important to consider intangible costs and benefits such as community confidence in the school and the value of student and staff comfort. It is also essential to analyze limited resources in a long-term context. In high-performance schools, discussed in chapter 23, an initial investment that may seem prohibitively expensive can pay for itself in a few years, so the frugal decision may at times call for spending more money. In any event, limited resources are a reality everywhere, and schools must nonetheless remain dedicated to improving school safety and health, using available funds strategically and wisely.

Important Benefits Sometimes Compete with Each Other

Setting priorities and making difficult decisions may also be necessary for reasons other than budget limitations. Sometimes two legitimate and valuable goals seem to collide. For example, getting to school on foot or by bicycle provides the enormous health benefits of physical activity, but in areas with heavy traffic and no sidewalks, those modes of travel may place children at risk of injuries from traffic (see chapters 21 and 22). On playgrounds, children need equipment and surfaces that minimize the risk of injuries, but if playgrounds are overly designed and regimented, children may miss out on developmentally important opportunities to explore and take risks (see chapter 8). In our quest to create safe and healthy school environments, real benefits sometimes compete with other real benefits, and the two need to be carefully and thoughtfully balanced.

Progress Occurs in Steps

Creating safe and healthy schools is a step-by-step process. If resource limitations prevent addressing all safety and health concerns immediately, schools should identify those issues that can be managed in the short term, deal with them, and plan for additional improvements over the long term. No school was built in a day, and no set of problems can be solved overnight, but with sustained dedication, we can achieve safe and healthy school environments.

Policymaking Is Complex

Many school districts and individual schools have policies that promote safe and healthy school environments. In some cases they develop these strategies independently, while in other cases policies are enacted to comply with state or federal mandates. According to the School Health Policies and Programs Study (SHPPS) 2000, conducted by the Centers for Disease Control and Prevention (CDC), some policies are far more common than others

Table 1.1. Proportion of schools with policies for regular inspection and maintenance of equipment and facilities

Type of policy	Schools (%)
Fire extinguishers	99.3
Inspection or maintenance of halls, stairs, and regular classrooms	96.6
Inspection or maintenance of indoor athletic facilities and equipment	95.5
Inspection or maintenance of kitchen facilities and equipment	96.6
Inspection or maintenance of outdoor athletic facilities and equipment	94.8
Inspection or maintenance of playground facilities or equipment	94.8
Inspection or maintenance of school buses or other student transport vehicles	98.4
Inspection or maintenance of special classroom areas (e.g., chemistry labs, workshops, art rooms)	80.8
Lighting inside the buildings	97.5
Lighting outside the buildings	94.6

From School Health Policies and Programs Study, 2000 (Everett Jones et al. 2003).

(Everett Jones, et al. 2003; see tables 1.1 and 1.2). For example, although the majority of schools have policies that call for regular inspection and maintenance of fire extinguishers, kitchens, and other facilities, few schools have programs that develop safe routes to school.

As schools determine the steps they need to take to ensure safe and healthy learning environments, they can enact relevant policies. Examples of such guidelines and sources of further information are provided throughout the chapters of this book. In January 2006, the EPA Healthy Schools web site (http://cfpub.epa.gov/schools/index.cfm) was expanded and now presents extensive information on many of these issues. We encourage concerned parents and school individuals to utilize the web site as a valuable complement to this book.

There Is Opportunity in Synergy

If actions produce many kinds of benefits, those actions are easier to justify, support, and fund. A safe and healthy school environment does more than benefit student health; it also improves academic performance and morale. It does more than-

Table 1.2. Proportion of schools with policies, programs, and facilities related to a healthy school environment

Policies, programs, and facilities	Elementary schools (%)	Middle/junior high schools (%)	High schools (%)
Requires uniforms or dress code	82.1	93.5	88.3
Uses communication devices	80.7	78.0	80.1
Designates a weapons-free school zone	24.4	21.2	25.8
Has a safe-routes-to-school program	16.4	13.0	8.1
Prohibits all tobacco use	47.8	41.9	49.4
Prohibits tobacco advertising	91.3	91.1	91.2
Designates a tobacco-free school zone	43.2	38.6	46.5
Designates a drug-free school zone	53.3	48.1	49.4
No junk food available before or during school hours	60.9	34.4	5.7
No soft drink contract or bans soft drink advertising	88.2	77.2	56.4
Does not promote junk food	66.2	65.8	59.3
Has a cafeteria	88.6	91.7	93.6
Cafeteria operates at or below capacity at peak mealtimes	98.5	96.0	92.6
Has a sickroom	84.8	75.4	78.6
Has supplies for universal precautions	36.9	34.6	36.8
Has a private room for providing mental health and social services	90.7	88.7	96.2
Has indoor or outdoor physical education facilities	100.0	100.0	99.6

From School Health Policies and Programs Study (2000); Everett Jones et al. (2003).

protect students; it also safeguards teachers and staff. If we extend this line of thought, it becomes clear that a high-performance school (chapter 23) does more than benefit the people in the school; it also contributes to the environment and helps control costs. It is important to recognize all the advantages of a safe and healthy school environment, to garner support from many stakeholders, and to promote beneficial policies and actions accordingly.

It's Not Just about Students

This is a key example of synergy. Much of the emphasis throughout this book is on students' health and performance, but the school environment affects teachers, administrators, and staff as well. In fact, the occupational health model (discussed in chapter 30) is based on the notion that people who go to work every day deserve the assurance of a safe and healthful workplace—a notion that is parallel to the goal of safe, healthy schools for students. Certainly, children bring special susceptibilities to school owing to their age and other factors, but so do adults. For example, teachers spend much of the day on their feet, are subject to high-stress demands, and may be exposed to noise, poor indoor-air quality, and other hazards, while custodians may have to handle unsafe chemicals or machinery. Safe and healthy schools offer important benefits not only for students but also for the adults who work there.

Common Problems Need More Attention

Catastrophic news sometimes seems to dominate the newspapers, radio, and television. For instance, the tragic shootings at Columbine High School (Littleton, Colorado, 1999) and at Red Lake Senior High School (Red Lake Reservation, Minnesota, 2005) were extensively discussed in news coverage and on the Internet in tones that at times suggested a tidal wave of school violence. However, statistical data tell a different story. As chapter 19 points out, schools are relatively safe havens from lethal violence. In contrast, less dramatic environmental challenges—poor air quality, inadequate lighting, carelessly applied pesticides, schools to which students cannot walk or bicycle—operate every day in thousands of schools across the country, and their cumulative burden is likely to be far higher than

that caused by catastrophes. It is important to keep environmental threats to health and safety in perspective. By doing so, we can select our investments wisely and work to make them maximally effective in protecting children, teachers, and staff.

Science Does Not Have All the Answers

In the medical world, we expect each medication, each surgery, and even each piece of advice to be supported by solid evidence. Ideally, health-care providers rely on randomized clinical trials—studies in which some patients receive a certain medication, others receive an alternative medication or a placebo, and both groups' responses are carefully monitored and compared. Although this standard of evidence is not always met, it remains the goal to which we aspire. Rigorous scientific evidence gives us confidence that medical guidelines are safe and effective.

In the world of school environments, we rarely have that kind of clear evidence. In some instances, of course, we have strong epidemiologic data and can draw firm conclusions. For example, statistics about the leading kinds of playground injuries helped guide the design of safer playgrounds, and follow-up data helped confirm that these changes had actually reduced injury rates (chapter 8). However, this is the exception. Scientific data on the effects of poor indoor-air quality, inadequate lighting, and low-level pesticide exposure are incomplete. No school-based clinical trials have compared different approaches to violence prevention, to food service, to soccer field design, or to school health services.

Nevertheless, school personnel need to make decisions every day, often on the basis of partial evidence and informed judgment. For example, the effects of poor indoor-air quality on performance have been extensively studied in adults but not in children, so school-based recommendations need to extrapolate from adult data to children (Mendell and Heath 2005). In other cases, recommendations must be based on expert opinion and almost no systematic data. In each of the topics this book covers, we present the available facts and figures and note their limitations. We then offer recommendations for achieving safe and healthy environments, based on data to the extent possible and on expert opinion otherwise, stating clearly which is which. In the long run, we need the most solid information possible to help make the best decisions, so further research on selected aspects of school environments remains a pressing need.

People with Disabilities Are a Part of Every School Population

In recent years, the recognition of how disabilities can undermine children's opportunities to learn, socialize, and ultimately be successful has grown. This understanding has led to environmental modifications, but, more important, it has also changed attitudes. There is a growing commitment to ensuring that everyone—children and adults—is included in every aspect of our society. This commitment is expressed through many different mechanisms, including public laws, beginning with the original PL 94-142 of 1974, which established the right of all children, regardless of nature and degree of disability, to a free and appropriate education in their local public school.

When limitations of mobility, vision, hearing, learning, attention, and other functions are taken into account, it is now recognized that large numbers of students, teachers, and staff have disabilities of some kind. Further, it is now acknowledged that these students, teachers, and staff deserve full inclusion in mainstream education to the extent possible, with reasonable accommodation, as both a matter of fairness and a matter of law. These realizations require changes in attitudes, in longstanding procedures, and, in many cases, in the physical environment of the school. Chapter 26 describes these changes in detail, but the inclusion of people with disabilities is a theme that recurs throughout the book. For example, when considering lighting (chapter 2), the needs of people with visual difficulties should be taken into account, and when designing acoustics (chapter 4), the needs of people with hearing difficulties must be considered. Schools need to be safe and healthful environments settings that foster learning, socializing, and thriving for everybody in them, regardless of level of ability.

Conclusion

We hope this book will be useful to parents, teachers, school administrators, facility managers, school board members, health-care providers, and public

health agencies. The commitment to great places for children—to schools where they can learn, grow, and thrive in safe and healthy surroundings—is a widely shared commitment, one that transcends differences in location, politics, and creed. It is a pledge that can inspire and propel us all.

References

Braza M, Shoemaker W, Seeley A. 2004. Neighborhood design and rates of walking and biking to elementary school in 34 California communities. Am J Health Promot 19(2):128–136.

Broughman SP, Pugh KW. 2005. Characteristics of private schools in the United States: Results from the 2001–2002 Private School Universe Survey. NCES 2005-305. Washington, DC: U.S. Department of Education, National Center for Education Statistics, 2005. Available: http://nces.ed.gov/pubs2005/2005305.pdf [accessed 8 April 2005].

Christina School District. 2003. Leisure Elementary Closed Due to Partial Roof Collapse. Available: http://www.christina.k12,de.us/en2/news_special/leasure_update.htm [accessed 14 January 2006].

Daisey JM, Angell WJ, Apte MG. 2003. Indoor air quality, ventilation, and health symptoms in schools: An analysis of existing information. Indoor Air 13:53–64.

Dellinger AM, Staunton CE. 2002. Barriers to children walking and biking to school: United States, 1999. Mortal Morbid Weekly Rep 51(32):701–704.

Edgewood Independent School District v. Kirby, No. 362, 516 (259th Dist. Ct., Travis Cty., TX, June 1, 1987), rev. 761 S.W. 2nd 859 (Ct. App. TX, 1988), rev. 777 S.W. 2nd 391 (1989).

Everett Jones S, Brener ND, McManus T. 2003. Prevalence of school policies, programs, and facilities that promote a healthy physical school environment. Am J Public Health 93(9):1570–1575.

Frumkin H, ed. 2005. Environmental Health: From Global to Local. San Francisco: Jossey-Bass.

Gitterman BA, Bearer CF. 2001. A developmental approach to pediatric environmental health. Pediatr Clin N Am 48(5):1071–1083.

Hoffman L. 2003. Overview of public elementary and secondary schools and districts: School year 2001–2002. NCES 2003-411. Washington, DC: U.S. Department of Education, National Center for Education Statistics. Available: http://nces.ed.gov/pubs2003/overview03/index.asp#a [accessed 8 April 2005].

Landrigan PJ, Kimmel CA, Correa A, Eskenazi B.

2004. Children's health and the environment: Public health issues and challenges for risk assessment. Environ Health Perspect 112(2):257–265.

Lanphear BP, Vorhees CV, Bellinger DC. 2005. Protecting children from environmental toxins. PLoS Medicine 2:e61. Available: http://medicine.plos journals.org/perlserv/?request=get-document&doi =10.1371/journal.pmed.0020061 [accessed 10 April 2005].

Mendell MJ, Heath GA. 2005. Do indoor pollutants and thermal conditions in schools influence student performance? A critical review of the literature. Indoor Air 15:27–52.

National Research Council (NRC), Committee on Pesticides in the Diets of Infants and Children. *Pesticides in the diets of infants and children.* Washington, DC: National Academies Press, 1993.

Okoben J. 2006. Roof collapse danger closes Cleveland school. Cleveland Plain Dealer. Available: http://www.cleveland.com/cuyahoga/plaindealer/ index.ssf?/base/cuyahoga/11365404674490.xml& coll=2 [accessed 14 January 2006].

Pauley v. Kelly, No. 75-C1268 (Kanawha County Cir. Ct., WV, May 1982).

Perry CL, Bishop DB, Taylor GL, Davis M, Story M, Gray C, et al. 2004. A randomized school trial of environmental strategies to encourage fruit and vegetable consumption among children. Health Educ Behav 31(1):65–76.

Saunders S. 1999. Mechanicville teacher hurt by ceiling collapse. New York Teacher. Available: http:// www.nysut.org/newyorkteacher/backissues/1998 -1999/990421mechanicville.html [accessed 14 January 2006].

U.S. Department of Education, National Center for Education Statistics. Condition of America's public school facilities: 1999. Washington, DC: U.S. Department of Education, 2000. Available: http:// nces.ed.gov/surveys/frss/publications/2000032/ [accessed 22 November 2005].

U.S. General Accounting Office (GAO). School facilities: Condition of America's schools. GAO/HEHS-95-61. Washington, DC: GAO, 1995. Available: http://www.gao.gov/archive/1995/he95061.pdf [accessed 8 April 2005].

U.S. General Accounting Office. 1996a. School facilities: America's schools report differing conditions. GAO/HEHS-96-103. Washington, DC: GAO. Available: http://www.gao.gov/archive/1996/ he96103.pdf [accessed 8 April 2005].

U.S. General Accounting Office. 1996b. School facilities: Profiles of school conditions by state. GAO/ HEHS-96-148. Washington, DC: GAO. Available: http://www.gao.gov/archive/1996/he96148.pdf [accessed 8 April 2005].

Weiss B. 2000. Vulnerability of children and the developing brain to neurotoxic hazards. Environ Health Perspect 108 (Suppl. 3):375–381.

Wirt J, Choy S, Rooney P, Provasnik S, Sen A, Tobin R. 2004. The condition of education 2004. NCES 2004-077. Washington, DC: U.S. Department of Education, National Center for Education Statistics. Available: http://nces.ed.gov/programs/coe/ 2004/pdf/04_2004.pdf [accessed 8 April 2005].

The Physical Environment of the School

Lorraine E. Maxwell

Crowding, Class Size, and School Size

■ *Summary*

- The number of students and teachers and their occupation of available space within a school are important considerations. The performance and well-being of both students and teachers are affected by overcrowding.
- Population issues relate to both class size and the size of the school.
- Regardless of school size, if the school is beyond its intended capacity, overcrowding is a concern.
- Crowding is both a subjective experience and a measurable condition.
- School size, class size, and furniture arrangements can be modified to alleviate crowded conditions. ■

This chapter discusses two separate but related aspects of the school environment: population, in relation to both class size and the size of the school, and crowding. A particular school may have a low, comfortable density. But if a school exceeds its capacity and has enrolled more students than the building was designed to accommodate, it may be crowded, regardless of its size. Both population and density play a role in school performance, health, and the well-being of students and teachers.

The Effects of Crowding

Crowding is both an objectively measurable condition and a subjective experience. The objective measure is density. *Social density* is the number of people in a space (e.g., 22 children per classroom), whereas *spatial density* is the amount of space available for each person (e.g., 25 square feet per child). In a residential setting, spatial density might be one room per person for a family of six in a six-room apartment (the ratio of one room per person is usually considered the threshold for a crowded home). In some school situations, social density may be low (e.g., 20 students per classroom), despite a high spatial density of perhaps 15 square feet per child.

Crowding is also a subjective experience, in that it relates to how a person feels in specific density situations. People feel crowded when their ability to control interaction with other people is affected or when other people interfere with their ability to conduct an activity such as reading, conversing, or studying. In other words, when either group size or spatial density creates a situation in which a person cannot control interactions with other people, that person is likely to feel crowded. People most often feel crowded in high-density situations but not always. For example, students attending sporting events are usually surrounded by large numbers of people, but they are not likely to feel crowded.

Two concepts help explain the experience of crowding: privacy and overstimulation. One reason that high density may result in feelings of being crowded is that people have a difficult time achieving privacy. Privacy is not necessarily the state of being alone; it is the perceived ability to control interactions with others. Privacy is often achieved by getting away from other people, but it is also attained by controlling the number of other people with whom one has to interact. Students who want to work on a group project may need space apart from the rest of the class to avoid interruptions or distractions. Children may ask to leave the classroom to use the toilet as a way of getting some time away from a crowded classroom and obtaining some privacy.

Overstimulation is a second aspect of crowding. A learning situation requires a high level of sustained attention; in the classroom, children must pay attention for extended periods of time. In addition to the lesson material, other sources of stimulation, (e.g., bulletin board displays, visuals on classroom walls, other students) are present in the classroom. Constant interaction with other people, a result of large group size or high spatial density, adds further stimulation. Classrooms offer the potential for conversation, interactive activities, and noise. High levels of stimulation require high levels of psychic energy. Maintaining an adequate level of concentration in a high-density classroom, especially for difficult or complex material, can lead to attentional overload or cognitive fatigue. Cognitive fatigue in turn inhibits learning—children are no longer able to continue paying attention to the material being taught (Evans 1994). Time away from a high-density classroom (e.g., for outdoor activities or for a trip to the school library) may help relieve cognitive fatigue. If an opportunity for restoration is not possible, children may opt for psychological privacy by just tuning out or daydreaming. Tuning out is a mechanism for coping with excessively high levels of stimulation. Although tuning out is effective, it also results in a loss of valuable learning time.

High density, or crowding, in primary environments is potentially more harmful than crowding in secondary environments. A *primary environment* is one in which someone spends a large amount of time, forms interpersonal relations with others, and has some level of personal investment—for example, the home, the workplace, and school. Because children spend a great deal of time in school, high density in this environment is of critical importance. A *secondary environment* is one in which the experience is transitory, interactions with others are generally with strangers, and people have little, if any, personal investment in the setting (e.g., public transportation, a department store, the beach). Even though people might experience a feeling of crowding in any of these settings, that response is not likely to have long-term effects. A child may have to ride a crowded bus to school every day; however, if the home and school are not crowded, the experience on the bus is not likely to have long-term negative consequences for the child. Based on these definitions, the school is a primary environment for both children and teachers. For teachers, clearly, school is a workplace.

In general, crowding has negative effects on human beings. In addition to cognitive fatigue, the perception of being crowded elicits an emotional response, with—feelings of stress, which may contribute to poor mental health. Feeling crowded may also elicit behavioral responses such as aggressive behavior in children and adults, disruptive behavior in children, social withdrawal, and/or departure (Gifford 2002; Saegert 1982). These psychological and behavioral reactions have implications for school performance. Finally, crowding is also associated with poor health, including high blood pressure and heart disease in both children and adults (Evans et al. 1998).

Crowding can have serious implications for children's psychological development. Children from crowded homes are at risk for developing motivational problems, which researchers call *learned helplessness* (Rodin 1976). When confronted with too much stimulation, such as the constant presence of and interaction with other people, children lose the motivation to pay attention or complete a task. This is more likely to happen when a task is complex or difficult. When confronted with a crowded situation for an extended period of time, children learn to be helpless; they simply give up when things get difficult.

Teachers are similarly affected. In crowded elementary school classrooms, teachers report that constant physical contacts are distracting and create difficulty in moving about (Ahrentzen 1981). The behaviors and attitudes of teachers are also likely to be positively affected by less crowded classrooms. In classrooms that provide adequate space for their occupants, teachers report that they can interact more with students, provide a more varied educational program, and encourage students to work together on projects (Moore and Lackney 1993). Teachers are less likely to feel stressed in an environment in which they can move about freely.

Similar emotional responses occur even with short-term exposure to crowding. In an experimental research setting, fourth-, eighth-, and eleventh-grade students reported feeling confined, tense, annoyed, frustrated, and uncomfortable because of proximity to other students in short-term, high spatial-density (fewer square feet per person) conditions (Aiello et al. 1979).

Moreover, crowding can affect children's interpersonal relations. Children in crowded situations are less likely to participate in cooperative ventures. They may be more aggressive with their peers or adults or socially withdraw from group activities. In contrast, children in low-density situations are more likely to avoid conflict (Aiello et al. 1979). Crowding is also related to poor parent–child relations, including harsh parenting styles and decreased responsiveness. Parents in crowded households are less likely to respond verbally to their children, which can have serious consequences for the development of children's early language and prereading skills (Evans et al. 1999). In child-care settings for preschool children, less space per child is associated with reduced social interaction (a critical part of learning at this age), more hostile and aggressive behavior, more time spent in solitary play, and less gross motor play (Burgess and Fordyce 1989; Loo 1979; Smith and Connolly 1980).

Children in crowded classrooms engage in more disruptive, aggressive, and hostile behaviors. Although boys show these responses more than girls, both boys and girls are affected (Maxwell 2003; Saegert 1982). In contrast, some children in crowded classrooms may withdraw from classroom participation (Loo and Smetana 1978) or become inattentive because of attentional overload (Evans 1994).

Given these effects, it comes as no surprise that crowding can undermine school performance. Lower reading scores are associated with less space per child, especially girls (range: 18.9–33.7 square feet per child; Maxwell 2003). Children, especially boys, from high-density homes (more than one person per room) are more likely to have lower academic achievement scores than their less-crowded peers (controlling for income) and to be rated by their classroom teachers as disruptive and aggressive (Evans et al. 1998; Saegert 1982). These behaviors can lead to academic difficulty for the student in question as well as others in the classroom as teachers may have to spend more time on discipline and classroom management than on instruction. If a child comes from a crowded home and is placed in a crowded classroom, these problems may intensify.

Students with special needs, including learning disabilities, attention deficit disorders (e.g., ADHD), intellectual and developmental disabilities, and chronic medical conditions may react differently to crowding in the classroom. These children may not be able to concentrate and therefore be unable to learn or perform well. Although some children with milder conditions may respond by withdrawing from engagement in activities and may have difficulty staying on task (Hutt and Vaizey 1966), others with more significant intellectual and developmental disabilities, including the autism spectrum conditions, may exhibit exacerbated aggressive and disruptive behaviors in response to either a decrease in space per child or an increase in class size (McFee 1987).

Class Size and School Size

Should schools be large or small? Should classes be large or small? For many school districts, economic considerations (and teacher shortages in some cases) have led to the consolidation of schools, with the result that many students are placed in large classes and schools. As of 2000, 33% of the students in the United States were in classes with 25 or more students, and 85% were in classes with 18 or more students (Cohen et al. 2000). Since then, many states have been working to reduce class size, and many of them have made the neediest schools (those with the largest class sizes, often in inner-city communities) their top priority when addressing class-size reduction. It is difficult, however, to track the success of their efforts (except for anecdotal case studies) because no state-by-state class-size data are available (National Educational Association 2004). Thus, although many school districts have made progress in reducing class size, crowding at the classroom level is still an issue worthy of discussion.

Small schools (i.e., elementary schools with fewer than 200 students, high schools with fewer than 500) offer several advantages. One is academic achievement: A positive relationship exists between academic achievement and smaller school size, especially for low-income, inner-city students (Fowler 1992; Summers and Wolfe 1977). In small schools, a higher proportion of students participate in extracurricular activities and assume leadership roles. Students exhibit greater personal responsibility, are more sensitive to the needs of their fellow students, and have greater self-esteem. Moreover, rates of crime, vandalism, and serious student misconduct are lower in small schools (Garbarino 1980). One reason for this may be that small schools seem to foster a sense of personal connection with the school. In large schools, relatively fewer students are likely to have an opportunity for meaningful participation. This lack of personal involvement in larger schools can be especially problematic for students who are having academic difficulties (Moore and Lackney 1993). The prosocial attributes (e.g., personal responsibility, cooperation among students) that small schools foster may play a role in improving learning and academic achievement.

Schools are a primary environment for children, and the classroom is the primary environment in a school setting. The majority of teaching and learning activities take place in the classroom, and this is where children form relationships with other students and with teachers. Therefore, the classroom environment is critical. The relationship of class size to student achievement has been the subject of much debate among researchers (see Schneider [2002] for a more detailed discussion of this debate). Much of the debate centers on methodology. For example, the student/teacher ratio is sometimes used as a measure for class size. However, this may not be an accurate representation of group size in the classroom, as all teachers (including librarians and part-time staff) are usually included in this calculation. Some research indicates no effect of class (group) size on student achievement but suggests that the range of class sizes may have been too narrow to produce any significant findings. Often effects are found only for large declines in class size (Johnson 2000). In addition, because student achievement is such a complex phenomenon, it may be hard to isolate a single variable such as class size.

Recent work has helped clarify this relationship. A longitudinal study in Tennessee known as Project STAR (Student/Teacher Achievement Ratio) found that elementary school-age children in smaller classes (13–17 students) outperformed their peers in the larger classes (22–26 students) on academic achievement measures. Positive effects of smaller class sizes were particularly pronounced for children from families of low socioeconomic status and for African American children (Ehrenberg, et al. 2001). Group size was used as a measure of class size, not student/teacher ratio.

In Project STAR, there was also sufficient variation in group size to test the effects of class size. Smaller class sizes seem to be especially important in the early grades (kindergarten through third grade), but it also appears that the more time spent in small classes, the greater the likelihood of positive benefits for academic achievement. Decreasing class size from the upper twenties or the low thirties to 21, 20, or even 18 students does not seem to be sufficient to make a difference in academic performance. Substantial differences in achievement are not observed until class size drops to about 15 or 16 students (Glass et al. 1982). In preschool-age children, a smaller group or class size has a positive effect on cognitive style. Children in larger classes (group size 16–23) were less thoughtful when trying to solve age-appropriate problems or tasks (Maxwell 1996).

Solutions

School Size

As noted earlier, optimal academic and behavioral outcomes are associated with elementary schools of

100–200 students and secondary schools with fewer than 500 students. Achieving these sizes, however, may be difficult for many districts.

Providing school facilities to meet these recommendations might mean first developing an updated capital master plan. Smaller schools will most likely result in more school buildings, and appropriate sites will have to be identified. Financial resources must also be considered. Because libraries, athletic and fitness facilities, food services, performance spaces, and high-tech/vocational services are expensive, school districts must consider the economies of scale when planning and building new facilities. Master planning can help districts develop ways to make sure that every student has access to high-quality support services without constructing megastructures.

Apparent school size can be reduced through careful physical and operational design. If larger buildings are necessary, they can be designed for subdivision into smaller functional units. Separate identifiable entrances, corridor systems, and other design features can give students and staff a sense that they are in a smaller school. Separate wings of the building are not enough. All aspects of the design should support the small-school concept, including the way students arrive at the school, staff parking, and offices. If these smaller units are also managed separately, students, teachers, and administrators can more closely identify with the smaller school. Certain facilities may have to be shared, but students' identification should be with the smaller school unit. Another alternative is to build schools near or in conjunction with certain community resources. For example, several small schools might share community athletic facilities or libraries.

Class Size

The greatest improvements in academic performance occur when classes accommodate 13–17 students. Improvements in student attitude and behavior may be achieved with slightly larger groups. Achieving these class sizes is an expensive undertaking, however. Additional teachers must be hired, and additional classroom space provided. New schools can be built to meet this goal if sufficient funds and other resources (i.e., qualified teachers) are available. Schools that are undergoing major renovations can also achieve these numbers.

Furniture and Spatial Arrangements

Districts that are not building new facilities or planning major renovations will find it more difficult to reduce class size. Attaining targeted class size goals may also be difficult because of financial constraints and shortages of qualified teachers. What options are available to teachers and administrators in these schools?

Classroom layout and design, including displays, can affect the perception of crowding in the classroom, even if the actual density remains the same. Aspects of the classroom such as furniture arrangement, layout, clutter, and displays can affect the occupants' sense of privacy, as well as the ability of students and teachers to control their interactions with others. Stimulus overload can also contribute to the perception of crowding. In general, recommended strategies involve the following:

- creating personal space
- subdividing the classroom into smaller work areas
- providing adequate learning resources
- avoiding clutter both in the room and on the walls
- reducing noise levels
- providing opportunities for restoration.

More specific recommendations are shown in box 2.1.

Furniture arrangements offer many options. A clustered grouping of chairs and tables is more supportive of student interaction than rows. However, row arrangements may better support learning-related behaviors such as paying attention and learning to use various materials. The important thing is that the classroom arrangement should fit the learning activity. If children are working on group projects and student interaction is necessary for the learning activity, the furniture arrangement should reflect this goal. Other arrangements may be necessary if the learning activity changes. A high-density classroom, especially a high spatial-density classroom where space is at a premium, may restrict the possible furniture and spatial arrangements.

Teachers and students may react differently to various furniture configurations. Their response seems to be related to the different ways that teachers and students use the classroom space. Teachers often move around during class sessions, but stu-

---

■ *2.1. Strategies for mitigating the effects of crowding in classrooms*

Provide personal space

- Be sure that each student has a personal work space. The work space should belong to the child the entire school year or semester. In crowded classrooms, establishing children's personal work spaces can help mitigate the negative effects of crowding on learning (Gifford 2002).

Create smaller work and activity areas

- If possible, change the furniture arrangement to fit the task: individual or small groupings when student concentration is required, and larger groupings when more interaction is required.
- When age appropriate, arrange the room around interest areas (e.g., science, art, language arts). To evenly distribute children around the classroom, avoid putting popular areas together.
- Create alcoves to provide students with small group and/or individual work spaces.

Provide adequate learning resources

- Plentiful play resources and equipment help avoid inappropriate behavior in crowded classrooms (Kantrowitz and Evans 2004).

Reduce clutter

- Use displays to exhibit classwork. Change displays to reflect the current study topics. Include children's input about what should be displayed and where. Keep displays at children's eye level. Avoid covering all of the wall space, however—too many displays are overwhelming, confusing, and distracting (stimulus overload).
- Store unused materials and supplies out of sight.
- Provide sufficient storage space for books and other learning supplies (built-in storage provides less flexibility for how the space can be used).

Reduce noise

- The acoustics should be appropriate to the activities that take place in the space.

Provide places for restoration

- Provide functional private spaces in the classroom; use rugs, screens, or bookcases to create an area that children can use when they need to be alone (having time to work in private can reduce cognitive fatigue).
- Provide space in the classroom for restoration (e.g., a private space near a window with a pleasant view or close to a fish tank or plants). ■

---

dents (beyond kindergarten or first grade) are usually seated for most of the lesson. In more crowded classrooms, teachers are more likely than children to report a feeling of being crowded and restricted movement. When classroom furniture is arranged in large clusters, students report feeling more crowded and distracted than teachers; however, the reverse is true when there are more but smaller clusters (Gifford 2002). More clusters are likely to restrict the teachers' ability to move around the classroom. If teachers feel distracted or crowded,

the way they teach or manage the classroom may be affected. Large clusters, in contrast, are more likely to put students in close contact with many other students and perhaps increase the level of distraction.

Providing personal space can be a useful approach to crowding. One elementary school teacher in a large urban public school district let children pick a specific spot in the classroom for independent reading time. The spot belonged to the child for the entire school year and was used each time the reading activity occurred. The classroom had a small sofa, several bean bag chairs, and a number of carpet squares and loose pillows that children could use in their personal reading spot. See box 2.1 for helpful strategies on reducing crowding in classrooms.

References

Ahrentzen S. 1981. The environmental and social context of distraction in the classroom. In *Design research interactions* (Osterberg AE, Tieman CP, Findlay RA, eds.). Ames, IA: Environmental Design Research Association, 241–250.

Aiello JR, Nicosia G, Thompson DE. 1979. Physiological, social, and behavioral consequences of crowding on children and adolescents. Child Dev 50: 195–202.

Burgess JW, Fordyce WK. 1989. Effects of preschool environments on nonverbal social behavior: Toddlers' interpersonal distances to teachers and classmates change with environmental density, classroom design, and parent-child interactions. J Child Psychol Psychiatry 30(2):261–276.

Cohen G, Miller C, Stonehill R, Geddes C. 2000. The class size reduction program—boosting student achievement in schools across the nation: A first-year report. Washington, DC: U.S. Department of Education.

Ehrenberg RG, Brewer DJ, Gamoran A, Willms JD. 2001. Class size and student achievement. Psychol Sci Public Interest 2(1):1–30.

Evans GW. 1994. Learning and the physical environment. In *Public institutions for personal learning: Establishing a research agenda* (Falk JH, Dierking LD, eds.). Washington, DC: American Association of Museums, 119–126.

Evans GW, Lepore SJ, Shejwal BR, Palsane MN. 1998. Chronic residential crowding and children's well-being: An ecological perspective. Child Dev 69(6): 1514–1523.

Evans GW, Maxwell LE, Hart B. 1999. Parental language and verbal responsiveness to children in crowded homes. Dev Psychol 35(4):1020–1023.

Fowler WJ Jr. 1992. What do we know about school size? What should we know? Paper presented at the American Educational Research Association Annual Meeting, San Francisco, April 18–22. Washington, DC: Office of Educational Research and Improvement, National Center for Educational Statistics, U.S. Department of Education.

Garbarino J. 1980. Some thoughts on school size and its effects on adolescent development. J Youth Adolesc 9:19–31.

Gifford R. 2002. *Environmental psychology: Principals and practices.* Victoria, British Columbia: Optimal Books.

Glass GV, Cahen LS, Smith ML, Filby NN. 1982. *School class size: Research and policy.* Beverly Hills, CA: Sage.

Hutt C, Vaizey M. 1966. Differential effects of group density on social behavior. Nature 209:1371–1372.

Johnson KA. 2000. Do small classes influence academic achievement? What the National Assessment of Educational Progress shows. Washington, DC: Heritage Foundation.

Kantrowitz E, Evans GW. 2004. The relation between the ratio of children per activity area and off-task behavior and type of play in day-care centers. Environ Behav 36(4):541–557.

Loo CM. 1979. A factor analytic approach to the study of spatial density effects on preschoolers. J Popul 2(1):47–68.

Loo CM, Smetana J. 1978. The effects of crowding on the behavior and perception of 10-year-old boys. Environ Psychol Nonverbal Behav 2(4):226–249.

Maxwell LE. 1996. Multiple effects of home and day-care crowding. Environ Behav 28(4):494–511.

Maxwell LE. 2003. Home and school density effects on elementary school children: The role of spatial density. Environ Behav 35(4):566–578.

McFee JK. 1987. Classroom density and the aggressive behavior of handicapped children. Educ Treat Child 10(2):134–145.

Moore GT, Lackney JA. 1993. School design: Crisis, educational performance, and design applications. Child Environ 10(2):99–112.

National Educational Association. 2004. Class size. Available: http://www.nea.org/classsize [accessed 24 June 2004].

Rodin J. 1976. Density, perceived choice, and responses to controllable and uncontrollable outcomes. J Exp Soc Psychol 12:564–578.

Saegert S. 1982. Environment and children's mental health: Residential density and low income children. In *Handbook of psychology and health* (Baum A, Singer JE, eds.), vol. 2. Hillsdale, NJ: Erlbaum, 247–271.

Schneider M. 2002. *Do school facilities affect academic outcomes?* Washington, DC: National Clearinghouse for Educational Facilities.

Smith PK, Connolly KJ. 1980. *The ecology of preschool behaviour.* Cambridge, MA: Cambridge University Press.

Summers AA, Wolfe BL. 1977. Do schools make a difference? Am Econ Rev 67:639–652.

3

Barbara Erwine

Lighting

■ *Summary*

• Good lighting design can improve health and learning as well as increase safety, reduce vandalism, lower energy use, and help students maintain visual connections with the environment. Bad lighting design, in contrast, contributes negatively to these issues.

• A holistic approach to optimal lighting includes provision of daylight and views in all classrooms and work areas, integration of daylight and electric lighting, and the addition of flexible lighting controls.

• Lighting problems result from numerous causes, including insufficient or unbalanced light, glare, unnatural lamp characteristics, and annoying side effects.

• Energy-efficient lighting accommodates seasonal changes and minimizes maintenance. Staff awareness of energy use can result in additional energy savings.

• A healthy lighting system results from careful planning early in the building design. Frequent system assessment ensures consistent performance. ■

A girl finds her state on a map the teacher displays before the class. A boy reads a math story-problem at his desk. These simple scenes are reenacted millions of times every day in classrooms around the world. Independent of whether these tasks are projected from a computer screen or are presented on a blackboard hanging on a bamboo wall, what connects the child to this magical information is the act of seeing (fig. 3.1). And what activates this ability to see, what makes it possible at all, is light. Light is the critical link, the messenger that brings us visual information about our physical world. Delivering information is crucial, but as researchers probe more deeply into the importance of light in our lives, they continue to uncover other important roles that light plays in the learning process. This chapter describes the breadth of the impact that lighting has on the health, well-being, and performance of schoolchildren and staff.

Lighting in Schools: A Brief History

In the early 1900s a typical classroom had large windows and depended mostly on daylight for lighting. Electric lighting was likely to be provided by a pendant incandescent luminaire—a fixture

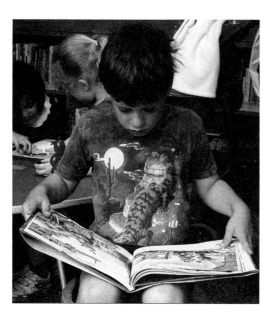

Figure 3.1. Good lighting is essential for a child who is reading. (Photo by Barbara Erwine.)

that became so common that it is now known as the "schoolhouse fixture" (fig. 3.2). In the 1950s, as fluorescent lighting grew in popularity, new classroom designs incorporated wraparound lensed fluorescent luminaires mounted on the ceiling or, later, lensed prismatic fluorescent luminaires recessed into the ceiling. These were much more energy efficient than the incandescent lights and rapidly replaced them. Later, as classroom computers grew in number, lighting designers became concerned about the reflections of these bright light sources on computer screens, so the lensed fixtures were often replaced by recessed parabolic luminaires with louvers to block direct views of the bright lamps. However, these recessed parabolic luminaires throw most of their light downward, directly onto desk surfaces, leaving the walls and ceilings relatively dark and imparting a rather gloomy atmosphere. Today, many newer classrooms instead use suspended fluorescent pendants ("direct/ indirect" fixtures), which direct light both upward toward the ceiling and downward toward the desks. Although direct/indirect fixtures require higher ceilings (minimum 9 feet), they provide bright, even illumination to all of the room surfaces. Most of these pendants also incorporate louvers or some other control strategy to minimize glare.

At the time this evolution in light fixtures was taking place, lamp (bulb) technology was also moving from incandescent to old-style T12 fluorescent lamps (commonly called warm white and cool white) with magnetic ballasts. The fluorescent-lamp technology was later improved with the development of newer, thinner lamps (T8 and T5) with electronic ballasts (see fig. 3.2). These newer lamps made colors appear more natural because of their higher color-rendering index (CRI). They did not impart the greenish tint that many people associate with fluorescent light. In addition, the move from magnetic to electronic ballasts increased the energy efficiency and changed the frequency of operation from 60 cycles per second to more than 20,000 cycles per second (well above the normal range of perception), eliminating both the flicker and the annoying buzz of earlier fluorescent lights.

Along with improvements in lamp technology, new lighting controls provided flexibility and greater energy efficiency for school lighting. Until the mid-1900s, the lights in most classrooms (and sometimes whole buildings) were controlled by a single switch that turned all the lamps on or off at the same time. Newer designs use multiple switches or automatic controls to turn off individual circuits or lamps within light fixtures to provide the correct light levels for different activities and to save energy when lights are not needed.

Our understanding of lighting quality has also changed over time. Although modern classrooms use only about 30–50 foot-candles (fc) (see box 3.1) of desktop illumination, past recommendations called for more than 100 fc. In 2000, the Illuminating Engineering Society of North America (IESNA), the industry organization that sets standards and lighting recommendations, adopted new standards for lighting quality that move beyond the simplistic approach of specifying only the amount of light needed above a desk. Recognizing that the whole visual environment contributes to our comfort and ability to see well, the *IESNA Lighting Handbook* (2000b) places less emphasis on horizontal light measurement and more emphasis on the illumination of walls and other vertical surfaces and the overall balance of light in an area. Lighting designs that continue to focus only on horizontal light levels miss the many benefits of a lighting approach that takes into consideration various types of surfaces.

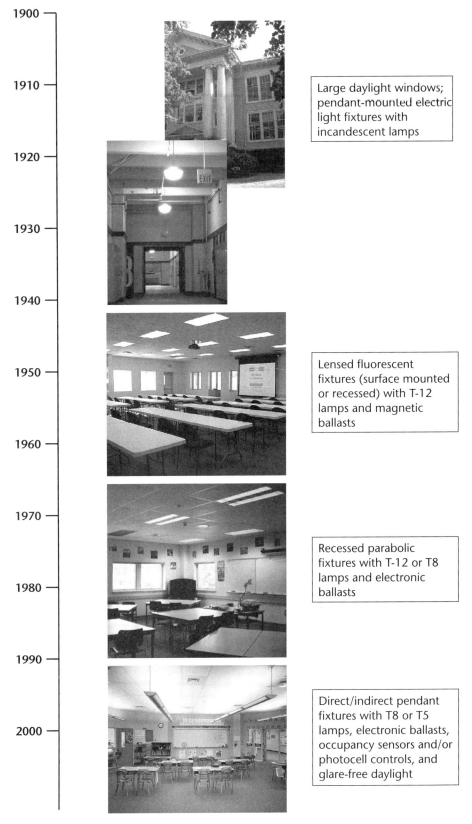

Figure 3.2. Lighting timeline in schools. (Photo of pendant fluorescent lights courtesy of Finelite and National Renewable Energy Laboratory Photographic Information eXchange, No. 03046.)

■ *3.1. Lighting vocabulary*

Light is energy, the part of the electromagnetic spectrum we can see. The wavelength of light ranges from 380 to 780 nanometers. The amount, or intensity, of light is measured in *lumens*.

The *foot-candle* (fc) is the unit of measure of the amount of light falling on a surface (lumens per square foot). Classroom lighting normally ranges from 30 to 50 fc on desktops. However, the quality of the lighting (e.g., brightness of wall and ceiling surfaces, balance of light across the room, absence of high contrasts) is often more important for vision than the quantity of light.

Sunlight (or direct sunlight) refers to the direct, parallel rays of the sun. It is very bright, casts strong shadows, and may cause glare in work areas. *Daylight* (or diffuse sunlight) refers to sunlight diffused by clouds, the earth's atmosphere, or reflection off a surface. Daylight is a soft, even source of light.

Electric light is provided by a variety of bulbs or lamps. In schools, the most common types are incandescent, fluorescent, and high-intensity discharge (HID) lamps such as metal halide and high-pressure sodium. Fluorescent and HID lamps require a ballast, which is a separate device that provides the necessary voltage and current for starting and operating the lamps. Linear fluorescent (tubular) lamps are designated with the letter "T," followed by a number that indicates the diameter of the lamp tube in eighths of an inch. T12 lamps are twelve-eighths of an inch (1.5 inches) in diameter; T8s are eight-eighths (1 inch); and T5s are five eighths of an inch. Light-emitting diode (LED) lamps have high energy efficiency but relatively low light output. Although they are currently used mostly for exit signs in schools, evolving research is likely to expand their use to other applications.

Color temperature refers to the relative yellowness or blueness of light produced by a lamp. Color temperature is measured in degrees Kelvin (K) and ranges from about 2,700 K for yellowish incandescent light to more than 5,500 K for more bluish daylight fluorescence. Fluorescent lamps can be purchased in a range of color temperatures.

Color rendering index (CRI) of a light source is a relative scale from 0 to 100 that indicates the ability of a lamp to make colors appear natural. The higher the CRI, the more natural colors appear. A CRI of 80–90 should be used in schools. ■

Why Is School Lighting Important?

Although we have long been aware of the need for sufficient quantities of light to move about safely and see the tasks at hand, we are just now beginning to understand the wide range of qualitative impacts that light has on health and well-being. Lighting has been credited with effects ranging from improving math scores on standardized tests to curing seasonal depression.

Learning Issues

Recent research by the Heschong Mahone Group (HMG) and others shows striking correlations between student learning rates and lighting quality. In a study of three school districts, HMG found that students with more daylight in their classrooms progressed more than 20% faster in math and reading skills than their counterparts in classrooms without daylight (HMG 1999). This study also showed a 7% increase in student performance when classroom windows were operable (providing natural ventilation).

Although we do not know exactly why students perform better in spaces that provide daylight, several reasons are worth considering. The quality of lighting affects our ability to see the information before us and sort through complex tasks more quickly. Daylight's potential for higher quality and quantity of light may give students the advantage of clear and precise sight. In addition to allowing better vision, lighting affects our moods and general health. The changes in performance may be explained at least in part by improvements in the health or mood of students or teachers (or both).

Daylight can also help reduce mental fatigue because it presents an ever-changing light source that reduces monotony. Windows that provide views to nature and activities provide additional mental stimulation. Surveys of work environments have shown that people prefer daylight to electric light, and the primary reason people prefer windows is the view they provide. A follow up study to the earlier HMG research on daylight and productivity in schools demonstrated that, when students have a better view from the windows (including vegetation, human activity, or objects in the distance), they also tend to perform better. In fact, in predicting student performance, variables such as the physical conditions of classrooms, most notably the window characteristics, have been shown to be as important as teacher characteristics, the number of computers, and attendance rates (California Energy Commission 2003a). Teacher and staff performance may also be affected by the availability of a view. A study by HMG found that office workers who had the best possible view performed 10–25% better on tests of mental function and memory recall than did those with no view (California Energy Commission 2003b).

In contrast, as one might expect, bad lighting can negatively impact learning (fig. 3.3). Both the HMG classroom studies showed that students do not perform as well when bad lighting conditions exist. The first study noted that, if skylights admit direct sun (glare) into the classroom, student learning rates drop by 21% (HMG 1999). This finding was reinforced in the second study, which found that variables describing window glare, sun penetration, and lack of visual control (operable blinds, etc.) correlate with lower performance on standardized tests (California Energy Commission 2003a).

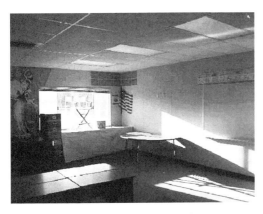

Figure 3.3. Direct sun in classrooms is distracting and reduces visibility. Exterior shading of the window or interior blinds could eliminate this problem. (Photo by Lisa Heschong.)

The HMG report on office workers also noted that, all other things being equal, "the greater the glare potential from primary view windows, the worse the office worker performance, decreasing by 15% to 21%" (California Energy Commission 2003b, p. vii).

Several recent research experiments on learning and electric lighting (Berman et al. 1993, 1994) noted improvements in small, precise vision with the use of high color temperature (5000°K or higher) fluorescent lamps, sometimes called daylight fluorescent. These results have been used to recommend high color temperature lamps for classrooms. However, the experiments showed improvements only for visual tasks at threshold levels (small image size, low contrast, or very low light level); the impact on classroom work at higher light levels is not yet clear. As this understanding is still evolving, school districts should watch for future research in this area and balance this information with other considerations of energy efficiency, cost, and appearance of the space. (Although higher color temperatures may make spaces appear brighter or more stimulating, they can also appear cold or harsh to some viewers.)

Effects on Health

Lighting can have both positive and negative impacts on the health of students and teachers over extended periods of time. The full extent of these effects is still being determined; however, we know that light and views have an impact on a wide range of health issues including the production of vitamin D, the regulation of our internal body clocks, relaxation, stress, moods, and reduction of headaches (Benya et al. 2003; Guzowski 2000). Some of these effects require the high light levels provided by exterior daylight; others are present at lower, interior levels.

A study by Judith Heerwagen at the University of Washington found that patients in hospital intensive care units (ICUs) with windows recovered faster than those in windowless ICUs (Guzowski 2000). Similarly, the HMG study of office workers noted earlier found that office workers' self-reports of better health conditions were strongly associated with better views (California Energy Commission 2003b). Many reasons, both physiological and psychological, may explain this association. In general, people find natural views to be calming. We also

■ *3.2. A word about full-spectrum fluorescent lighting*

Full spectrum is an imprecisely defined term that usually refers to a fluorescent lamp that simulates the spectrum of daylight. Compared with some standard fluorescent lights, a full-spectrum lamp has a higher color temperature (looks more bluish), has a higher CRI (ability to make colors appear natural), and produces more radiation in the ultraviolet (UV) range. Research in the 1980s comparing full-spectrum lamps with T12 lamps attributed a wide range of health benefits to the use of the former. Although the research procedure was questioned, manufacturers were quick to use this information to promote the sale of full-spectrum lamps. However, a major review of the research in this area by Veitch and McColl (1994) found no indication that full-spectrum fluorescent lighting was associated with increases in psychological well-being, health, or productivity. In addition, some of the performance characteristics of these lamps, such as higher color temperature and better color rendering, are now available from other, less expensive fluorescent lamps (e.g., T8 and T5 high-CRI lamps). ■

know that long-distance views reduce eyestrain by allowing the eye muscles to relax as they alternate between near and distant focus. When viewing close tasks, the eye muscles are contracted; looking at a distant view relaxes the eye muscles, possibly reducing the potential for headaches and other stress-related ailments.

In the past few years much attention has been directed to the link between light levels and symptoms of seasonal affective disorder (SAD). Light passing through the eye regulates the hypothalamus, a small but important part of the brain that controls many body functions including sleep, appetite, mood, activity, and circadian rhythms. It is now well documented that sustained periods of low light levels (such as those encountered at high latitudes in winter) can cause seasonal depression and reduced performance for some people (Benya et al. 2003). Clinical cases of SAD are frequently treated with specifically timed "doses" of very high light

levels (often in the blue wavelength range). Minor changes to classroom lighting cannot help students or teachers with clinical SAD symptoms, and those with this disorder should seek medical help. However, spending time outside or in a brightly lit outdoor space every day may have a positive effect on people with subclinical levels of SAD, and these practices should be encouraged.

Numerous studies (e.g., Benya et al. 2003) have also highlighted the importance of UV irradiation on the skin for the production of vitamin D in our bodies. Without sufficient UV exposure, vitamin D levels drop, causing widespread health effects including rickets and osteoporosis (Boyce et al. 2003). Both daylight and full-spectrum fluorescent lights (see box 3.2) contain UV radiation. However, most of the UV from daylight is blocked by window glass, and the UV content in a full-spectrum fluorescent light is far less than that of daylight. Exposure to sunlight outdoors is the simplest way to get an appropriate dose (20–30 minutes) of UV radiation—a requirement easily satisfied by outdoor recess. School designs and schedules should also foster time outdoors for older students and teachers who do not participate in recess.

Although good lighting has been shown to promote health, poor lighting design can do the opposite. Bright, uncontrolled light sources (glare) can cause squinting and may increase the incidence of headaches (see chapter 23 on high-performance schools). The flicker from magnetically ballasted fluorescent lights (120 cycles per second) is associated with several health issues (Benya et al. 2003). In the worst case scenario, flicker has the potential to initiate seizures in people with photosensitive epilepsy; one child in 4,000 may be affected (Harding 1984). In milder cases, flicker can cause increased headaches and stress.

Flicker has also been implicated in attention deficit hyperactivity disorder (ADHD). Although there is now general agreement that lighting flicker does not cause ADHD, it may cause discomfort and distractibility; therefore its elimination may reduce discomfort and distractibility and reduce the symptoms of ADHD. Several studies thus recommend minimizing environmental stimuli (especially visual and tactile) in the classroom (Thompson 1999). The hum of magnetic ballasts and the glare from poorly designed lighting can also be problematic for children with autism, sometimes causing painful distractions (Kluth 2004). All of these health concerns indicate the need to change from magnetic to electronic ballasts to eliminate flicker and buzz.

Increased Safety and Reduced Vandalism

During the day, well-lit school buildings help students navigate environmental hazards, thus reducing falls and other accidents. Well-placed windows also improve security by providing sightlines by which to monitor outside activities and identify visitors before they enter the school building.

Exterior security lighting can discourage theft, vandalism, and the unauthorized use of school grounds after hours. The goals of security lighting generally coincide with those for good vision: providing balanced illumination that keeps walls and other vertical surfaces bright and eliminates dark corners. Some schools have also experimented with a "dark campus" approach, using automatic occupancy sensors to control the lighting between midnight and 6:00 AM. If an area is unoccupied, all of the lights remain off; if someone enters the space, lights go on, signaling the intruder's location to the neighborhood and the police. When the Marion County, Florida, public schools implemented a dark campus approach, the district saved approximately $46,000 per year on energy expenses and reduced the cost of vandalism by more than 50% (Marion County Public Schools 2000). Chapter 19 provides further information and recommendations on security issues.

Lower Energy Use and Reduced Operating Budgets

Lighting constitutes a major use of energy in schools. In many school districts, energy costs are second only to salaries. Nationally, K–12 schools spend more than $6 billion annually on energy, and approximately 45% of that budget goes to lighting expenses. Daylight is a free light source that coincides with the hours of school operation. A good daylighting design, coupled with energy-efficient electric lights and automatic lighting controls that turn electric lights off when they are not required, can reduce overall lighting use by more than 50%. Savings may be even higher in gymnasia and other large spaces. One student shooting baskets in a gym can require the use of all of the lights, but a gym that makes use of daylighting may completely reduce the need for electric lighting. The heat from lights also adds to the cooling load for air-conditioning systems, further increasing energy use. The cost savings realized from the use of energy-efficient lighting can be funneled back into teachers' salaries and support material, contributing real value to the school's mission.

Greater Connections with Nature and the Environment

School buildings can provide continual lessons in environmental awareness. Windows maintain visual connections with the natural world. Good daylighting design encourages students to notice the movement of the sun and changing weather patterns, and efficient electric lighting can demonstrate the value of our nonrenewable resources. Numerous educational websites provide interactive student exercises for calculating building energy use and savings (see the resources list at the end of this chapter).

The Complex Challenge of School Lighting Design

Certainly the first consideration in any lighting design is to allow students to see the task at hand. This simple goal, however, is made more difficult to achieve by the complexity of the visual tasks, which are continually changing in both type and location. In the past, classroom activities might have been confined to students seated in rows, facing a blackboard, reading from textbooks, and writing in pencil on blue-lined paper. Many of today's classrooms have neither a clearly defined orientation nor any easily categorized visual tasks. Student learning occurs in both heads-up and heads-down positions. Students may be gathered facing a teaching wall or be dispersed about the classroom, working in small groups or on individual projects. The visual tasks are far and near, as well as large and small, and may appear on a blackboard, a whiteboard, printed paper, a three-dimensional medium, a computer screen, or a projected image. Compounding these variables are the relatively low budgets that school districts have to invest in quality lighting, both for initial building construction and for ongoing maintenance. Clearly, the complexity of these design elements can lead to lighting problems if not carefully considered.

Identifying Lighting Problems

Many complaints about lighting suggest that there is either too little or too much light. Within the lighting industry, the traditional, simplistic response to such concerns was to measure light levels (foot-candles) on the desk surface and ensure that the horizontal light level fell above an acceptable minimum. A range of standards was developed to specify required minimum light levels for specific tasks. Under these old criteria, classroom lighting schemes were expected to provide an average of 30–100 fc of light on each desk. Moreover, in these early analyses, the contribution of daylight was frequently ignored. However, visual tasks in a classroom are not confined to the desk surface. Recent research demonstrates that other attributes of a lighting design may be just as important as the quantity of light falling on the desk and perhaps even more so. Although most design standards still require a minimum light level on the horizontal work surface (usually 30–50 fc for today's classrooms), many other factors must also be evaluated to identify the lighting problems in a given area. Signs of these problems abound: blocked windows; permanently closed blinds; dark, unused corners; continuously burning electric lights; dirty windows and light fixtures; and unmatched lamps. Some of their common causes are discussed in the following sections:

Insufficient Lighting

A minimum light level is required to easily see and interpret visual information. The smaller the task, the more light required (up to a point of diminishing returns). Other factors may include the speed of the task, the contrast, or the age of the person performing the activity. The quality of the lighting design also strongly affects the perception of light levels in a space. High-quality lighting may provide good vision at lower levels of light on the horizontal plane, but no increase in the quantity of light can make up for poor-quality, unbalanced, or glaring light.

Unbalanced Lighting

The balance of light in a space refers to the way the light is distributed around the surfaces of a room. Although some situations benefit from dramatic directional lighting (e.g., theaters, restaurants, or retail displays), classrooms require a uniform, balanced distribution that illuminates tasks from several directions and eliminates strong shadows. Lighting the walls and ceiling, as well as the desks, both balances the light in the area and promotes a feeling of spaciousness (fig. 3.4).

Unbalanced lighting produces shadows that interfere with perception and draws often-inappropriate attention to the brighter areas. Even though some classrooms concentrate the work at the teaching wall and the desks, a strong focus on lighting only on these surfaces makes the room inflexible for activities in other areas.

Glare

A direct view of a strong light source, whether a fluorescent lamp, direct sunlight, or a very bright surface, creates glare and causes visual discomfort, fatigue, or even the inability to see at all. Even reflections of a bright light source may produce glare, such as patches of direct sun in a darker space or the shiny veiling reflections from windows and light fixtures that sometimes obscure information on computer screens and whiteboards. Some variation in brightness brings interest to a space, but brightness differences greater than 5:1 become distracting or possibly disabling, especially if they occur within students' and teachers' normal field of view. Glare moves attention away from the tasks at hand and can cause students to miss important information (like the page number for a homework assignment). The IESNA recommends that the luminance (brightness) of any surface normally viewed directly should not be greater than five times the luminance of the task (2000).

Monotonous Lighting

The converse of the problem of glare is the problem of monotony. Flat, directionless, uniform lighting becomes boring over long periods of time. Even at high light levels, flat lighting is often perceived as dim or dull.

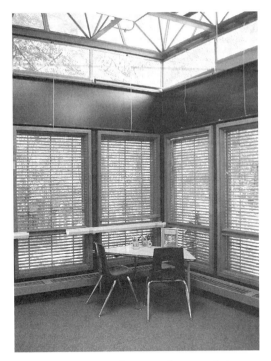

Figure 3.4. Lower windows provide screened views of nature; higher clerestory windows spread balanced daylight across the classroom. (Photo by Barbara Erwine.)

Gloomy Lighting

Diffuse ambient lighting that concentrates on one area and leaves others dark can make a space feel cavelike or gloomy. Although this type of lighting may sometimes be used for dramatic effect (e.g., in churches), it is not appropriate for classrooms. This cavelike effect can also be experienced when downlighting from parabolic fixtures or recessed cans provides the only light in a room, illuminating desktops but leaving the ceiling and walls dark.

Unnatural Lighting

If lamps have poor color characteristics (low CRI), colors and skin tones will appear unnatural (with the greenish tint associated with the old-style T12 fluorescent tubes).

Inflexible Lighting

Because classroom tasks vary greatly, the lighting design should be flexible enough to accommodate a variety of activities (audiovisual presentations, science demonstrations, creative writing, story time, performances, evening meetings, parent/teacher conferences). General classroom lighting should at least be flexible enough to be adjusted to half-brightness to allow students to see information projected on the teaching wall and still be able to take notes at their desks. Inflexible lighting can make it difficult to perform specific tasks and can consume excess energy.

Wasteful Lighting

Lights that burn unnecessarily waste valuable resources and consume budgetary dollars that could be directed to important educational activities. To minimize energy use, teachers and staff should be able to switch off or dim the lights when they are not needed. In addition, exterior lights that direct light into the sky or onto adjacent properties are both wasteful and irritating to neighbors.

Annoying Lighting Side Effects

The lighting system may be accompanied by annoying side effects. The buzzing and flickering of magnetically ballasted fluorescent lights can adversely affect concentration and health. In addition, if lamps are replaced only as they burn out, the older ones may show a spiraling "raccoon tail" of light or work only intermittently.

Lighting Design Recommendations

A holistic approach to lighting design both eliminates the aforementioned problems and ensures a healthy, safe, and stimulating environment (fig. 3.4). Holistic lighting design includes the following recommendations.

Prioritize Daylight Early in the Design

To capture the many benefits of daylight while avoiding the negative effects of poor daylight design, such as excessive heat gain or glare, daylighting must be considered early in the building design process. Daylight may even affect the choice of site and must be integrated with the overall building design. The orientation of the building, shading by adjacent landforms and vegetation, and the overall shape of the structure can have as much impact on when and where daylight is present as do the size and location of individual windows and skylights. The daylighting design should incorporate a plan to provide diffuse, usable daylight in every space where people will spend long periods of time (e.g., classrooms, administrative offices). Windows that face east or west bring low-angle sun that can cause overheating and glare and are therefore best avoided. The glare from direct sun penetration can be prevented by using diffusing skylights, orienting windows to the north or south, and fully shading south-facing windows.

Provide Views to the Outside

Views to the outside can provide a good connection to nature, allowing minds and eye muscles to relax. However, a single window cannot always serve as both a view window and a daylight window. Skylights or clerestory windows high in the wall work well to deliver daylight deep into a space; for views, smaller windows can be installed lower in the wall—at eye level.

Integrate Daylight and Electric Lighting

Daylight frequently supplies ambient lighting, but because it varies throughout the day and changes across the room, it must be supplemented with electric light. When the design team envisions the areas of high and low daylight in the room and integrates the electric lighting in similar zones that are separately switched or dimmed, electric light can be added in stages as daylight fluctuates. At night, in the absence of daylight, electric lights must provide good lighting across the entire space.

Light the Walls and Vertical Surfaces

In schools, the wall is the key learning surface, and occupants judge the light in a space by the brightness of the room surfaces. Lighting the ceiling, walls, and vertical surfaces and painting them with light colors imparts a bright, spacious appearance (fig. 3.5).

Avoid Direct Views of All Light Sources

Direct views of a bright light source (the sun, a bright sky, or an electric lamp) will create glare,

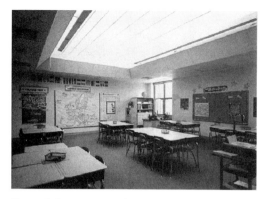

Figure 3.5. Louvers on this toplighting design diffuse and spread the light evenly in the space and prevent direct views of the sun. (Photo courtesy of Robert Flynn and National Renewable Energy Laboratory Photographic Information eXchange, No. 08834.)

causing visual discomfort and impaired performance. If bright window and skylight surfaces are in the normal field of view, baffles or blinds can help block a direct view of the glazing. Electric light fixtures should also be designed to block direct views of their lamps. Light-colored paint on the surfaces around windows and light fixtures reduces contrast with the adjacent surfaces and improves light distribution.

Provide Balanced, Low-Glare Daylight

Daylight from Two or More Directions

Diffuse daylight from multiple directions minimizes shadows, balances the light across the room, and reduces the need for electric lighting. A combination of view windows, high windows, skylights, and/or roof monitors allows daylight to enter the classroom from several directions.

Avoid Direct Sun in Classrooms and Work Spaces

Direct sun creates a distracting glare and has been shown to reduce performance (see "Learning Issues"). Diffuse light from north-facing windows or sunlight reflected off louvers or a lightshelf provides gentle, even lighting. The use of diffusing glazing or louvers in skylights spreads the daylight across the whole classroom, minimizing hot spots and glare (fig. 3.6). For additional control, teachers should have easy access to interior window shades or blinds to minimize potential glare conditions.

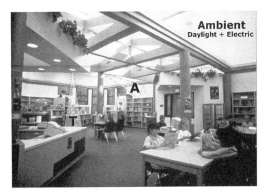

Figure 3.6. At Hunt Elementary in Puyallup, Washington, the library's diffuse (ambient) light comes from the clerestory windows and the indirect electric lighting high in the ceiling (turned off in this photograph). Additional task light (T) is provided by recessed compact fluorescent lighting above the reference desk. Accent lights (A) highlight wall displays. (Photo by Paul Rising, BLRB Architects.)

Design for Flexible, Low-Glare Electric Lighting

Direct/Indirect Pendants

Direct/indirect pendant lighting is the best choice to provide bright walls and ceilings without glare, but it usually requires a ceiling height of at least 9 feet. Lower ceiling heights require recessed or ceiling-mounted fixtures. Luminaires for lower-ceiling classrooms should deliver some light to the walls and ceilings. Use of recessed parabolic fixtures should be avoided unless they are combined with "wall wash" electric lighting that also brightens the walls.

Design with Lighting Layers

A general (ambient) lighting system provides light for routine classroom work. More demanding, focused work areas may need higher task lighting, and here, special accent lighting may be added to draw attention to displays. Good lighting design uses separate "layers" of light for ambient, task, and accent needs and provides switches to independently control each one. Additional controls that allow the teacher to dim or turn off some of the ambient lights for audiovisual presentations or for balancing daylight in the space also add flexibility.

Don't Waste Money on Excess Energy

Design Windows and Skylights to Deliver Light but Minimize Heat Gain in Summer and Heat Loss in Winter

Maximum energy savings can be realized by sizing window glazing appropriately and choosing energy-efficient glass and shading techniques suitable to the climate. Optimally, windows should be oriented to north and south, and those that face east or west should be avoided. Ander (2003), Benya et al. (2003), Heschong et al. (1998), and the U.S. Department of Energy (1997) provide additional design strategies to maximize the energy performance of windows and skylights.

Choose Energy-Efficient, Low-Maintenance Electric Lighting

For classrooms and staff spaces, T5 and T8 fluorescent lamps with electronic ballasts provide the highest-quality lighting and the greatest energy savings. High-output T5 fluorescent fixtures are gaining in popularity for use in gyms and other spaces with very high ceilings. Metal halide lamps are effective for lighting school grounds and parking areas. For lower-light applications, high-wattage compact fluorescent lamps are a good choice. Incandescent lights are best reserved for theatrical effects and special accents. The design of the light fixture also affects how efficiently it delivers light to an area. High-performance luminaries provide more light per luminaire and reduce the overall number of light fixtures needed, thus maximizing energy savings and minimizing installation cost and maintenance.

Turn Off Unnecessary Lights

Teachers should have easy access to light switches so that they can adjust light levels for different activities and respond to the balance of daylight in a particular area (fig. 3.7). Automatic controls can provide additional savings by ensuring that lights are off when they are not needed. In addition, occupancy sensors can turn off lights automatically when no one is in a room. Photocells sense daylight levels and automatically switch off or dim electric lights when daylight is plentiful. These techniques also extend the life of lamps by reducing the num-

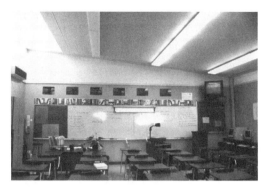

Figure 3.7. The linear skylight along the left wall of this classroom washes the wall with light and provides good daylight levels for about half the classroom space. One or two rows of electric lights can be turned off when daylight is plentiful. Note the reflections on the whiteboard from a bright window at back of classroom, which could have been prevented with window blinds. (Photo by Lisa Heschong.)

ber of hours of use, resulting in savings in both energy and maintenance expenditures.

Provide Emergency Egress Lighting

In emergencies, people must be able to see the egress route and any obstacles in their path. Egress lighting consists of both a system of general-area lights that remain on when the main power is lost and exit signs that indicate the way out. Local regulations specify brightness levels and other standards for these systems; energy-efficient lamps (e.g., LEDs) ensure minimal system operating cost. Well-placed windows and skylights can greatly enhance the available egress lighting during daytime hours.

Ensure an Efficient Lighting System

The following measures and frequent checkups will guarantee a healthy lighting system over time:

- Current operating procedures and manuals for all of the controls should be available.
- Commissioning the lighting system involves having the lighting designer or electrical engineer ensure that all electric lighting and controls are working properly at installation. A commissioning package may result in extra charges when the school is constructed, but it

will pay for itself in higher performance and reduced maintenance in the long run.
- Cleaning window glass and light fixtures on a regular schedule ensures that they will deliver the light they were designed to provide.
- A group schedule to replace electric lamps at the end of their useful life (but before they burn out) saves money in the long run and provides consistent performance from all the fixtures.
- Standardizing on a few lamp types for the school building minimizes stocking inventories and simplifies maintenance.
- Environmentally responsible measures include the use of low-mercury fluorescent lamps, as well as the recycling or proper disposal of lamps.

Develop a Lighting Plan and Set Priorities

In both new construction and the remodeling of an existing school, funds are usually limited and must be allocated among competing needs. For new construction, the highest lighting priority is the design of an integrated daylighting and electric lighting scheme that illuminates vertical surfaces and delivers balanced, low-glare light. This approach should include energy-efficient luminaires (with T5 or T8 lamps and electronic ballasts) zoned to match the areas of high and low daylight availability. If the budget does not allow for automated controls, manual controls for each of the light zones can be used, and automated lighting controls can be added later.

For remodeled facilities, the highest priorities are to remedy existing lighting safety problems and retrofit older T12 lamps and magnetic ballasts with T8 or T5 lamps and electronic ballasts. Such improvements increase both the quality and energy efficiency of the lighting system and reduce stress in occupants. Many local electric utilities and energy service companies have incentive programs to help defray part of the cost of these retrofits. If light fixtures are old, they may be replaced at the same time. This is an opportunity to improve the quality of the electric light by increasing the uniformity of light levels and the light on vertical surfaces. Finally, if the budget allows, automated lighting controls can be added to ensure energy savings.

If You Want to See a Specialist . . .

An important member of the architectural team is the lighting designer, who provides the expertise for an attractive, productive, and well-lit environment. Lighting designers with the initials "LC" after their name have passed the qualifying exam of the National Council on Qualification for the Lighting Profession. In North America, the IESNA and the International Association of Lighting Designers are the primary professional associations for lighting designers. These organizations develop industry standards and produce educational courses and reference materials. The following resources also offer information on healthy, high-quality, energy-efficient lighting design:

- *Lighting Handbook Reference and Application* (2000b): The IESNA publishes this primary resource for information about lighting technologies, the process of seeing, and the recommended practices of lighting design. It provides excellent discussions of all aspects of lighting design, health impacts, and currently available lamps and light fixtures and also includes a chapter on school lighting. The IESNA also publishes the Guide for Educational Facilities Lighting (2000a), which gives both a broad discussion of school lighting issues and specific recommendations for lighting a variety of learning spaces within the school environment (classrooms, gymnasia, libraries, laboratories, etc.).
- *Advanced Lighting Guidelines* is a comprehensive reference for information on lighting design practices and technologies. The goal of the guidelines is to provide a regularly updated document that will remain useful to lighting decision makers and encourage appropriate practices for lighting design in buildings. It is available online free of charge at http://www.newbuildings.org/lighting.htm or at a nominal charge for a paper or electronic copy at the same website.
- Collaborative for High-performance Schools (CHPS) includes a broad range of government, private industry, and nonprofit organizations whose goal is to facilitate the design of high-performance schools—environments that are not only energy efficient but also healthy, comfortable, and well lit. High-performance

schools achieve these goals by using a whole-building, integrated design strategy that incorporates the best of today's ideas and technologies. The integrated-design approach leverages the interactions among building components (windows, walls, building materials, air-conditioning, landscaping, etc.) to maximize the overall performance of the building. Much of this approach is described in chapter 23, and three Best Practices manuals (Planning, Design, and Criteria) are available online at no charge at http://www.chps.net/, along with design videos and other resources.

Resources

Lighting Design

The following websites provide information on good lighting design:

- http://www.CHPS.net (free download of Best Practices Manual)
- http://www.newbuildings.org/lighting.htm (free download of Advanced Lighting Guidelines)

Lighting and Energy Exercises for the Classroom

The following websites provide student exercises for measuring and evaluating energy performance in the classroom as part of an energy awareness curriculum:

- http://www.fsec.ucf.edu/ed/teachers/
- http://www2.nsta.org/energy
- http://www.ase.org/educators/index.htm
- http://www.rebuild.org/sectors/sectorpages/energyeducationlib.asp

References

Ander, GD. 2003. *Daylighting performance and design.* New York: Wiley.

Benya J, Heschong L, McGowan T, Miller M, Rubinstein F. 2003. Advanced lighting guidelines. White Salmon, WA: New Buildings Institute. Available: http://www.newbuildings.org [accessed 23 March 2005].

Berman SM, Fein G, Jewett DL, Ashford F. 1993. Luminance-controlled pupil size affects Landolt-C task performance. J Illuminating Eng Soc 22:150–165.

Berman, SM, Fein G, Jewett DL, Ashford F. 1994. Landolt-C recognition in elderly subjects is affected by scotopic intensity of surround illuminants. J Illuminating Eng Soc 23:123–130.

Boyce P, Hunter C, Howlett O. 2003. The benefits of daylight through windows. Sponsored by the Capturing the Daylight Dividend Program. Washington, DC: U.S. Department of Energy.

California Energy Commission. 2003a. Windows and classrooms: A study of student performance and the indoor environment. Technical Report P500-03-082-A-7. White Salmon, WA: New Buildings Institute.

California Energy Commission. 2003b. Windows and offices: A study of worker performance and the indoor environment. Technical Report P500-03-082-A-9. White Salmon, WA: New Buildings Institute.

Classroom Lighting Knowhow. 2002. Design Lights Consortium, Northeast Energy Efficiency Partnership, Inc., Lexington, MA. Available: http://www.designlights.org/downloads/classroom_guide.pdf [accessed 23 March 2005].

Guzowski M. 2000. Address Health and Well-Being. *In Daylighting for Sustainable Design.* New York: McGraw-Hill, 291–339.

Harding GFA. 1984. Photosensitive epilepsy. Volume 9, Issue 3. Available: http://www.epilepsytoronto.org/photo.html [accessed 23 November 2004].

Heschong L, Mahone D, Rubinstein F, McHugh J. 1998. Skylighting guidelines. Southern California Edison. Available: http://www.energydesignresources.com [accessed 16 July 2004].

HMG (Heschong Mahone Group). 1999. Daylighting in schools: An investigation into the relationship between daylighting and human performance. HMG Project No. 9803. San Francisco: Pacific Gas and Electric Company.

Illuminating Engineering Society of North America. 2000a. Guide for educational facilities lighting. Document no. IESNA RP-3-00, May 19. New York: IESNA.

Illuminating Engineering Society of North America. 2000b. *IESNA lighting handbook: Reference and applications,* 9th ed. (Rea M, ed.). New York: Wiley.

Kluth P. 2004. 2004. Autism, autobiography, and adaptations: Teaching exceptional children. Teach Except Child 36(4) (March/April):42–47.

Marion County Public Schools. March 2000. Principals' and directors' report. Ocala, FL. In *IESNA lighting handbook, Reference and applications,* 9th ed. (Rea M, ed.). New York: Wiley.

Myths and facts about energy in schools: Energy design resources. (2000, July). eNews 11 (July 21, 2000):3. Available: http://www.energydesignresources.com/docs/end-11.pdf.

Thompson S. 1999. Neurobehavioral characteristics seen in the classroom: Developing an educational plan for the student with NLD. Available: http://www.nldline.com/sue_educ.htm [accessed 23 November 2004].

U.S. Department of Energy. 1997. Tips for daylighting with windows. Building Technologies Program, Lawrence Berkeley National Laboratory. Available: *http://windows.lbl.gov/pub/designguide/copyright_tips .html* [accessed 24 June 2005]

Veitch J, McColl SL. 1994. Full-spectrum fluorescent lighting effects on people: A critical review. In *Full-spectrum Lighting Effects on Performance, Mood, and Health* (Veitch FA, ed.). Ottawa, Ontario: National Research Council Canada.

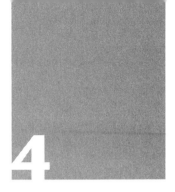

4

Lorraine E. Maxwell

Noise

■ *Summary*

- In a school setting, noise is any unwanted sound that interferes with classroom communication and is both disturbing and detrimental to the learning process.
- Noise sources can be external (e.g., roads, trains, aircraft) or internal (e.g., resulting from poor acoustic designs for classrooms, normal classroom activities, and ambient sources such as HVAC systems).
- Both acute and chronic noisy conditions influence learning. More specifically, noise affects communication between teachers and students, motivation, attention, memory, and thus academic achievement.
- Health issues related to classroom noise include stress and increased blood pressure and heart rates in children—conditions that may persist into adulthood. Teachers can also experience mental and voice fatigue.
- Most efforts to reduce noise are directed at the classroom. Additionally, careful school design and modification can alleviate noisy conditions in and around the building. ■

This chapter addresses the nonauditory effect of noise on children, that is, the effect of noise apart from hearing loss. Even when there is no damage to hearing, children's mental and physical health, as well as their ability to learn, can be affected by exposure to noise. A healthy learning environment supports all of a child's developmental needs—cognitive, emotional, social, and physical. Moreover, a noisy school environment can be a source of stress for both children and teachers.

To understand how noise relates to a safe and healthy school environment, we first examine how noise affects learning and academic achievement. A major goal of this book, and this chapter in particular, is to identify the factors that facility planners, designers, school administrators, and teachers can manipulate to help create a safe and healthy learning environment. Because building and acoustical standards can affect the level of noise in the classroom, it is important to consider how possible combinations of certain physical attributes (adjacencies, external noise, acoustical conditions) in a school setting are related to the effects of noise on children.

What Is Noise?

Noise can be defined as any unwanted sound. Therefore, because almost any sound can become noise, noise is largely a subjective experience (see table 4.1). Music played loudly and enjoyed by one person may be noise to the person in the next room who is trying to read or sleep. School settings present a myriad of sounds; schools are not meant to be silent places. So which sounds become noise, and what is too much sound?

More specifically, noise is "audible acoustical energy (sound) that is unwanted because it has adverse auditory and nonauditory physiological or psychological effects on people" (Kryter 1994, p. 1). It may also be "unwanted sound which may be hazardous to health, interferes with communication, or is disturbing" (Hirschorn 1989, p. A-3). These descriptions give us a more precise definition of noise: In a school setting, sounds that have an adverse physiological or psychological effect on learning become noise. In this environment, noise can come from intrusive outside sources, external to the school (road traffic, trains, or airports) or from internal sources inside the school building (speech from others nearby or ambient noise sources such as heating and air-conditioning systems).

In addition to having pitch and intensity, sound can be either intermittent or continuous. Loud noises can be tolerated by adults and children for brief periods but can become detrimental if they

---

■ *4.1. Properties of sound and noise*

Sound has *pitch* (high, low), measured in units called Hertz (Hz). Children and young adults can hear pitch tones between 20 and 20,000 Hz. Sound has *intensity* (loudness, softness), measured in decibels (dB). The unit dBA refers to the A-weighted scale for measuring intensity. Children and adults can hear between 0 dB (threshold of hearing) and 125–130 dB (threshold of pain) (Manlove et al. 2001).

For *acute noise,* exposure may be continuous or intermittent but does not occur over an extended period of time. For *chronic noise,* exposure may be continuous or intermittent and occurs every day over an extended period of time (months, years). ■

---

do not eventually cease. In general, the louder the sound, the briefer the exposure should be. For example, in the workplace, the maximum continuous exposure time at 85 dBA is 8 hours; at 100 dBA, the maximum exposure time is 1 minute, 29 seconds (National Institute for Occupational Safety and Health 1998). Exposure to loud noises for long periods of time can damage one's hearing. However, chronic exposure to noise at levels below 85 dBA, although not likely to damage hearing, can negatively affect learning.

Table 4.1. Noise levels of common sounds

Level (dB)	Example
10	Normal breathing
30	Soft whisper
50–75	Washing machine
60	Normal conversation
70	Television
75–85	Flush toilet
85	Heavy traffic, noisy restaurant
90	Shouted conversation
90–115	Subway
100	Woodworking class, boom box
110	Car horn, symphony concert
120	Chain saw, jet plane, band concert

Data from League for the Hard of Hearing (1996–2003).

Acoustics in the Classroom

The primary factors that affect classroom acoustics are reverberation, background noise levels, and signal-to-noise ratio (SNR). These factors, as well as the pitch and loudness of speech, help determine the quality of the learning experiences in the classroom in relation to noise. The amount of time a sound (or noise) persists once it has ceased is known as *reverberation time.* The reverberation time of a sound in a space such as a classroom is measured by the time required for the level of a steady sound to decay to 60 dB after the sound has been turned off (ANSI 2002). This *decay rate* depends on a number of factors, such as the frequency of the sound, the shape and volume of the room, the amount of sound-absorbing materials in the room, and the number of people present. Reverberation time is a critical element in speech intelligibility and therefore plays an important role in classroom activities. If reverberation is insufficient, sounds will not reach the listeners. However, reverberation can also contribute to the perception of a noisy classroom if sounds take a relatively long time to decay. The recommended reverberation time in unoccupied classrooms for school-age children is 0.4–0.7 seconds (ASHA 1995; ANSI 2002).

Background noise (also referred to as ambient noise) in classrooms is typically generated by fluorescent lighting, mechanical air-handling systems, or heating and cooling systems. It may also come from external sources such as a nearby street with constant heavy traffic. Recommended background noise levels for unoccupied classrooms for school-aged children is 30–35 dBA (ANSI 2002; Crandell and Smaldino 1994). When a classroom is occupied, noise levels increase, so it is important to keep background noise to a minimum. Ambient noise levels greater than 40 dBA can negatively affect speech intelligibility.

The SNR is a critical factor in assessing the acoustics of a classroom. The SNR is the difference in decibels between the level of a speaker's voice and the level of the background noise (Manlove et al. 2001). A positive SNR means that the speaker's voice is louder than the background noise; a negative SNR means the opposite. Speech intelligibility generally requires an SNR of 6–10 dB for normal-hearing adults. For normal-hearing children, researchers have found that the minimum SNR should be 15–20 dB (ASHA 1995). For children with hearing loss, for children with learning disabilities, or for children whom English is not their first language, the SNR should be higher (Hodgson 1999).

Typical Classroom Acoustics

We have just reviewed the major factors that affect classroom acoustics, including the recommended optimal conditions for reverberation time, background noise levels, and SNR. Optimal conditions are based on the requirements for speech intelligibility. Many classrooms in the United States, however, do not meet these conditions, which are summarized in table 4.2.

Noise in the School Building

A school usually has certain areas that are noisier than others, but all areas of a school may contribute to a noisy environment.

Areas for Congregation

Noise is likely to be an issue in corridors, stairways, and lunchrooms because large numbers of people usually occupy these spaces at the same time. The activities and the physical characteristics of the space generate noise. Because of the way classes are scheduled in most schools, large numbers of students move through the corridors and stairways at the same time. Although some schools may have policies about talking in the corridors, for many students the few minutes between classes is an opportunity to talk with classmates and friends. Even if students do not yell, corridors and stairways will become noisy. Bells announcing the change of classes also contribute to noisy corridors. The hard materials frequently used in the construction of stairways and corridors can withstand constant use but do not absorb sound well. A flexible class schedule that reduces the number of children in the corridors at the same time can potentially reduce the noise level.

Table 4.2. Typical classroom noise conditions

	Elementary school	Childcare	Recommended
Background noise	41–51 dBA	37–42 dBA	30–35 dBA
Noise in occupied room	52–62 dBA	58–94 dBA	45–55 dBA
Reverberation time (sec)	0.4–1.2	0.2–0.4	0.4–0.7
SNR	−7 to +5 dB	−3 to +12 dB	15–20 dB

Data from ANSI (2002); Manlove et al. (2001).

Mealtime should be a social time, so cafeterias are often very noisy places. Many schools have long tables that seat 20 or more children, making it difficult for children to talk to each other. Sometimes students complain that they cannot hear their conversations because the room is too noisy; as a result, children raise their voices. Round tables that seat six to eight students can help reduce noise levels, as children are seated closer together and can speak in more conversational voices.

Areas That Accommodate Noise-producing Activities

A noisy locker room or gymnasium is not likely to be a source of stress because children are usually not involved in difficult or complex mental tasks in either of these spaces. These areas are noisy because of the large numbers of students and the nature of the activities (conversation, games). The noise is usually expected and enjoyable. These spaces provide a respite from the more restrictive areas and activities of school life. However, unless the proper steps are taken, noise from gymnasiums and locker rooms can spill over into other areas of the school and become a source of distraction and annoyance.

In addition to the number of occupants and the activities that take place in these areas, the physical characteristics of gymnasiums and locker rooms contribute to the noise levels. Both hard surfaces and high-volume areas (e.g., rooms with high ceilings) increase reverberation time, thus contributing to a noisy environment.

Activity in music practice rooms is also a potential source of noise. However, these rooms do not have to contribute to a noisy school environment if they are designed to appropriately contain the sound generated in them. These spaces should shield the user from outside noise as well as control the transmission of sound to adjacent spaces.

Areas for Activities Requiring Concentration

Classrooms do not usually generate noise that affects other parts of the school. However, external conditions such as a nearby airport, a heavily traveled street, nearby train tracks can contribute to a noisy classroom. Noise is more problematic in classrooms than in other spaces such as gymnasi-

ums. Additionally, classroom noise can be generated by lighting, mechanical ventilation systems, and heating and cooling systems. Classroom activities and sounds from adjacent spaces such as the corridor can also create problems with noise.

Students and teachers are supposed to engage in dialogue in the classroom; however, if the acoustical design of the classroom is inappropriate, conversations can contribute to noise levels that detract from learning and teaching. In classroom settings, children report that the most annoying sources of noise are chatter from other students, scraping chairs, and sounds from the corridor (in that order) (Boman and Enmarker 2004).

A library is usually not a noise generator, but just as in the classroom, it can be adversely affected by noise. Noise from adjacent spaces such as music practice rooms, a busy corridor, or the cafeteria will adversely affect library activities if appropriate acoustical controls are not in place. Ideally, the library will not be immediately adjacent to noise-producing areas. However, external sources such as roads or airports can also contribute to noise in the school library. Mechanical systems should be designed to reduce noise levels in the library.

Noise and Learning

The relation between noise and learning is multi-faceted and depends on several conditions (Gifford 2002):

- the nature of the noise (loudness, continuity, meaningfulness),
- the learner's characteristics (age, gender, motivation, sense of control, personality, specific learning style or profile),
- the activity or task (listening, complex task, memorizing), and
- the type of learning that is being measured (performance of what has already been learned or learning that is in process).

Not all of these factors come into play in every situation, but each is important.

In the following sections, we look at the effects of noise exposure on various factors related to learning—namely, communication, attention and memory, motivation, and academic achievement. The most consistent finding is that the effects of chronic noise on learning are most pronounced when a task or activity is difficult or complex or when greater concentration is needed. Both chronic intermittent and continuous noise sources have a negative impact. The effects of chronic noise on learning are present even when children are removed for a short time from the noise source; permanent removal of the noise source can improve children's health and learning.

Communication

A critical part of knowledge acquisition is communication between teachers and students and among students. If the classroom environment makes it difficult for teachers and students to communicate with each other, learning will suffer. We already know that noise interferes with speech perception and children's ability to pay attention. It is clear that noisy classrooms make teacher–student and student–student communication difficult at best. As many teachers use small-group activities as part of their pedagogy, children must be able to communicate with each other in these small groups.

In addition to interfering with speech perception, noise is related to classroom communication through its effects on both student and teacher behavior. Students confronted with a noisy environment tend to resist interacting with other students. In noisy preschool classrooms, children withdraw socially, probably in an attempt to reduce the amount of stimulation they are experiencing. These children do not play or talk with other children, nor do they participate in play activities as much as their peers in quieter preschool classrooms. Older children also withdraw from communicating with their classmates in noisy environments. Although individual work is part of typical classroom activities, working with others helps students learn in different ways. When noise levels are high, teachers may discourage group projects, or students may withdraw from group activities, thus missing out on a potential source of learning.

Noisy classrooms also affect teachers' behavior and well-being. Teachers report lost teaching time due to significant interruptions from road, train, or airport-related noise. For example, one study in New York City found that 11% of teaching time was lost because of pauses in instruction during the noise from passing elevated subway trains (Bronzaft

and McCarthy 1975). Teachers also report high levels of irritation with these external sources of noise, as well as workplace dissatisfaction, mental fatigue, and difficulties in concentration (Ko 1979; Sargent et al. 1980). Teachers in noisy classrooms can also suffer from voice strain in an attempt to be heard by all of the students, adding to teachers' frustration and fatigue.

Anecdotal reports suggest that teachers' use of wireless microphones may facilitate classroom communication, but further controlled studies are needed before general recommendations can be made. In any event, use of these microphones facilitates communication in only one direction and does not eliminate other negative effects of chronic noise exposure.

Noisy classrooms make it difficult for teachers and students to communicate because of attention and speech perception issues. Noise has the potential to limit the amount of communication time teachers and students have with each other. In addition, students and teachers may withdraw from communicating in an attempt to reduce further stimulation or because it is too difficult to overcome the noise.

Attention and Memory

In school, children are often admonished to "pay attention." Attention involves the ability to concentrate on a specific task; noise is a source of distraction and thus interrupts voluntary attention. Teachers in noisy schools report that students have more trouble concentrating than do students in quiet schools, and students in noisy schools have difficulty staying on task. Noise exposure makes it especially difficult to learn or to focus on complex activities (Evans and Lepore 1993).

Noise has a negative effect on attention, in part because it interferes with auditory discrimination and speech perception. Short-term or acute noise exposure does not appear to have long-term negative consequences for children. Some children, especially boys, learn to concentrate in spite of noisy conditions. This adaptation, however, is short lived; eventually it becomes too difficult for children to block out the distraction of the noise, and they are unable to pay attention. Children who use the cognitive strategy of blocking out to deal with noise may generalize to all situations and tune out not only distracting background noise but also relevant material such as speech (Evans and Hygge 2006). Schoolchildren exposed to external noise sources or conversations from nearby classmates have difficulty sustaining attention, as well as understanding relevant speech. The SNR may be too low; that is, background noise may be interfering with the children's ability to pay attention to the classroom teacher or other pertinent input. If children become frustrated because they cannot understand the teacher, they may simply stop paying attention. Teachers who must consistently speak in a loud voice run the risk of becoming hoarse. Research further indicates that irrelevant conversations are more disturbing than conversations related to the task at hand (Knez and Hygge 2002). The effects of noise on attention and speech perception are found in children without hearing loss.

Chronic noise exposure interferes with long-term memory, particularly of complex or difficult material. Recognition memory, however, may not be adversely affected by chronic noise (Hygge 1993). For example, a child in a noisy classroom may have trouble answering an essay question about a social studies topic but may be able to answer the same question when given cues such as an image or certain words in multiple-choice answers. Thus, while steps should be taken to reduce noise levels in the classroom, teaching and testing methods can be altered to attempt to compensate for noisy conditions.

Motivation

Motivation is an important psychological process related to learning. A major feature of motivation is the belief that one can succeed at a task. A child who is consistently unable to complete or succeed at a task may become frustrated and eventually lose the motivation to continue trying.

Noise is related to motivation through lack of control and frustration. Children chronically exposed to noise who experience repeated frustration because of that exposure may become less motivated and less likely to feel in control. Chronic exposure to frustration and failure to achieve lead, in turn, to a lack of motivation and may eventually result in learned helplessness. Learned helplessness in children is manifested not only in their schoolwork but in other areas of their lives (Cohen et al. 1986). Girls appear to be more vulnerable than boys to feelings of learned helplessness in chronic

noise situations (Gifford 2002). Reducing chronic exposure to noise can improve a child's motivation and the ability to do well academically.

Academic Achievement

Noise in the classroom has negative effects on communication patterns and the ability to pay attention. Thus, it is not surprising that chronic exposure to noise is related to children's academic achievement, particularly in its negative effects on reading and learning to read. Maxwell and Evans (2000) found that, when preschool classrooms were modified to reduce noise levels, not only did the children speak to each other more often and in more complete sentences, but their performance on a prereading assessment measure improved. Research with older children suggests similar findings. On reading and math measures, elementary and high school students in noisy schools or classrooms consistently perform below their counterparts in quieter settings (Gifford 2002).

Short-term (acute) noise exposure in the classroom is unlikely to have long-term negative effects on reading or other academic skills. Chronic noise exposure is more detrimental. When children experience noisy classrooms every day over a period of months and years, the effects are likely to be highly detrimental. The good news is that, when children are permanently removed from these noisy settings, they can improve their academic performance.

Noise is most detrimental to academic achievement when children are exposed during the learning process. Researchers have been careful to distinguish between testing children in noisy and quiet situations. If noise at the point of testing were largely responsible for the negative effects on reading and math performance, the remedy would be less complicated. However, children from noisy schools have been tested in quiet settings along with children from quiet schools, and the noise-exposed children consistently performed below their peers from quieter settings. Noise appears to interfere with the way children process information and language, which may account for the findings related to reading (Evans and Maxwell 1997). Noise exposure is especially detrimental to children with lower aptitude and learning problems.

If children are generally exposed to environmental noise in the home and the community, then noise in the classroom only compounds their problems related to learning and academic performance. Children from noisy home environments (even those as young as 7 months) show deficits in cognitive development. Older children show deficits in reading performance. It is therefore essential that children from noisy environments do not have to contend with a noisy classroom as well.

The effect of acute noise on academic achievement may be related to gender or other personal characteristics or to the type of noise. Studies with children of elementary school age and with college students found that males performed better in acute noisy surroundings and that females performed better in quiet conditions (Gifford 2002). However, these differences largely disappear for chronic noise exposure. Meaningful noise, such as nearby conversation, is more disruptive to the performance of certain tasks than noise that does not have meaning (e.g., sounds from an air conditioner). When we hear speech, our attention is more likely to be diverted because we involuntarily attempt to make sense of the conversation.

Health Issues

In addition to effects on learning and academic achievement, noisy schools also pose a potential health threat to children. Noise can be a source of stress. One way of measuring the level of stress in people is to document blood pressure levels. Chronic elevated blood pressure levels are found in children chronically exposed to high-noise sources (those generally in excess of 70 dBA), such as airports or train traffic in residential or school settings (Evans et al. 2001). Children's health may also be compromised by everyday levels of environmental noise in the community such as road or train traffic. Elevated blood pressure levels and heart rates have been found in children who live in relatively noisier communities even when the noise levels did not approach the levels found in communities near airports (Evans et al. 2001). In all the studies that examined the health effects of noise on children, blood pressure and heart rates were taken at resting levels—in quiet conditions when children were not exposed to the noise levels of their communities—yet the blood pressure and heart rates were still higher than for children from quieter communities.

Children exposed to relatively higher levels of day-to-day community noise also have more self-reported symptoms of stress resulting from annoyance. As with adults, annoyance related to community noise does not seem to disappear over time (Haines et al. 2001).

We might expect blood pressure levels and heart rates to be elevated during exposure to a source of stress. However, research indicates that, even when children are removed from the noise source, their health can be threatened with chronic noise exposure in home or school settings (Evans et al. 2001). Although no longitudinal studies on this topic have followed children to adulthood, these higher blood pressure levels could persist to adulthood. Children's blood pressure levels do not habituate to noise exposure. Although the higher blood pressure levels do not suggest hypertension, when children age and remain in a noisy environment, they become potential candidates for stress-related health problems as adults. Equally important is the fact that children living in noisier communities reported symptoms of stress. Creating a quieter school environment can reduce stress and make it less likely that schoolwork will suffer because of noise.

Noise and Special Needs Children

Children with attention difficulties (e.g., ADHD), learning disabilities, developmental disabilities including sensory impairments (hearing or visual), conditions along the autism spectrum, or intellectual disabilities may require specialized environments in order to maximize their learning potential (see chapter 26). This is particularly relevant to sounds and noise because most instruction is verbal and therefore involves the auditory process. As an example, children with hearing impairments have special acoustical requirements (table 4.3). They generally require a space with less background noise.

Children with autism spectrum conditions may have problems distinguishing speech from background sounds, thus making their experience in a noisy classroom difficult (Alcántara et al. 2004). Given that children with autism may have greater difficulty in communicating with the teacher and other students, the presence of background noise will make this process even more problematic.

Table 4.3. Acceptable noise and reverberation times in enclosed classrooms by age for children with delayed speech processing[a]

Age (years)	Noise level in unoccupied or quiet occupied space (dBA)	Reverberation time (sec)
12+	33	0.5
10–11	32	0.5
8–9	27.5	0.5
6–7	21.5	0.5

[a]Includes children with hearing impairments, delayed language development, or nonnative speakers. Recommendations are based on enclosed space of approximately 10,000 cubic feet and voice level of 55 dBA, an average conversational level (Picard and Bradley 2001).

Children with intellectual disabilities also require less background noise because of their difficulty in understanding and processing information.

Many children with learning or developmental disabilities have associated auditory processing problems, which manifest in difficulties in a variety of functional areas of development and learning (National Center for Learning Disabilities 2004):

Preschool-age children
- learning to speak
- understanding spoken language
- separating meaningful language from background noise
- remembering stories or songs
- staying focused on a person's voice
- unusual sensitivity to noise
- confusing similar sounds.

School-age children
- remembering and following directions
- remembering people's names
- sounding out new words
- seeming to ignore others when engrossed in a nonspeaking activity
- understanding people who speak quickly
- finding the right word to use when talking.

It is therefore critical that each child who has difficulty in learning be assessed for his or her ability to hear and process auditory information so that appropriate accommodations can be made to ensure that the child receives maximum benefit from classroom instruction. (See chapter 26 on children and adults with disabilities for the determination of each child's Individual Education Plan.)

Long-term Effects

Chronic exposure to noise contributes to deficits in language acquisition in children. It reduces the ability to hear clearly and aggravates poor speech perception. Chronic exposure to noise can also exacerbate attentional deficits in children by reducing the ability to concentrate and pay attention. Furthermore, chronic exposure to noise decreases motivation and tolerance for frustration and often results in "learned helplessness." Chronic exposure to noise is also related to changes in physiological and psychological well-being, such as increased blood pressure levels, increased self-reports of stress in children, and increased mental and voice fatigue in teachers. Chronic exposure to noise also contributes to reading deficits in children. Some children initially perform well in noisy settings, but chronic exposure during the learning process leads to low achievement levels.

Addressing the Problem

A large part of what happens in the classroom relates to the ability of students and teachers to understand one another. Therefore, improving conditions for speech intelligibility is a critical step in reducing the harmful effects of noise. Schools can control noise by careful planning and by using appropriate building materials and surfaces. Those responsible for the building and maintenance of school facilities must take the necessary steps to eliminate and manage the noise generated within and outside schools and particularly in classrooms.

Controlling noise in the classroom, the primary learning space, is critical for dealing with the noise-related consequences for learning and academic performance. Therefore, most of the efforts to reduce noise in schools are concentrated on developing the ideal acoustical conditions in the classroom. The American National Standards Institute acoustical guidelines for schools recommend a maximum ambient (background) classroom noise level of 35 dBA, 0.7 seconds of reverberation time, and an SNR of 15–20 dB (ANSI 2002).

These standards are intended as guidelines to

assist school administrators, planners, and architects in the design and renovation of school buildings. The recommended decibel levels and reverberation time for learning spaces are based on conditions that promote a high degree of speech intelligibility. Nevertheless, these guidelines are only recommendations and are not required by any statute. School districts, local municipalities, or state education agencies, however, may choose to make these guidelines and recommendations mandatory for schools in their jurisdictions.

The ANSI guidelines are general recommendations and intended for all age levels. A "one-size-fits-all" guideline, however, may not be sufficient. Younger children, students whose native language is not English, and children with a hearing impairment may require different classroom acoustical conditions to achieve good speech intelligibility (Picard and Bradley 2001). These recommendations are based on individual differences related to speech processing (tables 4.3 and 4.4).

Noise Reduction

Appropriate noise measurements (reverberation time, SNR, and ambient noise level) in classrooms, corridors, cafeterias, music spaces, and other pertinent areas should be taken by licensed engineers.

Prevention

To achieve the recommended acoustical level for a learning space, designers must anticipate all likely sources of noise. Classrooms will require mechanical systems for air circulation and thermal comfort.

Table 4.4. Acceptable noise and reverberation times in enclosed classrooms by age for children with normal speech-processing ability[a]

Age (years)	Noise level in unoccupied or quiet occupied space (dBA)	Reverberation time (sec)
12+	40	0.5
10–11	39	0.5
8–9	34.5	0.5
6–7	28.5	0.5

[a]Recommendations are based on enclosed space of approximately 10,000 cubic feet and voice level of 55 dBA, an average conversational level (Picard and Bradley 2001).

Lighting systems and instructional equipment such as computers and projectors contribute to ambient noise. Finally, the activities proposed for the space will generate noise. Lecture spaces require acoustical considerations different from those needed in classrooms, where multiple simultaneous conversations occur.

Site Selection

Although new schools should not be sited near potential noise sources such as airports, railroads, and major roadways, neighborhood conditions often change. A new highway may be built, flight patterns can change, and runways may be added at a nearby airport. A school that was well sited when it was built can be exposed unexpectedly to a major external noise source. Certain site characteristics, such as trees and setbacks, can buffer a school somewhat from external noises.

Room Adjacencies

Reducing noise levels in primary learning spaces has certain design implications. In the planning stage for new schools or during renovations, care must be taken to locate learning spaces away from traditionally noisy areas such as cafeterias and athletic areas. Some spaces—music practice and athletic areas, for example—must be isolated to protect the rest of the school from the noise generated there. Unless initial building designs address these important issues, implementation may be difficult without major renovations. Other sound-attenuation steps will then have to be taken to reduce noise transmission.

Scheduling

All schools have to deal with a finite set of resources in both personnel and the use of space. Most schools are in a state of flux in dealing with students' changing needs, the demands of the curriculum, and the availability and flexibility of appropriate teachers and staff. Scheduled activities that may result in an increase in sound, such as band practice, drama classes, or gymnastics, must be considered in controlling sound and noise in the classrooms.

Building Materials

Appropriately designed walls, floors, ceilings, and roofs can significantly reduce noise transmission to adjacent spaces. In existing schools, walls, floors, and ceilings may require acoustical treatment to reduce noise levels. Teachers in preschool and early elementary school classrooms often use carpeting and other soft, sound-absorbent material on floors and walls to create better acoustical conditions. Carpeting alone, however, does not provide enough sound absorption to solve classroom noise problems (ANSI 2002). In addition, some sound-absorbent materials may present indoor air quality issues because of their porous or fibrous nature. Contact the U.S. Environmental Protection Agency for assistance with selection, installation, and maintenance of these materials (ANSI 2002).

The volume of the space also affects the noise level; therefore, ceiling height is an important part of managing classroom noise. Depending on activity in adjacent spaces, full-height walls will reduce noise transmission. It may be necessary to install acoustical materials in the ceilings, walls, and floors of appropriate areas of the school, including corridors and stairways, keeping indoor air quality in mind (see chapter 10).

Appropriate doors, windows, and skylights can diminish noise transmission from within the school and from external sources of noise. Well-designed doors and windows offer a measure of protection from changes in neighborhood conditions. It may be necessary to replace old windows and doors with newer types that reduce noise transmission from the outdoors and from adjacent internal spaces.

Finally, replacement of ventilation systems with less noisy equipment can also provide better air quality.

Furniture

Simple measures to reduce noise resulting from furniture can be helpful, such as placing chair leg tips on movable furniture to reduce scraping sounds.

Administrative and Behavioral Solutions

Speech, of course, is not the only activity in the classroom. Students must also concentrate on individual tasks. The proposed acoustical guidelines would not only reduce levels of frustration, irritability, and annoyance associated with noise but would also create a classroom environment that improves speech intelligibility and presumably helps improve the performance of teachers and students. School administrators and teachers may also want to consider factors in educational planning that could provide more than reduction in noise (e.g., smaller classes, more teachers per class, shorter and more interesting lessons, computer-aided lessons, and less talking during instruction; Boman and Enmarker 2004).

Classroom Accommodation

To reduce classroom noise, teachers can use several methods to focus the children's attention:

Visual reinforcement of oral instruction
- Use visual aides when talking to the whole class.
- Give written and oral instructions.
- Keep directions simple.

Voice amplification
- Consider using a voice amplification system with a microphone in the classroom.

Seating arrangements
- Seat students in small work groups. This reduces the amount of time the teacher has to address the whole class. The teacher can walk around and talk to small groups separately.
- Seat children in smaller groups in the cafeteria to reduce their need to speak loudly.

Environmental measures
- Do not play music as background (white) noise in the classroom.
- Reduce classroom ambient noise from lighting, ventilation, and heating and cooling equipment.
- Pay particular attention to the specific needs of children with learning disabilities, hearing impairments, intellectual disabilities, autism spectrum conditions, attention deficit disorder, and other medical or functional conditions.

Conclusion

We all learn through our senses and particularly through what we hear. Although much classroom

> ■ *4.2. What teachers can do to help children with auditory processing learning disability*
>
> - Keep directions simple.
> - Give directions both orally and written; use visual aids.
> - Speak slowly and maintain eye contact while speaking.
> - Seat child close to teacher.
> - Lecture less; work with children in small groups.
> - Assign older children a note-taking buddy.
> - Have child repeat the information or instructions to ensure comprehension.
> - Keep classroom background noise to a minimum.
>
> (National Center for Learning Disabilities 2005) ■

teaching is multimodal, most instruction is through the teacher's spoken word. It is therefore critical that the acoustic environment be optimal for the benefit of both teachers and students so that teaching and learning benefit everyone. We have looked at the elements of noise that play a part in compromising teaching and learning and discussed how these can be identified, examined, and modified to improve the quality of education in the school environment.

References

Alcántara JI, Weisblatt EJ, Moore BC, Bolton PF. 2004. Speech-in-noise perception in high-functioning individuals with autism or Asperger's syndrome. J Child Psychol Psychiatry 45(6):1107–1114.

ANSI (American National Standards Institute). 2002. Acoustical performance criteria, design requirements, and guidelines for schools. Melville, NY: Acoustical Society of America.

ASHA (American Speech-Language-Hearing-Association). 1995. Acoustics in educational settings. Subcommittee on Acoustics in Educational Settings of the Bioacoustics Standards and Noise Standards Committee of the American Speech-Language-Hearing-Association. ASHA 37 (Suppl. 14):15–19.

Boman E, Enmarker I. 2004. Factors affecting pupils' noise annoyance in school: The building and testing of models. Environ Behav 36(2):187–206.

Bronzaft A, McCarthy D. 1975. The effect of elevated train noise on reading ability. Environ Behav 7(4): 517–527.

Cohen S, Evans GW, Stokols D, Krantz DS. 1986. *Behavior, health, and environmental stress.* New York: Plenum Press.

Crandell CC, Smaldino JJ. 1994. An update of classroom acoustics for children with hearing impairments. Volta Rev 96:291–306.

Evans GW, Hygge S. 2006. Noise and performance in children and adults. In *Noise and its effects* (Luxon L, Prasher D, eds.). New York: John Wiley.

Evans GW, Lepore SJ. 1993. Nonauditory effects of noise on children: A critical review. Child Environ 10(1):31–51.

Evans GW, Lercher P, Meis M, Ising H, Kofler WW. 2001. Community noise exposure and stress in children. J Acoust Soc Am 109(3):1023–1027.

Evans GW, Maxwell LE. 1997. Chronic noise exposure and reading deficits: The mediating effects of language acquisition. Environ Behav 29(5):638–656.

Gifford R. 2002. *Environmental psychology: Principals and practice,* 3d ed. Victoria, British Columbia: Optimal Books.

Haines MM, Stansfeld SA, Job RFS, Berglund B, Head J. 2001. Chronic aircraft noise exposure, stress responses, mental health, and cognitive performance in school children. Psychol Med 31:265–277.

Hirschorn, M. 1989. *Noise control reference handbook.* Bronx, NY: Industrial Acoustics.

Hodgson M. 1999. Experimental investigation of the acoustical characteristic of university classrooms. J Acoust Soc Am 106:1810–1819.

Hygge S. 1993. Classroom experiments on the effects of aircraft, traffic, train, and verbal noise on long-term recall and recognition in children aged 12–14 years. In *Noise as a public health problem: Proceedings of the Sixth International Conference,* vol. 2 (Vallet M, ed.). Arcueil, France: Inrets, 531–538.

Knez I, Hygge S. 2002. Irrelevant speech and indoor lighting: Effects on cognitive performance and self-report affect. Appl Cognit Psychol 16:709–718.

Ko N. 1979. Responses of teachers to aircraft noise. J Sound Vib 62:277–292.

Kryter K. 1994. *The handbook of hearing and the effects of noise: Physiology, psychology, and public health.* New York: Academic Press.

League for the Hard of Hearing. 1996–2003. Noise levels in our environment fact sheet. Available: http://lhh.org/noise/decibel.htm [accessed 10 April 2004].

Manlove EE, Frank T, Vernon-Feagans L. 2001. Why should we care about noise in classrooms and child-care settings? Child Youth Care Forum 30(1):55–64.

Maxwell LE, Evans GW. 2000. The effects of noise on preschool children's pre-reading skills. J Environ Psychol 20:91–97.

National Center for Learning Disabilities. Auditory processing disorders. Available: http://www.ld.org/ldinfozone/infozone_factsheet_auditorypd.cfm [accessed 3 October 2004].

National Institute for Occupational Safety and Health. 1998. Criteria for a recommended standard: Occupational noise exposure. Publication 98-126. Cincinnati, OH: U.S. Department of Health and Human Services.

Picard M, Bradley JS. 2001. Revisiting speech interference in classrooms. Audiology 40:221–244.

Sargent, JW, Gidman, MI, Humphreys, MA, Utley, WA. 1980. The disturbance caused to school teachers by noise. J Sound Vib 70:557–572.

5

Jouni J. K. Jaakkola

Temperature and Humidity

■ *Summary*

- Thermal conditions—temperature, relative humidity, and air velocity—constitute the thermal environment and play an important part in the school environment.
- The thermal environment has direct effects on the human body and on functional outcomes such as performance, learning, and productivity.
- Thermal conditions can indirectly affect indoor air pollutant concentrations, as well as human exposure to these pollutants.
- Symptoms of the eyes, airways, skin, and central nervous system, the "sick building syndrome," are related to temperature and relative humidity.
- Regulation of the thermal environment is necessary to maintain optimal conditions and involves routine monitoring and adjustment of the temperature, relative humidity, and air movement. ■

This chapter describes the scientific parameters of temperature and humidity and the ways in which they affect comfort and health in schools. Some of these effects are direct, while others are indirect, mediated through environmental conditions such as microbial growth or emission and absorption of chemicals. Much of the available evidence comes from studies of other structures such as office buildings but can be readily applied to schools. Accordingly, we offer recommendations for maintaining temperature and humidity in schools to create an optimal environment for students and staff.

Historically, schools were situated in buildings that did not have the sophisticated temperature control mechanisms available today. Like other buildings in their environment, schools at best had stoves in the winter and open windows in the summer. Children and teachers dressed in clothing appropriate for the season. In schools in which uniforms were customary, students wore the uniforms were different for winter and summer months. Although this is still true for many schools around the world today, in the United States and other technologically developed countries, school buildings have heating and air-conditioning systems designed to create a uniform environment that makes the occupants as comfortable as possible. Some do not even have windows that open; in fact, some structures have a limited number of windows or windows that do not open in order to prevent heat loss and excessive heat accumulation.

Basic Concepts

Temperature, humidity, and air movement (velocity or flow) are central indoor air quality parameters. The range of both indoor temperature and relative humidity varies substantially according to season and climate. Structural and technical building characteristics and building materials influence thermal conditions. Air change in the building is also an important determinant of perceived temperature, humidity, and indoor air quality. Modern heating, ventilating, and air-conditioning (HVAC) technology can be used to control indoor temperature, humidity, and air exchange; however, complex HVAC systems may also have functional problems that can influence health and well-being.

Temperature is probably the most important indoor air quality parameter in schools and other buildings. Temperature can be considered suitable if the people in a specific environment feel comfortable and do not wish to be warmer or colder. Satisfaction with temperature depends on several factors, including indoor air temperature, radiation temperature from the sun and from cold and warm surfaces and equipment, and surface temperature, as well as an individual's particular tolerance.

Humans are homeothermic mammals, which means that normal body functions require a relatively constant internal body temperature (approximately 98.6°F/37°C). Temperature in the external parts of the body such as the skin and subcutaneous tissues may vary over a wider range without disturbing vital functions, but surprisingly small variations in temperature and humidity may feel uncomfortable and disturbing.

Body temperature is autonomically regulated in the hypothalamus based on blood temperature and sensory stimuli from the skin and internal organs. The body can control its temperature by constriction of blood circulation and muscular shivering when cold and by dilatation of the circulation and sweating when hot.

Thermal Environment in Schools

Thermal environment has received little attention in the literature on indoor air quality, ventilation, and building-related health problems in schools. In a systematic review of the main databases and conference proceedings, Shendell and colleagues

■ 5.1. Terminology

In the context of indoor environments, air humidity is usually expressed as relative humidity. *Relative humidity* expresses the percentage of water that remains in the air without condensing to liquid at a given temperature.

Absolute humidity refers to the concentration of water vapor in the air (gravimetric unit water/gravimetric or volumetric unit air). The absolute humidity of outdoor air varies according to temperature and season. Absolute humidity in cold air is low, although the relative humidity can be almost 100%. When cold air is heated, the relative humidity decreases. This explains why, in cold climates, the relative humidity of indoor air during the winter is often very low (10–20%), although the relative humidity of the outdoor air can be high. Respiration and perspiration of the occupants of an indoor space are important sources of indoor air humidity during the heating season. Air exchange removes humidity from the air, and high ventilation rates may contribute to the dryness of the air.

Air change refers to the introduction of new, cleansed, or recirculated air into a space. *Air change rate* describes the airflow in volume units per hour divided by the building space volume in identical volume units; it is expressed in air changes per hour. An air change rate of 1/hour corresponds to a complete air change within a particular space in 1 hour. Another measure of air change is the *ventilation rate*, which is expressed in cubic feet per minute (ft³/min) or liters per second (1/sec) per person or per room. ■

(2004a) identified 302 citations directly involving or closely related to school indoor environmental quality. Only three peer-reviewed papers and seven conference proceedings or abstracts provided information on the thermal environment of schools. Temperature, relative humidity, and air velocity in a space at a given point in time are easy to measure, but characterization of the thermal environment over time is more complicated. For example, vertical temperature difference, the presence of cold surfaces, or turbulent air flows may be perceived as uncomfortable and disturbing in a space where temperature and relative humidity at face level are within the recommended range.

The American Society of Heating, Refrigeration, and Air-Conditioning Engineers (ASHRAE 1992) has recommended an indoor thermal comfort range for different levels of relative humidity separately for winter (heating season) and summer (cooling season; table 5.1). Of importance for children is vertical temperature difference, measured as the difference between effective temperatures at 1.7 m and 0.1 m. Vertical temperature difference is an important determinant of thermal comfort. ASHRAE recommends a maximum temperature difference of 3 EC (effective temperature in degrees centigrade). ASHRAE Standard 55 was developed for adults in office environments; it is not known to what extent these standards are applicable for children in school environments.

The outdoor climate strongly influences indoor temperature and relative humidity. Problems related to thermal climate vary substantially according to different climatic conditions—from cold and dry to hot and humid. Thermal environments have been characterized in Danish (Thorstensen et al. 1990), Finnish (Kurnitski and Enberg 1997; Ruotsalainen et al. 1995b), and Swedish (Sahlberg et al. 2002; Smedje and Norbäck 1999) schools representing cold or moderate climate and in different climatic regions in the United States, including Las Vegas, Nevada (Shaughnessy et al. 1997), Santa Fe, New Mexico (Turk et al. 1997), and Los Angeles, California (Shendell et al. 2003a,b). The U.S. Environmental Protection Agency (EPA) conducted indoor air quality measurements in eight typical public schools in various U.S. climatic zones (Braganza et al. 2000). None of the schools studied had reported indoor air quality problems. Temperature and relative humidity were continuously monitored in 4 locations over 3 days during normal school hours. If average temperatures and relative humidity are considered, three of eight schools exceeded the thermal comfort envelope recommended by ASHRAE. Seven of the eight schools exceeded ASHRAE temperature and relative humidity recommendations at least occasionally.

A Finnish study of 56 classrooms in 10 schools describes thermal environments during the winter in a cold climate with outdoor temperatures varying from −20 to −10°C (−4 to 14°F; Kurnitski and Enberg 1997). The mean temperature was within recommended values (21.4°C; 70.5°F), but temperatures ranged from 17.2 to 25.4°C (63–77.7°F), covering levels that were both too cold and too warm. The mean relative humidity was typically low (22%; range 11–31%). The average ventilation rate was 3.5 l/seconds per person.

Framework for the Effects of Thermal Environment

The thermal environment, including temperature, relative humidity, and air velocity, may influence human health, well-being, and performance both directly and indirectly. The direct effects of the thermal environment can be readily understood in terms of temperature, humidity, and air velocity; however, it can also have indirect effects on humans in the environment by influencing sources, emissions, and indoor concentrations of indoor pollutants, as well as by possibly modifying the adverse effects of exposures. Figure 5.1 presents a theoretical framework for causal relations between thermal environment and human health and well-being.

According to the framework shown in figure 5.1, the thermal environment has direct and indirect effects on the human body and on functional outcomes such as performance, learning, and productivity. The indirect effects of thermal conditions involve indoor air pollutant concentrations, as well as human exposure to these pollutants, in several ways. High relative humidity combined with condensation of moisture creates suitable conditions

Table 5.1. Recommended thermal conditions

Relative humidity (%)	Winter season effective temperature (°C/°F)	Summer season effective temperature (°C/°F)
30	20.2–24.4 68.4–75.9	23.3–26.6 73.9–79.9
40	20.2–24.1 68.4–75.4	23.3–26.3 73.9–79.3
50	20.2–23.6 68.4–74.4	23.3–26.1 73.9–79.0
60	20.2–23.3 68.4–73.9	23.3–25.5 73.9–77.9

Data from ASHRAE (1992).

Table 5.2. Relative humidity (RH), temperature, and maximum vertical temperature in eight schools in the U.S. EPA school study

School location	RH (%) mean (range)	Temperature (°C/°F) mean (range)	Temperature difference (effective temperature, °C)	Outdoor temperature (°C/°F)	Outdoor RH (%)
Minnesota 1	25 (20–27)	23 (20–27) 73.4 (68–80.6)	2	18/73.4	33
Minnesota 2	46 (37–54)	23 (18–26) 73.4 (64.4–78.8)	3	20/68	66
Colorado	26 (17–35)	23 (18–27) 73.4 (64.4–80.6)	9	3/37.4	N/A
New Jersey	34 (25–45)	22 (18–23) 71.6 (64.4–73.4)	N/A	22/71.6	30
California 1	28 (19–40)	22 (19–24) 71.6 (66.2–75.2)	2	16/60.8	24
California 2	45 (41–58)	23 (21–26) 73.4 (69.8–78.8)	2	31/87.8	47
Texas	43 (34–52)	23 (20–27) 73.4 (68–80.6)	2	20/68	53
Florida	65 (51–78)	23 (20–25) 73.4 (68–77)	N/A	23/73.4	73

Data from Braganza et al. (2000).

for microbial growth. Changes in temperature and levels of relative humidity and air movement influence the emission and absorption of chemical compounds, gases, and particles from surface materials. The thermal environment also influences the conditions of particulate matter.

Direct Effects of the Thermal Environment

Thermal conditions within the range occurring in indoor environments directly affect the human body. The eyes, skin, and airways are in direct contact with indoor air. Thermal conditions, in combination with physical exercise and clothing, influence thermal balance and thus may affect subtle functions of the central nervous system such as concentration and subjective well-being.

Thermal Comfort

Thermal comfort can be defined as a state of satisfaction with the surrounding thermal conditions. The influence of temperature on the thermal comfort of healthy young adults has been studied ex-

tensively since the 1960s, but no systematic studies have been conducted on schoolchildren (Fanger 1967). It is reasonable to assume that determinants of thermal comfort are similar in schoolchildren and adults, but important factors such as metabolic rate, type of clothing, and level of exercise may result in differences in optimal conditions.

Thermal comfort is a function of the total body heat exchange with the environment. People vary substantially in their satisfaction with temperature, which means that in a given space it is nearly impossible to achieve conditions in which all of the occupants are satisfied. In an environment of 22°C (71.6°F) with negligible radiant temperature and reasonable air movement, approximately 80% of the occupants in sedentary work with light clothing feel comfortable. The remaining 20% would prefer a lower or higher temperature. A 100% satisfaction rate can be achieved only by personal control of the temperature.

The three most important environmental parameters affecting human thermal comfort include air and radiant temperature, humidity, and air movement (velocity), but physical activity and clothing also play an important role. A suitable room temperature depends on the ways in which

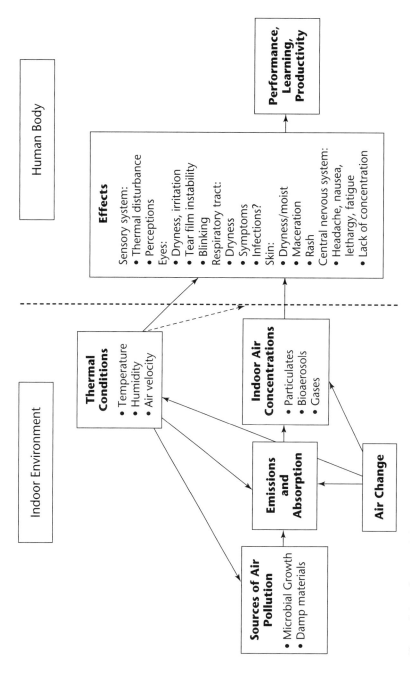

Figure 5.1. A framework for the association between the thermal environment and human health and well-being.

the space is used. The optimal temperature for classrooms is higher (21–23°C; 69.8–73.4°F) than for gymnasiums because of the level of exercise and the clothing customarily worn by the occupants. Physical exercise by the occupants affects temperature balance and thermal comfort through metabolism. Clothing is also important in achieving thermal comfort.

The thermal environment affects the mucous membranes and the skin, causing direct effects via the neural sensors of the tissues. The central nervous system is also indirectly affected by neurosensoral stimuli and changes in blood circulation.

Perceived Humidity and Temperature

Air dryness is a common complaint among school and office building occupants. In a cross-sectional study of 8853 Swedish high school students and 1023 employees in 16 high schools, 17% of the students and 32% of the employees indicated that dry air had often bothered them in the previous 3 months (Andersson et al. 2002). The corresponding 3-month prevalences were 8% and 9% for high temperature and 31% and 13% for low temperature. The prevalences of varying temperature problems were 20% and 13%. Draft was also considered a problem among 17% of the students and 15% of the personnel. Similar findings have been reported among office workers (Jaakkola and Miettinen 1995; Menzies et al. 1993) and among daycare

workers in cold climates (Ruotsalainen et al. 1995a).

Perceptions of dry air may be caused by low relative humidity, but such sensations may also be related to other indoor air parameters such as high temperature, airborne particles, and organic gases. Humans do not have a special sense to perceive humidity, and our perception of dry air is related to conjunctive, mucosal, and skin irritation. Andersen and colleagues (1973) assessed perceived humidity and temperature in relation to actual relative humidity and temperature in controlled experiments. Forty-eight young men were exposed to relative humidities of 70%, 50%, 30%, and 10% in 23°C (73.4°F) for 8 hours. No systematic association was found between perceived and actual relative humidity. Perceived temperature was strongly related to relative humidity: The sensation of warmth decreased in lower relative humidity.

A controlled crossover trial conducted with office workers in Helsinki, Finland, showed that perceived air dryness was alleviated by steam humidification of 29%–39% during the winter, when the relative humidity in nonhumidified periods varied between 12% and 28% (Reinikainen et al. 1992). In this study, a total of 169 office workers kept a daily diary of their thermal sensations for 6 weeks; both temperature and relative humidity were monitored (Palonen et al. 1993), and workers experienced consecutive weeks of humidification and no humidification. Figure 5.2 shows temperature acceptability ratings in different room temperatures.

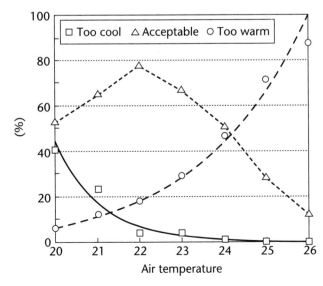

Figure 5.2. Percentage of office workers judging temperature acceptable, too cool, or too warm as a function of air temperature (in degrees centigrade) among Helsinki office workers. (From Palonen et al. 1993.)

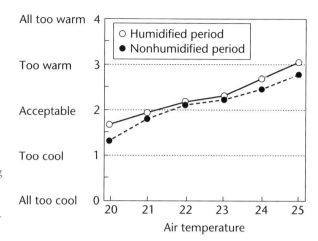

Figure 5.3. Mean value of temperature rating during humidified and nonhumidified conditions as a function of air temperatures (in degrees centigrade) among Helsinki office workers. (From Palonen et al. 1993.)

The percentage of satisfied study subjects was highest when the air temperature was 22°C (71.6°F). Average acceptability decreased in temperatures both below and above 22°C (71.6°F). At 22°C, an increase in relative humidity raised the mean thermal sensation only slightly.

Figure 5.3 shows the average acceptability rating between 20°C (68°F) and 25°C (77°F) in humidified and nonhumidified conditions. When the air temperature was an optimal 22–23°C (71.6–73.4°F), the mean values of the temperature ratings were almost identical during the humidified and nonhumidified periods. When the air temperature was low or high, workers felt the humidified room air was warmer than the nonhumidified room air.

Thermal Environment and Sick Building Syndrome

There is evidence that certain symptoms of the eyes, airways, skin, and central nervous system are related to temperature and relative humidity. The term "sick building syndrome" (SBS) has been used to describe a set of symptoms common among office workers in buildings with indoor air problems (World Health Organization 1983; see also chapter 10 in this book). The main components of SBS are nasal, eye, and mucous membrane symptoms, lethargy, dry skin, and headaches (Finnegan et al. 1984). The occurrence of SBS symptoms is related to temperature (Jaakkola et al. 1989; Menzies et al. 1993) and relative humidity (Reinikainen et al. 1991). In the Pasila Office Building study, Jaakkola

and colleagues first showed that the relation between the occurrence of SBS symptoms and temperature is U-shaped, with the lowest prevalence in temperature between 21 and 23°C (69.8 and 73.4°F; Jaakkola et al. 1989).

The concept of SBS has created some confusion. Some have argued that the SBS is a figurative concept of everyday language rather than a singular disease entity (Jaakkola 1995, 1998). Evidence from epidemiological studies clearly suggests that the symptoms of SBS at the individual level reflect a number of different health outcomes. Causative factors may range from physical, chemical, and microbiological exposure to social factors (Jaakkola 1995, 1998); therefore, it is more effective to consider separately the ways in which thermal conditions may influence the skin, eyes, airways, and central nervous system.

Skin

Exposure to extremes of heat and cold not usually encountered in indoor environments can lead to severe skin changes and skin diseases. However, evidence shows that thermal conditions in the range commonly occurring in schools contribute directly or indirectly to skin symptoms.

The optimal relative humidity for skin is 40–60%. Low relative humidity (<15%) results in dryness and laceration of the skin. High relative humidity (>90%) results in saturation of water on the skin surface and contributes to maceration and infection.

Few studies address the cutaneous effects of the

thermal environment among school children. However, Rycroft (1981) described various skin problems, including itching, irritation, and rash among office workers in a building where the temperature was increased and the relative humidity decreased temporarily. These symptoms disappeared when the relative humidity was increased to 35–55%. This type of reaction, which occurs during the heating season, is described as winter rash. In a controlled experiment, Rycroft (1985) showed that raising the relative humidity above 50% with concurrent use of moisturizing cream reduces the skin problems.

Several epidemiological studies conducted among office workers have shown an association between skin symptoms and low relative humidity (Bourbeau et al. 1997; Jaakkola and Miettinen 1995; Reinikainen and Jaakkola 2003). A six-period crossover trial conducted in Helsinki, Finland, showed that skin symptoms can be alleviated by steam humidification (Reinikainen et al. 1992).

Individual skin sensitivity to thermal climate varies substantially. People with atopic eczema or other dermatological problems experience indoor-related skin symptoms more frequently. They are likely to be more sensitive to both low and high relative humidity and temperature. In a German cross-sectional study of office workers, low skin sebum secretion and low hydration of stratum corneum were related to excessive occurrences of skin symptoms (Brashe et al. 2001).

Eyes

The outer eye, which consists of the conjunctiva and the cornea, is in direct contact with the environment. Unlike the skin and the airway mucosae, there is no vascularization of the cornea; therefore, nourishment and waste disposal occur either intraocularly or through the tear film. The surface cells of the cornea are covered by a thin layer of mucin, which consists primarily of glycoproteins secreted by the goblet cells of the conjunctiva. Tear fluid, produced by the lachrymal glands, combines with lipids and mucins to constitute the tear film, which covers the exposed part of the eye and continuously spreads by blinking. The tear film plays a major role in protecting the eyes against irritation and damage. It keeps the exposed parts moist and transports oxygen and nutrients to the cornea and carbon monoxide and other metabolic products away from the cornea. A stable tear film is central to the protection of the eyes. Paschides et al. (1998) presented evidence that people who live in warm, dry air conditions have a lower tear film stability compared with people in temperate, humid air conditions. This could be explained by the greater evaporation that occurs in warm, dry conditions. Air movement may also increase evaporation from the outer eye surface and thus decrease tear film stability.

Eye symptoms are common in nonindustrial workplaces such as offices and schools. Dryness of the eyes is one of the most common symptoms and is often combined with perceived dry air. In some epidemiological studies, relative humidity has been associated with dryness of the eyes and other eye symptoms such as irritation or itching (Bourbeau et al. 1997), but other studies found no such association (Reinikainen and Jaakkola 2003). In a six-period crossover trial conducted in Helsinki, Finland, during the winter, steam humidification alleviated eye symptoms (Reinikainen et al. 1992).

Exposure to several chemical and microbial indoor air pollutants also causes dryness of the eyes and other eye symptoms via mechanical irritation or allergic reaction. It seems likely that dryness of the eyes is often a result of several environmental factors.

Eye symptoms among office workers have been called "office eye syndrome" (Franck 1986, 1991). A fatty layer is essential for the continuity of the pericorneal tear film. However, Franck showed that office workers who suffer from eye symptoms have a thinner fatty layer, which causes a premature breakup of the film and leads to epithelia damage on the bulbar conjunctiva.

Respiratory Tract

Mucosal cilia in the airway are critical for the removal of microbes and other particulate matter, and the water content of mucosae influences ciliar function. Drying of the mucosae may increase the viscosity of the nasal mucus and thus interfere with ciliar movement; a thickening of the nasal mucus creates a suitable culture medium for bacteria (Lubart 1979). It has also been suggested that the inhalation of cool dry air increases the secretion of mucus (Richardson and Peatfield 1987). Dry air can increase the risk of infection by drying the airway surface. In cold climates, the incidence rate curve of respiratory infection is consistently inverse to the relative humidity of the indoor air in spaces where no air humidification is used.

It is difficult to assess the effect of dry air per se on the risk of respiratory infections because variation in relative humidity is often related to variation in a number of other indoor air quality parameters. A pragmatic approach is to determine whether humidification can reduce the incidence of respiratory infections. Eight studies in different settings were conducted in the 1960s and the 1970s to assess the effect of humidification on the occurrence of upper respiratory infections. Four of these studies involved children in schools or daycare centers. Green (1986) reviewed these studies and evaluated the findings. The preponderance of the evidence indicates that increasing the relative humidity from a level below 20–50% or more decreases the incidence of upper respiratory infections. The perception of risks related to nonhygienic humidification have probably decreased general interest in use of humidification in schools, although there is no comprehensive evidence-based assessment of the benefits and disadvantages of humidification.

In the nonexperimental (Reinikainen and Jaakkola 2001; Reinikainen et al. 1991) and experimental (Reinikainen and Jaakkola 2003; Reinikainen et al. 1992) epidemiologic studies conducted in office buildings in Helsinki, Finland, both upper and lower respiratory symptoms were related to low relative humidity. In a crossover trial, humidification alleviated upper respiratory symptoms, including throat and nasal dryness and irritation (Reinikainen et al. 1992).

Central Nervous System

General symptoms such as headaches, nausea, lethargy, and fatigue constitute a main component of SBS. Several epidemiological studies among office workers showed increased occurrence of these symptoms in ambient temperatures above 23°C (73.4°F; Jaakkola et al. 1989; Menzies et al. 1993). Sahlberg and colleagues (2002) studied staff members in 38 randomly selected schools in Uppsala, Sweden. Consistent with the findings from studies of office workers, the occurrence of the general symptoms was related to an increase in room temperature. The biological mechanisms are not known, but discomfort, nausea, and other symptoms are likely to be related to thermal control of the body. No similar studies have been conducted in schoolchildren, but it seems likely that they are affected similarly. Discomfort and lack of well-being caused by the thermal environment and indoor air pollutants are also likely to influence learning and intellectual performance. Again, this area needs to be investigated further.

Indirect Effects of Temperature and Humidity

Thermal conditions and their changes over time can influence microbial growth, as well as emissions from materials. The resultant change in the levels of microbiological and chemical pollutants may have adverse health effects.

Low relative humidity weakens paper and textile fibers, which leads to dust production and an increased concentration of particulate matter. Particles also remain longer in dry air, whereas humidity leads to the agglomeration of particles and their deposition on surfaces. Norbäck and colleagues (1999) studied indoor air quality over a 4-year period in six Swedish primary schools. Respirable dust, but not the concentration of volatile organic compounds, was enhanced at lower ventilation rates and high air humidity. Humid air increases emissions of organic gases such as formaldehyde. However, the use of formaldehyde in building surface materials has decreased substantially in Europe and North America since the 1980s, leading to reduced emissions.

Rapid changes in relative humidity and temperature may have an additional impact on emissions. The beginning and the end of the heating season are typically periods of change in thermal conditions. The impact of the changing thermal climate on indoor air and health warrants further investigation.

Humans present the chief source of bacteria and viruses in indoor air, and the high density of children in schools ensures abundant sources of infectious agents. Bacteria and viruses procreate in specific thermal conditions, which varies among species and influences the type of transmission. Airborne transmission may be enhanced in dry air.

Dampness and mold are common problems in schools and other indoor environments around the world. Although we know more about the occurrence of dampness problems in residential buildings than in schools, conditions in residential buildings are likely to reflect the situation in school environments. In the subtropical climate of Taiwan, where the relative humidity indoors is high most of the time, mold growth was reported in almost 60% of residences (Wan and Li 1999). In the northeastern United States, mold growth was reported in more than 50% of households with children (Maier et al. 1997), and across Canada, dampness or mold problems were found in 38% of homes (Dales et al. 1991). Residential dampness problems are also common in the United Kingdom and Central European countries; the estimates range from 13% to 51% (Brunekreef 1992; Jaakkola et al, 1993; Nowak et al. 1996; Williamson et al. 1997).

However, indoor dampness problems are also relatively common in colder climates. The estimated prevalence of residential dampness or mold in Sweden (Norbäck et al. 1999), Norway (Nafstad et al. 1998), and Finland (Jaakkola et al. 1993; Nevalainen et al. 1998) ranges from 4% to 82%. Relative humidity is usually low indoors (less than 40% for most of the year because of the cold outdoor temperatures) and should not cause dampness problems. Dampness results from construction problems (e.g., leaking pipes, construction defects in roofs or basements, tight buildings) combined with insufficient air exchange, which leads to the condensation of moisture (Nevalainen et al. 1998).

A Finnish survey investigated conditions representative of cold climates in 1164 schools. Serious water damage was reported in 20% of the schools, 60% had some damage, and 26% had visible mold or a moldy odor (Kurnitski et al. 1996). In a Swedish study of 38 randomly selected schools in Uppsala County, 19% of the classrooms had visible signs of dampness, mold growth, or a moldy odor (Sahlberg et al. 2002). The occurrence of ocular symptoms among the staff members was related to damp conditions.

Conclusions and Recommendations

Thermal conditions, which are defined as temperature, relative humidity, and air velocity, constitute an important part of the school environment. Relatively small changes in thermal conditions influence the thermal balance and comfort of the occupants and may impair their concentration and learning. Thermal conditions may also have health consequences, either through direct effects on susceptible surfaces or indirectly by influencing sources and emissions of chemical and microbiological air pollutants. Studies on office workers indicate that high temperature and low relative humidity increase symptoms of eye, skin, and mucosal irritation and general symptoms such as fatigue, lethargy, lack of concentration, and headache. It is likely that thermal discomfort can significantly affect academic performance. There is a need for further studies among schoolchildren.

The following are recommendations for controlling the thermal environment of schools:

- Indoor temperature, relative humidity, and air movement should be routinely monitored.
- Compliance with comfort-based temperature recommendations is important. The optimal temperature for office work is 22°C ± 2°C (71.6°F ± 3.5°F). This needs to be verified in school settings. In cold climates, people often tend to maintain indoor heat above 23°C (73.4°F), which results in a decrease in thermal comfort and an increase in mucosal symptoms and energy costs.
- Appropriate clothing and airing of classrooms are important ways to attain thermal comfort.
- Humidification of dry air in cold climatic conditions may reduce upper respiratory infections, although humidification equipment may lead to microbial pollution. Before humidification can be recommended, studies are needed to determine the beneficial effects and assess the risks for health problems. Optimal air exchange is an important part of the thermal environment. Besides increasing the level of indoor air pollutants, an air exchange rate that is too low will lead to condensation of humidity on cold surfaces. An exchange rate that is too high will critically reduce the relative humidity during cold climatic conditions when dry air (relative humidity below 20%) is a problem. A high air exchange rate will also result in increased air movement, which will be experienced as a draft.

References

Andersen I, Lundqvist GR, Proctor DF. 1973. Human perceptions of humidity under four controlled conditions. Arch Environ Health 26:22–27.

Andersson K, Stridth G, Fagerlund I, Aslaksen W, Rudblad S. 2002. Comparison of the perceived climate reported by students and personnel in sixteen senior high schools in Sweden. Proc Indoor Air 1:399–403.

ASHRAE. 1992. ASHRAE-55: Thermal environmental conditions for human occupancy. Atlanta, GA: American Society of Heating, Refrigeration, and Air Conditioning Engineers, Inc.

Bourbeau J, Brisson C, Allaire S. 1997. Prevalence of the sick building syndrome symptoms in office workers before and six months and three years after being exposed to a building with an improved ventilation system. Occup Environ Med. 54:49–53.

Braganza E, Fontana C, Harrison J. 2000. Baseline measurements of indoor air quality comfort parameters in eight U.S. elementary and secondary schools. Proc Health Build 1:193–198.

Brasche S, Bullinger M, Bronisch M, Petrovitch A, Bischof W. 2001. Eye and skin symptoms in German office workers: Subjective perception vs. objective medical screening. Int J Hyg Environ Health 203(4): 311–316.

Brunekreef B. 1992. Damp housing and adult respiratory symptoms. Allergy 47:498–502.

Carrer P, Bruinen de Bruin Y, Franchi M, Valovirta E. 2002. The EFA project: Indoor air quality in European schools. Proc Indoor Air 2:794–799.

Dales RE, Zwanenburg H, Burnett R, Franklin CA. 1991. Respiratory health effects of home dampness and molds among Canadian children. Am J Epidemiol 134:196–203.

Fanger PO. 1967. Calculation of thermal comfort: Introduction of a basic comfort equation. ASHRAE Trans 73(2):3.4.1–3.4.20.

Finnegan MJ, Pickering CAC, Burge PS. 1984. The sick building syndrome: Prevalence studies. Br Med J 289:1573–1575.

Franck C. 1986. Eye symptoms and signs in buildings with indoor climate problems ("office eye syndrome"). Acta Ophthalmol (Copenhagen) 64:306–311.

Franck C. 1991. Fatty layer of the pericorneal film in the "office eye syndrome." Acta Ophthalmol (Copenhagen) 69:737–743.

Green GH. 1986. The effect of relative humidity on absenteeism and colds in schools. ASHRAE Trans 92:131–141.

Jaakkola JJK. 1995. Sick building syndrome: The phenomenon and its air-handling etiology. Helsinki University of Technology, Laboratory of Heating, Ventilating, and Air-Conditioning, Report A2, Espoo, Finland.

Jaakkola JJK. 1998. The office environment model: A conceptual analysis of the sick building syndrome. Indoor Air 9:7–16.

Jaakkola JJK, Heinonen OP, Seppänen O. 1989. Sick building syndrome, sensation of dryness, and thermal comfort in relation to room temperature in an office building: Need for individual control of temperature. Environ Int 15:163–168.

Jaakkola JJK, Jaakkola N, Ruotsalainen R. 1993. Home dampness and molds as determinants of respiratory symptoms and asthma in preschool children. J Expos Environ Epidemiol 3 (Suppl. 1):9–23.

Jaakkola JJK, Miettinen P. 1995. Types of ventilation systems in office buildings and the sick building syndrome. Am J Epidemiol 141:755–765.

Kurnitski J, Enberg S. 1997. Indoor climate and moisture problems in Finnish schools. Proc Healthy Build 1:111–116.

Kurnitski J, Palonen J, Enberg S, Ruotsalainen R. 1996. Koulujen sisailmasto: rehtorikysely ja sisailmastomittaukset. Espoo, Finland: Helsinki University of Technology, Faculty of Mechanical Engineering, B43.

Lubart J. 1979. Health care cost containment. Am J Otolaryngol 1:81–83.

Maier WC, Arrighi HM, Morray B, Llewellyn C, Redding GJ. 1997. Indoor risk factors for asthma and wheezing among Seattle schoolchildren. Environ Health Perspect 105:208–214.

Menzies R, Tamblyn R, Farant JP, Hanley J, Nunes F, Tamblyn R. 1993. The effect of varying levels of outdoor-air supply on the symptoms of sick building syndrome. N Engl J Med 328:821–827.

Nafstad P, Øie L, Mehl R, Gaarder PI, Lødrup-Carlsen KC, Botten G, et al. 1998. Residential dampness problems and development of bronchial obstruction in Norwegian children. Am J Respir Crit Care Med 157:410–414.

Nevalainen A, Partanen P, Jaaskelainen E, Hyvarinen A, Koskinen O, Meklin T, et al. 1998. Prevalence of moisture problems in Finnish houses. Indoor Air 55 (Suppl. 4):45–49.

Norbäck D, Björnsson E, Janson C, Palmgren U, Boman G. 1999. Current asthma and biochemical signs of inflammation in relation to building dampness in dwellings. Int J Tuberc Lung Dis 3: 368–376.

Norbäck D, Torgren M, Edling C. 1990. Volatile organic compounds, respirable dust, and personal factors related to prevalence and incidence of sick building syndrome in primary schools. Br J Ind Med 147:733–741.

Nowak D, Heinrich J, Jörres R, Wassmer G, Berger J, Beck E, et al. 1996. Prevalence of respiratory symptoms, bronchial hyperresponsiveness, and atopy among adults: West and East Germany. Eur Respir J 9:2541–2552.

Palonen J, Seppänen O, Jaakkola JJK. 1993. The effects of room temperature and relative humidity on thermal comfort in the office environment. Indoor Air 3:391–397.

Paschides CA, Stefaniotou M, Papageorgiou J, Skourtis P, Psilas K. 1998. Ocular surface and environmental changes. Acta Ophthalmol Scand 76:74–77.

Reinikainen LM, Jaakkola JJK. 2001. Effect of temperature and humidification in the office environment. Arch Environ Health 56:365–368.

Reinikainen LM, Jaakkola JJK. 2003. Significance of temperature and humidity on symptoms of skin and upper airways. Indoor Air 13:344–352.

Reinikainen LM, Jaakkola JJK, Heinonen OP. 1991. The effect of air humidification on different symptoms in an office building. Environ Int 17:243–250.

Reinikainen LM, Jaakkola JJK, Seppänen O. 1992. The effect of air humidification on symptoms and the perception of air quality in office workers: A six-period cross-over trial. Arch Environ Health 47:8–15.

Richardson PS, Peatfield AC. 1987. The control of airway mucus secretion. Eur J Respir Dis (Suppl. 153):43–51.

Ruotsalainen R, Jaakkola N, Jaakkola JJK. 1993. Ventilation and indoor air quality in Finnish daycare centers. Environ Int 19:109–119.

Ruotsalainen R, Jaakkola N, Jaakkola JJK. 1995a. Dampness and molds in daycare centers as an occupational health problem. Int Arch Occup Environ Med 66:369–374.

Ruotsalainen R, Teijonsalo J, Seppanen O. 1995b. Ventilation and indoor air quality in Finnish schools. In *Proceedings of indoor air quality in practice: Moisture and cold climate solutions* (G. Flatheim, ed.). Oslo: Norwegian Society of Chartered Engineers, 489–493.

Rycroft RJG. 1981. Occupational dermatoses from warm dry air. Br J Dermatol 105:29–33.

Rycroft RJG. 1985. Low humidity and microtrauma. Am J Ind Med 8:371–375.

Sahlberg B, Smedje G, Norbäck D. 2002. Sick building syndrome among school employees in the county of Uppsala, Sweden. Proc Indoor Air 3:494–499.

Shaughnessy RJ, Turk B, Casey M, Harrison J, Levetin E. 1997. Use of energy recovery ventilators to provide ventilation in schools and the impact of indoor air contaminants. Proc Healthy Build 1:161–166.

Shendell DG, Barnett C, Boese S. 2004a. Science-based recommendations to prevent or reduce potential exposures to biological, chemical, and physical agents in schools. Available: http://www.healthyschools.org [accessed 8 March 2004].

Shendell DG, Winer AM, Weker R, Colome SD. 2004b. Evidence of inadequate ventilation in portable and traditional classrooms: Results of a pilot study in Los Angeles County. Indoor Air 14:154–158.

Smedje G, Norbäck D. 1999. Factors affecting the concentration of pollutants in school buildings. Proc Indoor Air 1:267–272.

Thorstensen E, Hansen C, Pejtersen J, Clausen GH, Fanger PO. 1990. Air pollution sources and indoor air quality in schools. Proc Indoor Air 1:531–536.

Turk B, Powell G, Casey M, Fisher E, Ligman B, Marquez A, et al. 1997. Impact of ventilation modifications on indoor air quality characteristics at an elementary school. Proc Healthy Build 1:155–160.

Wan GH, Li CS. 1999. Indoor endotoxin and glucan in association with airway inflammation and systemic symptoms. Arch Environ Health 54:172–179.

Williamson IJ, Martin CJ, McGill G, Monie RDH, Fennerty AG. 1997. Damp housing and asthma: A case-control study. Thorax 52:229–234.

World Health Organization (WHO). 1983. Indoor air pollutants: Exposure and health effects. EURO Reports and Studies No. 78. Copenhagen: WHO Regional Office for Europe.

Cheryl Bennett, Andree Woodcock,

and Diane Tien

Ergonomics for Students and Staff

■ *Summary*

- Ergonomics is the science of fitting a workstation, product, or task to the person.
- A good fit between people and the objects they use or the tasks they perform can make them more comfortable and help them build important life skills.
- A bad fit can result in discomfort, dissatisfaction with the item, or disorders of various muscles, tendons, and ligaments (musculoskeletal disorders).
- Topics of ergonomic importance in schools include furniture, information and communication technology, and school bags.
- General physical fitness, posture, back pain, and back care are related to furniture, information and communication technology, and school bags.
- Ergonomic practices are often cost effective; many can be implemented through education, procedural changes, or adjustments to existing equipment or furniture. ■

Ergonomics is the science of taking human characteristics into account when we design and use things. Drawing upon scientific knowledge from

fields such as physiology, psychology, biomechanics, and engineering, ergonomics attempts to make systems, the environment, and the objects in it compatible with the users. Ergonomics has become a central part of occupational health, in which awkward workstations, repetitive motions, and similar design flaws are recognized as threats to workers' health and well-being in a variety of ways. Ergonomics is also well recognized in daily life. Although drivers come in many shapes and sizes, when ergonomics has been considered, all but the very smallest and largest can assume the steering wheel will not block the view of important gauges on the dashboard and expect to be able reach the controls easily. When we get into a car, the first thing we do to be comfortable and safe is adjust the seat and mirrors. These elements of car design represent daily encounters with ergonomics, and it is evident to us when these issues have not been addressed.

It is important to consider ergonomics in schools for at least three reasons. First, good ergonomic design can protect the health and well-being of children and teachers. Second, good ergonomic design can enhance learning and teaching. Third, behaviors learned at school, especially during the early years, can have a major impact on later life and cross over into home life (Woodcock 2003b).

Until recently, however, not enough attention has been focused on the need for ergonomic assessment and intervention in schools. In the past, children and teachers have endured ill-fitting furniture, a situation made worse by lesson plans that require children to remain virtually immobile for long periods of time. Teachers have often been required to sit on furniture designed for children or bend over for long periods of time to look at a child's work. The resulting discomfort they feel may reduce their concentration and create unnecessary physical strain, contributing to joint and back pain and other symptoms.

Applying ergonomics in schools helps make school life simpler and safer. Can all the children see and hear the teacher or monitor for computer classes (fig. 6.1)? Are the chairs and desks comfortable (fig. 6.2)? Does the teacher have to assume poor posture when talking to the children? Schools and equipment should be designed to accommodate the characteristics of both children and teachers and provide an optimum teaching and learning environment for everyone. The role of ergonomics within schools is not only to optimize new design but also to improve existing practices, spaces, and equipment to enhance comfort, safety, and usability.

For the ergonomist, a learning environment in a school, library, or home can be represented as a complex system of interactions between physical–environmental factors and human–organizational

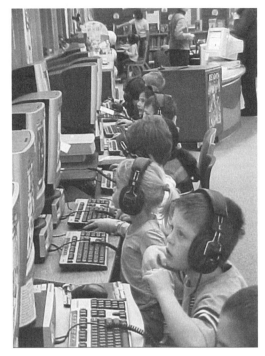

Figure 6.2. In this multiage library, these third-graders may have to assume uncomfortable positions or strain to use the computers. (Photo by Diane Tien.)

factors (Caterina 2003). Included in the system are the relationships among the teachers, children, parents, and educators and their work, workplace, equipment, materials, and rules. In designing a school as a successful teaching and learning environment, many factors should be considered including:

- building design (color of the walls, lighting sustainability, noise levels)
- interior play areas
- desks (size, shape), computer learning stations, arrangement of the teaching and learning space
- design modification for differently abled students and staff
- jobs of teachers and other support staff in the school (are they overworked? do they have appropriate furniture and equipment?)
- teaching methods (are both children and teachers engaged? is there a balance between physical and mental activities?)
- interface between home and school
- playgrounds
- school buses.

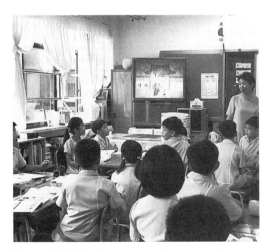

Figure 6.1. This big-screen monitor connected to a computer is visible to every student. (Photo by Cheryl Bennett.)

Architects, environmental psychologists, and teachers all recognize that the school environment can affect a child's predisposition to learn. The colors and proportions of buildings and spaces affect both physical and psychological comfort. Rooms of different proportions can produce different effects; for example, low ceilings produce feelings of intimacy. Attaianese (2003) reviewed some of the issues ergonomists consider in the school environment; they range from class size and seating arrangements to the teacher's abilities.

Much of this chapter is common sense, but empowerment also plays a role. From an early age, students can learn and apply ergonomic concepts in their learning environment (e.g., in the safe use of computers) and thus internalize healthy behaviors for lifelong use. Parents can promote the consideration of ergonomics when selecting schools, volunteering, or serving in parent-teacher associations. Educators can use ergonomic principles to help them adopt a more holistic approach to the design of lesson plans and classroom space. Administrators can take an ergonomic approach in their assessment of furniture and classroom design for new and renovated facilities. Building design, furniture choices, staff training, classroom layout, and materials used throughout the building can all be positively impacted by the basic principles of ergonomics.

Certain important areas of ergonomics such as lighting (chapter 3) and noise (chapter 4) are covered elsewhere in this book. This chapter focuses on furniture, information and communication technology (ICT), and school bags, three topics of special concern for ergonomists not only in U.S. schools but worldwide. Chile has produced guidelines for school furniture design (UNESCO-MINEDUC 2001), large prospective studies of ICT use by children are under way in Australia (Straker 2001), and children use school bags everywhere.

Furniture in the School Environment

Classroom Furniture

Furniture in classrooms is usually utilitarian and uniform. Children, however, come in different sizes, grow throughout the school year, and use furniture in many different ways. One size of furniture cannot be expected to fit all students com-

fortably, even if they are all the same age. Anthropometry is the measurement of human dimensions and capacities such as grip strength. The application of anthropometric data in a conventional way (designing for the 95th percentile) is not expected to meet the needs of the largest and smallest children. In practice, unfortunately, school furniture fits far fewer than 95% of children (fig. 6.3). Anthropometric studies in schools have found that classroom furniture is mismatched with large numbers (sometimes as many as 80–100%) of students, and research has indicated that learning may be affected as a result (Legg et al. 2003; Parcells et al. 1999).

Ethnicity, gender, and individual differences are associated with different body proportions that are important in the selection of furniture. This anthropometric variation can make even two people of the same height experience a chair-table combination quite differently. For example, students of Asian, African, and Latin heritage may differ in their trunk and leg proportions. Anthropometric data derived 30 years ago are also likely to be outdated. The average height of children since that time has increased with better nutrition, and the mix of ethnic groups has become much more complex. Furniture design is related to issues such as back pain, posture, and obesity and should be understood as one aspect of a multidimensional issue.

Seating

Children spend the overwhelming majority of school time in a sitting position. They may sit for 60 minutes (Storr-Paulsen and Aagaard-Hensen 1994) or even longer without a break. The total time spent sitting may be as much as 1260 hours per year (Jones 1981), although this estimate might be lower today because of changes in classroom procedures. Maintaining the same posture for long periods is hard on the human body. Static postures create compression force on the lumbar spine (McGill 2002), static loading, or pressure on the soft tissues and often cause discomfort. Sitting for an extended length of time has been associated with back pain (Pope et al. 2002). The high incidence of student reports of back pain and discomfort or pain in other parts of the body must be considered along with other factors in relation to classroom seating.

Recent research in biomechanics indicates that

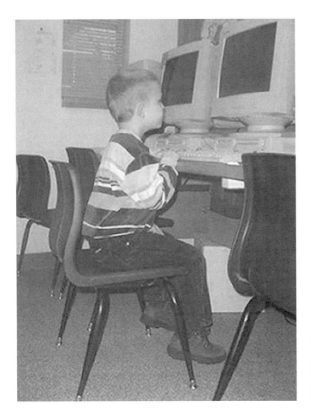

Figure 6.3. This computer lab is equipped with fixed-height furnishings. Note the boy's hanging legs and the awkward angles required to view the screen and use the keyboard. (Photo by Diane Tien.)

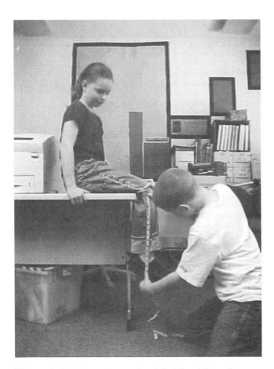

Figure 6.4. Measuring popliteal height. (Photo by Diane Tien.)

the ideal sitting posture is one that continually changes and thus prevents the accumulation of too much strain on any single tissue (McGill 2002). Seats are often too high or too low. In addition, they may also be too deep (from back of seat to front edge), which prevents the chair back from being used as a backrest or, if the backrest is used, the seat edge puts pressure on the legs. Such pressure can reduce circulation in the blood vessels and restrict the nerves close to the surface in the sensitive area behind the knee.

The distance from the floor to the back of the knee when sitting is called the popliteal height (fig. 6.4). This distance is a better measure of the appropriate seat height than the standing height of a person because of variation in the trunk/leg ratio (Molenbroek, Kroon-Ramaekers, Snijders 2003). When the seat height exceeds the popliteal height, the feet do not reach the floor (see fig. 6.3). As part of a science-of-math lesson plan, students can take measurements of popliteal height and seat depth on each other. Anthropometric data gathered by students are ideal for statistical analyses and graphing. Summaries of the data can also be supplied to personnel purchasing school furniture to give them more information about the size range of students who need to be fit.

Tables and Desks

Tables and desks provide the writing and work surfaces necessary for schoolwork. Some schools are structured around group-seating tables with flat work surfaces, encouraging more collaborative activity. Individual seats with attached work surfaces are generally referred to as desks. Desks encourage more individual work. If the work surfaces are low, students lean or hunch forward as they work. This forward flexion of the trunk puts considerable stress on the lower spine, while forward flexion of the head increases tension in the neck and shoulder area. Tables that are too high require elevation of the upper arms and can make the fine motor coordination required by writing more difficult. A general guideline for writing tasks is a table height that allows the upper arms to be relaxed at the sides with elbows bent to about 90°.

When school desks were designed to be individual seating stations, sloping surfaces were often provided for writing and reading. Surfaces with a higher slope are associated with a more upright posture and less forward flexion of the neck (Mandal 1981). Ergonomists who encourage the use of forward-tilted seats recommend a table about 2 inches (4–6 cm) higher than elbow height (Bendix and Bloch 1986). Some desks have writing surfaces designed for right- or left-handed writers. The requirements of left-handed students should also be considered when hand-specific furniture or objects are being used.

When reading from paper, common locations for discomfort are the eyes, neck, midback, and head (Straker 2001). Musculoskeletal symptoms may be related to leaning forward, as would occur with reading a book. To provide an inexpensive raised reading surface, three-ring binders can be placed on a desk or table, with the higher edge away from the student. An adjustable table can assist in maintaining more efficient anatomical alignment when students are sitting and writing (Marschall et al. 1995).

Knee clearance (the distance between the knees and the underside of the desk or table) is particularly important for taller students (Bennett 2002). If the knees cannot fit comfortably beneath the

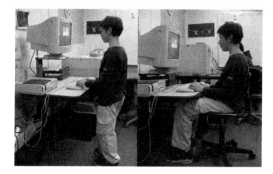

Figure 6.5. Motorized adjustable table in a computer lab used by K–12 students. This arrangement permits a student to assume different positions, as shown, and different students to use the same equipment. (Photo by Diane Tien.)

writing or computer keyboard surface, students tend to lean and reach forward, which causes tension in the neck and shoulders and stresses the lower back.

When students use computers, it is important to provide a surface wide enough for both keyboard and pointing device (mouse or trackball) to be on the same level. Keyboard trays or adjustable tables can readily allow students to position these input devices at the appropriate height (fig. 6.5).

The Future of Furniture

The chair that has become common in schools, with a backward-sloping or horizontal seat accompanied by a backrest, is not the only chair design available. In Denmark a higher, 10°–15° forward-sloping seat has been developed to allow a more open (90°) hip-to-trunk angle and to position the pelvis and spine so as to promote natural spinal curvature (Mandal 1981). Some schools in Europe are using furniture that incorporates this design.

Adjustable tables and chairs have been rated as significantly more comfortable for students. Such furniture with controls easy enough for a child to operate is commercially available. After such furniture has been provided, students need instructions on how to adjust it. Adjustable furniture may be an excellent ergonomic option that provides long-term benefits (Linton et al. 1994).

Purchases of adjustable chairs may be more feasible if combined with other, less costly seating options, such as allowing children to sit on the floor. A substantial proportion of the world's population is more accustomed to sitting on the floor and squatting than to sitting in chairs (Gurr et al. 1998). Children are very comfortable sitting on the floor and adapt well to alternative seating solutions.

Therapy balls offer another option for short-term sitting. Children quickly can become adept at using them, and the active engagement of the muscles required for stable posture can build core strength. A study of students with attention deficit-hyperactivity disorder (ADHD) who were seated on therapy balls showed improved in-seat behavior and legible word production. Both students and teachers preferred the therapy balls (Schilling et al. 2003).

The stability of therapy balls presents some challenges, however, and teachers should exercise caution, especially at the time of introduction. Clear limits should be set on acceptable behavior, and sharp objects that could puncture the balls should be removed from the area. The ball height, which can easily be varied by adjusting the volume of air, should allow the feet to be planted solidly on the floor. At present, no studies of long-term sitting on therapy balls have been conducted. The

use of therapy balls should probably be restricted to short periods of time (30 minutes maximum per session).

School furniture has been used to keep students in place and to minimize distracting interactions (Knight and Noyes 1999). However, continuous sitting in any position—in a chair, on a therapy ball, or on the floor—is not recommended for more than about 30 minutes at a time. To vary children's posture throughout the day, teachers should encourage alternative options for sitting or standing. Young children should have time to "shake out the wiggles." Older students can be offered stretch breaks or a change of activity. In fact, there may be advantages to encouraging students to move around the classroom. In an experiment in which a classroom was organized to facilitate movement rather than fix students in place, children did not run through the classroom, and there was no reduction in the time spent reading or writing (Cardon et al. 2004). The healthy tendency to wriggle, shift position, and move is inherent in children. Even the practice of rocking back in a chair can be seen as an attempt to release the spine from

---

■ *6.1. Classroom furniture*

- Find ways to organize the classroom so that students are free to move around as much as possible.
- Make some part of the floor attractive and available for sitting or reclining during portions of the school day.
- Ensure that students have stretch breaks or vary their activities so they do not sit for more than 30 minutes at a time.
- Encourage those who purchase furniture for the school district to consider the anthropometry (physical dimensions) of students. A representative sample of the range of popliteal heights of the school populations is a better measure of appropriate chair height than student height. Sitting elbow height or a little higher is a reasonable approximation for table height.
- Purchase adjustable chairs and tables for high-use computers whenever possible.
- Keyboard trays can be attached to fixed tables and provide an adjustable surface. When keyboard trays are used, make sure the surface is wide enough for the tray and the pointing device to be at the same level.
- Have more than one chair size in classrooms. Educate students about fit in chairs: Feet should contact the floor while the person is sitting against the backrest; a proper fit allows a space the width of least three fingers between the back of the knee and the edge of the chair.
- Make sure that the knees of the tallest students in a classroom fit under tables and desks.
- Provide footrests (boxes or other inexpensive objects) for the smaller children if their feet do not touch the floor when seated in a chair. Provide cushions or large books for students to sit on if a reading or writing surface is more than about 2 inches (4–6 cm) above elbow height.
- Tables, computer desktops, and built-in shelves should have rounded edges. ■

stressful tension. The psychosocial aspects of a sense of autonomy can be enhanced by the perception of having freedom to move. Teachers who are well informed about the benefits of dynamic posture will be better motivated and able to find safe practices that accommodate the urge to move.

The purchase of furniture for schools is too often based upon cost, expedience, and tradition. Administrators who make decisions about buying furniture may be willing to consider alternatives if they are aware of the impact of mismatched furniture on students. Those who select furniture are likely to apply criteria that emphasize cost and durability unless given specific guidance. Obtaining measurements that include the range of popliteal heights of a representative sample of the largest and the smallest students for whom chairs are being purchased allows a more strategic selection.

The design, size, and orientation of school furniture provide structure in the classroom and can affect student comfort and behavior. For example, seating students in rows favors informative communication because the students are more passive; a circular layout encourages interaction. A comparison of classroom furniture arranged in rows and furniture arranged in grouped tables found that 10- to 11-year-old students spent more time on task when seated in rows (Wheldall 1982). Different seating arrangements can be chosen for various types of activities.

As schools continue to be renovated and rebuilt, planners have an opportunity to consider ergonomics in their design and purchasing. Teachers, information technology specialists, and students can be valuable partners in designing schools and classrooms. To facilitate a participatory process, building contracts can stipulate meetings between architects and designers and the intended users of the areas under consideration.

Information and Communication Technology

We are relying increasingly on ICT to support all aspects of our lives. Children are now required to be more ICT literate than their parents, and increasingly, products are being developed for this growth market. This situation gives rise to several concerns. First, we do not know the effects of early or long-term computer use, as this is a relatively new

phenomenon. What are the psychological and physical effects of sitting at a computer 8 hours a day for 30 years? Second, much of the computer hardware has been developed for adults and adopted by children. It has therefore not been appropriately designed for its final and possibly chief user group. Third, the child and youth market for computer leisure products is a growth area, yet little academic research has been conducted to determine the effects of prolonged game play on psychological, physiological, and social development. For example, some games and parts of the Internet may have addictive features designed into them. Finally, what design features (assistive technologies) are needed to ensure that all children, including those with disabilities, have full access to ICT?

The increase in the length of time that children spend in front of computers and television ("screen time")—sedentary activities—coincides with the decline in physical activity. This tendency, together with unhealthy dietary trends (see chapter 17), has contributed to an increase in obesity in children. This is especially worrisome because obesity in children has adverse health and social effects during childhood and on into adulthood.

Computers

Computers are a prominent part of children's lives. In the United States, 90% of children between the ages of 5 and 17 use computers at home, school, or both (Bennett and Tien 2003). Children and teenagers use computers and the Internet more than any other age group (U.S. National Telecommunications and Information Administration 2002), yet in many cases, the computer and the environment in which it is used have been designed for adults. Typical computer setups may expose students to acute and chronic risks such as musculoskeletal disorders (MSD) or visual impairments.

The computer learning station is one important concern. Like other school furniture, computer workstations need to be designed to accommodate children of different shapes and sizes. Failure to do this (e.g., by placing a computer on a desk designed for reading and writing) may require children to adopt suboptimal postures when they are working on the computer. This in turn places stress on the neck, back, arms, and shoulders. A study of more than 1400 high school students in Canada and Australia found that workspaces were consistently poorly rated (Zandvliet and Straker 2001). Additionally, classrooms designed for non-ICT lessons may not have adequate room to support prolonged activity at the computer. A study of 95 primary schools by Oates et al. (1998) showed a marked lack of suitably designed facilities.

Psychological and social issues represent a second area of important computer-related concerns. The cognitive impact of computer use on children has yet to be determined. Much may depend on the home and school environment, that is, the situation in which the computer is used, why it is used, and how it is incorporated into the syllabus. Some research (Macfarlane et al. 2000) has suggested an increase in attributes such as motivation, critical thinking, writing, math skills, and social interaction (Burgess and Trinidad 1991), whereas other studies (Moseley and Tse 2001) have suggested a negative impact. Clearly, children who use computers regularly will benefit later from higher computer literacy, and computers are one way of helping shy children to participate in discussions.

Vision is a third computer-related concern. Staring at a computer screen for long periods of time may cause eye strain, including symptoms such as eye twitching; tired, burning, itching, or dry eyes; blurred or double vision; and increased sensitivity to light. Formal testing may reveal changes in accommodation (focusing), binocular vision (coordination of the two eyes), and eye movements (tracking). These symptoms are of special concern because they can interfere with school performance and reduce athletic ability. For example, a child with visual problems may not be able to read small print comfortably, have difficulty completing reading or homework assignments, and be easily distracted or inattentive. Visual problems should be promptly ruled out in children with reading problems, learning disabilities, or dyslexia.

A fourth concern related to computer use is musculoskeletal disorder. MSD is common in children (box 6.3) and may relate not only to computers but also to heavy backpacks, poorly designed furniture, and other factors. Computer use may be a contributor through poorly designed workstations that require awkward postures and repetitive movements in using the mouse and the keyboard. Box 6.4 offers recommendations for preventing and managing these disorders in children.

■ *6.2. Vision at computer workstations*

- Ensure proper lighting of the classroom and computer areas (see chapter 3).
- If possible, position computers away from the glare from windows or provide blinds.
- Monitor students for reading difficulty, distractibility, or a tendency to lean forward to see, which can signal vision difficulties. An eye examination may be warranted, according to the American Optometric Association Consensus Panel (Cooper et al. 2001).
- Computer users should look away from the computer periodically and focus on something in the distance. A good guide is the 20-20-20 rule: Every 20 minutes, look 20 feet away for 20 seconds. ■

Laptops

The current trend is to provide children with laptop computers for use in lessons at school and at home (fig. 6.6). Because not all families can afford laptop computers, some municipal or state organizations have provided them for students (such as for all seventh-grade students in the state of Maine).

The benefits of using individual laptops include greater flexibility, fun, access to information resources, and independent learning. However, their use has also been associated with increases in MSD related to carrying laptops and the postures that

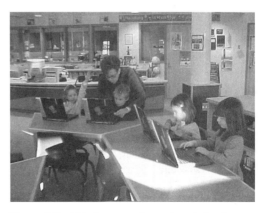

Figure 6.6. A kindergarten class using wireless laptops in a library. What ergonomic issues are evident in this photo? (Photo by Diane Tien.)

■ *6.3. Musculoskeletal disorders in children*

Musculoskeletal disorders (MSD) include a variety of conditions of the muscular and skeletal system, including associated soft tissues and nerves. They involve pain and inflammation, typically in the neck, shoulders, back, arms, and hands, with various levels of severity. These disorders are prevalent among children (Milanese and Grimmer 2004; Murphy et al. 2004). For example, among children 12–18 years of age, 50% report occasional neck and upper limb pain; 20% of girls and 10% of boys have recurrent pain (Niemi et al. 1996). MSD symptoms include stiffness, tingling, numbness, and pain in an affected joint, sometimes spreading to nearby parts of the body.

Although children report MSD symptoms when asked by researchers, it has been noted they often do not complain to parents (Royster 1999) or doctors unless asked. Pediatricians usually do not inquire about MSD symptoms unless there is an acute injury.

An important potential contributor to MSD is placing too much stress on joints and associated muscles, tendons, and other soft tissues. Examples include repetitive motions at the computer (e.g., overuse of the mouse, hitting the same keys for hours on end), overuse injuries in sports or in playing musical instruments, and carrying heavy school bags. Poor physical fitness, known as deconditioning, may also be a risk factor. On the other hand, preventive strategies such as maintaining good body position, avoiding repetitive motions, and avoiding overload may help.

If a child complains of excessive fatigue or stiffness in the neck or back, it is advisable to seek medical care. Treatments vary but may include rest, cold treatments to the affected area, and anti-inflammatory medication. When inflammation subsides, rehabilitation may include a stepwise return to full activity, exercises, and modifications in work or practice activities. ■

---

children adopt when using them (Fraser 2002; Harris and Straker 2000). As they do with desktop computers, children may use laptops for extended periods of time without giving thought to posture, and this situation occurs during critical stages of skeletal growth. Harris and Straker (2000) have proposed the following guidelines for laptop use:

• Avoid use in places with glare and reflections (see fig. 6.6).
• Use a high-quality screen.
• Where possible, provide low-weight laptops.
• Consider how the laptop is transported (wheeled or in a two-strap backpack).
• Provide an external keyboard, mouse, or even monitor to allow independent adjustment of keyboard and screen and a more natural wrist and hand posture.
• Take frequent breaks, and promote a routine of posture stretches.
• Encourage good working postures, with support aids where possible.

Internet Safety

Ergonomists are concerned about all dimensions of health and safety with respect to product or system use. With respect to the World Wide Web, computer games, and other computer activities, health and safety include not only the physical aspects of computer use but also the quality of the experience or service that children receive after they have logged on. Children learn by conducting their own research for school reports, sending and receiving e-mail, and playing educational games. Indeed, homework assignments now often require children to search out information on the Web. However, the Internet was designed primarily for adults and is mostly unregulated. Inappropriate content is readily available, and in the extreme, encounters with dangerous predators can occur. Parents are advised to monitor their children's computer use carefully, use blocking or filtering software, and teach their children precautions such as not responding to certain messages and telling parents about any frightening or threatening messages (Dowshen 2002).

Information and Communication Technology at Home

Computer use as a leisure activity has replaced many less sedentary pursuits. Roberts et al. (1999),

◼ *6.4. Working at the computer*

- A chair with adjustable height, seat depth, back angle, and armrest is ideal. Adjustable seat height and depth are the features that allow a chair to fit a wider range of body sizes.
- The top of the monitor screen should roughly align with the child's eye level, allowing a view of the entire screen while the child remains in a neutral position without extending or flexing. It should be directly in front of the child, not at an angle.
- The monitor should be about 2 feet from the computer user. Leaning forward to see should not be necessary.
- The height and tilt of the monitor should be easily adjustable.
- The keyboard should be about elbow height and adjustable for taller or shorter people.
- The angle of the elbows should be 90° relative to the upper arms or slightly more open (100°–110°). The elbows should be close to the side of the body so the upper arms do not have to reach out to the side when typing.
- Wrists should be in a neutral position for typing or using the mouse, not overly flexed (bent down), extended (bent up), or bent to the side when typing. A wrist rest can keep the hands in the neutral position; only the palm should rest on it but not while typing.
- Fingers and wrists should remain level while typing.
- Legs should be positioned comfortably, with the legs and hips perpendicular or at a more open angle (between 90° and 110°) relative to the trunk.
- The natural curvature of the spine should be maintained as much as possible, and the small of the back should be supported. An adjustable lumbar support or cushion can provide support if the seat is too deep for the backrest to be contacted when the knees are over the front edge of the seat.
- Feet should rest comfortably on the floor. A raised footrest can help smaller children attain an ergonomically correct position.
- Frequent breaks and a routine of posture stretches should be promoted.
- Children should be familiar with the dangers of incorrect posture and positioning and MSD.
- Pounding on the keyboard is unnecessary and can hurt both the student and the keyboard.
- Maximum adjustability in the workstation setup is important. In addition, all students should know how to adjust the furniture for themselves and do so routinely. ◼

in a study of U.S. children 2–7 years of age, found that 20% had used a computer during the previous day. Just a few years later 31% of children younger than 3 years of age and 70% of those 4–6 years of age had used computers (Rideout et al. 2003). As noted earlier, this may contribute to a more general shift toward a sedentary lifestyle. In Australia, one response has been a campaign to encourage parents to limit their children's sedentary activities, such as television viewing and computer games (Bauman et al. 2002). As with computer use for work, prolonged engagement in computer games can be dangerous and lead to MSD, especially when the same actions are repeated in the same position for hours. Many games draw children into a so-called video game trance, and they may not realize that they have spent hours in front of the screen. In an extreme example in Hong Kong (Szeto 2003), chil-

dren suffered from exhaustion and dehydration after many hours of nonstop computer games.

The following recommendations are from HealthyComputing.com and are similar to those relating to more general computer use:

- Hold the game pad (joystick) lightly, and do not hit the keys too hard.
- Take regular breaks to relax the muscles, especially when using force-feedback game pads. (Program developers could be advised to develop prompts or other integrated methods to remind users to take a break and stretch after each level is completed.)
- Use programmable features to group common functions or key sequences.
- Regularly change position at the computer.
- Check posture to ensure that you are not

slumped over the screen and that the wrists are in a neutral (unbent) position.

Educating Children about the Use of Computers

Schools are ideal venues in which to teach children about safe computer use. However, when equipment is available at home, children spend more time using computers and electronic games at home than at school. In a study of primary school children, Dockrell, et al. (2003) concluded that, although children of this age did not spend long periods of time on the computers at school, it was at this stage that habits were acquired that would continue into adulthood. However, Sotoyama et al. (2002) noted that few schools actively incorporate ergonomics information into computer training.

The most successful approach to teaching computer ergonomics has been its introduction into a variety of areas of the curriculum, including physical education, music, and mathematics, as well as in conjunction with ICT courses (Bennett and Tien 2003). Accordingly, a program relating to the safe use of computers should be incorporated in the curriculum of primary schools. Current secondary school students may not have been introduced to ergonomics in primary school. Ergonomics instruction should also be provided in high schools because some students will not have received this training in elementary school and because those who are college bound will soon be using computers extensively.

Audiovisual Equipment in the Classroom

Ideally, audiovisual (AV) equipment should be designed as an integral part of the classroom rather than added later. For maximum effectiveness, AV design and planning should begin with the architectural phase of building. However, much can be done with the arrangement of existing interiors. Specific recommendations, adapted from the Ergonomics for Children and Educational Environments (ECEE) technical committee of the International Ergonomics Association, appear in box 6.5.

Overall, ICT presents important challenges for children's health. Summary guidelines and recommendations for healthy computer use are listed below:

◼ *6.5. Classroom audiovisual equipment*

- Teachers must be able to see the monitor projections they are using for class discussions. The optimal arrangement would include a projection screen or monitor large enough to be seen from all student seating areas. The projection screen should also be connected to a monitor that is oriented so the teacher can see both the screen and the students without turning around.
- Projection monitors should be free from glare and visible without darkening the classroom.
- Images and text should be large enough for students sitting farthest away to see clearly.
- Students with visual impairments should be seated where they can see images without straining.
- A sound system allows teachers to vary the volume of the audio presentation. Special equipment enhancements may be necessary for students with hearing impairments. ◼

- Ensure that children have regular eye tests.
- Get in the habit of taking brief breaks or changing activities every 20 minutes.
- Establish a healthy routine that mixes physical and sedentary activities.
- Encourage everyone who uses a computer at home and at school to adjust the workspace for comfort and health. Make sure everyone knows how to use the features of adjustable furniture. Online resources can help.
- Promote healthy ergonomics as part of basic computer skills. Improve awareness, and respond early to body symptoms such as aches in the neck, shoulders, or wrists. Determine the cause of the problem and correct it.
- Provide training on the proper use of the keyboard and the mouse.

School Bags

Children carry a variety of items to and from school. In addition to books, laptop computers, and sports equipment, they may carry other electronic devices, lunch or a snack, musical instruments, and a variety of personal items. These items are commonly carried in some type of bag, such as a book bag, backpack, computer bag, athletic bag, or satchel (see fig. 6.7). Here we refer to them generically as school bags.

Elementary students usually carry bags to and from school and store items in their lockers or cubbyholes for most of the school day. In contrast, middle and high school students often carry their school bags with them as they change classrooms throughout the day. For these older students, lockers may be unappealing or unavailable, and many schools have eliminated them. In one study of secondary students, the children carried school bags for a mean time of 84.8 minutes, and 25% of the students who had access to lockers never used them. Only 35.7% used a locker on a daily basis (Whittfield et al. 2001). Inconvenience, lack of time between classes, and fear of locker break-ins were cited as reasons for not using them. When lockers are used, other ergonomic considerations can arise. Short children should not be assigned high lockers, and children who have difficulties with fine motor skills should not be given locks that are difficult to manipulate.

The weight of school bags is a growing concern. The spine matures later than the rest of the skeletal structure and continues to develop during adolescence. During the peak growth ages (around 13 in girls and around 15 in boys), the spine may be more vulnerable to heavy loads (Grimmer and Williams 2000). The American Academy of Pediatrics (2001) recommends carrying no more than 10–20% of body weight in a backpack, but many stud-

ies have found that students use school bags exceeding this limit. The American Chiropractic Association (n.d.) recommends a more conservative range of 5–10% of body weight. However, in a study in three Texas elementary schools (Forjuoh et al. 2003a), student backpacks weighed an average of 8.2% of their body weight, increasing from 6.2% among kindergarteners to 12.0% among fifth graders, and more than one in four students carried backpacks that weighed at least 10% of their body weights. Students, teachers, and even parents are often unaware of the weight being carried in school bags. When the parents of 188 students identified as carrying more than 10% of their body weight were contacted, 96% of the parents had never checked the weight, and 34% had never checked the contents (Forjuoh et al. 2003b).

The following tips on how to identify a backpack that is too heavy are adapted from the Backpack Intelligence program (Goodgold and Nielsen 2003):

- struggling to get the backpack on or off
- pain when wearing the backpack
- tingling or numbness
- red marks
- changes in the natural curvature of the spine.

Among other factors, heavy loads carried in school bags are associated with widespread reports of back pain and other musculoskeletal discomfort among students. In a 2003 study of 1122 backpack users between 12 and 18 years of age, 74.4% suffered from back pain (Sheir-Neiss et al. 2003). Back pain is not the only effect of heavy loads; students also report shoulder pain and numbness (Pascoe et al. 1997).

A study of data from the National Electronic Injury Surveillance System of the U.S. Consumer Product Safety Commission focused on backpack-related injuries (Wiersema et al. 2003). This database derives from emergency room visits and thus reveals more about acute injuries than chronic symptoms. In this study, 77% of all backpack injuries treated in emergency rooms were related to nonstandard uses of a backpack (e.g., tripping over it, reaching into it, or getting hit with one). The remaining 23% of the injuries related to standard use (e.g., wearing, lifting, taking off; Wiersema et al. 2003).

School bags may also affect health and safety in ways other than causing back and shoulder pain.

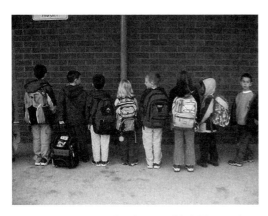

Figure 6.7. Seven- and eight-year-old children with backpacks. (Photo by Diane Tien.)

For example, heavy loads in backpacks restrict lung function (Lai and Jones 2001). In a study of university students, a load weighing 13.2 pounds (6 kg), representing just 6.9–12.8% of body weight, reduced lung function (Legg et al. 2002). Backpacks also cause a forward-inclined trunk posture and affect gait (Hong and Cheung 2003). Finally, straps and other hanging objects may be caught in doors or escalators and present potential safety hazards.

Design and Portage

Students who wear backpacks engage in a variety of motions and positions, including climbing stairs, entering vehicles, riding bicycles, and walking over rough terrain. Backpacks with two shoulder straps are the most common design. However, students sometimes suspend the bag from one shoulder, dispensing with the use of the second strap. A comparison of double- and single-strap bags found that wearing a double-strap bag and using both straps was generally superior in terms of preference, practicality, comfort, balance, and ease of walking and produced less neck discomfort and shoulder pressure and lower perceived exertion (Legg et al. 2002). Carrying school bags in one hand has been reported to be the most inefficient method, as it requires an energy expenditure of more than twice that of the backpack method (Malhotra and Gupta 1965). Few students use only one hand to carry their school bags.

Wheeled Bags

Wheeled bags such as wheeled backpacks, computer bags, or small luggage can be used to transport school items. Wheeled bags eliminate the need to support the weight of a school bag with the body. Concern about backpack weight is often cited as a reason for using wheeled bags. However, when entering or exiting vehicles and negotiating stairs or uneven terrain, the user must lift the wheeled bags. The result may be a heavier intermittent load that must be handled in an awkward posture. The torque exerted on the shoulder and arm may also be a concern when curbs or other impediments are encountered, particularly unexpectedly. The wheels of such bags should rotate 360° to reduce binding on turning. For older students, it is im-

■ *6.6. Using backpacks*

- Students, their parents, and teachers should know the approximate weight of the typical full bag. Weigh students' school bags in the morning when they are likely to be heaviest. Next determine the percentage of the body weight it represents.
- Encourage backpack weights of ≤ 10% of body weight.
- Read and follow the adjustment labels for the straps on the backpacks.
- Parents should encourage students to empty their school bags once a week to eliminate nonessential items.
- If school bags are carried, pack heavier items (e.g., books) toward the back and in the lower sections of the bag.
- Parents and teachers should work together to minimize the number of heavy items students transport to and from school.
- If economically possible, a duplicate set of textbooks can be purchased so that students can keep one set at home.
- If laptops are transported to and from school, provide wheeled, padded bags or a separate bag to distribute the load. Introduce the bags with educational information about ergonomics and how to reduce the health and safety risks.
- Schools should provide areas for storing school bags. Backpacks and satchel-type bags can be hung on hooks, but other arrangements may be necessary for wheeled bags.
- Policies should be established to make hitting others with a school bag or tampering with another student's bag serious discipline issues. ■

portant that the handle extend high enough to allow the user to stand upright while pulling the bag.

Research is needed to assess the relative benefits and risks of wheeled bags. The benefits may outweigh the risks, but this has not yet been documented. If wheeled school bags are promoted in educational campaigns as a way to prevent strain on the body, information about both benefits and risks should be provided.

Back Pain in Students: The Role of Ergonomics

Back pain is a common affliction and a leading cause of disability in adults, but only recently has back pain been documented in large-scale studies in children and adolescents (Grimmer and Williams 2000; Jones et al. 2003; Troussier et al. 1994). Back pain in students is a serious concern. For adults, the strongest predictor of future back pain is previous back pain, so having back pain in childhood could have serious future implications. The prevalence of nonspecific back pain during the previous month increases from 10% in the preteenage years to 50% in 15- to 16-year-olds (Sheir-Neiss et al. 2003). Children and adolescents rarely seek medical care for back pain, and parents are not always aware that their children are experiencing back or other musculoskeletal pain or discomfort.

Studies of back pain in children have implicated numerous causative factors, including heavy backpacks (Grimmer et al. 1999), psychosocial issues (Watson et al. 2003), and poor furniture design (Troussier et al. 1994). Ironically, both sedentary lifestyles and involvement in competitive sports are associated with higher incidence of back pain (Murphy et al. 2004).

Ergonomics awareness and posture training may offer an important preventive approach to back pain and should therefore be incorporated into physical education programs. Children can readily recognize what major muscles might be working in different tasks if they are asked to give it thought. It is important that they learn about the structure of the spine and back care. Recognizing the natural curves of the neutral spine and learning to maintain the natural curves while lifting and sitting may help reduce the risk of MSD.

Posture and back care are not currently emphasized in educational curricula, and posture education may not be included in the standards required by individual states. For instance, in 2002, posture was included as a specific topic in the standards for Washington State but not in those for California.

Back care education has been evaluated in a number of studies (Balagué et al. 1996; Cardon et al. 2001). The efficacy of the training, which was measured by videotaped observation of students' movements, was improved when a physical education teacher or physical therapist was present and when classroom teachers were also present and subsequently reinforced the training. However, when teachers were not trained, results were variable.

Ergonomics for Staff Members

Teachers

Ergonomic issues are equally important for both teachers and students, and it is essential that school systems include ergonomics in their approach to occupational safety and health for teachers.

Teaching can impose significant physical stress, but the teaching profession has been little studied from the perspective of ergonomics. At the elementary school level, teachers are working in a physical world that has been designed more for children than for adults. At all grade levels, the physical demands of teaching are likely to include bending, stooping, inclined trunk postures, walking, and sitting.

Two hundred teachers surveyed in Oregon spent 1–2 hours per day on computers at school, usually in short 15-minute periods for lesson plans and Internet access, and 2–3 hours per day on computers at home, preparing lessons and doing other tasks. In both environments they experienced an equal amount of pain, especially related to the neck, shoulders, back, wrists, and eyes (Williams 2001). This is a distribution similar to that found in office workers who use computers for extended periods of time. Both at home and at school, the design of the workstation and the chair were the teachers' main concerns. Seventy-one percent thought a computer ergonomics program for teachers would be a good idea.

An ergonomic orientation to teaching benefits both students and teachers. Teachers serve as role models, sources of information, and class managers. If they are aware of the importance of ergonomic concerns, they may be more likely to encourage children to pay attention to these issues, thus contributing to long-term health benefits for students. Ergonomics has not traditionally been a part of the educational preparation for teaching (Woodcock 2002). Teaching colleges and universities are beginning to include technology in the curriculum of teacher certification programs. However, ergonomics has been included in only a few teaching programs thus far, leaving school jurisdictions responsible in most cases for training teachers and students.

The work of a teacher includes many different activities: lecturing, correcting papers, meeting with students, speaking on the telephone, reading, and, increasingly, computer use. The teacher's workspace includes the classroom and any office, preparation area, computer area, or other location in which teachers work. Frequently a variety of activities is conducted in the same physical space, which may be the classroom. Each workspace in which a teacher routinely spends more than 30 minutes doing the same activity should be evaluated for appropriate design. Support, training, and communication can help teachers recognize the need to consider their work practices and to develop habits such as regular breaks from long sessions grading papers or working on the computer.

Because discomfort from poor positioning usually does not occur immediately, teachers may initially consider economy of space and convenience rather than ergonomic issues when they set up their computer area. When using a computer, the teacher should be supported in a comfortable posture that maintains the natural curvature of the spine without twisting. If possible, an adjustable chair should be available. A teacher whose computer or preparation area is in the classroom may use tables or desks that were designed for students. Using a small student chair can mean that a teacher's knees are higher than hip level, restricting circulation. Using low student desks or tables requires a teacher to bend forward and thus increases compression force on the lower back. If a traditional fixed-height desk is used, it should be appropriately sized for the teacher. Adjustable furniture easily fits any user and is ideal when budgets allow. If teachers are provided with laptop computers, workstation design and methods of carrying the computer should be addressed.

Adequate storage space is important for teachers, as placement of objects can affect safety and efficiency. Heavier items should be stored between shoulder and hip height (rather than above the shoulders) or on the floor for the best mechanical advantage in lifting. Ideally, frequently used items are readily accessible, and items used infrequently are stored in a separate space.

■ *6.7. Ergonomics for teachers*

To provide teachers with the tools to create a comfortable and healthy workspace, it is important to do the following:

- Include ergonomic training during orientation for new teachers. Include and emphasize neutral posture, the need for stretching, taking vision breaks from computers, and learning how to use adjustable furniture, if provided. Provide guidance for appropriate adjustment.
- Make sure the desk and computer areas have adequate space. Provide a height-adjustable surface for the computer if possible. Instructions for adjustment should be affixed to the furniture and pointed out to new users.
- Provide an appropriately sized or adjustable chair (for height and depth of seat) for writing and computer use. A stool can be helpful for elementary school teachers since it allows them to interact with students without having to bend over.
- Place the monitor screen where reflection and glare are minimized.
- Keep feet supported on the floor or with a footrest. Avoid crossing legs for extended periods of time. The use of ICT may constitute a health risk; ergonomics should be integrated into continuing professional development for teachers and staff.
- Ergonomics should be a part of the design process for new schools and major ICT purchases. ■

Guidelines and recommendations for ergonomics appear in box 6.7.

Other Staff

Administrative personnel use computers routinely and have needs and risks similar to those of most office workers. A study in New Zealand (Kai 2000) found that school office staff used computers 5.1 hours per day and did not take regular breaks. Although aware of the potential risks, few people took active preventive measures or participated in professional development to reduce the health risks. Only 54% of teachers and 49% of principals monitored their posture, and only about 60% considered the lighting. Very few teachers and principals had ergonomically designed furniture. Only 49% of secondary school and 33% of primary school administrators had asked for specific items to make their computer use safer. The investigator concluded that the introduction of ICT had emphasized equipment purchase rather than health and safety.

An adjustable chair is important for those who are sitting most of the day. If one's feet do not comfortably reach the floor, a footrest is needed; the keyboard should be at a comfortable height, usually at or below elbow level. An adjustable work surface provides optimal flexibility, but a keyboard tray can be useful if a surface of an appropriate height is not available. The monitor should be directly in front of the user, and the top of the viewing screen at approximately eye level. Training should be provided for any adjustable furniture. It is important to emphasize the need for rest breaks and to create a culture in which breaks are encouraged.

Principals can model ergonomic practices by supporting the training of staff and students. The principal can also work with the purchasing staff to identify needs such as adjustable chairs, teacher space, and accommodations for differently abled people. The parent community may include experts from the health profession who are capable of supporting the school's efforts to promote an ergonomics program.

Custodial work includes lifting and other manual tasks that require additional safety and ergonomic training to prevent disorders and encourage high productivity. Job rotation, tool maintenance, and checklists are important elements of any ergonomics program.

School librarians handle many books and frequently use a pinch grip. Taking rest breaks, rotating jobs, and limiting work sessions may help prevent discomfort. In many schools the librarian may evolve into a media specialist when ICT is adopted as a standard research tool. Students from all classes, of all ages, and of all sizes in a school usually use the same facility. Thus, the media center or library may be an opportune environment for introducing ergonomics to students.

Building Support for Ergonomics in Schools

Developing and maintaining an effective school ergonomics program requires broad-based awareness and support. Several groups of people must be involved, including parents, administrators, teachers, and students.

Parents are powerful advocates for children and thus can encourage the school system to promote ergonomics. Parents first of all need to protect their own children by being aware of the weight of their children's school bags, monitoring their children's screen time, and ensuring sufficient physical activity. Asking children whether they have any painful joints or muscles rather than waiting for them to offer this information is prudent. In addition to monitoring screen time, parents need to set limits and find ways to make sure their children develop good habits, such as taking breaks and arranging computer stations to fit.

Parents can also become active in the school. As observers in the classroom, they can determine whether the furniture is a good match for the students, find out how backpacks are stored, and learn whether computer stations can be adjusted to fit students of different sizes. Through parent-teacher organizations and school board meetings, parents can urge schools to include ergonomics education in the curriculum. Backpack safety programs can be developed at a grassroots level. Parents may identify ergonomists in the community who can be invited to speak to classes or act as consultants for the school. Much of the neglect of ergonomics in schools is a result of lack of awareness of the issues or knowledge of what to do about them.

Active participation by teachers and administrators is essential to a successful ergonomics program. As noted earlier, ergonomics has not been part of teacher training, although this is changing. Training of teachers and administrators and ongoing reinforcement will help solidify these programs. Teachers and administrators can serve as role models and local experts. Principals, school boards, and administrators should encourage consideration of ergonomics when furniture purchases are planned. Students can gather anthropometric data and supply purchasing personnel with the range of sizes the furniture needs to fit.

Finally, students must also be active participants in an ergonomics program. Children understand ergonomic concepts that are presented to them in a way that makes sense and draws upon their current knowledge base (Woodcock 2003a). Fraser (2002) outlines a long-term ergonomics education program involving children in the assessment of their use of laptop computers. The following guidelines can assist those who wish to adopt this approach in tackling ergonomics issues in their schools:

- Develop a program of ergonomics in which children understand the basic principles and are empowered to effect change.
- Provide an introduction to the concepts.
- Ask children to identify and measure problems (e.g., location, severity, type of discomfort).
- Ask children and others to develop feasible solutions to problems (e.g., if feet do not touch the floor, provide boxes or footrests).
- Make visual records of the experience to discuss and serve as reminders and to share with others.
- Allow everyone to see and assess the interventions that have been made.

Conclusion

This chapter has reviewed three pressing ergonomic concerns in schools—furniture, ICT, and school bags—to illustrate the role of ergonomics in promoting the long-term health of the next generation and in making school environments safer. Where possible, we have supplemented the text with guidelines and recommendations. Readers who desire more information may consult the authors or one of the web sites in the Resources section.

Acknowledgments

The authors extend their thanks to Rick Goggins and Barbara Silverstein.

Resources

- Ergonomics 4 Schools. Created by the UK Ergonomics Society to promote learning about ergonomics among secondary school students

and their teachers:
http://www.ergonomics4schools.com
- Ergonomics for Children and Educational Environments. An International Ergonomics Association technical committee. Includes information and research; will be adding more guidelines and tips for teachers, parents, and students:
http://www.ergonomics4children.org
- CergoS. Computer Ergonomics for Elementary Schools. Designed by the Oregon Public Education Network (OPEN) and now a part of the Oregon Occupational Safety and Health Division (OR-OSHA):
http://www.orosha.org/cergos/index.html
- HealthyComputing.com:
http://www.healthycomputing.com
- Ergonomics for Kids. Includes sections on computers, backpacks, and gaming:
http://www.healthycomputing.com/kids/index.html
- Childata. Comprehensive source of anthropometric data for children:
http://www.virart.nott.ac.uk/pstg/childata.htm
- CUErgo. Cornell University website. Includes school ergonomics programs; links to pages with ergonomics information:
http://ergo.human.cornell.edu/MBergo/intro.html
- KidsHealth/Dowshen. Internet use guidelines:
http://www.kidshealth.org/parent/firstaid_safe/home/net_safety.html

References

American Academy of Pediatrics. Backpack Safety Fact Sheet. 2001. http://www.aap.org/advocacy/backpack_safety.pdf [accessed 16 January 2006].

American Chiropractic Association. n.d.. Backpack misuse leads to chronic back pain, doctors of chiropractic say. http://www.acatoday.com/pdf/backpacks02.pdf [accessed 16 January 2006].

Attaianese E. 2003. Effects on learning performances of emotional and affective components: Human factor affective design contribution. In Proceedings of the Triennial Congress of the International Ergonomics Association [CD-ROM]. August 25–29, Seoul, South Korea.

Balagué F, Nordin M, Gonazage D, Waldburger M. 1996. Primary prevention, education, and low back pain among school children. Bull Hosp Joint Dis 55(3):130–134.

Bauman A, Bellew B, Vita P, Brown W, Owen N. 2002. Getting Australia active: Toward better practice for the promotion of physical activity. no. 3015. Melbourne, Australia: National Public Health Partnership.

Bendix T, Bloch I. 1986. How should a seated work-place with a tiltable chair be adjusted? Appl Ergon 17(2):127–135.

Bennett C. 2002. Computers in the elementary school classroom. Work 18(3):281–285.

Bennett C, Tien D. 2003. Introducing ergonomics in two U.S. elementary schools. In Proceedings of the Triennial Congress of the International Ergonomics Association [CD-ROM]. August 25–29, Seoul, South Korea.

Burgess Y, Trinidad S. 1991. Perceptions of computers: What do five-year-olds think? Aust Educ Comput J 6(1):16–18.

Cardon G, Clercq DD, Bourdeaudhuij ID, Breithecker D. 2004. Sitting habits in elementary schoolchildren: A traditional versus a "moving school." Patient Educ Couns 54(2):133–142.

Cardon G, De Bourdeaudhuij I, De Clercq D. 2001. Back care education in elementary school: A pilot study investigating the complementary role of the class teacher. Patient Educ Couns 45(3):219–226.

Caterina G. 2003. School interactive workstation for the improvement of children's learning performances. In Proceedings of the Triennial Congress of the International Ergonomics Association [CD-ROM]. August 25–29, Seoul, South Korea.

Cooper JS, Burns CR, Cotter SA, Daum KM, Griffin JR, Scheiman MM. 2001. Optometric clinical practice guideline care of the patient with accommodative and vergence dysfunction. Reference guide for clinicians (no. CPG18). St. Louis, MO: American Optometric Association.

Dockrell S, Fallon E, Kelly M, Masterson B, Shields N. 2003. An investigation of primary school teachers' education on computer-related ergonomics. In Proceedings of the Triennial Congress of the International Ergonomics Association [CD-ROM]. August 25–29, Seoul, South Korea.

Dowshen S. 2002. Internet Safety. KidsHealth for Parents. The Nemours Foundation. Available: http://www.kidshealth.org/parent/firstaid_safe/home/net_safety.html [accessed 16 January 2006].

Ergonomics for Children and Educational Environments (ECEE). 2004. ECEE web site. International Ergonomics Association Technical Committee. http://www.ergonomics4children.org [accessed 16 January 2006].

Forjuoh SN, Lane BL, Schuchmann JA. 2003a. Percentage of body weight carried by students in their school backpacks. Am J Phys Med Rehabil 82(4):261–266.

Forjuoh S, Little D, Schuchmann J, Lane B. 2003b. Parental knowledge of school backpack weight and contents. Arch Dis Child 88(1):18–19.

Fraser M. 2002. Ergonomics for grade-school students using laptop computers. In Proceedings of the Sixteenth International Occupational Ergonomics and Safety Conference [CD-ROM], June 10–12, Toronto.

Goodgold S, Nielsen D. 2003. Effectiveness of a school-based backpack health promotion program: Backpack intelligence. Work 21:113–123.

Grimmer K, Williams M. 2000. Gender-age environmental associates of adolescent low back pain. Appl Ergon 31:343–360.

Grimmer K, Williams M, Gill T. 1999. The relationship between adolescent head-on-neck posture, backpack weight, and anthropometric features. Spine 24(21):2262–2267.

Gurr K, Straker L, Moore P. 1998. Cultural hazards in the transfer of ergonomics technology. Int J Ind Ergon 22(4–5):397–404.

Harris C, Straker L. 2000. Survey of physical ergonomics issues associated with school children's use of laptop computers. Int J Ind Ergon 26(3):337–346.

HealthyComputing.com. Ergonomics for Kids. Available: http://www.healthycomputing.com/kids/index.html [accessed June 29, 2005].

Hong Y, Cheung C. 2003. Gait and posture responses to backpack load during level walking in children. Gait Posture 17(1):28–33.

Jones A. 1981. A new breed of learning consultant. In *Designing learning environments* (Sleeman PJ, Rockwell DM, eds.). New York: Longman. 48–66.

Jones G, Watson K, Silman A, Symmons D, Macfarlane G. 2003. Predictors of low back pain in British schoolchildren: A population-based prospective cohort study. Pediatrics 111(4 Pt. 1):822–828.

Kai K-W. 2000. Health risks with computer use in New Zealand schools. In Proceedings of the Eighth International Conference on Computers in Education and the International Conference on Computer-assisted Instruction (ICCE/ICCAI), Taipei, Taiwan, November 22.

Knight G, Noyes J. 1999. Children's behavior and the design of school furniture. Ergonomics 42(5):747–760.

Lai JP-H, Jones AY. 2001. The effect of shoulder-girdle loading by a school bag on lung volumes in Chinese primary school children. Early Hum Devel 62:79–86.

Legg S, Cruz C, Chaikumarn M, Kumar R. 2002. Efficacy of subjective perceptual methods in comparing between single- and double-strap student backpacks. In Proceedings of CybErg 2002 [CD ROM]. Johannesburg: International Ergonomics Association Press, September–October.

Legg SJ, Pajo K, Marfell-Jones M, Sullman M. 2003. Mismatch between classroom furniture dimensions and student anthropometric characteristics in three New Zealand secondary schools. In Proceedings of Triennial Congress of the International Ergonomics Association [CD ROM]. August 25–29, Seoul, South Korea.

Linton SJ, Hellsing A-L, Halme T, Akerstedt K. 1994. The effects of ergonomically designed school furniture on pupils' attitudes, symptoms, and behavior. Appl Ergon 25(5):299–304.

Macfarlane A, Harrison C, Somekh B, Scrimshaw P, Harrison A, Lewin C. 2000. Establishing the relationship between networked technology and attainment. London: British Educational Communications and Technology Agency.

Malhotra MS, Gupta JS. 1965. Carrying of schoolbags by children. Ergonomics 8:55–60.

Mandal AC. 1981. The seated man (Homo sedens). The seated work position: Theory and practice. Appl Ergonom 12(1):19–26.

Mandal, A.C. 1997. Changing standards for school furniture. Ergon Design 5(2): 28–31.

Marschall M, Harrington AC, Steele JR. 1995. Effect of workstation design on sitting postures in young children. Ergonomics 38(9):1932–1940.

McGill S. 2002. *Low back disorders: Evidence-based prevention and rehabilitation.* Champaign, IL: Human Kinetics.

Milanese S, Grimmer K. 2004. School furniture and the user population: An anthropometric perspective. Ergonomics 47(4):416–426.

Molenbroek JFM, Kroon-Ramaekers YMT, Snijders CJ. 2003. Revision of the design of a standard for the dimensions of school furniture. Ergonomics 46(7): 681–694.

Moseley DMM, Tse N. 2001. Using computers at home and in the primary school: Where is the value added? Educ Child Psychol 18(3):31–46.

Murphy, S., Buckle, P. and Stubbs, D. 2004. Classroom posture and self-reported back and neck pain in schoolchildren. Appl Ergon 35(2): 113–120.

Niemi S, Levoska S, Kemila J, Rekola K, Keinanen-Kiukaanniumi S. 1996. Neck and shoulder symptoms and leisure time activities in high school students. J Orthop Sports Phys Ther 24(1):25–29.

Oates S, Evans GW, Hedge A. 1998. The effect of computer workstation design on student posture. J Res Comput Educ 31(2):173–188.

Parcells C, Stommel M, Hubbard RP. 1999. Mismatch of classroom furniture and student body dimensions: Empirical findings and health implications. J Adolesc Health 24:265–273.

Pascoe DD, Pascoe DE, Wang YT, Shim DM, Kim CK. 1997. Influence of carrying book bags on gait cycle and posture of youths. Ergonomics 40(6):631–640.

Pope MH, Goh KL, Magnusson ML. 2002. Spine ergonomics [review]. Annu Rev Biomed Eng 4:49–68.

Rideout VJ, Vandewater EA, Wartella EA. 2003. Zero to six: Electronic media in the lives of infants, toddlers and preschoolers (No. 3378). Menlo Park, CA: Kaiser Family Foundation.

Roberts DF, Foehr UG, Rideout VJ, Brodie M. 1999. Kids and the media at the new millennium: Executive summary. Menlo Park, CA: Kaiser Family Foundation.

Royster L, Yearout R. 1999. A computer in every classroom–are school children at risk for repetitive stress injuries? In Lee G. (Ed.), *Advances in occupational ergonomics and safety.* Amsterdam: IOS Press, 407–412.

Schilling DL, Washington K, Billingsley FF, Deitz J. 2003. Classroom seating for children with attention deficit hyperactivity disorder: Therapy balls versus chairs. Am J Occup Ther 57(5):534–541.

Sheir-Neiss GI, Kruse RW, Rahman T, Jacobson LP, Pelli JA. 2003. The association of backpack use and back pain in adolescents. Spine 28(9):922–930.

Sotoyama M, Bergqvist U, Jonai H, Saito S. 2002. An ergonomic questionnaire survey on the use of computers in schools. Ind Health 40(2):135–141.

Storr-Paulsen A, Aagaard-Hensen J. 1994. The working positions of school children. Appl Ergon 25(1): 63–64.

Straker L. 2001. Are children at more risk of developing musculoskeletal disorders from working with computers or paper? In *Advances in occupational ergonomics and safety* (Bittner AC, Champney PC, Morrissey SJ, eds.) Amsterdam: IOS Press, 344–353.

Szeto GPY. 2003. Potential health problems faced by an Asian youth population with increasing trends for computer use. In Proceedings of the Triennial Congress of the International Ergonomics Association [CD-ROM]. August 25–29, Seoul, South Korea.

Troussier B, Davoine P, de Gaudemaris R, Fauconnier J, Phelip X. 1994. Back pain in school children: A study among 1178 pupils. Scand J Rehabil Med 26:143–146.

UNESCO-MINEDUC. 2001. Guia de recomendaciones

para el diseño de mobiliaro escolar. Santiago: Ministario de Education.

U.S. National Telecommunications and Information Administration. 2002. A nation online: How Americans are expanding their use of the Internet. http://www.ntia.doc.gov/ntiahome/dn/anation online2.pdf. [accessed 16 January 2006].

Watson KD, Papageorgiou AC, Jones GT, Taylor S, Symmons DP, Silman AJ, et al. 2003. Low back pain in schoolchildren: The role of mechanical and psychosocial factors. Arch Dis Child 88:12–17.

Wheldall K. 1982. Seating arrangements and classroom behaviour. Assoc Child Psychol Psych News 10:2–6.

Whittfield J, Legg SJ, Hedderley DI. 2001. The weight and use of schoolbags in New Zealand secondary schools. Ergonomics 44(9):819–824.

Wiersema BM, Wall EJ, Foad SL. 2003. Acute backpack injuries in children. Pediatrics 111(1):163–166.

Williams IM. 2001. Elementary school teachers' working comfort while using computers in school and at home. Available: http://education.umn.edu/kls/ecee/pdfs/ElementarySchoolTeachersinger.pdf [accessed 29 June 2005].

Woodcock A. 2002. Ergonomics in the secondary school curriculum. In *Contemporary ergonomics 2002* (McCabe PT, ed.). London: Taylor and Francis, 558–563.

Woodcock A. 2003a. Developing material for encouraging 4–7 year old children to consider ergonomics. In Proceedings of the Triennial Congress of the International Ergonomics Association [CD-ROM]. August 25–29, Seoul, South Korea.

Woodcock A. 2003b. Teaching ergonomics to 4–6 year olds. In *Contemporary ergonomics* (McCabe PT, ed). London: Taylor and Francis, 519–524.

Zandvliet D, Straker L. 2001. Physical and psychosocial aspects of the learning environment in information technology rich classrooms. Ergonomics 44(9):838–857.

7

Jerome A. Paulson and Chinonye Harvey

Animal Safety

■ *Summary*

- The presence of animals in school settings is controversial. Some experts argue that animals have no place in schools, whereas others contend that animal contact is beneficial.
- Animals in school settings raise three major health and safety concerns: infectious diseases, allergies, and bites.
- Infectious diseases that can be transmitted from animals to humans are called zoonoses. Some of these are theoretically risky, but transmission from animals to humans is actually very uncommon.
- People with lowered immune function, such as those on chemotherapy or with diseases of the immune system, may be at special risk.
- Allergies affect 10–15% of children and may be aggravated by animal contact. Both domestic and wild animals can bite people, and precautions are necessary. Accommodations need to be made for people who use service animals. ■

Some experts argue that animals have no place in schools, whereas others contend that animal contact is beneficial and that there are no good health reasons for not allowing dogs and other animals that are properly cared for in schools (Delta Society 2002). Animals are commonly seen in schools' science laboratories. Animals may also have a role as classroom pets, service animals, or transient visitors intentionally brought to school. Animals can also be unintended visitors to the school—bats that find their way in, rodents between the walls, or dogs, cats, foxes, deer, raccoons, squirrels, or other animals making their way across school grounds. The animals themselves may not be a problem, but their interaction with students, staff, and administrators can present challenges for school personnel.

To date, no extensive scientific studies of the impact of animals on the health of people in schools have been published. However, we have enough information about the impact of animals, both pets and wild animals, on people in other settings to make some useful recommendations to school personnel regarding the presence of animals in schools.

Animals in School Settings

The decision about whether to have animals in schools should be made by weighing the risks of their presence, both to the animals and to people, against the benefits they might provide (fig. 7.1).

Classroom Pets

For adults, pets offer many benefits. At home or in health-care settings, pets lower blood pressure and blood lipids and decrease feelings of loneliness and stress. Pet owners tend to get more exercise and socialize with other pet owners (Banks and Banks 2002; Kingwell et al. 2001; Rew 2000; Zasloff and Kidd 1994). For children, the presence of animals can reduce the anxiety associated with medical and dental exams (Havener et al. 2001; Nagengast et al. 1997). However, there is no evidence linking any of these benefits to the presence of pets in the classroom.

Experience with classroom pets can help children increase their understanding of animals and human-animal relationships, provide opportunities to observe reproduction and growth, instill and reinforce a sense of responsibility, and give lonely children an object of affection (Russell 1980). However, some people and organizations have signifi-

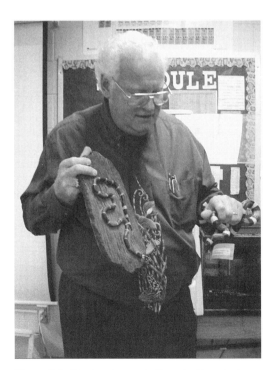

Figure 7.1. Teacher demonstrating adaptive mimicry using a classroom pet, a snake. (Photo by Lynwood Ward.)

cant concerns about the presence of animals in schools. Are the animals appropriately housed and adequately fed? Are teachers and students knowledgeable about the needs of the animals? Is competent veterinary care provided? Animals may be left alone in school buildings for extended periods without food and water or taken to multiple homes with variable levels of care for weekends or vacations. Children may cause unintentional injury to the animals, and lack of appropriate year-end planning can lead to abandonment of the animals (American Humane Association, n.d.; Russell 1980). Multiple issues must be considered in formulating a policy regarding pets in the classroom.

In addition, every effort should be made to minimize any health risks to children and adults who care for, observe, or handle classroom animals (based on recommendations of Adams [1998]):

- There should be no poisonous animals in the school (poisonous snakes, poisonous spiders, venomous insects).
- Younger children (perhaps less than age 8) should not handle animals at school.
- Older children should handle animals at school only under close supervision.
- Children and adults who handle animals or their waste should wear gloves.
- Children and adults who handle animals or their waste should wash their hands afterward.
- There should be no kissing or nuzzling of animals.
- If a classroom animal should get sick or die, a veterinarian should be contacted to determine the cause of illness or death and whether the children or adults in the school are at risk.
- Pregnant women should not have contact with cat feces, as it can transmit toxoplasmosis to the fetus.
- Food for people should be stored away from animal food.
- Animal food should be stored in closed containers so as not to attract vermin.
- Animal waste, vomitus, or blood that is spilled should be cleaned by an adult wearing gloves and using an appropriate disinfectant.

Household Pets Visiting the School

On occasion, pets may be brought to school for brief visits, such as for show-and-tell. Although this obviates some of the concerns about the long-term presence of animals in schools, the primary risk in this situation is likely to be bites, especially from dogs. Ensuring that the owner is the only one to handle the animal is likely to minimize this risk. However, visiting animals may still present some of the risks associated with allergic reactions and infections.

Laboratory Animals

Biology and life science classes with associated laboratory activities may involve live and preserved animals (fig. 7.2). In one school district in which data were collected, a variety of animals was used in the schools: fish (catfish, goldfish, guppies, minnows, sunfish), other aquatic organisms (tadpoles, brine shrimp, crayfish), mammals (gerbils, hamsters, rabbits, rats, mice), and other organisms (crickets, earthworms, silkworms) (Adams 1998). The National Science Teachers Association (1991) and the National Association of Biology Teachers (1995) have developed guidelines for the appropriate use of animals in educational settings. If these guidelines and the recommendations made in this chapter are followed, health risks to the children can be minimized.

Service Animals

The term "service animal" is a legal term defined in the Americans with Disabilities Act (ADA) of 1990. A service animal is any animal individually trained to do work or perform tasks for the benefit of a person with a disability. Title III of the ADA mandates that, under most circumstances, people with disabilities must be allowed access with their service animals into places of public accommodation, including restaurants, public transportation, schools, and health-care facilities. Service animals may include guide dogs, hearing or signal dogs, seizure-alert cats, mobility dogs, and emotional support cats (Duncan 2000).

A discussion of legal issues related to the presence of service animals in schools is beyond the scope of this chapter. However, service animals are likely to be well trained and represent a minimal risk of biting. They are also generally well cared for and have regular veterinary visits and are thus less likely to be a source of infection. If faculty, staff, and students are well informed about the role of service animals and their benefits to the people who depend on them, the risk of animal-associated problems is further reduced. Nevertheless, problems with allergies may still occur.

Health Problems Associated with Animals

Infectious Diseases

Zoonoses are diseases that are communicable from animals to humans under natural conditions. The Centers for Disease Control and Prevention (CDC) of the U.S. Department of Health and Human Services maintains an extensive web site, "Healthy Pets, Healthy People," which provides information about multiple zoonoses associated with dozens of different animals (http://www.cdc.gov/healthypets). This section focuses on a limited number of animals and diseases.

Before we delve into specific diseases, it is important to recognize that there are people in schools who are immunocompromised. These people are generally more susceptible to infections and are likely to have more serious problems as a result of a specific infection than people who have a normal immune system. Immunocompromised individuals may be children with inborn deficiencies of their immune system or children or adults with acquired immune deficiencies. These acquired problems can occur as a result of medications for the treatment of cancer or some autoimmune diseases or for the

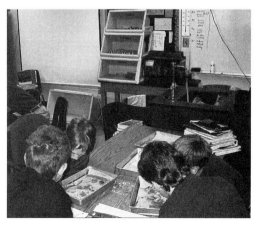

Figure 7.2. Children learning anatomy by dissecting frogs in biology class. (Photo by Lynwood Ward.)

treatment of patients who have had organ transplants; diabetes; removal of the spleen; acquired immune deficiency syndrome (AIDS); or the long-term use of high-dose steroids for the treatment of certain diseases.

A number of animals have been associated with the transmission of salmonella to humans, including reptiles (lizards, snakes, turtles), amphibians (frogs, toads, newts, salamanders), and baby ducks and chicks (Anonymous 2000; CDC 2003b). Salmonella may cause vomiting and diarrhea in children and adults and, less commonly, may cause a serious infection.

Hamsters, gerbils, and other rodents will bite, particularly if they are not handled gently. Although there is no risk of the transmission of rabies from these animals, like all animals and humans, they do have bacteria in their mouths. Therefore, anyone bitten by one of these animals is at risk for the development of a bacterial infection at the site of the bite.

Cat scratches and bites can result in cat scratch disease, an infection caused by the *Bartonella henselae* bacteria. This infection can cause swollen lymph nodes ("swollen glands"), fever, and other symptoms.

Most school personnel probably think of ringworm as an infection spread from child to child, but this fungal infection (not really a worm) can also be transmitted from cats, dogs, rabbits, and guinea pigs to humans. It causes a round rash on the skin and hair loss on the scalp.

Psittacosis is a bacterial disease caused by *Chlamydia psittaci* and transmitted to humans from parrots, parakeets, cockatiels, canaries, pigeons, turkeys, ducks, and other birds. Symptoms include cough, fever, chills, and muscle aches.

Four parasitic diseases deserve mention here:

- Toxocariasis is caused by intestinal infection with the dog roundworm (*Toxocara canis*) or cat roundworm (*Toxocara cati*). These can be contracted from animal feces if the animals are in the classroom or, more likely, from feces on the school grounds.
- Tapeworm infections (*Dipylidium canium*) are also transmitted from dogs and cats. Tiny segments of the worm are ingested by fleas, and, if the flea is accidentally swallowed by a human, that person can become infected.
- *Cryptosporidia* is a parasite that is associated with cats, dogs, and farm animals. The most common route of transmission to humans is through drinking water. In a school-related setting, a person is most likely to become infected on a school-sponsored camping trip when drinking unpurified water from a contaminated stream, river, or lake.
- Toxoplasmosis is an infection caused by the *Toxoplasma gondii* parasite. This parasite, often present in cat feces, can cause a spontaneous abortion in pregnant women or brain damage and other problems in infants born to the infected woman. For this reason, pregnant women should never handle cat waste.
- *Mycobacterium avium* complex and *Microsporidia* parasites are associated with fish and aquarium water. In healthy children, the *Mycobacterium avium* complex is most likely to cause swelling of the lymph nodes that ultimately resolves. In immunocompromised individuals, serious infections of the *Mycobacterium avium* complex or *Microsporidia* can spread throughout the body.

Problems Related to Asthma and Allergy

Both children and adults are affected by the challenges of asthma and allergies, and chapter 28 provides a detailed discussion of the issues associated with asthma. Asthma affects approximately 4.8 million children in the United States (Mansour et al. 2000) and accounts for 14 million days of school missed annually for children 5–17 years of age and for 14.5 million missed work days annually for adults 18 years of age and older (Mannino et al. 2002). Asthma and allergies often coexist, and 10–15% of all children have some kind of allergy.

Environmental factors that contribute to the development of allergies and asthma or that trigger asthma attacks in children can be found in places where children spend most of their time, that is, at home, at school, and on the playground. In this chapter we focus on allergens from pets in schools. Exposure to dog, cat, and mite allergens occur in schools where these animals are kept as pets or for education (Carrer et al. 2001). Mite allergen is primarily a problem at home, but cat and dog allergens are found in high concentrations in schools and daycare centers, even when the pets are not kept in the school. Therefore, children attending school can be exposed to the types of allergens that can induce asthma or sensitization in children who are allergic to furry animals (Berge et al. 1998).

Animals shed hair and dander (flakes of skin and dried saliva) that can attach to dust or clothing and be spread within the place of origin and beyond. Allergens can be carried from homes with pets to schools without animals and from schools to homes without pets. Animal allergens are routinely present in the schools at levels that are at least as high as those found in homes without pets (Wood 1999). Children without cats in their homes carry those allergens home from school, as evidenced by the fact that they have cat allergens in their mattress dust samples (Epstein 2001; Wood 1999). Therefore, the animals do not have to come in direct contact with a child or even be in the same place as a child for an allergic reaction or asthma trigger to occur (Dybendal et al. 1989; Epstein 2001).

In five Norwegian schools studied, the most common allergens in classroom dust that caused allergic reactions were from cats and dogs (Dybendal et al. 1989). According to a research study conducted in Swedish schools, dog and cat allergen levels were high enough to cause sensitization or induce asthma in schoolchildren who had existing allergies to cats and dogs (Almqvist et al. 1999; Munir et al. 1993).

Researchers found that some schoolchildren with no pets in their homes were allergic to animal dander and developed severe asthma as a result of exposure to cat and dog allergens in classrooms (Almqvist et al. 1999). People who do not own pets can become sensitized through secondhand exposure to their pet-owner counterparts, and the levels of cat allergens found in classrooms are sufficient to cause an allergic reaction in children with cat allergies (Smedje and Norback 2001).

Sensitization in children with asthma results from multiple factors in their environment (Amr et al. 2003), among which is the fact that children tend to spend most of their time indoors. They tend to play closer to the ground, where they are more likely to become exposed to contaminated dust on floor surfaces. The floors of classrooms can be covered with rugs, wall-to-wall carpet, or linoleum, or they can remain smooth, bare surfaces. Smooth-surfaced floors are relatively easy to clean. Conversely, carpets and rugs, as well as upholstered furniture and textiles, serve as reservoirs for cat and dog allergens. Allergens have a tendency to stick closer to the bottom of the carpet, making it difficult to clean effectively (Dybendal 1989). In an analysis of allergens found in settled dust samples in 12 Baltimore public elementary schools, the concentrations of dust mites and cat and dog allergens were much higher in rooms with carpet or rugs than in classrooms with bare floors (Amr et al. 2003). When children play on surfaces covered with rugs or carpet, they become exposed, and this may trigger asthma and allergic responses.

In school, children or adults who have allergies severe enough to substantially limit one or more major life activities would have a disability as defined by the ADA. Those people would be entitled to protection under the ADA, and a conflict could arise between the needs of someone with a disability who has a service animal and someone else who has a disability related to an allergy to some component of that animal.

Encountering Animals on Field Trips

If the decision is made to ban or restrict animals in school buildings, should field trips be considered as an alternative that would still allow students to interact with animals? Significant illness associated with field trips to petting zoos or farms have been reported, although rarely. For example, outbreaks of *Escherichia coli* O157:H7 infection have occurred with these types of visits (CDC 2001). The bacteria spreads from the animals to the hands of the children and then to their mouths, where it enters the gastrointestinal tract. *E coli* can cause vomiting and diarrhea and may trigger a very serious medical problem known as hemolytic uremic syndrome (HUS). Children with HUS present with bleeding in their skin and develop kidney failure. The use of hand-washing facilities at the zoo or farm can significantly limit the risk of this problem.

The CDC, in collaboration with the Zoonoses Working Group, National Association of State Public Health Veterinarians, U.S. Department of Agriculture, Animal and Plant Health Inspection Services, and other groups, has drafted the following recommendations to reduce the risk for farm animal–human transmission of enteric infections (CDC 2003a):

- Information should be provided. Those who offer public access to farm animals should inform visitors about the risk for transmission of enteric pathogens from farm animals to humans and strategies for preventing such transmission. This should include public information and training of facility staff. Visitors should be made aware that certain farm animals pose a greater risk of transmitting enteric infections to humans than others. Such animals include calves and other young ruminants, young poultry, and ill animals. When possible, information should be provided before the visit.
- Venues should be designed to minimize risk. Farm animal contact is not appropriate at food service establishments and infant care settings, and special care should be taken with school-aged children. At venues where farm animal contact is desired, layout should provide a separate area where humans and animals interact and an area where animals are not allowed. Food and beverages should be prepared, served, and consumed only in animal-free areas. Animal petting should occur only in the interaction area to facilitate close supervision and coaching of visitors. Clear separation methods such as double barriers should be present to prevent contact with animals and their environment other than in the interaction area.
- Hand-washing facilities should be adequate. Hand-washing stations should be available to both the animal-free area and the interaction area. Running water, soap, and disposable towels should be available so that visitors can wash their hands immediately after contact with the animals. Hand-washing facilities should be accessible, sufficient for the maximum anticipated attendance, and configured for use by children and adults. Children younger than 5 years should wash their hands with adult supervision. Staff training and posted signs should emphasize the need to wash hands after touching animals or their environment, before eating, and on leaving the interaction area. Communal basins do not constitute adequate hand-washing facilities. Where running water is not available, hand sanitizers may be appropriate, but the CDC makes no recommendations about the use of hand sanitizers because of a lack of independently verified studies of efficacy in this setting.
- Hand-to-mouth activities (e.g., eating, drinking, smoking, carrying toys and pacifiers) should not be permitted in interaction areas.

People who are at high risk for serious infections should observe heightened precautions. Farm animals should be handled by everyone as if the animals were colonized with human fecal pathogens. However, children younger than 5 years, elderly people, pregnant women, and immunocompromised persons (e.g., those with HIV/AIDS) are at higher risk for serious infections. These people should weigh the risks for contact with farm animals. If allowed to have contact, children younger than 5 years should be supervised closely by adults, and the precautions should be strictly enforced.

Lyme disease must be considered if a school trip involves hiking or camping in the woods. This infection is transmitted to humans by ticks that have previously bitten animals. In the United States, Lyme disease is a risk primarily in states in the northeastern, mid-Atlantic, and upper north-central regions of the country and in several counties in northwestern California. Lyme disease can cause a skin rash, but its more serious manifestations include joint pain and inflammation of the heart and nerves.

Encountering Animals on School Property

It can be safely said that most wild animals on school property will avoid children and adults, but if they do not, they are probably ill and should be avoided (CDC 2000). Rodents can transmit hantavirus and plague. Ticks can transmit Rocky Mountain spotted fever and Lyme disease. Mammals such as raccoons, skunks, foxes, coyotes, and bats can transmit rabies. If a wild animal arrives on school property and appears to be sick or does not move away promptly, the local animal control resources should be called. Children and adults should be kept away from the animal.

Neighborhood animals that are loose on the school grounds should also be avoided because of the potential for bites, especially from dogs. Depending on the breed of animal, these can be very serious. The Humane Society of the United States (HSUS) has developed the following guidelines for preventing dog bites and coping with a threatening situation (HSUS, n.d.)

- Never approach a strange dog, especially one that is tied or confined behind a fence or in a car. Do not pet a dog—even your own—without letting the animal see and sniff you first.
- Never turn your back to a dog and run away.
- Do not disturb a dog while it is sleeping, eating, chewing on a toy, or caring for puppies.
- Always assume that a dog who does not know you may see you as an intruder or a threat.

If you are approached by a dog that may attack you, follow these steps:

- Never scream and run.
- Remain motionless, hands at your sides, and avoid eye contact with the dog.
- Once the dog loses interest in you, slowly back away until it is out of sight.
- If the dog does attack, "feed" it your jacket, purse, bicycle, or anything that you can put between yourself and the dog.
- If you fall or are knocked to the ground, curl into a ball with your hands over your ears and remain motionless. Try not to scream or roll around.

Conclusions

The presence of animals in school settings is common, and the balance of benefits and risks remains controversial. Carefully collected scientific evidence to address this disagreement remains scarce. This chapter presented evidence that addresses both the benefits and the risks of animals in schools and makes recommendations to maximize the benefits and minimize the risks of animal contact in the school setting.

Resources

- Centers for Disease Control and Prevention www.cdc.gov
- Delta Society www.deltasociety.org
- Humane Society of the United States www.hsus.org
- National Association of Biology Teachers www.nabt.org
- National Science Teachers Association www.nsta.org
- National Service Dog Center www.deltasociety.org/dsb000.htm
- U.S. Department of Justice ADA Information Line 1-800-514-0301

References

Adams RM. 1998. Animals in schools: A zoonosis threat? Pediatr Infect Dis J 17(2):174–176.

Almqvist C, Larsson PH, Egmar AC, Hedren M, Malmberg P, Wickman M. 1999. School as a risk environment for children allergic to cats and a site for transfer of cat allergen to homes. J Allergy Clin Immun 103(6):1012–1017.

American Humane Association. n.d. The classroom pet: Considerations for teachers. Englewood, CO: Author.

Amr S, Bollinger ME, Myers M, Hamilton RG, Weiss SR, Rossman M, Osborne L, Timmins S, Kimes DS, Levine ER, Blaisdell CJ. 2003. Environmental allergens and asthma in urban elementary schools. Ann Allerg Asthma Immunol 90(1):34–40.

Anonymous. 2000. Salmonellosis associated with chicks and ducklings: Michigan and Missouri, Spring 1999. Mortal Morbid Weekly Rept 49(14):297–299.

Banks MR, Banks WA. 2002. The effects of animal-assisted therapy on loneliness in an elderly population in long-term care facilities. J Gerontol A, Biol Sci Med Sci 57(7):M428–M432.

Berge M, Munir AK, Dreborg S. 1998. Concentrations of cat (Fel d1), dog (Can f1) and mite (Der f1 and Der p1) allergens in the clothing and school environment of Swedish schoolchildren with and without pets at home. Pediatr Allergy Immunol 9(1):25–30.

Carrer P, Maroni M, Alcini D, Cavallo D. 2001. Allergens in indoor air: Environmental assessment and health effects. Sci Total Environ 270(1–3):33–42.

Centers for Disease Control and Prevention (CDC). 2000. An ounce of prevention: Keep the germs away. Avoid contact with wild animals. Available: http://www.cdc.gov/ncidod/op/animals.htm [accessed 29 June 2005].

Centers for Disease Control and Prevention (CDC). 2001. Outbreaks of *Escherichia coli* O157:H7 infections among children associated with farm visits—Pennsylvania and Washington, 2000. Morbid Mortal Weekly Rept 50(15):293–297.

Centers for Disease Control and Prevention (CDC). 2003a. Recommendations: Farm animal contact. Available: http://www.cdc.gov/foodborneout breaks/publication/recomm_farm_animal.htm [accessed 29 June 2005].

Centers for Disease Control and Prevention (CDC). 2003b. Reptile-associated salmonellosis: Selected states, 1998–2002. Morbid Mortal Weekly Rept 52(49):1206–1209.

Centers for Disease Control and Prevention (CDC). 2005. Outbreaks of Escherichia coli O157:H7 Associated with Petting Zoos—North Carolina, Florida, and Arizona, 2004 and 2005. Morbid Mortal Weekly Rept 54(50):1277–1280.

Delta Society. 2002. Program for animal-assisted activities and therapy: Reducing risk. In *Pet partners team training course manual,* 5th ed. (Howie AR, ed.). Renton, WA: Author, 172–173.

Duncan SL. 2000. APIC State-of-the-art report: The implications of service animals in health-care settings. Am J Infect Control 28(2):170–180.

Dybendal T, Hetland T, Vik H, Apold J, Elsayed S. 1989. Dust from carpeted and smooth floors: Comparative measurements of antigenic and allergenic proteins in dust vacuumed from carpeted and noncarpeted classrooms in Norwegian schools. Clin Exp Allergy 19(2):217–224.

Epstein BL. 2001. Childhood asthma and indoor allergens: The classroom may be a culprit. J Sch Nurs 17(5):253–257.

Havener L, Gentes L, Thaler B, Megel ME, Baun MM, Driscoll FA, Beiraghi S, Agrawal S. 2001. The effects of a companion animal on distress in children undergoing dental procedures. Issues Compr Pediatr Nurs 24(2):137–152.

Humane Society of the United States. N.d. Stay dog bite free! Available: http://www.hsus.org/pets/pet _care/dog_care/stay_dog_bite_free/ [accessed 29 June 2005].

Kingwell BA, Lomdahl A, Anderson WP. 2001. Presence of a pet dog and human cardiovascular responses to mild mental stress. Clin Auton Res 11(5):313–317.

Mannino DM, Homa DM, Akinbami LJ, Moorman JE, Gwynn C, Redd SC. 2002. Surveillance for asthma: United States, 1980–1999. Surveillance Summaries. Mortal Morbid Weekly Rept 51(1):1–13.

Mansour ME, Lanphear BP, DeWitt TG. 2000. Barriers to asthma care in urban children: Parent perspectives. Pediatrics 106(3):512–519.

Munir AK, Einarsson R, Schou C, Dreborg SK. 1993. Allergens in school dust: The amount of the major cat (Fel d1) and dog (Can f1) allergens in dust from Swedish schools is high enough to probably cause perennial symptoms in most children with asthma who are sensitized to cats and dogs. J Allergy Clin Immunol 91(5):1067–1074.

Nagengast SL, Baun MM, Megel M, Leibowitz JM. 1997. The effects of the presence of a companion animal on physiological arousal and behavioral distress in children during a physical examination. J Pediatr Nurs 12(6):323–330.

National Association of Biology Teachers. 1995. The use of animals in biology education. Available: http://www.nabt.org/sub/position_statements/animals.asp [accessed 31 December 2003].

National Science Teachers Association. 1991. Guidelines for the responsible use of animals in the classroom. NSTA position statement (July). Available: http://www.nsta.org/159&psid=2 [accessed 31 December 2003].

National Science Teachers Association. 1991. Responsible use of organisms in precollege science. Available: http://www.nsta.org/organisms/ [accessed 31 December 2003].

Rew L. 2000. Friends and pets as companions: Strategies for coping with loneliness among homeless youth. J Child Adolesc Psychiatr Nurs 13(3):125–132.

Russell HR. Classroom pets? 1980. Nature Study 33:10–11, 19.

Smedje G, Norback D. 2001. Incidence of asthma diagnosis and self-reported allergy in relation to the school environment: A four-year follow-up study in schoolchildren. Int J Tuberc Lung Dis 5(11):1059–1066.

Wood RA. 1999. Animal allergens: Looking beyond the tip of the iceberg. J Allergy Clin Immun 103(6):1002–1004.

Zasloff RL, Kidd AH. 1994. Loneliness and pet ownership among single women. Psychol Rept 75(2):747–752.

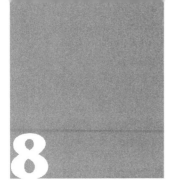

8

Robin Moore

Playgrounds
A 150-Year-Old Model

■ *Summary*

- Current playground design reflects changing recreational philosophies and institutional commitments over the last 150 years.
- Effective playgrounds provide a safe environment for active play, learning, exploration, and physical activity, which are crucial for healthy development.
- Mortality is extremely rare in school playgrounds. In contrast, injuries, although improved in some areas, continue to be a major concern. Falls from equipment remain the most frequent cause of injury on school grounds.
- In addition to playground equipment, designed landscape settings provide a viable strategy for safe, health-promoting playgrounds.
- Successful playground design or renovation is likely to result from a master plan and the collaboration of school and community. ■

Webster's defines a playground as "a piece of ground for and usually having special features for recreation, especially by children" (Gove 1961, p. 1737). This definition is helpful. Special recreational features, designed and constructed according to a plan, distinguish a children's playground from a vacant lot or a forest. The character and extent of those features and the type of recreation the area supports have taken many forms in the last 150 years, reflecting changing philosophies of children's recreation and varying institutional commitments to supporting children's recreational needs.

This chapter begins by tracing the history of playgrounds and exploring the philosophies behind the changes. Two major themes emerge. First, playgrounds should be places where children can play without incurring serious injury. Second, playgrounds should be spaces that support healthy child development through the process of active play, learning, and exploration. With regard to playground safety, this chapter reviews trends in injuries and fatalities and presents prevention strategies. Finally, case studies of community-based efforts to create playgrounds and school parks that meet both sets of goals are discussed. With a focus on elementary schools serving children 4–12 years of age (prekindergarten to sixth grade), the chapter offers suggestions on how to optimize playgrounds as educational and developmental settings that are safe for all children.

Playgrounds through History

Playgrounds as Pedagogy

Equipped playgrounds have a long history. The first fully illustrated publication of this concept appeared in 1848, authored by Henry Barnard (Brett et al. 1993). Barnard's playground was conceptually a pedagogical space centered on play. In the image from the original book (fig. 8.1), teachers are shown joining with students in traditional games as the core of childhood cultural transmission, and modern innovations such as wooden blocks are also introduced. Small carts are shown as toys to play with and as storage for blocks at the end of the day. There are large shade and fruit trees against a high wall surrounding the play yard. The only items of anchored equipment are two rotary swings—one for girls, the other for boys. Ropes hang from swivels on the top of tall poles. The children grab the ropes, run in a circle, and thrust themselves outward to ride airborne for a few moments propelled by centrifugal force—a pedagogical benefit.

By the end of the nineteenth century, variations on this model, influenced by German playground concepts developed in the 1880s, had spread to schools and settlement houses in Boston, Chicago, and New York. The Playground Association of America, founded in 1906, helped promote the playground concept at a municipal level as a means of attracting young people to a safe place away from the perceived social and physical dangers of city streets. Organized playgrounds, informed by prevailing theories of child development, were used to socialize urban youth into prosocial, cooperative, physically active lifestyles in a community context away from the influence of parents.

Industrial versus Natural Settings

By the early twentieth century, playgrounds were increasingly outfitted with industrial products. Manufactured steel slides, swings, seesaws, and jungle gyms were anchored in threadbare turf and later in asphalt, the ultimate no-maintenance solution (fig. 8.2). Sometimes a covering of thin rubber tiles softened the surface immediately underneath the structures. However, severe injuries occurred with disturbing frequency when children fell from a height onto a hard surface or otherwise suffered the consequences of poorly designed and maintained equipment.

Over time, the approaches to manufactured

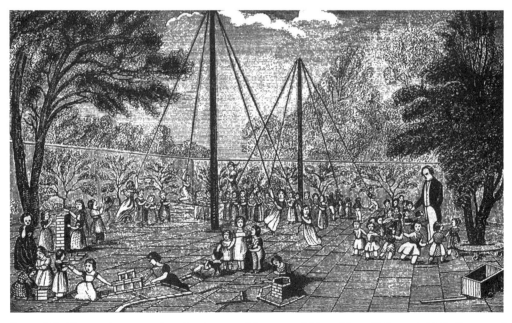

Figure 8.1. Nineteenth-century view of a playground for young children. (From H. Barnard, 1848. Courtesy of University of Michigan, Making of America.)

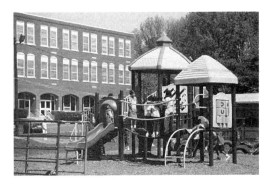

Figure 8.2. Typical, standardized, manufactured equipment playground. (Photo by Robin Moore.)

playground equipment evolved. Safety modifications were introduced, and individual structures—a swing set here, a jungle gym there—gave way to extensive composite structures, some approaching small play villages in complexity and size (fig. 8.3). Finally, some groups replaced conventional, boring equipment and asphalt with community-built structures. These areas included commercial playground equipment together with custom settings installed through a participatory community process. Natural settings were sometimes included, along with other expressions of local history, culture, and the arts.

In fact, the growing use of playground naturalization reflects a return to an earlier pedagogical approach. The schoolyard is viewed as a curricular resource—a multifaceted outdoor setting that supports mandated curricular objectives, as well as children's social and physical development. Such a naturalized schoolyard might include commercial

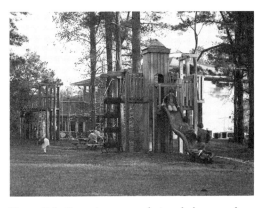

Figure 8.3. Extensive custom-designed playground equipment in a natural setting. (Photo by Robin Moore.)

playground equipment set within a larger area of open space planted with trees. Figures 8.4 and 8.5 show the transformation of rural and urban school play areas through naturalization.

Across the United States and Canada—and more strongly in Europe—a grassroots naturalization movement is growing in strength, including coalitions of educators, environmental advocacy groups, parents, and children involved in helping to define their own everyday environment. The most successful of these initiatives are substantial partnerships between school systems, university departments, natural science museums, botanical gardens, parent–teacher organizations (PTOs), wildlife organizations such as Audubon and the National Wildlife Federation, and a multitude of community-based organizations. A small but growing number of schoolyards are being deliberately designed to serve educational ends. Environmental educators see this as a key strategy for exposing urban children to the educational richness of the natural world through play, discovery, and formal learning.

The Concept of Recess

In addition to explicit curricular goals, some educators and parents have emphasized children's need to "let off steam" for short periods each day. The assumption is that school-aged children need to run around and clamber on structures to expend pent-up energy before returning to their classroom studies. In recent years, as academic performance accountability pressures have risen, many school systems have curtailed or abandoned recess altogether. Now, however, parent groups across the country are pressuring local school boards to restore recess. This counterattack puts forth three arguments: Children have a right to play, rest, and relaxation (United Nations 1989); recess helps children perform better academically; and recess is a significant factor in physical and mental health and healthy socialization (Clements 2000; American Association for the Child's Right to Play 2005).

Recess, at this basic level of consideration, means a minimum amount of time outside. It says nothing about the quality of that time, which for children is associated with the quality of the physical surroundings and the extent to which they provide a broad range of play and learning opportunities.

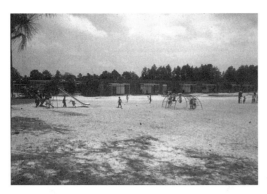 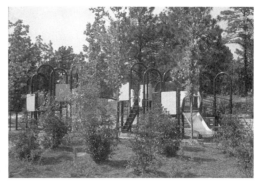

Figure 8.4. (Left) Bland, featureless, rural school grounds before renovation. (Right) The same school grounds after renovation. The manufactured equipment has been naturalized by the addition of a grove of shade trees and shrubs. (Photos by Robin Moore.)

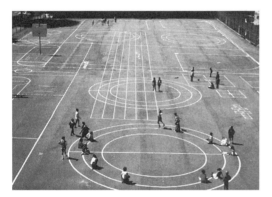 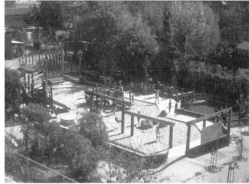

Figure 8.5. (Left) Hard, asphalted, urban school yard before renovation. (Right) The same school yard after renovation. Asphalt has been replaced for diversified play and learning opportunities in naturalized settings. (Photos by Robin Moore.)

In recent years, obesity has reached epidemic proportions in the United States, and children are very much affected (Strauss and Pollack 2001). This epidemic relates to both gluttony and sloth— to excess consumption of calories and sedentary lifestyles that do not burn off sufficient calories (Prentice and Jebb 1995). Children need to be more physically active. Public health researchers have become increasingly aware that the school site is one of several community settings with potential for antiobesity interventions (Baranowski et al. 2000). From this perspective, playgrounds that offer pleasurable and meaningful physical activity can be viewed as an intervention aimed at changing children's daily behavior.

Outdoor spaces are ideal for this purpose. Although school gymnasiums provide an alternative space for physical activity, they generally serve as places for formal physical education classes and organized sports and are less likely to establish a lifelong pattern of freely chosen physical activity.

Summary: Playgrounds That Serve Many Purposes

This brief history shows that the goals of playgrounds have evolved over the last 150 years. At the dawn of the twenty-first century, we can identify four crucial agendas for playgrounds:

- safety
- educational success through engagement with diverse, living environments
- healthy social and psychological development through deep, creative play
- active living (i.e., at least a minimal amount

of sustained physical activity during the school day).

Playgrounds and schoolyards should be designed, managed, and programmed to integrate all of these objectives. This implies an expanded view of playgrounds beyond mandated, structured time on manufactured equipment to creative time in nontraditional equipment and settings. This view of the playground as an educational resource can serve all four of these goals. Moreover, it offers the added advantage of engaging teaching staff in meaningful educational roles outdoors together with children. If the outdoor environment is designed to serve the needs of teachers, as well as those of children, they too will find the experience pleasurable and meaningful. This strategy can be effective (Moore and Wong 1997).

An irony in playground design is that both safety and risk, seemingly opposing goals, are desirable. Safety interventions can prevent serious injuries. However, in *Risk and Our Pedagogical Relations to Children: On the Playground and Beyond* (1998), Stephen Smith points out that taking chances (and therefore incurring risk) is a component of healthy development. The optimal balance of safety and risk is a pedagogical issue that implies intentional relationships between teachers and children. This is very different from the simplistic view of adult supervision, which places adults in the role of watchdogs that control behavior while doing little to teach children responsible behaviors. For Smith, play is about learning through risk-taking behaviors that motivate children continually to push the frontiers of their own development, not just physically, but psychologically and socially as well.

Jay Beckwith (2003), one of the pioneer industrial designers of the new breed of playground equipment, suggests that the balance of safety and risk has tipped too far toward safety. He cites two reasons: the constraints imposed by the Americans with Disabilities Act Guidelines for Play Areas (U.S. Access Board 2000) and the focus on legal liability. Beckwith argues that an unintended consequence of the Americans with Disabilities Act (ADA) may be the removal of appropriate levels of challenge from play environments for the large majority of able-bodied children. He also maintains that risk avoidance has seriously compromised the play value of playgrounds now being installed. A bal-anced approach would reconcile the value of play in healthy child development, with choice of environmental accessibility and an appreciation of the importance of safety.

Elements of Playground Safety

Data on injuries in school playgrounds come from several sources, including death certificates, emergency room records, and surveys of health-care providers. Although the data are not perfect, they reveal a consistent pattern. Fatal injuries (mortality) on school playgrounds are extremely rare, but nonfatal injuries (morbidity) such as bruises, cuts, and broken bones are common.

Playground-related Mortality and Morbidity at School and Other Locations

Mortality

A major source of data regarding safety in schools is the comprehensive publication, *Risks to Students in School*, from the U.S. Congress, Office of Technology Assessment (1995), which analyzed unintentional, as well as intentional (homicide and fighting), injuries of children 5–19 years of age. Overall, the Office of Technology Assessment (OTA) study establishes the fact that schools are relatively safe places for children. The two leading causes of death to children overall are motor vehicles and firearms. Together with cancer, they account for more than eight in ten deaths in children. Very few deaths are associated with schools.

Tinsworth and McDonald (2001) analyzed the U.S. Consumer Product Safety Commission (CPSC) data files related to 147 deaths associated with playground equipment (the CPSC gathers only product-related data) that occurred between 1990 and 2000. Although these records did not include all playground-associated deaths and did not constitute a statistically valid sample, the data are a valuable source of information about the circumstances surrounding playground deaths. Sixty-eight percent of the deaths were of children 5–14 years of age, which represents about 10 deaths per year in all locations. Of the 128 cases where the location was specified, 38 incidents (30%) occurred at public playground equipment locations, and the remaining 70% occurred at home. This means that at public playgrounds, including both schools and parks, about four deaths per year were reported over the 10-year period. One may assume that the bulk of these playgrounds were at schools, reflecting the estimate by Phelan et al. (2001) that approximately four times more nonfatal injuries occurred on school and daycare playgrounds than in parks. Three causes of death predominate: strangulation (54%), falls to nonresilient surfaces such as asphalt (21%), and tip-over or collapse of equipment (16%). Strangulation usually results from clothing or cords becoming entangled or caught on the equipment, especially slides. Given these fatality statistics, efforts at reducing death on playgrounds should focus on three areas: appropriate clothing (no protruding cords), adherence to the CPSC guidelines, and good maintenance of equipment.

The death of a child, particularly from unintended injury, is always a tragedy, but these four annual playground equipment deaths represent a far smaller toll than the estimated 37 children killed each year by vehicles while waiting for school buses, the 20 sports injury–related deaths each year, or the 44 school homicides annually (Office of Technology Assessment 1995).

Morbidity

Morbidity presents a somewhat different picture. There is a considerable body of research on playground-related injuries (MacKay 2003), but assembling a clear picture of these events is a challenge. Different studies use differing age and location categories and inconsistent definitions of injury and severity. Another problem is that the CPSC collects only equipment-related injury data, rather than data associated with whole play areas or school grounds. Despite these limitations, it is clear that playground injuries are a leading cause of injury to elementary and junior high students, ages 5–14 years, while at school. The policy task requires first establishing a sense of perspective on the issue by assessing the magnitude of playground injuries relative to other domains of childhood injury, then isolating school playground injuries and describing them in sufficient detail to guide appropriate responses.

Based on published studies, the OTA concluded that the most common locales for unintended school injuries were playgrounds, gymnasiums, and athletic fields. Injuries associated with

playgrounds were the most prevalent and accounted for 30–45% of unintended school injuries.

Using data gathered through the National Electronic Injury Surveillance System (NEISS), the CPSC study of playground deaths also analyzed playground equipment–related injury covering a 12-month period from November 1998 to October 1999 (Tinsworth and McDonald 2001). During the target year, an estimated 205,850 playground equipment–related injuries were treated in U.S. hospital emergency rooms. Of these, 156,040 (78.8%) were associated with equipment designed for public use, of which 70,218 (45%) were associated with playground equipment in schools. Figure 8.6 shows the distribution of the playground injury data by location.

In their study of injuries caused by playground *falls*, Phelan et al. (2001) used data from the National Hospital Ambulatory Medical Care Survey (NHAMCS) gathered between 1992 and 1997 for children and youth under 20 years of age. Children 5–9 years of age (kindergarten to fourth grade) were three times more likely to visit the emergency room as the result of a playground fall than were 10- to 14-year-olds. The rate of playground fall injuries did not vary between girls and boys or between white and black children. The most frequent location of playground falls was at school; however, the data also included daycare locations. School and daycare playground falls accounted for 40% of such injuries, home playground falls for 25%, and public parks and other recreational areas for 9%. Playground falls accounted for a greater proportion of all falls at school.

Phelan et al. (2001) analyzed data for motor vehicle and bicycle emergency room visits to compare them with playground falls. In the 6-year period of the study, motor vehicle–related visits were 10 times more frequent than playground fall visits. Schwebel et al. (2002) used diaries completed each day by 6- and 8-year-olds and their parents to gather information about commonly occurring minor injuries. They found that twice as many injuries occurred at home as on playgrounds, in the streets, or on athletic fields. The vast majority of injuries were either cuts and scrapes or bumps and bruises in roughly equal proportions. The authors found that relatively few injuries occurred at school. Logically, injuries occur in places where children spend the majority of their time. Children spend 15–20% of their waking hours in school. Homes and motor

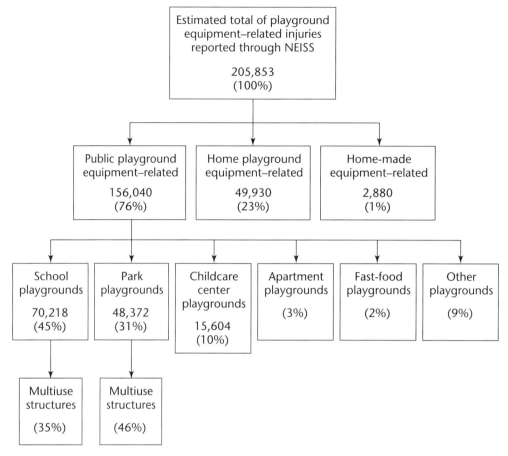

Figure 8.6. Distribution of playground equipment injuries by location. (From Tinsworth and McDonald 2001.)

vehicles expose children to far more risk of injury than do schools (Schwebel et al. 2002). However, within the school setting, playgrounds expose children to more risk of injury than other school locations. In other words, playground safety is a logical focus for efforts to reduce school-related injuries.

An earlier CPSC study, using 1988 adjusted data, estimated that about 170,000 playground equipment–related injuries resulted in emergency room visits (Office of Technology Assessment 1995). Of these, 70% (about 120,000) involved public playground equipment. The OTA (1995) calculated that approximately 30% (36,000) of these injuries occurred on school playgrounds. Of these, only 36% (approximately 13,000) occurred during school hours, representing about 8% of all public playground equipment injuries. This finding is an important reminder that school playgrounds function as significant play locations for children even outside of school hours. Most of the injuries sustained on school playgrounds occur outside of school hours.

Tinsworth and McDonald (2001) compared the 1988 and 1998–1999 NEISS/CPSC data (though neither data set is directly comparable to the 1988 OTA data just discussed). Comparison between the 1988 and 1999 data shows an increase in public playground equipment–related injuries from 70% of playground injuries requiring emergency room care in 1988 to 76% in 1999, despite the substantial advances in safety standards. Falls accounted for 79% of injuries related to public play equipment in 1999, compared with 74% in 1988. This increase may reflect a proportional drop in other injuries such as impact with moving or stationary equipment and contact with hardware, pinch points, and sharp edges, reflecting substantial design improvements made by the play equipment industry during the last 10 years. The difference may also indicate the additional exposure resulting from increases in after-school care. Moreover, it may reflect the propensity of children to take greater risks in play environments that they perceive as being safe.

Types of Playground Injury and Parts of the Body Affected

The types of playground injuries (all ages) reported by Tinsworth and McDonald (2001) were fractures (39%), lacerations (22%), contusions and abrasions (20%), and strains and sprains (11%). The large majority of fractures (almost 80%) involved the elbow, lower arm, or wrist. Body areas most frequently affected (school-aged children only) were the arm and hand (43%) and head and face (34%). About 15% of injuries to the face and head were diagnosed as concussions, internal injuries, and fractures. These injuries accounted for only about 5% of all surface fall–related wounds.

Types of Injury and Playground Equipment

An analysis of NEISS data for 1990–1994 concluded that, for the 5- to 14-year age group, "approximately 35% of injuries associated with public playground equipment were severe (concussions, dislocations, fractures, internal injuries, amputations, crushing injuries). Seventeen percent were moderately severe (ingestions, foreign bodies, hematoma, dental injuries, punctures, strains, sprains, hemorrhage, avulsion, dermatitis, conjunctivitis), and 48% were relatively minor" (Mack et al. 1997, p. 101).

Tinsworth and McDonald (2001) reported that 79% of injuries that occurred on all public equipment involved falls. Falls to the surface below accounted for 68%. Falls to other parts of the equipment (steps, rungs, horizontal climbing bars, or vertical poles) accounted for 10%. They indicated that the great majority of public playground–related injuries were associated with just three types of equipment: climbers (53%), swings (19%), and slides (17%). Eighty-six percent of injuries associ-

ated with climbers were fall related. Equivalent rates for swings and slides were 80% and 69%, respectively (fig. 8.7). Fifty-nine percent of the injuries associated with other equipment (seesaws, merry-go-rounds, etc.) were falls. All injuries that required hospitalization (although they constituted only 3% of all playground injuries) resulted from falls. Falls thus present the greatest risk to children using playground equipment and account for a disproportionate number of severe injuries. Injuries to the arms and hands are the most frequent.

Looking more closely at injuries associated with climbers, of the 75% of records that included details of the type of element, 60% were associated with horizontal ladders, 6% with hand-over-hand rings or triangles, and 2% with arch climbers. In other words, two-thirds (68%) of injuries associated with climbers involved elements of overhead equipment (Tinsworth and McDonald 2001).

The most frequently reported causes of falls were the children losing their grip (40%; most often related to climbing bars or swing chains), skipping or tripping (16%; most often on slides), and jumping or dismounting intentionally (10%; most often on swings). The types of falls that were least often reported occurred when a child was pushed by another child or reached for a part of the equipment and missed the grip. Tinsworth and McDonald (2001) note that in school settings, more than a quarter (28%) of play equipment incidents involved other children.

The 1988 and 1999 CPSC studies show that falls continue to account for the majority of injuries associated with public playground equipment. In 1988, the conditions of safety surfaces were not reported. The OTA (1995) reported that, in every study of safety surfacing on public playgrounds, high proportions of unsafe conditions were found, some as high as 99%. In contrast, the 1999 CPSC special study reported that, in locations where public equipment was installed, 80% had a protective surface under the equipment, most often bark mulch or wood chips. Dramatic improvements in safety surfacing under play equipment have apparently been achieved. The few cases of falls involving serious head injury occurred where either there was no protective surface or it was too shallow.

Rigorous maintenance protocols for safety surfacing and playground equipment must remain a top priority. However, in almost 80% of the inci-

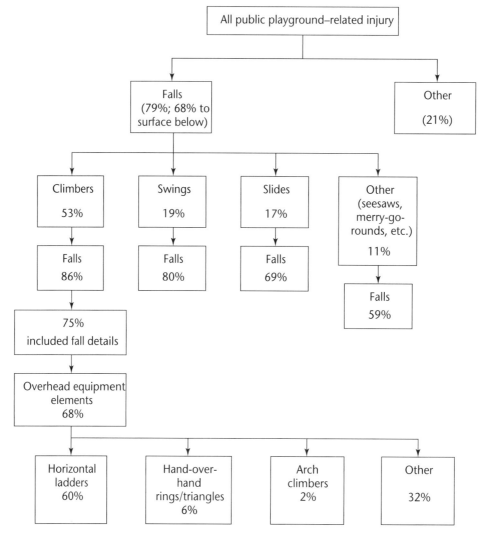

Figure 8.7. Distribution of public playground equipment fall injuries by type of equipment. (From Tinsworth and McDonald 2001.)

dents involving public playground equipment, no information was available concerning regular maintenance or safety inspection programs.

Playground Injury by Age and Gender

Tinsworth and McDonald (2001) reported the distribution of playground injuries by age and incidence by age group per 10,000 for the 1999 U.S. population as a whole (table 8.1).

Girls were injured somewhat more frequently than boys (55% vs. 45%). Because of the dominance of the 5- to 14-year-old group, the Tinsworth and McDonald data (2001) were adjusted for this chapter to show the association between this age

Table 8.1 Distribution of playground injuries by age and by incidence, United States, 1999

Age group	% of injuries	Incidence per 10,000 injuries/year
All children	100	7.5
< 5 years	30	29
5–9 years	56	
5–14 years		35
10–14 years	14	
> 15 years		1

Table 8.2. Type of equipment and associated injuries for children age 5–14 years

Type of equipment	Number (percentage of total injuries)
Climbers	66,161 (57)
Swings	26,980 (23)
Slides	12,998 (11)
Seesaws	4,541 (4)
Merry-go-rounds	187 (1)
Other	4,590 (4)
	115,457 (100)

Data from Tinsworth and McDonald (2001).

group and specific items of playground equipment (table. 8.2). More than half (57%) of all public playground equipment–associated injuries were related to climbers; about one-quarter (23%) were related to swings; one-tenth (11%) were related to slides, 4% were related to seesaws, and 1% to merry-go-rounds. Other injuries (4%) were related to other equipment such as sandboxes, trapeze bars, ball pits, and track rides.

Children with Disabilities

None of the playground equipment safety studies mention safety issues related to children with disabilities. Common sense tells us that children with disabilities are playground users, especially given the energetic push in recent years toward educational integration, social inclusion, and accessible playgrounds.

Adaptive physical education is now integrated into the general school curriculum and should be used in all aspects of the playground. Children with and without disabilities should interact within the same setting, enhancing socialization and increased acceptance of children with different strengths and limitations. Playground equipment builds muscle tone, provides kinesthetic movement, and improves coordination and balance, all of which are beneficial. Because the playground may also serve as a community recreation area, it affords all children, with and without disabilities, access to well-designed equipment.

Every school playground should be accessible to all students. Within the playground, there should be some well-designed play equipment available for use by able-bodied children, as well as by children using wheelchairs or other supportive devices.

Prekindergarten Programs on School Sites

Prekindergarten programs are increasingly available. Children between 3 and 5 years of age are attending these programs, either because they are recognized as being at high risk for developmental disabilities or because they are part of a comprehensive program to increase school achievement. The elementary school setting in use for pre-K programs may or may not have been renovated to meet the needs of smaller children. No guidelines have been established that specifically address playgrounds for children of this age group. However, the use of poorly implemented play yards, defined by chain-link fencing, surfaced with turf or mulch, and furnished with plastic play items, clearly does not meet the program goals for these children. These children, many of whom come into pre-K programs already labeled "at risk," need environments with a health-promoting focus that offers the sensory, physical, and social stimulation that has been lacking in these children's lives.

Applicable Standards and Guidelines

Key government publications and other sources of standards and guidelines for the design and management of school grounds are described below.

- U.S. Consumer Product Safety Commission Handbook for Public Playground Safety (1981). This document presents a set of guidelines that covers most items of manufactured playground equipment, safety surfacing, and maintenance protocol recommendations. The handbook was first issued in 1981 and is the most commonly referenced and applied standard of care for manufactured playground equipment. The intended audience includes playground designers, purchasers, installers, and consumers.
- American Society for Testing and Materials, ASTM F 1487 Standard Consumer Safety Performance Specification for Playground Equipment in Public Use (1993). This more technical publication is intended as a guideline for manufacturers and represents a voluntary

standard. The ASTM also publishes relevant voluntary standards for surface systems under and around playground equipment (ASTM F 1212, 1991) and for drawstrings on children's upper outerwear (ASTM F 1816, 1997). Falls from equipment remain the most frequent cause of injury. The most important protection against injury from falls is the presence of a shock-absorbing safety surface below the equipment within the use zone. These ASTM voluntary standards describe appropriate safety surfaces for playgrounds.

- Rigorous maintenance protocols for safety surfacing must remain a top priority. Kutska et al. (1998) provide guidance on the development of public playground safety and maintenance programs.
- *Play for All Guidelines: Planning, Design, and Management of Outdoor Play Settings for All Children* (Moore et al. 1992). First published in 1987 as the result of an extensive national consultation and interdisciplinary conference, this volume has become a standard reference for playground designers by combining best practices for safety and accessibility with designs that support the developmental needs of school-aged children. The book covers site planning, design of specific settings for playing and learning, design programming, and risk management.
- The Architectural and Transportation Barriers Compliance Board (U.S. Access Board 2000) is in the process of issuing final accessibility guidelines that are intended to serve as the basis for U.S. Department of Justice standards for new construction and alterations of play areas covered by the ADA. The guidelines include scoping and technical provisions for ground-level and elevated-play components, accessible routes, ramps and transfer systems, ground surfaces, and soft, contained play structures. The guidelines will ensure that newly constructed and altered play areas are readily accessible to and usable by people with disabilities.

Beyond the Conventional Playground

Much progress has already been made in reducing the hazards of playground injury:

- Slide-related injuries have decreased, most likely because of the lowered heights and preventive design features added in recent years. The lowered heights and slower speeds of plastic compared with stainless steel slides are problematic for children, however, in that they may seek more stimulating, unconventional, and therefore potentially hazardous ways of using the equipment.
- Swing-related deaths have been dramatically reduced in the last 15 years, probably because heavy, solid seats are no longer used. However, swing-related falls and other injuries still account for almost one-fourth of play-equipment injuries. Swing-related injuries may be declining because few schools are installing swings, although it is the most popular item of play equipment in the opinion of users (Moore and Young 1978; Moore 1989).
- Installation of shock-absorbing safety surfaces under and around climbing structures has reduced the rates of both serious and fatal head injuries resulting from falls onto concrete or asphalt. However, the major source of playground equipment–related injuries at schools remains falls from climbers, which result mostly in arm injuries.
- Self-imposed design standards for the playground equipment industry have almost eliminated injuries from protrusions, crush points, and sharp edges that were frequent causes of injury 20 years ago.
- Entrapment injuries are rare because the causes have been "designed out" of equipment. Equipment is now more sturdily constructed with higher-grade materials, and moving parts are engineered to higher standards. The longevity of equipment has been increased, and wear-and-tear hazards reduced.

Children's Compensatory Behavior

This progress is confounded by a fundamental, predictable characteristic of children's behavior: If the environment is insufficiently challenging, children will find ways to make it more stimulating by inventing new behaviors. On climbing structures, children commonly balance on the tops of railings or clamber along their outer edges. Children will always experiment with going headfirst down slides. They need to test every possible combination of tire swing use. Successful "bailouts" on to-and-fro swings remain a childhood rite of passage demonstrating exquisitely timed interactions with gravity. Designers must anticipate these behaviors, try to predict the consequences, and propose design and management responses. Most professional playground designers would probably agree that the guidelines already in place represent the limits of what can be done with respect to manufactured playground equipment. An additional strategy, which de facto has been in effect for decades, is rooted in what used to be the community-built approach to playgrounds: Widen the range of play choices by providing designed landscape settings in addition to playground equipment settings.

Safe, Health-Promoting Playgrounds and School Grounds

This landscape design strategy is viable in both new construction and playground renovation projects. The approach most directly addresses health promotion criteria by extending the range of options for social, physical, and cognitive behaviors. The following concepts are useful in designing or renovating playgrounds to maximize the benefits of an extensive, health-promoting landscape:

- Provide play opportunities for children who are intimidated by manufactured playground structures because of inadequate physical skills or personality traits that do not match the high-energy behavioral style of play structure users.
- Reduce behavioral pressures, especially on multiuse structures where overcrowded conditions can increase the risk of slipping or tripping incidents that can cause falls.
- Spread out the behavior horizontally across the play area, using the space to better advantage. Playground equipment tends to attract behavior in dense clusters that makes ineffective use of the overall space of the schoolyard.
- Increase levels of moderate and vigorous activity across the population of children by dispersing behavior settings. Children tend to run between settings. More complex landscapes encourage chasing games such as hide-and-seek. School grounds that incorporate topographical variety and are naturalized with

shrubs and shade trees provide increased stimuli for ground level, horizontal active play in addition to the vertical play of manufactured play equipment (thereby also reducing the risk of falls associated with equipment).

- Offer an extensive landscape with a variety of additional settings and behavioral options to more effectively meet the individual needs of children according to stages of development, personality types, and friendship patterns.
- Encourage spending class time outdoors, enabling students to reap the health benefits of increased physical activity in fresh air and sunlight.
- Provide numerous opportunities for teachers to extend learning processes into the outdoors and thus increase options for meeting state-mandated curricular objectives. This wider range of educational settings will better match the variety of learning styles in an average class of students.
- Help schools move away from curtailing or abandoning recess on the assumption that recess reduces classroom time for academic study.
- Engage children with nature both through play and curricular activity, thus encouraging an emotional attachment to the natural world and increasing their understanding about how the natural world works and how to care for it.
- Offer teachers a break from the intensity of classroom teaching with a move to stimulating natural surroundings. Development of interpersonal relations around cooperative learning activities outdoors offers teachers an opportunity to establish alternative relationships with their students, especially with "difficult" students, who may respond positively to the freedom of hands-on learning beyond the restrictions of classroom space.

School Grounds as Community Resource

Viewing school grounds as potentially health-promoting environments moves the discourse to a higher plane. To meet this potential, all stakeholders must be engaged in a joint educational endeavor. These stakeholders include students, teachers, parents, school administrators (at site and system level), other sectors of government (e.g., parks and recreation), and organizations with similar goals.

School sites occur in a broad range of socioeconomic, cultural, geographic, and urban contexts. They can be old, renovated, or new, as well as inner city, urban, suburban, or rural. Schools exhibit many degrees of cultural diversity. School grounds can be large, small, and in between, and they are located both north and south of the frost line. They may be spread out over flat or hilly terrains, and they may be situated in the forest or on the plains. A standardized approach to playground provision cannot possibly respond to this diversity of dimensions. Nonetheless, design strategies based on landscape diversification and health promotion

can respond to these opportunities in myriad ways to create environments that offer a sense of place and belonging for students, teachers, and the community (Grant and Littlejohn 2001).

Naturalization also responds to an important issue largely missing from the safety literature: shade. Shade obviously provides comfort, particularly for children in the southern states. Sunlight presents a classic case of the need to balance health protection and health promotion. Too much sun can be harmful and cause serious, life-threatening disease. (See box 8.1 for safety recommendations for sun exposure.) On the other hand, lack of sunlight can cause rickets, a serious disease, as well as other negative health effects such as seasonal affective disorder (SAD) (Rosenthal 1998).

▨ *8.1. Safety in the sun*

Outdoor play provides exercise and promotes physical fitness. However, cumulative sun exposure over a lifetime increases the risk of the most common skin cancers (basal cell epithelioma and squamous cell epithelioma) and may also increase the risk of the rarer but more life-threatening type of skin cancer called malignant melanoma. Sun exposure increases the risk of skin cancer even when actual sunburn is avoided (Scherschun and Lim 2001). As much as 80% of a person's lifetime sun exposure occurs before the age of 18 years. Reducing sun exposure involves the use of protective clothing (ultraviolet [UV]-blocking sunglasses, hats, and garments made of tightly woven cloth) and sunscreens. Both UVA (315–400 nm) and UVB (290–315 nm) rays from the sun penetrate the atmosphere and pose a threat of sun-induced skin damage. Sunburn can occur even on cloudy days, as the cloud cover blocks only a small part of UVA and UVB rays.

Sunscreens should block both UVA and UVB rays to minimize skin damage from the sun. Products blocking both UVA and UVB rays are described as "broad spectrum." Various ingredients may be blended in a sunscreen to achieve this goal; common constituents include oxybenzone, octyl salicylate, and octyl methoxycinnamate. Some people may find that a particular ingredient irritates the skin or causes an allergic reaction; those people should avoid products containing that ingredient.

Products are rated by their ability to prevent sunburn when applied at a uniform thickness. This ability is measured as the sun protection factor (SPF). A product with an SPF of 30 reduces UVB penetration by 97%, whereas a product with an SPF of 15 filters 93% of UVB when applied at the recommended thickness (U.S. EPA 2001). Leading authorities recommend the use of broad-spectrum, water-resistant products with an SPF of 15 or higher (American Academy of Pediatrics 2000; Moloney et al. 2002; Scherschun and Lim 2001). Sunscreen should be reapplied at least every 2 hours during continuous sun exposure (American Academy of Pediatrics 2000; U.S. EPA 2001).

Appropriate sunscreen application involves the use of 30 ml (1 ounce) over the whole body of a typical adolescent or adult. Most people normally apply half of this amount or less, and this thinner application reduces the stated SPF by half or more (Moloney et al. 2002).

(Robert J. Geller) ▨

Improvement Models for Playgrounds and School Grounds

Recognition of the potential of school playgrounds and school grounds as educational resources, rather than as just places to let off steam at recess, revived in the late 1960s and early 1970s. Slowly but steadily the school playground development movement has been growing in many countries, including the United States. Most notably in the English-speaking world, Canada (Evergreen Foundation) and the United Kingdom (Learning through Landscapes) have well-established national advocacy, technical assistance, and training organizations with impressive achievements on the ground (details in the list of resources at the end of this chapter).

In the United States, a substantial, dispersed grassroots movement has been gathering momentum for many years. A search of Internet sites under "schoolyards" provides an excellent impression of the many local, state, and national organizations involved. Some of those groups currently most relevant are listed at the end of this chapter in "Resources," including the Schoolyard Habitat listserv.

Citywide Initiatives

Citywide initiatives to rebuild school grounds are under way in many locations across the country, including Berkeley, Boston, Denver, and San Francisco.

Berkeley

Since the late 1960s, Berkeley, California, has had a rich history of improving the grounds of its public schools as a collaborative effort between the schools, parks and recreation agencies, and local groups. Models of success include the Environmental Yard at Washington Elementary School (Moore and Wong 1997) and the Edible Schoolyard at Martin Luther King Junior High School (www.edible schoolyard.org).

Boston

The Boston Schoolyard Initiative (BSI; http://www .schoolyards.org/overview.htm) was launched in 1995 to respond to the condition of Boston's public schoolyards and to encourage public and private sectors to cooperate in revitalizing these neglected spaces. BSI has since tackled more than 64 projects (Howard 2004).

Denver

The Learning Landscape Alliance (LLA; http:// thunder1.cudenver.edu/cye/lla/home.) started in 1998 as a collaboration between Denver Public Schools and the Department of Landscape Architecture at the University of Colorado, Denver. The 6-year involvement of parents, students, staff, neighbors, and local businesses produced the first learning landscape at Bromwell Elementary School. The LLA has resulted in the development of more than 50 integrated traditional and nontraditional settings.

San Francisco

The San Francisco Green Schoolyard Alliance (http://sfgreenschools.org/index.html) was formed in 2001 to promote inclusive, community-driven processes that create and maintain healthy, environmentally sustainable learning environments in San Francisco schools.

School Parks

In reality, any well-developed schoolyard can be considered a neighborhood park for those families living close by. Official or not, school grounds will be used when school is not in session. However, the term "school parks" usually means that the school grounds are a joint enterprise of the school system and the parks and recreation department. School parks are a well-established method of capturing the full social value of school grounds as a public resource, especially in neighborhoods where community parks are scarce. Implementation requires transparent legal relationships and clearly defined management responsibilities. Although any developed school ground can serve as a neighborhood park, when a local school board agrees to implement a systemwide transformation with a city or county parks system, the impact can be far greater.

Some individual schools have renovated their school grounds to such a high standard that they attract after-school and weekend use by the community and have become de facto neighborhood parks. Blanchie Carter Discovery Park (Southern

Pines Primary School, Southern Pines, NC) and Kids Together Park (a community park in Cary, NC) both demonstrate how manufactured equipment, including low-to-the-ground equipment, can be creatively naturalized to provide a range of community play settings. The American Planning Association Parks Forum publication (2003) contains several case examples.

Participatory Design Programming: A Key to Success

The participation of the school community (children, teachers, administrators, parents, neighbors) in school ground renovation is essential for success. The outcome of this process is a design program and a master plan that together provide the school with both a long-term vision and a detailed description of learning and play settings—their physical content and programmatic objectives (Moore and Wong 1997; Moore et al. 1992).

The master plan offers a guidance system for site development, without which wasteful mistakes are likely to be made. Without a master plan, it is unlikely that the site will be used to the best advantage. Important aspects of the master plan process are circulation (how will users move through the site comfortably?), grounds maintenance (service entrance, storage of materials and tools), and location of the most substantial, popular settings (play equipment, water play, drinking fountains, social gathering spaces).

A master plan, in essence, is a system of learning and play settings. Each setting provides a predictable type of activity. In renovating existing schoolyards and in new construction, any number of play and learning settings can be specified during the design-programming phase and integrated into the master plan for developing the outdoor environment. Setting descriptions also provide a common vocabulary to help the school community develop an implementation strategy in accordance with budget limitations. This approach allows improvements to be implemented in one setting at a time as resources become available. Improvements implemented with local volunteer labor can be differentiated from projects requiring skilled professional assistance. Settings can be ranked according to cost.

A PTO teamed with a college class or student organization can execute naturalization projects such as the installation of a vegetable garden, perennial flowering plants, shrubs, trees, or a reforestation zone. These costs are low. Projects can be implemented in a single workday or distributed over several workdays. Naturalization projects may be easier to implement in rural towns where people are closer to the soil and where the necessary equipment, expertise, and instruction are at hand. In contrast, installation of play equipment settings requires substantial, "lumpy" up-front costs, skilled professional help, and volunteer assistance spread over several days.

Conclusion

Playgrounds at school are an important part of the learning environment. How playground features are programmed, managed, and maintained inevitably reflects the play values of the adults who manage the institutions they have created to care for and educate our children. Schools designing playground spaces should consider the multiple potential opportunities for learning life skills that can occur in a playground setting.

Playgrounds are also the site of many injuries and occasionally even deaths. Playgrounds should be designed to permit exploration and appropriate risk-taking behavior while also minimizing the risk of injury. Appropriate equipment design and maintenance and careful attention to walking and landing surfaces help minimize the risk of injury.

Resources

- American Association for the Child's Right to Play. The U.S. chapter of the International Play Association promotes children's right to play as guaranteed by the International Convention on the Rights of the Child (United Nations 1989), article 31. IPA-USA launched a national initiative to promote recess and outdoor activity in elementary schools and has advocated strongly against the reduction and abandonment of recess. The organization's web site contains valuable resources on this issue.
  http://www.ipausa.org/
- Antioch New England Institute, Center for Environmental Education. Publishes guide-

lines that provide a comprehensive definition of what a "green school" can be. The guidelines can also be used as an assessment tool to evaluate individual schools in the greening process.
http://www.schoolsgogreen.org/

- Boston Schoolyard Initiative
  http://www.schoolyards.org/overview.htm
- EE (environmental education) in Georgia has a Green and Healthy Schools program, including schoolground development.
  http://eeingeorgia.org/
- Evergreen Foundation. EF is a Canadian national advocacy organization that was founded in 1991 with a mandate to bring nature to Canadian cities through naturalization projects. This nonprofit foundation motivates people to create and sustain healthy, natural outdoor spaces and gives them the practical tools to be successful through one of its core programs, Learning Grounds, which is devoted to transforming school grounds. For EF, naturalization is a collective, community effort that includes people from all walks of life in the revitalization of their schools, homes, and communities and ultimately in the environmental, social, and economic functioning of cities. EF has produced a large number of publications (details on their web site) about all aspects of school ground development. See details of the EF video below.
  http://www.evergreen.ca
- Georgia Native Plant Society. Provides schoolyard gardening resources.
  http://www.gnps.org/SCHOOL2.HTM
- Georgia Wildlife Federation offers an on-line schoolyard wildlife habitat planning guide.
  http://www.gwf.org/swhguide.htm
- Landscapes for Learning. LFL is based at Clemson University Cooperative Extension Service, South Carolina. LFL sponsors projects at schools across the state and produces a newsletter that presents practical information for school grounds naturalization.
  http://business.clemson.edu/Lflearn/
- Learning through Landscapes. LTL is a national campaign that promotes the right of children to have decent school grounds and to help make school grounds better places for learning and play. LTL contends that many children and young people in the United

Kingdom do not have access to well-designed school grounds and are therefore not getting the best start in life. For LTL, high-quality school grounds are essential because they provide unique opportunities for healthy exercise, creative play, and socialization. School grounds are places for learning by doing and for putting children in touch with the natural world. Since it was launched in 1990, LTL has developed numerous programs and has worked with 8,000–10,000 schools. Visit the Natural Leaning Initiative (http://www.naturalearning.org and link to publications) to download an in-depth 2004 Times Educational Supplement article about the trials and tribulations of school ground development in the United Kingdom.
http://www.ltl.org.uk

- Long Term Ecological Research. LTER is a schoolyard program.
  http://schoolyard.lternet.edu/
- Maryland Association for Environmental Outdoor Education, Green School Program. Uses the environment as an integrating context for instruction, promotes the use of best environmental practices in operation and design of schools, and extends learning into the community to address local environmental issues. Research report on association of green school designation with educational achievement.
  www.maeoe.org
- National Playground Safety Institute. This program of the National Parks and Recreation Association (NPRA) offers training courses and playground safety inspector certification for those who pass the exam.
- National Program for Playground Safety. This program was established in 1995 with support from the Centers for Disease Control and Prevention at the School of Health, Physical Education, and Leisure Studies, University of Northern Iowa. The program promotes playground safety, conducts studies, and presents national training events.
  http://www.uni.edu/playground/home.htm
- National Wildlife Federation Schoolyard Habitat Program. Encourages schools and other educational facilities to build wildlife-friendly school grounds.
  http://www.nwf.org/schoolyardhabitats
- North American Association for Environmen-

tal Education. NAAEE lists selected school-yard examples.
http://eelink.net/eeactivities-schoolyardecology
.html

- Schoolyard Habitat Listserv. To subscribe, send a blank e-mail to syh-exchange-sub
scribe@igc.topica.com.
- Schoolyard Habitat Network. SHN is a Connecticut-based collaborative effort dedicated to promoting hands-on environmental education on school property. Established in 1998, this group of educators, natural resource professionals, and consultants functions as a central resource for educators and administrators who wish to design and develop outdoor classrooms on school grounds and incorporate multidisciplinary activities into the curriculum. http://www.ctwoodlands.org/shn.html
- South Carolina Wildlife Federation. Promotes schoolyard developments.
http://www.scwf.org/about/index.php
- The central government of the United Kingdom has launched a major program to harness the full potential of the "outdoor classroom" as a teaching and learning resource.
http://www.teachernet.gov.uk/teachingand
learning/resourcematerials/growingschools
- Wallace Floyd Design Group. Provides examples of projects completed by the Boston Schoolyards Initiative.
http://www.asbj.com/lbd/2003/honors.html
- Wild Bird Trust of British Columbia. Provides information on its green school grounds program.
http://www.greengrounds.org/guide.html

Videos

- The Evergreen Foundation has produced a pair of fine videos called "A Crack in the Pavement" in partnership with the National Film Board of Canada (2000). The two programs are "Digging In" (19 min.) and "Growing Dreams" (19 min.). Call 1-800-276-7710; order number C 9100 116.
- The Canadian Biodiversity Institute has released a video about involving children in school ground development, *Asking Children, Listening to Children*, produced by Ann Coffey, coordinator of the CBI School Grounds Transformation Program.

References

American Academy of Pediatrics. 2000. Protecting your child from the sun. Available: http://www.aap.org/family/protectsun.htm [accessed 4 August 2004].

American Association for the Child's Right to Play. 2005. Available: http://www.ipausa.org/recess_proceedure.htm [accessed 4 November 2005].

American Planning Association. 2003. How cities use parks to help children learn. City Parks Forum Briefing Paper #6. Available: http://www.planning.org/cpf/briefingpapers.htm [accessed 22 January, 2005].

American Society for Testing and Materials. 1993. ASTM F 1487 standard consumer safety performance specifications for playground equipment in public use. Available: http://www.astm.org/DATABASE.CART/PAGES/F1487.htm [accessed 4 November 2005].

Baranowski T, Mendlein J, Resnicow K, Frank E, Cullen K, Baranowski J. 2000. Physical activity and nutrition in children and youth: An overview of obesity prevention. Prev Med 31:S1–S10.

Barnard H. 1848. *School architecture; or contributions to the improvement of school-houses in the United States.* New York: A. S. Barnes. Available from Digital Library Production Service, University of Michigan, Ann Arbor, MI.

Beckwith J. 2003. The challenging playground: How the law of unintended consequences has diminished children's play. Landsc Archit Specif News 19(09):78–82.

Brett A, Moore R, Provenzo E. 1993. *The complete playground book.* Syracuse, NY: Syracuse University Press.

Clements R, ed. 2000. *Elementary school recess: Selected readings, games, and activities for teachers and parents.* Boston: American Press.

Gove PB (ed.). 1961. *Webster's third new international dictionary of the English language unabridged.* Springfield, MA: Merriam-Webster, Inc.

Grant T, Littlejohn G. 2001. Greening school grounds: Creating habitats for learning. Toronto: Green Teacher Magazine (Gabriola Island, British Columbia: New Society Publishers).

Howard J. 2004. Extreme makeover. Landsc Archit 94(7):118–127.

Kutska K, Hoffman K, Malkuska A. 1998. Playground safety is no accident: Developing a public playground safety and maintenance program, 2d ed. Alexandria, VA: National Recreation and Parks Association.

Mack M, Hudson S, Thompson D. 1997. A descriptive analysis of children's playground injuries in the United States 1990–1994. Inj Prev 3:100–103.

MacKay M. 2003. Playground injuries. Inj Prev 9:194–296.

Moloney FJ, Collins S, Murphy GM. 2002. Sunscreens: Safety, efficacy, and appropriate use. Am J Clin Dermatol 3(3):185–191.

Moore R. 1989. Playgrounds at the crossroads. In *Public spaces and places*, vol. 10. *Human behavior and the environment* (Altman I, Zube E, eds.), New York: Plenum Press, pp. 83–120.

Moore R, Goltsman S, Iacofano D. 1992. *Play for all guidelines: Planning, design, and management of outdoor play settings for all children*, 2d ed. Berkeley: MIG Communications.

Moore R, Wong H. 1997. *Natural learning: The natural history of an environmental schoolyard*. Berkeley, CA: MIG Communications.

Moore R, Young D. 1978. Childhood outdoors: Toward a social ecology of the landscape. In *Children and the environment* (Altman I, Wohlwill J, eds.), vol. 3. New York: Plenum Press, pp. 83–130.

Office of Technology Assessment. September 1995. Risks to students in school. OTA-OTA-ENV-633. Washington, DC: U.S. Government Printing Office.

Phelan K, Khoury J, Kalkwarf H, Lanphear B. 2001. Trends and patterns of playground injuries in United States children and adolescents. Ambul Pediatr 1(4):227–233.

Prentice AM, Jebb SA. 1995. Obesity in Britain: Gluttony or sloth? Br Med J 311(7002):437–439.

Rosenthal N. 1998. *Winter blues: Seasonal affective disorder: What it is and how to overcome it*. New York: Guilford Press.

Scherschun L, Lim HW. 2001. Photoprotection by sunscreens. Am J Clin Dermatol 2(3):131–134.

Schwebel D, Binder S, Plumert J. 2002. Using an injury diary to describe the ecology of children's daily injuries. J Safety Res 33:301–319.

Smith S. 1998. *Risk and our pedagogical relation to children: On the playground and beyond*. Albany: State University of New York Press.

Strauss RS, Pollack HA. 2001. Epidemic increase in childhood overweight, 1986–1998. J Am Med Assoc 286(22):2845–2848.

Tinsworth D, McDonald J. 2001. Special study: Injuries and deaths associated with children's playground equipment. Bethesda, MD: U.S. Consumer Product Safety Commission.

United Nations. 1989. Convention on the Rights of the Child. New York: UNICEF.

U.S. Access Board. 2000. Americans with Disabilities Act (ADA) Accessibility Guidelines for Play Areas. Available: http://www.access-board.gov/play/finalrule.htm [accessed 4 November 2005].

U.S. Consumer Product Safety Commission. (1981). Handbook for public playground safety. Publication No. 325 Available: http://www.cpsc.gov/CPSCPUB/PUBS/325.pdf [accessed 5 August 2004].

U.S. Environmental Protection Agency. 2001. The burning facts. EPA 430-F-01-015. Available: http://www.epa.gov/sunwise [accessed 4 August 2004].

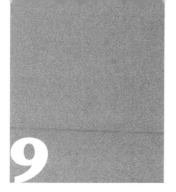

Sandra S. West, Hope Jackson,

Robert J. Geller, and Howard Frumkin

Injury Prevention

■ *Summary*

- Long considered "safe havens" for children, schools are now recognized as the site of a substantial number of childhood injuries.
- Injury prevention, including eliminating or reducing exposure to hazards and the probability of injuries from them is an important goal for schools. This involves striving for optimal balance between minimizing risk and maximizing student involvement in classroom activities.
- Safety requires the creation of a conducive environment, through facility design, supportive policy, and adherence to safe practices. Teachers, staff, and students all play important roles.
- Classroom design should anticipate and support the intended use of the space, including rooms for science labs, creative arts, and vocational arts and technical skills.
- Injury risk may be increased during certain activities, such as construction or renovation at the school, and during specific weather conditions (such as icy or rainy conditions). Policies should be designed to anticipate these risks and establish strategies to address them. ■

Safety is generally understood as freedom from injuries, and safety programs in schools (as in other places) have two general aims: preventing injuries and minimizing the consequences of those that do occur. However, in a broader sense, safety extends beyond preventing and controlling injuries. When parents send their children to school, they expect the environment to be secure and conducive to learning and growth. Safety is the sense of security that results from a carefully designed and maintained environment.

Injuries remain a major problem for children, both in and out of school. The majority of childhood injuries occur in places other than schools, but an hour a child spends at school is no safer than an hour out of school, despite the greater supervision available at schools and the opportunities for safety interventions (Miller and Spicer 1998). According to data from the National Health Interview Survey, of the more than 20 million childhood injuries each year that require medical care and/or limit a child's activity, about 4 million (one in five) occur at school. This corresponds to a school injury incidence rate of about one injury per 20 children per year (Miller and Spicer 1998; Danseco et al. 2000). Less severe injuries are more common; one study estimates that four in five elementary school children visit the school nurse for an injury-related complaint (Nader and Brink 1981).

This burden of school injuries does more than hurt children and undermine learning. It is also costly. The economic impact is estimated at $3 billion in direct medical costs, $10 billion in lost future earnings, and $34 billion in reduced quality of life (corresponding to reduced mobility, reduced cognition, pain, cosmetic disfigurement, and other outcomes of injury), for a total cost of $47 billion (in 1994 dollars; Danseco et al. 2000). This equates to an average cost of $11,800 per injured child, or $600 when averaged over all children.

Although there is no national data collection system on schools (Office of Technology Assessment 1995), there are many sources of information about school injuries. In some cases, researchers have collected data on injuries within individual school systems, such as those in Tucson, Arizona (Boyce et al. 1984), or across entire states, such as Hawaii (Taketa 1984). An especially valuable source of information is the Utah Student Injury Reporting System (SIRS), a registry that has been operating since 1984 (Spicer et al. 2002). In addition, national databases, such as the National Pediatric Trauma Registry, have provided useful information (Di Scala et al. 1997). Many of the available data on school injuries have been summarized in review articles (Gratz 1992; LaFlamme et al. 1998).

The incidence of school injuries in these studies has roughly paralleled the incidence reported in the National Health Interview Survey—approximately 5 injuries per 100 students per year, with a range from 1.7 to 7.5 injuries (Gratz 1992). This is equivalent to about 1 injury for every 20 children per year. Put differently, over the 12 years of school from kindergarten to high school graduation, the average student's probability of sustaining an injury at school is greater than 50%. The different findings across studies may reflect diverse definitions of injury, different approaches to detecting injuries, and/or varying environments in different schools.

Both personal and environmental factors seem to play a role in school injuries. Boys generally have higher injury rates at school than girls. The effect of age is not consistent; younger children are at higher risk in some studies, whereas others suggest higher risk for older children. Some students seem to be "accident prone" (Boyce and Sobolewski 1989), perhaps because of poor locomotor skills (Angel 1975) or difficult interpersonal relations (Bremberg and Gerber 1988).

Environmental factors are also important. For example, rates of injury among individual schools vary markedly, with schools differing in their injury rates by as much as 25-fold. Higher overall injury rates occur in schools with longer hours, alternative educational programs, less experienced school nurses, and lower student-to-staff ratios, as well as during unsupervised activities. It is also likely that specific environmental conditions at some schools increase the risk of injuries.

Studies also reveal some of the particulars of school injuries. Intentional acts of violence account for only about 1 in 10 school injuries (Boyce et al. 1984), even in studies that focus on more severe injuries (Di Scala et al. 1997). Falls are a common form of school injuries. Two kinds of falls predominate—falls on level surfaces, probably from tripping or slipping, and falls from playground equipment—but in some cases children fall down stairs or from heights (including obviously unsafe places such as upper-floor windows, rooftops, and bleachers; Di Scala et al., 1997). Sports injuries are also a common category, with the pattern of injuries varying by sport. For example, handball injuries are more likely to involve the hands and arms, soccer injuries the ankles and feet, and gymnastics injuries the head and spine (Jackson et al. 1980).

Because school injuries fall into many categories and occur in many parts of the school, they are

---

■ *9.1. A science lab injury*

On October 12, 2001, a flash fire burned seven students in a chemistry classroom at Genoa-Kingston High School in Dekalb County, Illinois. One of the students was critically injured, with second-degree burns to his upper body. The fire occurred when the chemistry teacher was demonstrating the use of flame tests to identify certain salts dissolved in methanol.

(Wronski and Keilman 2001) ■

discussed throughout this book. Intentional injuries that result from acts of violence are discussed in chapter 19. Two particular environments with special injury risks—playgrounds and sports fields—each merit their own chapters (chapters 8 and 18, respectively). Transportation-related injuries are discussed in chapter 21. Joint and soft tissue injuries that develop gradually, such as back pain, are discussed in the ergonomics chapter, chapter 6. And an unusual category of injuries—those related to animal bites—is discussed in chapter 7.

This chapter is about all the other kinds of injuries that may occur throughout schools—on the walkways, in hallways, in general classrooms, and in specialized settings such as vocational arts shops, biology and chemistry labs, and theaters. The first part of the chapter focuses on general classroom hazards, and the next part focuses on specialized classrooms. Next, we discuss the control of injuries in schools, review relevant regulations, describe the elements of effective school safety programs, and offer practical strategies to enhance safety.

A common theme in this chapter is that safety is a mindset. The safety mindset requires both that school administrators and teachers exercise leadership and set an example and that students behave appropriately in following that lead. The safety mindset requires school architecture that plans for a safe environment and school maintenance that eliminates hazards when they begin to develop.

An optimal school environment can set the climate for safety, while a poorly designed and haphazardly maintained school environment can predispose students to injuries. However, even an optimal school environment cannot overcome the results of human misbehavior or rare combinations of events. Some injuries may be inevitable, but the safe school will make such injuries rare.

General Classroom Hazards

Classrooms range from the generic classroom, where subjects such as math are taught, to specialized rooms for computer labs, vocational arts and technology, photography, fine arts, and science.

Overcrowding

Overcrowding is a potentially serious hazard in any classroom (see chapter 2). The association between overcrowding and increased risk of injury has been documented in both safety research and field reports for many years (Macomber 1961; Young 1972, 1997; West et al. 2002). Science teachers cite overcrowding as their greatest safety concern (West et al. 2002) Classes that are too large for the teacher to see all the students adequately make it difficult to supervise students' activity. Teachers experience the same difficulty when students do not have adequate individual workspace. Professional organizations such as the National Science Teachers Association (NSTA) offer best practice recommenda-

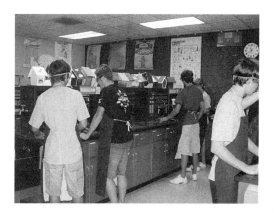 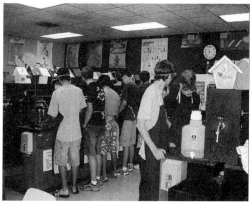

Figure 9.1. Uncrowded versus crowded school laboratories. (Left) Each student has adequate space in which to work safely (58 square feet per student). The teacher has adequate space to monitor activity. (Right) Students do not have enough individual space in which to work safely (43 square feet per student). (This is not a recommended design for a science lab.) Students are working too closely; the teacher cannot see what the students are doing. (Photo by Sandra S. West.)

tions for some school settings. For example, the NSTA recommends that science classes be limited to 24 students and that science laboratories—defined as rooms that accommodate science activities and/or contain science furniture or equipment—should have at least 45 square feet per middle or high school student in a pure science laboratory and 60 square feet per middle or high school student in a combination laboratory/classroom (see fig. 9.1). An internet-based tool that may be useful in planning science lab space is available (see West in resources list for more details).

Electrical Hazards

Electrical hazards may be found in all classrooms, although some activity-based content courses, such as fine arts, vocational, technology, and science, may pose greater risks. Safe classrooms feature an adequate number of properly wired and grounded electrical outlets, particularly where students are using electrical equipment.

Electrical systems in older schools may be inadequate to handle the current use patterns of electrical devices. Evidence of electrical problems such as carbon soot on electrical outlets or periodically tripped circuit breakers should alert the staff and administration to inadequate wiring that constitutes a potential fire hazard.

In activity-based classrooms, a minimum of two duplex outlets per student workstation and three duplex outlets on the instructional wall are generally recommended to reduce the need for extension cords. All outlets, particularly those in activity classrooms, should be protected by ground fault circuit interrupters and tested periodically to ensure that they are wired correctly.

In lab settings, all power sources should be turned off when setting up circuits or repairing equipment. Student setups should be checked before the power is turned on. Do not use metal articles such as rulers or metal writing utensils, and do not wear metal jewelry when working with electrical equipment. Box 9.2 provides additional pointers on electrical safety.

Good Housekeeping

Good housekeeping is a safety issue, not a lifestyle choice. Trips and falls are a leading cause of school injuries, and good housekeeping practices can help

---

■ *9.2. Electrical safety tips*

- Ensure that repairs, maintenance, and installation work is completed by competent professionals.
- Arrange periodic school inspections to test the safety of equipment and outlets.
- Maintain electrical equipment regularly, and identify and deal with any electrical hazards immediately.
- Implement and maintain safety procedures for all electrical equipment in use.
- Never connect, disconnect, or operate a piece of electrical equipment with wet hands or while standing on a wet floor.
- Locate outlets above floor level and away from water sources, and make sure they have safety caps.
- Use caution when handling electrical equipment that has been in recent use, as it may be hot or retain an electrical charge.
- Use only equipment that has been approved by Underwriters Labs (UL) or Canadian Standards Association (CSA), preferably operating at 120 volts or less.
- Electrical cords should be in good condition. They should not be frayed or loosely connected to the plug.
- If an extension cord is needed, it should be heavy-duty and not placed where people are moving around. ■

---

prevent them. Aisles and work surfaces should be kept clear of anything that is not being used in an activity. Books, papers, materials, and equipment should be clean, organized, and stored out of sight, conveying a message that the environment is structured and disciplined and that students can safely enjoy active learning.

Other Hazards

Many other classroom hazards are also associated with an increased risk of injury. For example, schools should make sure that light fixtures are securely mounted, furniture is durable and kept in good repair, and exits can be easily accessed. Such safety features help ensure a safe learning and work environment for faculty, students, and staff.

Specialized Classrooms Hazards

Specialized classrooms are often used for art, vocational education, and science.

Fine Arts

The fine arts, including painting, ceramics, metalworking, and theater, may present a number of injury risks. Exposures to hazardous chemicals such as some lacquers, paint removers, and ceramics glazes are well recognized (see chapter 15). However, cutting and grinding introduce a risk of lacerations and abrasions, welding and the use of kilns pose the risk of burns, and some theater props, catwalks, light stations, and costumes may introduce a risk of falls. Each of these hazards requires appropriate safety training, procedures, and equipment. For example, welding requires protection against impact and the intense light and heat produced, which calls for appropriate goggles and protective clothing (Rossol 2001a, Rossol 2001b).

Construction activities, such as those that occur in building theater sets, require impact-resistant (ANSI Z87.1) safety glasses. Construction activities also pose risks of falling from elevated structures while they are being assembled or used. Such hazards can be minimized by careful attention to guard rails and appropriate flooring design. Protective headgear that meets OSHA standards for construction areas is prudent when students are working where materials may fall from overhead.

Vocational Classes

Vocational training includes traditional types of courses, such as automotive mechanics and woodshop, as well as advanced technology courses. Some new vocational courses incorporate components of the science curriculum such as physics to form courses called "Principles of Technology".

Information on injuries in vocational classes is available from the Utah Student Injury Report database (Knight et al. 2000). During the five-year period from 1992 to 1996, 7.1% of school injuries in Utah (1,008 of 14,133) occurred in shop class. Equipment use accounted for 88.4% of these injuries. Of these, nearly one in three was attributed to three kinds of equipment: band saws (11.9%), table saws (11.6%), and sander/buffers (7.4%). Other types of equipment associated with injuries

included other types of saws (7.2%), other cutting equipment (6.4%), drills (3.8%), welders (3.7%), and routers (2.8%). The equipment-related injuries were far more likely to result from improper use of the equipment than from equipment malfunction (37.9% versus 3.5%). The type of injury varied depending upon circumstances; equipment-related injuries included lacerations (70.9%), burns (6.0%), and abrasions (4.6%), while injuries that were unrelated to equipment included lacerations (45.4%), fractures (9.2%), and pain or tenderness (presumably sprains and strains) (6.7%). Equipment injuries most commonly affected fingers/thumbs (64.0%), hands/wrists (12.8%), and eyes (5.6%), while injuries unrelated to equipment most often affected the eyes (19.3%), fingers/thumbs (17.6%), and hands/wrists (10.9%).

Indeed, vocational classes use a variety of hazardous equipment and chemicals. Power equipment poses risks from electricity, hot surfaces, cutting edges, and projectiles. Missing covers for belts of belt-driven equipment and missing blade guards are common hazards in vocational shops. Appropriate safeguards include training, close supervision, selection of safe equipment including covers and guards, and meticulous maintenance of equipment.

Biology Classrooms

Animals, both living and preserved, are commonly found in elementary and secondary life science classrooms and labs. Animals are typically used to help students learn science, either by long-term observation or by dissection. Living animals pose some safety problems (see chapter 7).

Safety precautions for the use of dissection equipment include training, close supervision, proper use of equipment, and sanitation. Personal protection including chemical splash goggles and gloves should be used during dissections. To dissect properly, students should practice the following:

- Do not hold the specimen in the hand while dissecting.
- Cut down toward the specimen.
- Do not stab at the specimen.

Insects can be collected as part of an insect or ecological study. Most insects can be anesthetized by freezing them in a jar for up to an hour. Do not use ether; it is flammable and may produce explosive peroxides. Triethylamine, although safer than ether, is flammable, toxic if ingested, and corrosive to the skin and eyes.

Dangerous equipment, such as centrifuges and syringes with needles, should be used only by students who have been instructed in their safe use. The teacher must monitor closely the students' use of syringes with needles. Puncture wounds are potential sources of foreign bodies and infections. Always follow safe needle-handling practices, including disposal of syringes in a "sharps" container. Never try to recap a needle. Keep all syringes, scalpel blades, and containers of biological specimens in locked storage when not in actual use.

Physics and Earth Science Classes

Projectiles, falling objects, and heated objects are common hazards in physical science classes, although these dangers can also be present in other specialized classrooms.

Projectiles and Welding Hazards

Because projectile hazards can be present in physical science, theater, and vocational activities, eye protection is needed. Physics assignments that may result in flying objects or debris require the use of impact-resistant (ANSI Z87.1) safety glasses by all occupants of the room. Earth science activities that involve chipping, breaking rock, or grinding also require the use of safety glasses.

Hot Objects

Heated objects, such as hot glassware in science, hot bulbs in theater, hot ceramics in art, and hot metal in vocational classrooms, require that students use body protection. Appropriate clothing includes lab coats and aprons, welding aprons, and leather gloves or oven mitts. The school should supply these types of protective clothing in sufficient quantity to enable both students and faculty to participate in learning activities safely. In addition, polyester and other synthetic fibers that will melt and adhere to the skin should generally be avoided. Fine arts activities such as glassblowing may also produce intense heat and sharp pieces of glass.

Noise

Many physical science investigations, fine arts activities, and vocational courses can generate loud noise, which is also a potential hazard. Noise abatement techniques should be followed, and ear protectors that meet OSHA standards should be used whenever applicable. Further discussion about noise and its impact on the school can be found in chapter 4.

UV or Infrared Energy

Protective goggles should be worn whenever either ultraviolet (UV) or infrared energy is present. UV light is recognized as a cause of eye damage and even skin cancer after intense or prolonged exposure. UV sources include sunlight, welding, and carbon arc lamps. Infrared is produced whenever metals are heated until they glow.

Chemistry Classrooms and Chemical Storage

Chemicals may be dangerous in two ways. The toxic effects of chemicals, such as liver damage, are discussed in chapter 15. Safety risks, such as chemical burns and eye splashes, are discussed here, together with ways to reduce the risk of such injuries (Young 1997a, Young 1997b).

Chemical Inventory

Always complete a chemical inventory before ordering new chemicals. Order no more chemicals than can be used within a school year. It is extremely expensive to properly dispose of excess or unwanted hazardous chemicals. To minimize hazards, teachers should always use the safest chemicals available to teach the concepts being studied.

Working with Chemicals

All chemicals sold in the United States are required to be supplied with the applicable material safety data sheet (MSDS). Read the MSDS on each chemical before using it to obtain information on safe handling, proper storage, and disposal. The MSDS for each chemical identifies the type of hazard and describes the safe use, storage, and disposal of the chemical. Wear appropriate personal protection as indicated by the MSDS. Match the correct glove to the substance to be used, according to reliable information such as that provided by the glove manufacturer or qualified industrial hygiene experts. Potential hazards from inappropriate glove selection include the chance that a glove may be dissolved by contact with a chemical or that a chemical may diffuse through a glove, increasing exposure as the glove holds the chemical against the skin.

Chemical Storage

Chemicals must be stored properly by compatible families in either separate, secure chemical store-rooms or in secure locked chemical storage cabinets in storerooms—not in classrooms. They should not be stored in fume hoods or in a preparation or equipment storeroom. To avoid the theft of chemicals, teachers should never allow students or other unauthorized people to access these store-rooms.

The chemical storeroom door should be labeled "Authorized Personnel Only," with the appropriate National Fire Protection Association (NFPA) label so that, in an emergency, fire or hazardous materials personnel will know what types of chemicals are stored there. The school office and the local fire marshal should have an annually updated chemical inventory by room. Chemical store-rooms should have appropriate forced air ventilation with adequate air changes per hour, and the storeroom exhaust should be vented directly to the outdoors.

The storage cabinets and shelves must be resistant to corrosion and securely attached to the walls. Chemicals should be stored in an upright position and no more than two containers deep. Shelves should have lips to prevent spilled chemicals from dripping over the edge or accidentally sliding off the shelf. Chemicals should not be stored above eye level and never kept on the floor. The storeroom must be adequately lighted and equipped with smoke detectors. Chemicals must be maintained at the correct temperature all year; if necessary, the air-conditioning must remain on during the summer.

Chemicals can be classified as one of four types of hazards: corrosive, flammable, toxic, and reactive or oxidizer. They should usually be stored by their type and reactivity, rather than alphabetically, to reduce the risk of adjacent chemicals inadvertently reacting with one another.

Corrosives are chemicals that can injure body tissues or damage metal by direct chemical reaction. Corrosives other than acids and bases include substances such as iodine and ferric chloride. They must be stored in cabinets that are properly de-signed to hold them (i.e., without metal shelves or shelf supports). Acids and bases must be stored separately. Nitric acid should be kept separate from other acids.

Flammable solids and liquids include solvents, as well as other chemicals, such as glacial acetic acid. Liquids do not usually burn, but they produce vapors that do. Vapors from flammable solids are as dangerous as vapors from liquids. Flammables must be stored in an approved flammable cabinet that is not vented. Do not accumulate more flammables than the storeroom size and flammable cabinet can legally accommodate. Contact your local fire marshal for specific information.

Oxidizers and reactives are chemicals that can explode, violently polymerize, and form explosive peroxides; they are also pyrophoric. Pyrophoric substances, such as calcium carbide, sodium, and magnesium powder, may ignite spontaneously when exposed to water or oxygen. Oxidizers include substances such as nitric acid, hydrogen peroxide, and potassium nitrate. Hazardous polymers may form upon prolonged storage of certain compounds. Explosive peroxides can form within months from some substances such as ethers and vinyl compounds. Water-reactive chemicals should be stored where they will remain dry.

Classroom Safety Regulations

Several federal regulations apply to classroom safety. The Occupational Safety and Health Act applies to private schools and to public schools in states that have chosen to apply the act in this way. The Americans with Disabilities Act (1990) (see chapter 26) requires schools to ensure that students with disabilities are not excluded from participation or denied the benefits of their services, programs, and activities. Therefore, modifications in the design of certain school facilities, such as science labs, may be necessary to accommodate students with disabilities so that they may safely participate in learning activities.

State and local requirements can include laws, rules, and regulations that cover the use of eye protection and space and may exceed federal requirements. Fire codes for devices such as sprinkler systems or areas such as exits apply to schools. Regular fire drills that train both employees and students maximize the chance of safe egress in various fire situations.

Other state or local statutes can address school facilities standards that delineate construction requirements for schools. State and local facility regulations are often based on guidelines provided by expert professional organizations such as the National Fire Protection Association Life Safety Code and the National Electrical Code.

The NFPA Life Safety Code 101 was developed "to establish minimum requirements that will provide a reasonable degree of safety from fire in buildings and structures." If adopted by a state or local entity, rooms such as science labs are impacted by the code with regard to areas of egress, fire extinguishers, smoke alarms, and water sprinkler systems. The code requires two clearly marked, unobstructed, emergency exits in each lab and preparation/equipment room. It also requires public school science classrooms, including the support rooms that are in the class C hazardous lab group, to have a second exit for any laboratory of at least 1000 square feet. Fire extinguishers should be placed at each exit. Rooms for subjects such as science, art, and vocational arts should have an ABC extinguisher. A functioning general fire alarm system throughout the building is required. Fire drill procedures must be posted and practiced. If there is no outside window, an emergency light should be available in the science labs, prep rooms, and art and vocational rooms.

Electrical fires are one of the most frequent types of fires and typically result from the overuse of electrical circuits or the use of extension cords. Compliance with the National Electrical Code (NFPA 70) is the best means of eliminating potential electrical fires. Once again, facilities design plays an important role in providing sufficient electrical outlets for various types of equipment for instruction, such as microscopes in science classes and hot plates in art.

Safety guidelines are also available for science labs. For example, the National Science Teachers Association published the *NSTA Guide to School Science Facilities* (Biehle et al. 1999), which provides guidelines for the construction of safe science labs. The Council of State Science Supervisors also provides guidance through its publications, which are directed at both secondary and elementary schools. Some states, such as Texas, have adopted many of these recommendations in their school facility standards (Texas Education Agency 2003).

Elements of Effective School Safety Programs

An effective school safety program should create a safe school environment that supports both academic and extracurricular achievement. While a safety program focused on prevention will help minimize emergency or hazardous situations, it is also important to understand that mishaps can occur in even ideal safety conditions. It is thus necessary to have a response component to the safety program. This response should be well coordinated and planned in advance to minimize confusion and enhance the response. Achieving such a program requires a collective effort by faculty, administrators, and staff, coupled with support from parents and students.

Establishing an Environment That Encourages Safety

Features of the overall school environment—high academic standards, strong administrative leadership, students' feelings of connectedness to the school, and clear policies and expectations—do much to create a safety culture. The Centers for Disease Control and Prevention (CDC 2001) refer to this as establishing a social environment that promotes safety. A person with overall responsibility for coordinating safety activities should be designated. Injury prevention should be practiced in all school activities. Disciplinary policies that support safety should be clearly enunciated and enforced.

Teachers' Roles and Responsibilities

Teachers play a critical role in creating a safe classroom environment. Teachers who have undergone appropriate safety training are less likely to have hazardous events occur (Ward and West 1990). In the "Safety Makes Sense" program to prevent unintentional injuries in New York public schools, teachers were trained during staff development workshops to understand that the procedure for teaching and reinforcing safety skills is similar to that for teaching most other skills, including solving an equation, reading, playing an instrument, and dribbling a basketball (Eichel and Goldman 2001). The workshops acknowledged that children are quick to pick up inconsistencies between what adults say and do, so modeling consistent, safe, and caring behavior is important. In addition, it is important for teachers to provide feedback and encouragement to students while they are learning to make safety a priority.

Policy

Policy, a critical safety component, should be carefully researched and well thought out. To be maximally effective, policy should be written in advance, rather than worked out in reaction to a problem. Policy should meet or exceed federal, state, and local requirements and incorporate the findings of safety research and best practice recommendations. Accountability for lack of compliance should be built into the policy statement. Student and staff misbehavior should be dealt with in an effective way to prevent incidents. The policy should cover all aspects of safety, including student discipline, reporting of incidents and injuries, eye protection, and the use of chemicals.

Safety Inspections of the Building and Classrooms

Safety inspections of the entire school campus, including all buildings and classrooms, should occur at least annually. Procedures for these inspections are described in chapter 25. Additional safety inspection surveys and audit forms are available from many professional organizations, school board associations, insurance companies, and state departments of health and education. Examples are provided in the resource list at the end of this chapter.

Safety Training

Schools should schedule annual safety training for all employees, including teachers. No one should

---

■ *9.3. Safety training*

Many good examples of school safety training programs are available:

- In San Diego, eight elementary schools were selected to receive the Think First for Kids (TFFK) program in grades 1–3, and eight comparison schools without such training were identified. The TFFK curriculum integrates information on the major causes of injury associated with math, reading, and science classes and covers six topics: (1) violence prevention, gun safety, and conflict resolution; (2) playground, recreation, and sports safety, (3) bicycle safety, (4) water safety; (5) vehicle and pedestrian safety, and (6) brain and spinal cord anatomy. In a pretest-posttest assessment, the children who participated in TFFK demonstrated improvements in their safety knowledge and behavior that were significantly greater than those of nonparticipants (Gresham et al. 2001).
- In New York City, the New York Academy of Medicine and the Board of Education partnered in an initiative called "Safety Makes Sense," beginning in 1998. This program included extensive teacher and staff training, curriculum innovations in health courses, and a range of administrative, environmental, and regulatory changes. A unique feature was the use of music; children learned songs such as "Walk with Your Pencil Pointing Down" and "Hey, Look Where You're Going, Don't Clown Around. You Don't Want to Trip and Fall on the Ground." A CD was produced that included many safety songs (Eichel and Goldman 2001).
- In Vancouver, a peer-driven injury prevention program was targeted at alternative school students in grades 9–11, based on information that this group faced a high risk of injury. The program included an introductory lecture called SAFETY (statistics, anatomy, friends, effects, talk, you), a visit by a sports star, a video, and extensive peer-led discussion. Although evaluation of the program did not show changes in knowledge or behaviors, the students' attitudes and behavioral intent seemed to improve significantly (Tenn and Dewis 1996). ■

be exempt from this training for any reason, including extracurricular duties. Additionally, in-depth mandatory safety training that is specific to individual duties should be conducted at least yearly. If the hazards change or increase, then additional safety training is needed. When new activities or equipment are introduced into the classroom, specific safety training on the hazards associated with them is needed. Science teachers who have a better content background and more specialized training and experience in their teaching field are less likely to have adverse events occur in their science classroom or laboratory and during field activities (Macomber 1961; Young 1972), whether in agriculture, art, photography, welding, auto mechanics, theater, chemistry, physics, geology, or biology.

Safety training for students, at a grade-appropriate level, has been shown to increase awareness and decrease risk of injury. Many successful models are available (see box 9.3). While safety training should permeate the curriculum, it is especially important to integrate it into hands-on courses such as theater and science. The training should include practical information such as fire safety, which may be broadly applicable, given that many fires occur in the home.

Scheduling

Inappropriate class scheduling can create unsafe conditions. Examples include allowing too much or too little time between classes and not scheduling hands-on classes such as science, vocational skills, or art with adequate time for materials and equipment to be set out before or at the beginning of class and then dismantled at the end of class. Student movement from classroom to classroom can also create congested hallways if all of the students change classes at the same time.

Materials Management

Administrative activities must be coupled with practical steps to minimize hazards and implement a climate that values safety. Materials management is a challenging organizational logistics problem. Adequate time should be allotted for teachers to attend to the safe and proper management of their instructional materials. Widely used guidelines for organizing include cleaning out unused materials annually, sorting by activity or general use, and properly labeling equipment, shelves, or containers. Adequate space for storage should be addressed in designing new or renovated school facilities.

In addition to general organization principles, each discipline has its own unique sets of materials and equipment with discipline-specific space and storage requirements. Even within a discipline such as the fine arts, the areas of theater, art, and photography, for example, use very different sets of equipment, materials, and chemicals. Theater makes use of large sets, equipment such as lights, set decorations, costumes, and dressing and painting areas. Photography classes need specialized rooms and equipment that may include a darkroom with hazardous chemicals, as well as technical equipment such as digital cameras and computers for digital manipulation and enhancement. Because instruction in art and science makes use of many kinds of materials, both types of classes often need storage areas for large and small pieces of equipment. Therefore, adequate and appropriate storage space should be provided for each discipline, with well-maintained egress routes and doors large enough to permit the movement of the largest piece of equipment.

Facilities

Safe facilities are the foundation of safe active learning in schools. Facilities that are designed and built correctly for safe and effective learning provide the first line of defense against problems. For example, a phone with at least one outside line should be installed in each classroom to expedite requests for help in emergencies.

Many schools do not provide adequate space to meet the needs for active learning, technology, ADA requirements, and multiple uses in the same room. Additionally, many schools have inadequate numbers of specialty rooms, perhaps because of unanticipated changes in student interests. For example, a school builds one art room, but there are more students than anticipated who can and want to take art classes. The school is then left with undesirable choices: Students are either denied the opportunity to study art, or the classes are over-crowded and therefore potentially unsafe, or art is scheduled in a room not designed for the subject, which may also be unsafe.

Personal Protection

In many settings, items for personal protection, including chemical splash goggles, face shields, eyewashes, showers, aprons, and gloves, are required and must be supplied by the school. The equipment must be worn if there is any chance of exposure to harmful substances.

Eye Protection

Eye protection is critical because the eyes can be seriously injured in a very short time. The eyes must be protected from splashes, contaminated fingers touching the eyes, vapors, dust, and impact throughout an activity (including clean-up). Any classrooms or outside areas in which hazardous chemicals are used, such as vocational skills, art, photography, theater, home economics, and science, must have a set of splash-protective chemical goggles for each class participant. Face shields are not a substitute for goggles; goggles must usually be worn even with the use of face shields.

The eyewear must fit properly. The goggles should be large enough to protect and form a seal around the eyes. If worn with eyeglasses, the goggles should be able to form a seal around the glasses without affecting the eye correction afforded by the eyeglasses.

The wearing of contact lenses in these settings is controversial. Each setting poses different risks for the contact lens wearer, and the lens prescriber should discuss these risks with the wearer. It is universally true, however, that contact lenses *never* replace other eye protection. The American Optometric Association reports that there is no reason to prohibit the use of contact lenses when chemical splash goggles are also worn (Cullen 1998). Of course, this assumes that the air is not contaminated by chemical vapors or mists that would require more extensive eye protection for everyone. Check your local and state regulations for specific requirements regarding the preferred eye protection, which may be inscribed as a code on the frames and lenses.

Goggles can be sanitized by using germicidal (UV) cabinets or 10% sodium hypochlorite (bleach) solutions. If using the UV method, the UV intensity needs to be checked yearly with a cali-brated UV meter. The lamp needs to be cleaned weekly to remove dust or dirt, which will affect the intensity of the lamp. If bleach is used, the person who cleans the item must wear goggles. The goggles that are being sanitized should be dipped into the bleach solution, rinsed first with tap water and then distilled water, and then air dried. Hair lice nits are not usually transferred from goggles unless the headband is frayed and hair can be pulled out when removing the goggles.

Areas in which projectile hazards are present, such as in some vocational, technology, or theater activities, can use impact-resistant (ANSI Z87.1) spectacles. Specific activities such as welding require even more specialized eye protection, which must be worn during the entire activity. Laser goggles are rated for the wavelength and power of a particular laser. One type of goggles is not automatically usable with every laser. Chemical splash goggles are not suitable for use with lasers.

Eyewashes

An eyewash must meet applicable building code and OSHA requirements, which generally call for a hands-free water flow that starts within 1 second of activation and can flush both eyes simultaneously. The water should be tepid (60°–95°F), and the flushing should continue for at least 15 minutes. The water should spray 2–3 inches above the eyewash holes and arc so that both eyes are gently washed simultaneously. "Hands free" means that no hands are required to keep the water flowing, thus leaving both hands free to hold the eyes open against the reflexive urge to close them. Students must be able to use the eyewash without assistance. Small bottle washes do not meet the safety standard for use as eyewashes in any way and should be immediately replaced with adequate eyewashes. Portable eyewashes can be obtained that meet these standards.

The eyewash should be accessible to every user in the room within 10 seconds. It must be ADA compliant as well. The pathway, as well as the eyewash, must be unobstructed, with nothing stored or placed in front of or beneath the eyewash. The eyewash should be flushed weekly long enough to remove particulate, physical, or biological contaminants. A wall chart for logging the eyewash flushing should be posted and maintained to ensure the eyewash is operating properly for emergency use.

Safety Showers

Safety showers should be available where hazardous chemicals are used, including technology, vocational, art, and science areas. Like eyewashes, showers must meet applicable building code standards, including accessibility to every user within 10 seconds and with a 15-minute duration of flow. A deluge shower should deliver at least 20 gallons of tepid water per minute at 30 PSI. Handheld sprayers generally do not meet these standards. Monthly flushing should be carried out to confirm that showers work properly.

The safety shower must be ADA compliant. It must be large enough to accommodate both the injured person (perhaps in a wheelchair) and an adult assisting with the emergency. No protruding floor edges should pose any impediment to wheelchair entry into the shower.

Gloves

Gloves should be used to protect the hands against chemicals, heat, sharp objects, body fluids, and other hazards. The type of glove needed must match the hazard. For example, polyethylene gloves protect the hands against light corrosives and irritants. There are both latex and hypoallergenic nonlatex gloves that protect against biological materials. Nitrile gloves are resistant to solvents, punctures, and abrasions. Oven mitts should be used when dealing with heat sources and heated materials.

Garments

Body-protecting attire, such as flame-retardant lab aprons and coats, is worn to protect the skin and clothing from spilled materials that might be hazardous. Aprons should have bibs that tie the material closely to the lower part of the neck, cover

---

■ *9.4. Helpful hints for glove use*

• Discard any glove with holes or cracks.
• When removing gloves, peel them off your hand, starting at the wrists and working toward the fingers.
• Do not allow the outside surface of the gloves to touch the skin while removing gloves. ■

---

the body to the knees, and work with clothing that covers the arms. General rules that prohibit the wearing of unsafe clothing and dress, including loose clothing, long loose hair, loose jewelry, opentoed shoes, shorts, and highly flammable fabrics such as rayon, continue to be important safety measures.

Housekeeping in Specialized Classrooms

Clean surfaces reduce the risk of contaminating body parts and clothing with hazardous chemicals and disease-causing organisms. Food and drinks should not be consumed in areas where biology or chemical hands-on activities occur or where chemicals are stored. The application of any kind of makeup should not be allowed at any time in any classroom where chemicals are used.

Waste disposal containers that are properly labeled with added safety icons should be available in every area where waste might be produced. Separate labeled waste containers are needed for paper, broken glass, biohazard materials, toxic or caustic waste, and so forth. The containers may be specialized for the hazard, such as a puncture-proof container for biohazardous sharp objects. Proper containers may be ordered from equipment supply companies. Students should be educated on the proper disposal of hazardous materials. Any specimens or materials contaminated with body fluids should be placed in red biohazard containers and disposed of properly.

Exits should be kept clear, and emergency equipment such as the eyewash should be ready for use, easily visible, and have unobstructed access.

Safety during School Renovations and Construction

School renovations and construction, especially when the building is occupied, may create safety and health risks for students, faculty, and staff.

Construction and Demolition Work

Construction and demolition work usually create nuisance dust, with the greatest amount generated during dry dusting and sweeping. Because excessive dust in the work area may cause health-related problems for the building's occupants, dry dusting

> ■ *9.5. Potential health hazards often associated with school renovation and construction*
>
> - dust and debris
> - asbestos
> - lead
> - air pollutants such as paints, sealers, glues, varnishes, urethanes, and roofing materials
> - diesel exhaust, carbon monoxide
> - mold
> - accumulated bird droppings
> - noise.
>
> (New Jersey Public Employees Occupational Safety and Health Program, March 2004) ■

and sweeping should either be avoided or conducted in a manner that controls dust generation (New Jersey Public Employees Occupational Safety and Health Program 2004). Construction can also create excessive noise that can be disruptive to students and staff. See chapter 4 for more information on noise and its effects in schools.

Other safety problems related to construction may include the following:

- dangerous traffic patterns
- open construction areas

- falling objects
- unattended construction equipment
- blocked exits
- disabled fire alarms, detection systems, and emergency lights.

Reduction of Safety and Health Hazards during Renovation

The key to preventing or controlling health and safety problems during and after renovation and construction is to consider these issues in the planning phase of the operation (New Jersey Public Employees Occupational Safety and Health Program 2004). For information on protecting students and staff from renovation pollutants, see table 9.1. Below are some suggestions that should be implemented before and during school renovations:

- Before construction begins, inspect designated areas of the school to evaluate potential problems.
- Establish a health and safety committee that meets regularly to monitor health issues that may arise during the renovations and designates steps to be taken to address these issues.
- Evaluate the school evacuation plan to ensure that exits that were used prior to renovation still provide a safe exit or that alternate exits are provided and well marked.

Table 9.1. Techniques for protecting occupants from renovation pollutants

Technique	Suggestion
Testing	Before performing any demolition, check for lead-based paints, asbestos, and mold-based contaminants.
Timing	When possible, perform work at times when the occupants are not in the building, such as vacation breaks, weekends, or evenings.
Barriers	Install temporary barriers (e.g., plastic sheeting) to seal off the work areas from the occupied areas. Cover all supply and return air grilles if the HVAC system in the renovation area also serves occupied areas so that the air ducts will not spread pollutants to occupied areas. Exhaust air from the construction area so that pollutants cannot flow from the construction area to the occupied areas.
Containment	When possible, keep pollutants confined to as small an area as reasonably possible, rather than allowing them to spread. Examples include wet sanding or vacuum sanding drywall to prevent the spread of dust, misting asbestos with water to prevent it from easily becoming airborne during demolition, and keeping containers of chemicals such as solvents, adhesives, paints, and other coatings closed as much as possible. Do not operate the heating/cooling equipment when work is causing dust to be visible in the air.
Cleanup	At least daily, construction debris, dust, and scraps should be adequately cleaned up to lessen the chance that these pollutants will enter occupied areas.

From the U.S. Environmental Protection Agency (http://www.epa.gov/iaq/schooldesign/renovation.html).

• Keep parents, students, faculty, and staff regularly informed of the progress of the renovation process.
• Maintain strict control of access to construction sites to avoid injuries to students and staff.
• Investigate ongoing health symptoms in students and staff.

Conclusion

The myriad activities occurring in a vibrant school program pose the potential for many different types of injury. The risk of injury must be balanced against the opportunities these activities afford the learners. Risk of injury should be minimized wherever practical.

Students learn best and achieve their full potential in safe and orderly schools and classrooms. Teachers and staff can provide meaningful experiences to students in environments that are conducive to work. With commitment from parents, students, staff, administrators, and communities at large, we can begin to decrease classroom injuries, crime, and violence and thereby encourage the growth of productive, safe, and informed school communities.

Resources

• Centers for Disease Control and Prevention (CDC). One of the most thorough and authoritative guides to preventing school injuries is the CDC's school health guidelines to prevent unintentional injuries and violence, published in 2001 (Morbidity and Mortality Weekly Report 50[RR22]:1–46).
http://www.cdc.gov/mmwr/PDF/RR/RR5022.pdf.
• Arts, Crafts, and Theater Safety. This not-for-profit corporation provides a variety of health and safety services for artists. Its web site has free fact sheets on specific hazards in the arts areas, and the group provides several books that offer safety information for participants in the arts. The ACTS is located at 181 Thompson Street, Suite 23, New York, NY 10012. Telephone: 212-777-0062.
http://www.artscraftstheatersafety.org/.
• Association for Career and Technology Education. This association has multiple resources for safely using the hazardous equipment and materials typically found in vocational shops. The ACTE is located at 1410 King Street, Alexandria, VA 22314. Telephone: 703-683-3111 and 800-826-9972.
http://www.acteonline.org.
• Council of State Science Supervisors. Science education safety: Key issues in school laboratory safety.
http://www.csss-science.org/safety.shtml
• West S. Science Lab Needs Calculator.
http://www.bio.txstate.edu/%7escied/Science

Safety inspection protocols and audit forms are widely available; this topic is covered in chapter 25. Content-specific organizations such as the National Science Education Leadership offer guides to help schools assess science safety. Another excellent reference is the NSTA guide to school science facilities (Biehle et al. 1999; Gerlovich et al. 2001; Young 1997). Others sources include the Laboratory Safety Institute(http://www.labsafety.org) and Texas State University, San Marcos, Texas, http://www.bio.txstate.edu/%7escied/Safety.

References

Americans with Disabilities Act. 1991. Accessibility guidelines for buildings and facilities. Fed Reg 56(144).

Angel CR. 1975. Locomotor skills and school accidents. Pediatrics 56:819–822.

Biehle J, Motz L, West S. 1999. NSTA guide to school science facilities. Arlington, VA: National Science Teachers Association.

Boyce WT, Sobolewski S. 1989. Recurrent injuries in schoolchildren. Am J Dis Child 143(3):338–342.

Boyce WT, Sprunger LW, Sobolewski S, Schaefer C. 1984. Epidemiology of injuries in a large, urban school district. Pediatrics 74(3):342–349.

Bremberg S, Gerber C. 1988. Injuries at school: Influence of schoolmate interaction. Acta Paediatr Scand 77:432–438.

Centers for Disease Control and Prevention. 2001. School health guidelines to prevent unintentional injuries and violence. Mortal Morbid Weekly Rept 50 (RR22):1–46.

Council of State Science Supervisors. Science and safety: It's elementary! Available: http://www.csss-science.org/downloads/scisaf_cal.pdf [accessed 29 December 2005].

Council of State Science Supervisors. Science and safety: Making the connection. Available: http://www.csss-science.org/downloads/scisafe.pdf [accessed 29 December 2005].

Cullen AP. 1998. American Optometric Association. Guidelines for the use of contact lenses in industrial environments. Available: http://www.aoa.org/x1879.xml [accessed 29 December 2005].

Danseco ER, Miller TR, Spicer RS. 2000. Incidence and costs of 1987–1994 childhood injuries: Demographic breakdowns. Pediatrics 105(2):E27.

Di Scala C, Gallagher SS, Schneps SE. 1997. Causes and outcomes of pediatric injuries occurring at school. J School Health 67(9):384–389.

Eichel JDS, Goldman L. 2001. Safety makes sense: A program to prevent unintentional injuries in New York City public schools. J School Health 71(5):180–183.

Emergency Eyewash and Shower Equipment (ANSI Standard Z358.1-1990). New York: American National Standards Institute.

Fire Protection for Laboratories Using Chemicals (NFPA Standard 45). 1996. Quincy, MA: National Fire Protection Association.

Gerlovich J, Parsa R, Wilson E. 1998. Safety issues and Iowa science teachers. J Iowa Acad Science 105(4):152–157.

Gerlovich JA, Whitsett J, Lee S, Parsa R. 2001. Surveying safety: How researchers addressed safety in science classrooms in Wisconsin. Science Teacher (April):31–35. Available: http://www.nsta.org/main/news/pdf/tst0104_31.pdf [accessed 5 February 2005].

Gratz RR. 1992. School injuries: what we know, what we need. J Pediatric Health Care 6(5 Pt 1):256–262.

Gresham LS, Zirkle DL, Tolchin S. 2001. Partnering for injury prevention: Evaluation of a curriculum-based intervention program among elementary school children. J Pediatr Nursing 16:79–87.

Jackson DS, Furman WK, Berson BL. 1980. Patterns of injuries in college athletes: Retrospective study of injuries sustained in intercollegiate athletics in two colleges over a two-year period. Mt Sinai J Med 47:423–426.

Junkins EP Jr, Knight S, Lightfoot AC, 1999. Epidemiology of school injuries in Utah: A population-based study. J School Health 69:409–412.

Junkins EP Jr, Knight S, Olson LM, Lightfoot AC, Keller P, Corneli HM. 2001. Analysis of school injuries resulting in emergency department or hospital admission. Acad Emerg Med 8(4):343–348.

Knight S, Junkins EP, Lightfoot AC, Cazier CF, Olson LM. 2000. Injuries sustained by students in shop class. Pediatrics 106:10–13.

Laflamme L. Menckel E. Aldenberg E. 1998. School-injury determinants and characteristics: developing an investigation instrument from a literature review. Accid Anal Prev 30(4):481–495.

Life Safety Code (Standard 101). 1997. Quincy, MA: National Fire Protection Association.

Macomber RD. 1961. Chemistry accidents in high school. J Chem Ed 38:367–368.

Miller T, Spicer R. 1998. How safe are our schools? Am J Public Health 88:413–418.

Nader PR, Brink SG. 1981. Does visiting the school health room teach appropriate or inappropriate use of health services? Am J Public Health 71:416–419.

National Association of Biology Teachers. 2005. Role of laboratory and field instruction in biology education. Position statement. Reston, VA: National Association of Biology Teachers. Available: http://www.nabt.org/sub/position_statements/laboratory.asp [accessed 29 December 2005].

National Institute for Occupational Safety and Health. 1984. *Manual of safety and health hazards in the school science laboratory.* Cincinnati, OH: U.S. Department of Health and Human Resources.

National Science Teachers Association. 2000. Safety and school science instruction. Position statement. Available: http://www.nsta.org/positionstatement&psid=32

National Science Teachers Association. 2005. Responsible Use of Live Animals and Dissection in the Science Classroom. Position statement. Arlington, VA: National Science Teachers Association. Available: http://www.nsta.org/positionstatement&psid=44 [accessed 11 January 2006].

New Jersey Public Employees Occupational Safety and Health Program. 2004. Renovation and construction in schools: Controlling health and safety hazards. Available: http://www.state.nj.us/health/eoh/peoshweb/schoolsren.pdf [accessed 14 April 2005].

Office of Technology Assessment. 1995. Risks to students in school. Publication OTA-ENV-633. Washington, DC: U.S. Government Printing Office.

Rossol M. 2001a. *The artist's complete health and safety guide,* 3d ed. New York: Allworth Press.

Rossol M. 2001b. *The health and safety guide for film, TV, and theater.* New York: Allworth Press.

Spicer RS, Cazier C, Keller P, Miller TR. 2002. Evaluation of the Utah student injury reporting system. J School Health 72(2):47–50.

Taketa S. 1984. Student accidents in Hawaii's public schools. J School Health. 54(5):208–209.

Tenn L, Dewis ME. 1996. An evaluation of a Canadian peer-driven injury prevention programme for high-risk adolescents. J Advanced Nursing 23:329–337.

Texas Education Agency 2003. School Facilities Standards and Guidelines. http://www.tea.state.tx.us/school.finance/facilities/stg.html [accessed 11 January 2006].

Ward S, West S. 1990. Accidents in Texas high school chemistry labs. Texas Science Teacher 19(2):14–19.

West S. 1990. Science laboratory safety survey. Texas Science Teacher 19(2):9–13.

West S. 1991. Lab safety. Texas Science Teacher. 58(6):46–59.

West S, Westerlund JF, Nelson NC, Stephenson AL, Nyland CK. 2002. What the safety research says to Texas science teachers. Texas Science Teacher 31(1):11–15.

West S, Westerlund JF, Stephenson AL, Nelson NC, Nyland CK. 2002. Texas science safety profile, 2001. Texas Science Teacher 31(1):16–18.

Wronski R, Keilman J. 2001. Seven students burned in chemistry class: Demonstration goes awry at Genoa-Kingston. *Chicago Tribune.* October 12, 2001.

Young JA. 1997a. Chemical safety, Part 1. Science Teacher (March):43–45. Available: http://www.nsta.org/main/news/pdf/tst9703_43.pdf [accessed 5 February 2005].

Young JA. 1997b. Chemical safety, Part 2. Science Teacher (March):40–43. Available: http://www.nsta.org/main/news/pdf/tst9704_40.pdf [accessed 5 February 2005].

Young JR. 1972. A second survey of safety in Illinois high school laboratories. J Chem Ed 49(1):55.

Air Quality
in Schools

10

Robert Axelrad

Indoor Air Quality

■ *Summary*

- Indoor air quality (IAQ) in schools, as in other buildings, can have an important impact on health. Poor IAQ is a problem that has worsened with modern construction techniques.
- Four factors determine IAQ in schools: sources of indoor air pollution; heating, ventilating, and air-conditioning systems; pollutant pathways; and the people themselves.
- IAQ problems may be recognized and diagnosed using EPA's Tools for Schools program.
- IAQ problems may be mitigated and managed with a variety of strategies including controlling sources and exposures and educating teachers, staff, and students. ■

In 1999, one in five schools in the United States reported unsatisfactory indoor air quality (IAQ); one in four reported inadequate ventilation (General Accounting Office 1995, 1996; NCES 2000, 2003). Good IAQ is an important component of a healthy indoor environment and can help schools reach their primary goal of educating children.

Why Indoor Air Quality in Schools Is Important

Most people are aware that outdoor air pollution can damage their health, but many do not know that indoor air pollution can also have significant harmful effects. U.S. Environmental Protection Agency (EPA) studies of human exposure to air pollutants indicate that indoor levels of pollutants may be 2 to 5 times—and occasionally more than 100 times—higher than outdoor levels. These indoor levels may be of particular concern because it is estimated that most people spend about 90% of their time indoors. Comparative risk studies performed by the EPA and its science advisory board have consistently ranked indoor air pollution among the top five environmental health risks to the public.

Indoor air problems can be obvious, as in the case of a spill or other sudden event, or they may be more subtle because they do not always produce easily recognized impacts on health, well-being, or the physical plant. Nevertheless, failure to prevent and respond promptly and effectively to IAQ problems can have serious health, cost, and educational consequences.

Although IAQ is a critical aspect of operating

and maintaining school facilities, special attention to IAQ is also important in the design of new schools and the renovation of existing ones. Many communities are embracing the concept of designing high-performance schools, which are based on an integrated whole-building approach, to address a myriad of important (and sometimes competing) priorities such as energy efficiency, IAQ, daylighting, materials efficiency, and safety—all within the context of tight budgets and limited staff (see chapter 23).

Failure to prevent indoor air problems or to respond promptly when they occur can have consequences such as:

- increasing the potential for long-term and short-term health problems for students and staff
- affecting the student learning environment, comfort, and attendance
- reducing performance of teachers and staff because of discomfort, sickness, or absenteeism
- accelerating deterioration and reducing efficiency of the school physical plant and equipment
- increasing the potential that schools will have to be closed or occupants temporarily relocated
- straining relationships between school administration, parents, and staff
- creating negative publicity that could damage the image and effectiveness of a school or an administration
- creating potential liability problems.

Understanding Indoor Air Quality Problems and Solutions

Over the past several decades, exposure to indoor air pollutants is believed to have increased because of a variety of factors, including the construction of more tightly sealed buildings, reduced ventilation rates to save energy, the use of synthetic building materials and furnishings, and the use of chemically formulated personal care products, pesticides, and housekeeping supplies. In addition, some activities and decisions, such as deferring maintenance to save money, lead to problems from sources and ventilation (U.S. EPA 1995).

Four basic factors determine IAQ and its effects on the students and staff in a school: sources of indoor air pollutants; heating, ventilation, and air-conditioning (HVAC) systems; pollutant pathways; and the people themselves (U.S. EPA 1995).

Sources of Indoor Air Pollutants

Indoor air contaminants can originate within the building or can be drawn in from outdoors (table 10.1). If pollutant sources are not controlled, IAQ problems can arise, even if the HVAC system is operating properly. Air pollutants consist of numerous particulates, fibers, mists, bioaerosols, and gases. It may be helpful to think of air pollutant sources as fitting into one of the categories in table 10.1.

In addition to the number of potential pollutants, another complicating factor is that concentrations of indoor air pollutants can vary by time and location within the school building or even a single classroom. Pollutants can be emitted from point sources such as science storerooms or from area sources such as newly painted surfaces. Pollutants can vary with time, such as only once each week when floor stripping is done, or continuously, as with fungi growing in the HVAC system.

Mold

Concern about indoor exposure to mold has been increasing as the public becomes aware that exposure to mold can cause health problems. A report of the Institute of Medicine of the National Academy of Sciences (2004) concluded that mold and other factors related to damp conditions in homes and buildings are associated with asthma symptoms in some people with the chronic disorder and with coughing, wheezing, and upper respiratory tract symptoms in otherwise healthy people.

Schools have not been exempt from mold concerns (see chapter 11). In brief, the key to mold control is moisture control. Moisture problems in buildings can have many causes, including uncontrolled humidity. Some moisture problems in buildings have been linked to changes in construction practices in the 1970s, 1980s, and 1990s. Some of these changes have resulted in buildings that are tightly sealed but may lack adequate ventilation, potentially leading to moisture buildup. Building materials such as drywall may not allow moisture to escape easily. Moisture problems may stem from a leaky roof, landscaping or gutters that

Table 10.1. Typical indoor air pollutants and sources

Outside sources	Building equipment	Components and furnishings	Other indoor sources
Polluted outdoor air • pollen • dust • mold • Industrial and vehicle emissions Nearby sources • loading docks • fumes from dumpsters • unsanitary debris or building exhausts near outdoor air intakes Underground sources • radon • pesticides • leakage from underground storage tanks	HVAC equipment • microbiological growth in drip pans, ductwork, coils, and humidifiers • improper venting of combustion products • dust or debris in ductwork Non-HVAC equipment • emissions from office equipment (volatile organic compounds, ozone) • emissions from shops, labs, or cleaning processes	Components • microbiological growth on soiled or water-damaged materials • dry drain traps that allow the passage of sewer gas • materials emitting volatile organic compounds, inorganic compounds, or damaged asbestos • materials that produce particles (dust) Furnishings and finishes • emissions from new furnishings and finishes such as flooring • microbiological growth on or in soiled or water-damaged furnishings	• science laboratories • vocational arts areas • copy/print areas • food prep areas • smoking lounges • cleaning materials • emissions from trash • pesticides • fumes and volatile organic compounds from paint, caulk, adhesives • occupants with communicable diseases • dry-erase markers and similar pens; insects and other pests • animals in classrooms • personal care products

direct water into or under the building, and unvented combustion appliances. Delayed and insufficient maintenance are also associated with moisture problems in schools and large buildings. Moisture problems in portable classrooms and other temporary structures have frequently been associated with the growth of mold.

The EPA and a number of other organizations have developed guidelines for the remediation and cleanup of mold and moisture problems in schools and commercial buildings. These guidelines include measures designed to protect the health of building occupants and remediators (U.S. Environmental Protection Agency 2001; (see chapter 11).

Radon

The EPA and other major national and international scientific organizations have concluded that radon is a human carcinogen and a serious public health problem. A person's risk of developing lung cancer from radon increases with the level of radon, the duration of exposure, and the person's smoking habits. The EPA estimates that 20,000 lung cancer deaths in the United States each year are attributable to radon. Because many people spend much of their time at home, the home is likely to be the most significant source of radon exposure. For most schoolchildren and staff, the second largest

contributor to their exposure to radon is likely to be their school. As a result, the EPA recommends that school buildings as well as homes be tested for radon.

Asbestos

Asbestos is a fibrous mineral that has been widely used in construction materials such as roofing and siding shingles, pipe and boiler insulation, and floor and ceiling tiles. Asbestos is a problem because, as a toxic substance and a known carcinogen, it can cause several serious diseases in humans. Symptoms of these diseases typically develop over a period of years after exposure to asbestos.

Asbestos-containing materials in buildings do not always constitute a hazard to occupants and workers in those buildings. Asbestos is a problem when the fibers get into the air and are inhaled, that is, when there is human exposure. Intact, undisturbed asbestos-containing materials generally do not pose a health risk. They may become hazardous and pose an increased risk when they are damaged or disturbed in some manner or as they deteriorate over time and thus release asbestos fibers into the indoor air.

The EPA's asbestos program for schools implements a 1986 federal law, the Asbestos Hazard Emergency Response Act (AHERA). This program, like the EPA's guidelines for owners of other buildings, is founded on the principle of in-place management of asbestos-containing materials. This approach is designed to keep asbestos fiber levels low by teaching people to recognize asbestos-containing materials and to actively manage them. Removal of these materials is not usually necessary unless the material is severely damaged or will be disturbed by a building demolition or renovation project.

HVAC System Design and Operation

The HVAC system includes all heating, cooling, and ventilating equipment serving a school. A properly designed and functioning HVAC system

- controls temperature and humidity to provide thermal comfort
- distributes adequate amounts of outdoor air to meet the ventilation needs of school occupants
- isolates and removes odors and pollutants through pressure control, filtration, and exhaust fans.

Not all HVAC systems are designed to perform all of these functions. Some buildings rely on natural ventilation only. Others lack mechanical cooling equipment, and many function with little or no humidity control. The two most common HVAC designs used in schools are unit ventilators and central air-handling systems. Both can perform the same HVAC functions, but the central air-handling unit serves multiple rooms, whereas the unit ventilator serves a single room.

Pollutant Pathways and Driving Forces

Airflow patterns in buildings result from the combined forces of mechanical ventilation systems, human activity, and natural effects. Air-pressure differences created by these forces move airborne pollutants from areas of higher pressure to areas of lower pressure through available openings in walls, ceilings, floors, doors, windows, and the HVAC system. An inflated balloon can serve as an example to illustrate this driving force. As long as the opening to the balloon is kept shut, no air will flow, but when the balloon is open, air will move from inside (area of higher pressure) to the outside (area of lower pressure). Even if the opening is small, air

will move until the pressures inside and outside are equal.

Building Occupants

The occupants of schools include the staff, students, and other people who spend extended periods of time in the building. They may be exposed to readily identifiable sources of indoor air contamination, such as chemicals (e.g., a mercury spill, cleaning solvents), high levels of radon, asbestos fibers, or lead paint dust, to name just a few. However, the effects of IAQ problems on occupants are often nonspecific symptoms rather than clearly defined illnesses. Symptoms commonly attributed to IAQ problems include

- headache, fatigue, and shortness of breath
- sinus congestion, coughing, and sneezing
- eye, nose, throat, and skin irritation
- dizziness and nausea.

All of these symptoms, however, may also be caused by other factors and are not necessarily due to air quality deficiencies. Environmental stressors such as improper lighting, noise, vibration, overcrowding, poor ergonomics, and psychosocial problems (such as job or home stress) can produce symptoms similar to those associated with poor air quality but require different solutions.

Because of varying sensitivity among people, one person may react to a particular IAQ problem while surrounding occupants do not display ill effects. In other cases, complaints may be widespread. In addition to different degrees of reaction, an indoor air pollutant or problem can trigger different types of reactions in different people. Groups that may be particularly susceptible to the effects of indoor air contaminants include but are not limited to (1) people with allergies or asthma or people with sensitivity to chemicals; (2) people with respiratory disease; (3) people whose immune systems are suppressed or impaired because of radiation, chemotherapy, or disease; and (4) contact lens wearers.

An Ounce of Prevention

Taking steps to implement a preventive IAQ management program can significantly reduce the likelihood that schools will experience major IAQ or other environmental incidents (U.S. Environmental Protection Agency 2002). Many schools across the country have observed health-related benefits from implementing the EPA's Tools for Schools program:

- Little Harbour School in Portsmouth, New Hampshire, experienced a dramatic decrease in absenteeism, fewer bronchitis cases reported by school staff, an increase in comfort, and a 25% reduction in the number of visits to the school nurse with complaints of stomachaches and headaches within the first 5 months of implementing the kit.
- Hamden Public Schools in Connecticut reported a decrease in the number of complaints from staff and students of headaches and sinus infections, the number of trips to the school nurse for asthma and asthma treatments, the use and storage of students' inhalers at school, and symptoms of chronic respiratory illnesses.
- G. W. Carver Elementary School in San Francisco experienced a 50% reduction in visits to the office for the use of asthma inhalers.
- The Okaloosa County School District in Florida reported a reduction in the number of complaints related to health and faulty equipment from 75 in 1994 to fewer than 15 in 1999.
- Since implementing the program in 1998, the Hillsborough County Public School District in Florida has spent only $400 on IAQ consultants, compared with an estimated $250,000 before 1997.
- Nearly all IAQ complaints were resolved in-house at Monmouth Junction Elementary School in New Jersey at a total cost of less than $1,000. The improvements focused on preventive maintenance, integrated pest management, and the use of environmentally preferable cleaners.

In January 2006, the EPA Tools for Schools web site was expanded to present information about Healthy Schools in addition to its original content (http://cfpub.epa.gov/schools/index.cfm), and will prove to be an even more valuable resource.

Diagnosing Indoor Air Quality Problems

Diagnosing symptoms that relate to IAQ can be tricky. Acute (short-term) symptoms of IAQ problems typically are similar to those of colds, allergies, fatigue, or influenza. Nevertheless, certain clues can serve as indicators of a potential indoor air problem:

- The symptoms are widespread within a class or the school as a whole.
- The symptoms disappear when the students or staff leaves the school building for a day.
- The onset is sudden, particularly after some change at school, such as painting or pesticide application.
- People with allergies, asthma, or sensitivity to chemicals have symptoms indoors but not outdoors.
- A doctor has found that a student or staff member has an indoor air–related illness.

However, an absence of symptoms does not ensure that the IAQ is acceptable. Symptoms from long-term health effects (such as lung cancer due to radon) often do not become evident for many years.

The goal of diagnosing an IAQ problem is to discover the cause of the problem so that an appropriate solution can be implemented. Often more than one problem will be present, thus likely requiring more than one solution. The IAQ diagnostic process begins when a complaint is registered or an IAQ problem is identified. Many problems can be simple to diagnose because they require only a basic knowledge of IAQ and some common sense. Not all complaints about IAQ are caused by poor indoor air. Other factors such as noise, lighting, and job-, family-, or peer-related psychosocial stressors can individually and in combination contribute to a perception that the IAQ is poor.

The EPA's Tools for Schools kit includes a problem-solving checklist and a problem-solving wheel, both of which can assist in identifying and resolving problems. They serve to lead the investigation in the right direction and offer suggestions for other areas to evaluate.

Start with the problem-solving checklist and enlist the assistance of school staff members to answer questions or perform activities suggested by the checklist and the wheel. Consider that pollutant sources and the ventilation system may act in combination to create an IAQ problem.

If the investigation identifies a potential problem (e.g., you find a blocked vent), remedy the situation to see whether the symptoms stop. You may find problems unrelated to the symptoms or a number of potential causes. Resolve as many problems as is feasible, and make note of any problems that you intend to fix later.

Spatial and Timing Patterns

As a first step, use the spatial pattern (locations) of complaints to define the complaint area. School lo-cations where symptoms or discomfort occur define the rooms or zones that should be given particular attention during the investigation. However, the complaint area may need to be revised as the investigation progresses. Pollutant pathways can cause complaints in parts of the school that are far removed from the source of the problems (see table 10.2).

After a location or group of locations has been defined, look for patterns in the timing of complaints. The timing of symptoms and complaints can indicate potential causes and provide direction for further investigation. Review the data for cyclic patterns of symptoms (e.g., are they worst during

Table 10.2. Spatial patterns

Complaints	Suggestions
Widespread, no apparent spatial pattern	• Check ventilation and temperature control for entire building • Check outdoor air quality • Review sources that are spread throughout the building (e.g., cleaning materials or microbiological growth inside the ventilation system) • Check for distribution of a source to multiple locations through the ventilations system • Consider explanations other than air contaminants
Localized (e.g., affecting individual rooms, zones, or air-handling systems)	• Check ventilation and temperature control within the complaint area • Check outdoor air quality • Review pollutant sources affecting the complaint area • Check local HVAC system components that may be sources or distributors of pollutants
Individuals	• Check for drafts, radiant heat (gain or loss), and other localized temperature control or ventilation problems near the affected people • Consider that common background sources may affect only susceptible people • Consider the possibility that individual complaints may have different causes not necessarily related to the building (particularly if the symptoms differ among the individuals)

Table 10.3. Timing patterns

Complaints	Suggestions
Symptoms begin and/or are worst at the start of the occupied period	Review HVAC operating cycles. Pollutants from building materials or from the HVAC system itself may build up during unoccupied periods
Symptoms worsen over course of occupied period	Consider that ventilation may not be adequate to handle routine activities or equipment operation within the building or that temperature may not be properly controlled
Intermittent symptoms	Look for daily, weekly, or seasonal cycles or weather-related patterns, and check linkage to other events in and around the school
Single event of symptoms	Consider spills and other unrepeated events as sources
Symptoms relieved on leaving the school, either immediately, overnight, or (in some cases) after extended periods away from the building	Consider that the problem may be associated with the building, though not necessarily due to air quality. Other stressors (e.g., lighting, noise) may be involved
Symptoms never relieved, even after extended absence from school (e.g., vacations)	Consider that the problem may not be related to the building

periods of minimum ventilation or when specific sources are most active?) that may be related to HVAC system operation or to other activities in and around the school (see table 10.3).

Resolving Indoor Air Quality Problems

A solution should be selected based on the data gathered during diagnostics. The diagnostics may have determined that the problem was either a real or a perceived IAQ problem or a combination of problems. For each problem the diagnostics identify, develop a solution using the six basic control methods for lowering concentrations of indoor air pollutants. Often only a slight shift in emphasis or action using these methods is needed to more effectively control IAQ. Specific applications of these basic strategies can be found in each team member's checklist.

Source management includes source removal, source substitution, and source encapsulation. Source management is the most effective control method when it can be practically applied. Source removal is very effective. Policies and actions that keep potential pollutants from entering the school are the best approach to preventing IAQ problems. Examples of source removal include not allowing buses to idle near outdoor air intakes, not placing garbage in rooms where HVAC equipment is located, and banning smoking within the school.

Source substitution includes actions such as selecting a less toxic art material or interior paint than the products currently in use. Source encapsulation involves placing a barrier around the source so that it releases fewer pollutants into the indoor air.

By exhausting the contaminated air outside, local exhaust is very effective in removing point sources of pollutants before they can disperse into the indoor air. Restrooms and kitchens typically use local exhaust. Other examples include science labs and housekeeping storage rooms, printing and duplicating rooms, and vocational/industrial areas such as welding booths.

Ventilation, through the use of cleaner (outdoor) air to dilute the polluted (indoor) air that people are breathing, is often a solution. The ventilation system, when properly designed, operated, and maintained, will automatically take care of normal amounts of air pollutants. For emergency situations such as quick removal of toxic fumes, increased ventilation can be useful, but when considering long-term operating costs, employing "dilution as the solution" is best applied after attempts have been made to reduce the source of the pollutant.

Exposure control includes adjusting the time, amount, and location of use to reduce exposure. Try not to use a pollutant source when the school is occupied. For example, strip and wax floors on Friday after school is dismissed. Floor products will then have a chance to off-gas over the weekend, reducing the level of pollutants in the air when the school is reoccupied on Monday. If less of an air-polluting source is used, less of it will end up in the air. Move the polluting source as far as possible from occupants, or relocate susceptible occupants.

Air cleaning primarily involves the filtration of particulates from the air as it passes through the HVAC equipment. Gaseous pollutants can also be removed, but these removal systems must be engineered on a case-by-case basis.

Education of school occupants regarding IAQ is critical. If people are provided information about the sources and effects of pollutants and about the proper operation of the ventilation system, they can act to reduce their personal exposure.

Some solutions, such as major ventilation system modification, may not be practical to implement because of lack of resources or because of the need for long periods of nonoccupancy to complete the work safely. Employ temporary measures to ensure good IAQ in the meantime.

Evaluating the Effectiveness of a Solution

Two kinds of indicators can help school authorities evaluate the success of an effort to correct an indoor air problem: a reduction in the number of complaints and measurement of the properties of the indoor air.

Reduction or elimination of complaints appears to be a clear indication of success, but that is not necessarily the case. Occupants who realize that their concerns are being heard may temporarily stop reporting discomfort or health symptoms, even if the actual cause of their complaints has not been corrected. On the other hand, lingering complaints may continue after successful mitigation if people have become upset over the handling of the problem. A smaller number of ongoing complaints may indicate that there were multiple IAQ problems and that one or more problems are still unresolved.

Measurements of airflows, ventilation rates, and air distribution patterns can help school officials assess the results of their control efforts. Airflow measurements taken during the investigation can identify areas with poor ventilation; later, they can be used to evaluate attempts to improve the ventilation rate, distribution, or direction of airflow. Studying air distribution patterns will show whether a mitigation strategy has successfully prevented a pollutant from being transported by airflow.

Although the measurement of pollutant levels can sometimes serve as a means of determining whether IAQ has improved, this approach may be difficult to implement and/or prohibitively expensive. Concentrations of indoor air pollutants typically vary greatly over time; further, the specific contaminant measured may not be causing the problem. The EPA does not recommend sampling for pollutants as a routine part of an IAQ investigation because the results can be extremely difficult to interpret and require costly measurement equipment and significant training and experience in using the equipment. However, under certain circumstances, measurement of a specific pollutant by a professional is appropriate, for example, when a problem is known to be associated with a particular pollutant.

Persistent Problems

Even the best-planned investigations and mitigation actions may not produce a resolution to the problem. You may have made a careful investigation, found one or more apparent causes of a problem, and implemented a control system. Nonetheless, your correction strategy may not have caused a noticeable reduction in the concentration of the contaminant or an improvement in ventilation rates or efficiency. Worse, the complaints may persist even though you have been successful at improving ventilation and controlling all of the contaminants you could identify. When you have pursued source control options and increased ventilation rates and efficiency to the limits of your expertise, you must decide how important it is to pursue the problem further.

If you have made several unsuccessful efforts to control a problem, it may be advisable to seek outside assistance. The problem may be complex, occur only intermittently, or cross the borders that divide traditional fields of knowledge. It is even possible that poor IAQ is not the actual cause of the complaints. Bringing in a new perspective at this point can be very effective.

Hiring Professional Indoor Air Quality Assistance

Some IAQ problems are simple to resolve when school personnel understand the building investigation process. Many potential problems will be prevented if staff and students do their part to maintain good IAQ. However, a time may come when outside assistance is needed. For example, professional help might be necessary or desirable in the following situations:

- If you suspect that you have a serious building-related illness that is potentially linked to biological contamination in the building, mistakes or delays could have serious consequences (e.g., health hazards, liability exposure, regulatory sanctions). Contact your local or state health department.
- Testing for a public health hazard (such as asbestos, lead, or radon) has identified a problem that requires a prompt response.
- The school administration believes that an independent investigation would be better received or more effectively documented than an in-house investigation.
- Investigation and mitigation efforts by school staff have not relieved an IAQ problem.
- Preliminary findings by staff suggest a need for measurements that require specialized equipment and skills not available in-house.

As you prepare to hire professional services for a building investigation, be aware that IAQ is still a developing area of knowledge. Most people who are working in IAQ received their primary training in other disciplines. It is important to define the scope of work clearly and discuss any potential consultant's proposed approach to the investigation, including plans for coordinating efforts among team members. The school's representatives must exercise vigilance in overseeing diagnostic activities and corrective action. Performance specifications can help to ensure the desired results.

With the exception of lead and asbestos remediation, no federal regulations cover professional services in the general field of IAQ, although some disciplines (e.g., engineering, industrial hygiene) whose practitioners work with IAQ problems have licensing and certification requirements. Ask questions of individuals and groups that offer services in this evolving field about their related experience and their proposed approach to your problem. In addition, request and contact their references.

Local, state, or federal government agencies (e.g., education, health, or air pollution agencies) may be able to provide expert assistance or direction in solving IAQ problems. If available government agencies do not have personnel with the appropriate skills to assist in solving your IAQ problem, they may be able to direct you to firms in your area with experience in IAQ work. You may also be able to locate potential consultants by looking in the yellow pages (e.g., under Engineers, Environmental Services, Laboratories Testing, or Industrial Hygienists) or by asking other schools for referrals. Often a multidisciplinary team of professionals is needed to investigate and resolve an IAQ problem. The skills of HVAC engineers and industrial hygienists are typically useful for this type of investigation. Input from other disciplines such as chemistry, architecture, microbiology, or medicine may also be important.

If problems other than IAQ are involved, experts in lighting, acoustic design, interior design, psychology, or other fields may be helpful in resolving occupants' complaints about the indoor environment.

Evaluating Potential Consultants

As with any hiring process, the better you know your own needs, the easier it will be to select individuals or firms to service those needs. The more clearly you can define the project scope, the more likely you are to achieve the desired result without paying for unnecessary services. An investigation strategy based on evaluating building performance can be used to solve a problem without necessarily identifying a particular chemical compound as the cause. Some state regulations call for the involvement of a professional engineer for any modifications or additions to a school's HVAC system. Whether or not this is legally mandated for your school, the professional engineer's knowledge of air handling, conditioning, and sequencing strategies will help design ventilation system modifications without creating other problems. In some situations, proper engineering can save energy while improving IAQ. An example of this might be the redesign of outside air-handling strategies to improve the performance of an economizer cycle.

Before starting to take measurements, investigators need a clear understanding of how the results will be used. Without this understanding, it is impossible to plan appropriate sampling locations and times, instrumentation, and analysis procedures. Non-routine measurements, such as relatively expensive sampling for volatile organic compounds, should not be conducted without site-specific justification.

The idea of testing the air to learn whether it is safe or unsafe is very appealing. However, most of the existing standards for airborne pollutants were developed for industrial settings, where the majority of occupants are healthy adults. Concentrations low enough to comply with occupational standards could still be harmful to children or other school occupants. In addition, industrial IAQ problems tend to arise from high levels of individual chemical compounds, so these standards set limits for individual contaminants or contaminant classes. Exposure standards of this type are rarely exceeded in schools. Instead, IAQ investigators often find a large number of potential sources contributing low levels of many contaminants to the air.

Building Better Schools: Integrated, Whole-building Design

Many jurisdictions and organizations are embracing the concept of designing high-performance schools, based on an integrated "whole-building" approach, to address a myriad of important (and sometimes competing) priorities such as energy efficiency, IAQ, daylighting, materials efficiency, and safety—all of which are within the context of tight budgets and limited staff (Collaborative for High-performance Schools 2002). For example, a typical 450-student elementary school today pays more than $45,000 annually for energy-related utilities. Incorporating energy-efficient design improvements into the design and building of the school could save that school $13,000 per year. These savings do not include the potential benefits of improved occupant health, productivity, and performance from integrating high-performance design features. A full discussion of high-performance schools appears in chapter 23.

The IAQ component of high-performance school design encompasses factors such as maintenance of acceptable temperature and relative humidity, control of airborne contaminants, and distribution of adequate ventilation air. It requires deliberate care on the part of the entire project team. Achieving thermal comfort begins with good design, continues with proper building management, and seeks to avoid uneven temperatures, radiant heat gains or losses (e.g., from window areas), draftiness, stuffiness, excessive dryness, or high relative humidity (which can promote the growth of mold).

Through careful selection of materials, designers can avoid introducing potential pollutant sources. Mechanical engineers and allied tradespeople must select and install reliable ventilation systems that dilute the by-products of occupant activities and, to the greatest extent possible, supply fresh air on demand in the right quantities and in the right locations. During construction, air passageways need to be protected, and mechanical systems must be balanced and commissioned to achieve optimal operation. Facility managers and custodial and maintenance staff also play a role in keeping areas clean while minimizing the use of irritating cleaning and maintenance supplies.

Even if all of a school's objectives are met, attaining an IAQ acceptable to everyone may be difficult because of the diversity of sources and contaminants in indoor air, occupants' perceptions, and individual susceptibility.

The EPA has developed detailed recommendations for incorporating IAQ into the design, construction, and renovation of new schools in its web-based guidelines, Indoor Air Quality Design Tools for Schools (2003). These design tools provide voluntary guidance for school personnel, architects, engineers, builders, contractors, parents, and the community on key school construction and renovation issues:

- incorporating high-performance building features into the design process
- controlling pollutants and their sources
- selecting and designing HVAC systems
- controlling moisture to prevent mold growth and damage to building materials and systems
- specifying and maintaining portable classrooms
- renovating existing schools
- providing links to resources on a wide range

of high-performance construction issues such as acoustics, daylighting, life-cycle costing, and commissioning.

IAQ Design Tools for Schools is intended to help school districts and facility planners design the next generation of learning environments so that the school facility will help rather than hinder schools in achieving their core mission of educating children.

References

Asbestos Hazard Emergency Response Act of 1986. 1986. Public law 99-519.

Collaborative for High-performance Schools (CHPS). 2002. Best practices manual. Available: http://www.chps.net [accessed 3 February 2005].

General Accounting Office. 1995. School facilities: Condition of America's schools. GAO/HEHS-95-61. Washington, DC: U.S. General Accounting Office.

General Accounting Office. 1996. School facilities: America's schools report differing conditions. GAO/HEHS-96-103. Washington, DC: U.S. General Accounting Office.

National Academy of Sciences. 2004. Damp indoor spaces and health. Institute of Medicine, Committee on Damp Indoor Spaces and Health. Washington, DC: National Academy of Sciences.

National Center for Education Statistics, U.S. Department of Education. 2000. Condition of America's public school facilities: 1999. Washington, DC: National Center for Education Statistics, 15, 2.

National Center for Education Statistics, U.S. Department of Education. 2003. Digest of education statistics. Washington, DC: National Center for Education Statistics, 12–14.

U.S. Environmental Protection Agency. 1995. Indoor air quality tools for schools. Available: http://www.epa.gov/iaq/schools [accessed 3 February 2005].

U.S. Environmental Protection Agency. 2001. Mold remediation in schools and commercial buildings. EPA 402-K-01-001. Washington, DC: U.S. Environmental Protection Agency.

U.S. Environmental Protection Agency. 2002. Indoor air quality tools for schools program: Benefits of improving air quality in the school environment. EPA 402-K-02-005. Washington, DC: U.S. Environmental Protection Agency.

U.S. Environmental Protection Agency. 2003. Indoor air quality design tools for schools. Available: http://www.epa.gov/iaq/schooldesign [accessed 3 February 2005].

11

Robert J. Geller

Mold

■ *Summary*

- Mold frequently grows in schools and other buildings when warm, humid conditions are present indoors.
- Many different mold species can be found indoors. No particular species has been demonstrated to pose a higher risk to the public than any other.
- People with allergies to mold can suffer adverse effects, but the ability of mold to cause other human illness is controversial and not well established.
- The two main strategies for managing mold are removing the sources of moisture and cleaning up the mold.
- The extent of mold contamination in an area will determine how extensive the remediation should be and how much it will cost. ■

Alarming reports of mold infestations have appeared in the press and the media in recent years. A highly publicized outbreak of a rare illness in several infants in Cleveland, Ohio, was initially attributed to mold (Etzel et al. 1998). Despite these reports, our knowledge of the effects of mold on humans is incomplete.

The cost of dealing with a mold problem can be astronomical. School districts have spent from $200,000 to $13.1 million to correct severe mold problems in school buildings (U.S. Environmental Protection Agency 2001), so it is important to identify the problem in its early stages, when damage is limited. We are left with the need to act prudently, utilizing our current knowledge, to eradicate mold where appropriate and to protect health.

Mold spores are usually present in the air. These spores are a dormant but very hardy form of living fungi. Humid, warm settings favor regrowth of mold from the spores. Many schools and homes have such warm and humid conditions, particularly in poorly ventilated areas and after flooding or water leaks. The presence of visible mold is frequently a marker of excess humidity. These circumstances also favor the development of other medical issues, leading to concern that the mold may be causing the medical problems (Storey et al. 2004). Studies to date are of inadequate quality to determine whether such is the case.

This chapter reviews some of the existing information behind these issues and suggests practical approaches to the evaluation of a building and its occupants.

What Is Mold?

The terms "mold," "fungus," "spore," and "mildew" are frequently used in similar ways. The *Random House Dictionary of the English Language* (1987, p. 776) defines a fungus as "any of a diverse group of eukaryotic single-celled or multinucleate organisms that live by decomposing and absorbing the organic material in which they grow, comprising the mushrooms, molds, mildews, smuts, rusts, and yeasts." Mold is the "growth of minute fungi forming on vegetable or animal matter, commonly as a downy or furry coating, and associated with decay or dampness" (p. 1238). A spore is a protected form of the fungus (or other organism) capable of giving rise to another organism, under suitable conditions (p. 1844). Mildew is the discoloration caused by mold growth on fabric, leather, paper, or similar materials under damp conditions (p. 1219).

Airborne mold spores are found throughout most of the world. Fungi thrive in warm, moist climates where lighting conditions are favorable and food is available. Fungi perform an important function in the global ecosystem by breaking down larger carbon-containing compounds into smaller molecules. These smaller molecules can then be reused as building blocks for the production of new compounds. Once a mold starts growing, it produces spores that become airborne and permit the mold to spread.

More than 100 species of fungi have been recognized. The visual appearance of mold varies both by the specific species and by the conditions in which the mold is growing, particularly the surface on which growth is occurring. The species of fungi prevailing in a specific area vary, depending both on the climate and on the use of the land in that area. For example, the fungi that are predominant over grasslands will likely be different from those found over forests in the same climate. Fungi inside buildings generally have entered from outside the building, so local outdoor fungal patterns are likely to be important in understanding indoor mold patterns (Burge 2002; table 11.1).

Factors That Favor Indoor Mold Growth

In buildings where the moisture content is high and the room temperatures are warm, mold may thrive, even to the point of visible growth on exposed surfaces. Porous materials such as wallboard and composition tile are particularly favorable to the growth of mold (figure 11.1).

Mold spores present in the circulating air will germinate and begin to grow when such favorable conditions are encountered. The fungal organisms obtain their nutrition from both the air and the surface on which they are growing, and both wallboard and composition ceiling tile provide suitable surfaces for growth. In some circumstances, mold may grow rapidly. After water penetrates into concealed spaces, mold species may also grow, hidden inside walls and other indoor spaces.

Health Effects of Mold

The effects of mold on human health are poorly understood; so the subject is open to much controversy. We know that some people are allergic to molds, and serious diseases have sometimes occurred soon after exposure to mold. Molds release chemicals, including mycotoxins and other organic chemicals, that may be toxic to humans. However, none of these circumstances fully explains the patterns of disease that some attribute to mold exposure. We discuss these topics further below.

Table 11.1. Mold species commonly encountered indoors[a]

Species	Human health impact
Actinomyces	Actinomycosis, a rare infection
Alternaria	Allergic sensitivity to *Alternaria* in patients with asthma has been recognized as a risk factor for severe asthma
Aspergillus	Allergic bronchopulmonary aspergillosis, a rare condition in which infection of the lungs with aspergillus results in bodywide symptoms
Cladosporium	None specifically identified
Curvularia	None specifically identified
Penicillium	Allergic sensitivity to penicillium may result in allergy to penicillin-class drugs
Stachybotrys	A possible cause of lung bleeding in infants, as discussed in the text

Data from U.S. EPA (1997).

[a]No specific species has been shown to cause a higher hazard than any others to the public at large, although certain people may be sensitive to a specific species of fungus.

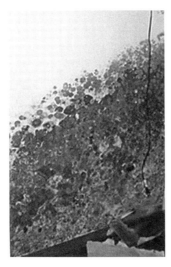

Figure 11.1. Mold on a wall surface, indicative of water damage. (Photo courtesy of Disaster Contractors Network; www.DCNonline.org.)

Mold as an Allergen

Inhaling mold spores, even at low concentrations, can produce hypersensitivity (allergic) reactions in predisposed individuals, such as those with previously diagnosed asthma or allergic rhinitis. Some people react to many different mold species, whereas others react to only certain ones. These reactions include many nonspecific symptoms:

- stuffy or runny nose
- difficulty breathing
- worsening of asthma
- chest tightness
- headache
- altered sense of smell or seeming to smell unusual odors
- fatigue.

Mold as a Toxin

Mold also frequently produces various chemicals as part of its growth. Some of these are large chemical molecules called mycotoxins. Some of these mycotoxins produce toxic reactions in rats and other selected species. Aflatoxin B (found on moldy peanuts and to a lesser extent in grains and other ag-

ricultural products which have been stored damp) is recognized as a cause of human liver cancer. However, it is not clear whether mycotoxins other than aflatoxin B cause cancer in people (Burge 2002; McConnell et al. 2003) Aflatoxin has caused jaundice and liver failure after consumption of maize that had been stored under damp conditions (Nyikal et al. 2004).

Mycotoxin compounds are generally large molecules that do not evaporate easily. They are too large to penetrate through intact skin after contact. To date, it has not been shown that these mycotoxins become airborne in quantities sufficient to cause toxic effects in humans after inhalation (Burge 2002).

Toxic illnesses were suspected in some studies of subjects after exposure to concentrated fungal trichothecene mycotoxins during the Vietnam War ("yellow rain"; Sudakin 2003). Investigators with the U.S. Centers for Disease Control and Prevention (CDC) initially attributed pulmonary hemorrhage (bleeding into the lungs) in several infants in Cleveland, Ohio, to the presence of *Stachybotrys chartarum* in the homes of these infants (CDC 1994). It was never clearly established whether these illnesses were due to toxins produced by *Stachybotrys,* to infection, or to other factors. Subsequently, other experts who reviewed these data disagreed with the conclusions of the original investigators. The study was eventually withdrawn by a CDC review panel because of problems with experimental design, though the investigators continue to express confidence in their original findings (CDC 1999, 2000; Montana et al. 1997). The Institute of Medicine (IOM) of the National Academy of Sciences, an organization well regarded for its intellectual rigor and credibility, was asked to investigate the matter independently. In its draft report, a study committee of the IOM concluded that the available data did not provide enough evidence to confirm that *Stachybotrys* had caused the children's illnesses (Institute of Medicine 2004).

Fungal Infection

Human skin infections caused by fungi are common, especially under persistently moist conditions. Common names for these infections are athlete's foot, jock itch, and thrush. These infections rarely spread beyond the skin and are caused by different species of fungi from those commonly encountered in indoor air.

People with cancer, HIV infection, or other immune abnormalities are at higher risk of fungal infection after exposure to mold spores. Before any infection within the body can occur, the fungus must penetrate the body's first line of defense. The skin provides an excellent barrier and prevents spores that land on the skin from entering the body. The nasal passages and airways make it difficult for particles larger than 10 microns to enter the lungs, and fungal spores are generally large enough for these defenses to work effectively (Kuhn and Ghannoum 2003).

Symptoms Reported after Mold Exposure

Many people in homes and schools where mold is visible complain of multiple symptoms, including musty odor, a general feeling of illness (malaise), irritability, headaches, deteriorated school performance, lack of concentration, and digestive problems. Several studies have demonstrated a higher incidence of breathing problems in people who live in moist homes, with or without identified mold growth (McConnell et al. 2003; Stark et al. 2003). On the basis of this and other evidence, the IOM concluded that mold and other factors related to damp conditions in homes and other buildings are associated with a worsening of asthma symptoms in sensitized people, as well as to coughing, wheezing, and upper respiratory tract symptoms in otherwise healthy people. However, the IOM committee did not find sufficient evidence to support or refute mold as the cause of these findings (Institute of Medicine 2004).

Given our current state of knowledge, we cannot clearly show that molds cause other effects on human health. One group of health-care providers, sometimes known as clinical ecologists, attribute numerous health problems to mold, ranging from immune dysfunction to heart disease to altered intellectual function. Some of these providers treat such patients with large doses of antifungal medications and diet modifications, which they believe will reduce fungal growth. Not only do these practices have potential adverse effects of their own, but there is also no evidence to support this nonstandard approach.

It remains to be determined whether these clinical effects are caused by the various mold species capable of producing toxins. It is possible that mold is actually the cause of the health problems, but it is also possible that the problems are caused by other factors present in buildings (Hardin et al. 2003). For example, conditions that are frequently observed in such indoor settings might include viral illnesses, irritant illnesses caused by high particulate levels in the air, poor air quality due to inadequate fresh air intake, and problems created by vehicles idling near the fresh-air intakes of buildings. Determining the exact cause of illness is difficult when multiple factors are present.

Concerns about Long-term Effects

Information about the long-term effects of mold exposure is lacking. In many cases, patients with asthma-like symptoms triggered by mold need long-term management for asthma. Their condition seems to remain stable or gradually improve with ongoing treatment.

Recognizing and Managing Mold Overgrowth

The checklist in box 11.1 offers an overview of our recommended approach to a mold problem (U.S. Environmental Protection Agency, 2001).

Mold overgrowth may be noted visually. Given that mold is ubiquitous in the air in most climates, it is not unusual to find small areas of mold growth in damp settings such as showers or baths. However, the presence of extensive mold is not expected, and visible patches of mold on walls, ceilings, or floors indicate a need for further evaluation and management of the situation. Investigation of the cause of unusual odors or assessment of people with symptoms may also disclose the presence of high concentrations of mold.

The EPA and a number of other organizations have developed guidelines for the remediation and cleanup of mold and moisture problems in schools and commercial buildings. These guidelines include measures designed to protect the health of both building occupants and remediators (U.S. Environmental Protection Agency 2001). The guidelines have been designed primarily for building managers, custodians, and others responsible for commercial building and school maintenance and should serve as a reference for potential mold and moisture remediators. When a substantial mold problem is discovered in a school or home, outside assistance may be warranted. Consultants may offer to evaluate the severity of the problem, as well as mitigate the mold overgrowth. The EPA mold-remediation document and other sources can help those with little or no experience with mold remediation to make a reasonable judgment as to whether a situation can be handled in house. These resources help those in charge of maintenance to evaluate an in-house remediation plan or a plan for services submitted by an outside contractor.

Before hiring an outside contractor, school officials should decide whether they want advice only, abatement of the problem, or a strategic plan for resolving the problem, which often includes participation in the process of addressing the issues with impacted groups. Consultant services may offer spore counts, identification of the mold species present, or comparison of indoor and outdoor mold conditions.

Before deciding which, if any, of these services should be performed, school administrators should decide how the data will affect the actions to be taken. It is important to recognize that there are no well-established standards for interpretation of these data; there is as yet no clearly established threshold above which too much mold is present. Mold spore counts within a building are often compared with counts taken immediately outside the building at the same time. However, it is unclear how outdoor weather conditions at the time of the sampling affect the validity of this comparison. For example, measuring spore counts during or immediately after a rainstorm may not provide the same results as those obtained several days after the last rain. Similarly, it is not clear how indoor values can be appropriately compared with outdoor counts obtained in winter in colder climates versus those obtained in summer. Moreover, there is at present no pathway for certification or licensure of contractors who offer to measure, identify, or eradicate mold (U.S. Environmental Protection Agency 2002).

Mold Abatement

Regardless of whether mold is the cause of these problems, there is clearly no benefit in having it present. The best approach to mold is to clean it up and dry out the building.

Particularly where mold is a problem, indoor humidity should be reduced to less than 50–60%, and adequate airflow throughout the structure should be established. Mold growing on nonporous surfaces such as tile or rock can generally be eradicated by the application of household bleach or several other household cleaners according to their label directions. On porous surfaces, it is difficult, if not impossible, to permanently remove mold infestations once they are established. The entire area may need to be removed and replaced (California Department of Health Services 2003; New York City Department of Health and Mental Hygiene 2002; U.S. Environmental Protection Agency 2001). Here, too, there is variation among published mold-removal strategies.

More extensive cleanup may extend to air-handling ducts if they are also involved in the problem. It seems reasonable that removal of mold from the ductwork near the site of the infestation would be helpful, but the health impact of this practice is unproven (U.S. Environmental Protection Agency 1997). The likely benefits decrease, and the costs mount, as the distance from the site of the problem increases.

The topic of mold control in schools is addressed in the EPA's Tools for Schools publication (2000). In a school setting, the school management must respond quickly to complaints of mold issues. The appropriate response will depend on many factors, including the extent of the problem, its location, and other damage that may have occurred to the building. For example, if a recently flooded area becomes moldy, it must be dried out well and the damaged area repaired; at the same time, remaining patches of mold should be cleaned or removed. The area of damage should be closed to further use and its ventilation separated from the occupied part of the school until all of these goals are accomplished. On the other hand, in a school gym shower, mold on tile should be removed by the use of appropriate cleaners, and ventilation should be improved, but the area can generally return to routine use quite soon.

In a home situation, the family may have vacated its home during remediation. In a school setting, such decisions are made more difficult by the large number of people potentially impacted. If abatement of visual mold can be quickly accom-

▨ *11.1. Checklist for mold remediation*

Investigate and evaluate moisture and mold problems:

- Assess size of moldy area (square feet).
- Consider the possibility of hidden mold.
- Clean up small mold problems, and fix moisture problems before they get worse.
- Consider selecting a remediation manager for medium-to-large mold problems.
- Investigate areas associated with occupants' complaints.
- Identify source or cause of water or moisture problems.
- Check inside air ducts and air handlers.
- Obtain professional assistance where desired or necessary.

Communications with involved individuals:

- Designate contact person for questions and comments.
- Share information about problem and planned approach with involved staff, parents, and students, as appropriate.

Plan remediation

- Adopt or adapt remediation guidelines to fit the specific circumstances.
- To prevent mold growth, dry the wet material within 48 hours of its becoming wet, as per EPA guidelines,.
- Clean up moldy items, as per EPA guidelines and/or other expert advice.
- Contain extensive mold outbreaks to prevent further spread and to protect building occupants.
- To implement the remediation plan, select personnel who have the necessary skills, training, and experience.

Carry out remediation

- Fix moisture problems.
- Carry out repair plans as appropriate.
- Dry wet materials before they become moldy (within 48 hours).
- Clean and dry materials that are already moldy, or remove and discard them if they cannot be cleaned.

(Adapted from U.S. Environmental Protection Agency 2001) ▨

---

plished, and if airflow can be adjusted and filtration established to reduce the circulating mold to a tolerable level, vacating the building may not be necessary. Where the mold infestation is substantial, it is wise to cordon off the area under renovation until remediation is substantially completed. When considerable mold is present, it is also prudent to ensure that the ventilation for the affected area is separate from the air circulating through the remainder of the school building.

Prevention

Helping people who complain of various symptoms attributed to mold is challenging. There are currently no specific diagnostic tests to confirm or refute the role of mold. In addition to avoidance of directly affected areas, those who are experiencing symptoms must seek medical care after ruling out other causes. For example, symptoms that are thought to be allergen mediated can be managed with antihistamines, asthma control drugs (such as inhaled corticosteroids and leukotriene antagonists), and bronchodilators, as appropriate.

Conclusions

Our knowledge of the effects of mold on humans is incomplete. Currently we are aware of potential risk and no potential benefits of mold in schools and other buildings. When substantial indoor mold growth is noted, steps should be taken to eliminate the conditions that led to its development and to eradicate the mold to the extent practicable. People who become ill after exposure to mold should seek medical care to address their symptoms, even if it is unclear whether the mold infestation or other factors may have caused the illness. Additional epidemiologic and clinical research is needed to address the multiple issues associated with mold infestation.

References

Burge HA. 2002. An update on pollen and fungal spore aerobiology. J Allergy Clin Immunol 110: 544–552.

California Department of Health Services. 2003. Mold in my school: What do I do? National Clearinghouse for Educational Facilities. Available: http://www.edfacilities.org/pubs/mold.html [accessed 29 December 2005].

Centers for Disease Control and Prevention. 1994. Acute pulmonary hemosiderosis among infants, Cleveland, January 1993–November 1994. Mortal Morbid Weekly Rept 43:881–883.

Centers for Disease Control and Prevention. 1999. Reports of members of the CDC External Expert Panel on Acute Idiopathic Pulmonary Hemorrhage in Infants: A synthesis. Available: http://www.cdc.gov/mold/pdfs/aiphi_report.pdf [accessed 29 December 2005].

Centers for Disease Control and Prevention. 2000. Update: Pulmonary hemorrhage/hemosiderosis among infants, Cleveland, Ohio, 1993–1996. Mortal Morbid Weekly Rept 49(9):180–184.

Etzel RA, Montana E, Sorenson WG, Kullman GJ, Allan TM, Dearborn DG, Olson DR, Jarvis BB, Miller JD. 1998. Acute pulmonary hemorrhage in infants associated with exposure to *Stachybotrys atra* and other fungi. Archives of Pediatrics and Adolescent Medicine 152(8):757–762.

Hardin BD, Kelman BJ, Saxon A. 2003. Council on Scientific Affairs, American College of Occupational and Environmental Medicine evidence-based statement: Adverse human health effects associated with molds in the indoor environment. J Occup Environ Med 45:470–478.

Institute of Medicine, Committee on Damp Indoor Spaces and Health. 2004. Damp indoor spaces and health. Washington, DC: National Academy of Sciences, 1–14.

Kuhn DM, Ghannoum MA. 2003. Indoor mold, toxigenic fungi, and *Stachybotrys chartarum:* Infectious disease perspective. Clin Microbiol Rev 16:144–172.

McConnell R, Berhane K, Gilliland F, Molitor J, Thomas D, Lurmann F, et al. 2003. Prospective study of air pollution and bronchitic symptoms in children with asthma. Am J Respir Crit Care Med 168: 790–797.

Montana E, Etzel RA, Allan T, Horgan TE, Dearborn DG. 1997. Environmental risk factors associated with pediatric idiopathic pulmonary hemorrhage and hemosiderosis in a Cleveland community. Pediatrics 99:117–124.

New York City Department of Health and Mental Hygiene, Bureau of Environmental and Occupational Disease Epidemiology. 2002. Guidelines on assessment and remediation of fungi in indoor environments. Available: http://www.ci.nyc.ny.us/html/doh/html/epi/moldrpt1.shtml [accessed 29 December 2005].

Nyikal J et al. 2004. Outbreak of Aflatoxin Poisoning–Eastern and Central Provinces, Kenya, January–July 2004. Mortal Morbid Weekly Rept 53: 790–793.

Random House Dictionary of the English Language, 2d ed. 1987. New York: Random House.

Stark PC, Burge HA, Ryan LM, Milton DK, Gold DR. 2003. Fungal levels in the home and lower respiratory tract illnesses in the first year of life. Am J Respir Crit Care Med 168:232–237.

Storey E, Dangman KH, Schenck P, DeBernardo RL, Yang CS, Bracker A, Hodgson MJ. 2004. Guidance for clinicians on the recognition and management of health effects related to mold exposure and moisture indoors. Farmington, CT: University of Connecticut Health Center. Available: http://oehc.uchc.edu/clinser/MOLD%20GUIDE.pdf [accessed 3 December 2004].

Sudakin DL. 2003. Trichothecenes in the environment: Relevance to human health. Toxicol Lett 143:97–107.

U.S. Environmental Protection Agency. 1997. Should you have the air ducts in your home cleaned? EPA-

402-K-97-002. Washington, DC: U.S. Environmental Protection Agency. Available: http://www.epa.gov/iaq/pubs/airduct.html [accessed 29 Dec 2005].

U.S. Environmental Protection Agency. 2000. Indoor air quality tools for schools program. Second Edition. EPA 402-K-95-001. Washington, DC: U.S. Environmental Protection Agency.

U.S. Environmental Protection Agency. 2001. Mold remediation in schools and commercial buildings. EPA 402-K-01-001. Washington, DC: U.S. Environmental Protection Agency. Available: http://www.epa.gov/iaq/molds/mold_remediation.html [accessed 11 February 2004].

U.S. Environmental Protection Agency. 2002. Indoor air—mold/moisture: Mold resources. Washington, DC: U.S. Environmental Protection Agency.

U.S. Environmental Protection Agency. 2003. Indoor air quality design tools for schools. Washington, DC: U.S. Environmental Protection Agency. Available: http://www.epa.gov/iaq/schooldesign/index.html [accessed 29 December 2005].

Andrea Hricko

Outdoor Air Pollution

■ *Summary*

- Outdoor (ambient) air pollution presents a number of issues in the school environment, including exposure of children to diesel exhaust from older buses, potential risks for students who play or exercise outdoors on smoggy days, and exposure to emissions from nearby traffic and industrial facilities.
- The current asthma epidemic raises additional concerns since air pollution exacerbates and may even cause asthma.
- There are a variety of ways to assess air pollution in the area surrounding the school and there are steps that school administrators can take to protect children and address pollution. ■

Outdoor air pollution continues to present a serious public health problem, especially for children, a vulnerable population (see box 12.1). Exposure to air pollution, even at levels that the government currently allows, is linked to a variety of adverse respiratory health effects in children, among them decreased lung function, increased symptoms of and hospitalizations for respiratory illnesses, and aggravation of asthma. Because children (as well as

teachers and staff) spend so much of their day at school, the air in that environment can affect their health. If the air pollution levels are high, precautions must be considered for children who are playing or exercising outdoors. Travel to and from school can also present special concerns, as can school siting.

Background

Ambient air refers to the outdoor air in a neighborhood or community, as opposed to the air inside buildings such as homes and schools. Children spend part of many school days outdoors, whether during recess or in walking between school buildings. However, outdoor air does not simply stay outside. It can get into a building through open windows and doors and penetrate in other, more subtle, ways, including through openings, joints, and cracks in walls, floors, and ceilings, and around windows and doors.

Air pollution in communities with high ozone levels is often referred to as smog. Two of the key constituents of smog are ozone and particles (particulate matter). Under the federal Clean Air Act, both ozone and particles are regulated, along with

141

four other key pollutants: carbon monoxide, lead, nitrogen dioxide, and sulfur dioxide. Other pollutants are found in the air from vehicle exhaust, road dust, fires, fuel combustion, industrial facilities, power plants, consumer products, and other sources. Some of these pollutants are considered air toxics and are subject to regulation.

Key Air Pollutants

Ozone

Ozone is formed by chemical reactions that occur primarily from the action of sunlight on hydrocarbons and nitrogen oxides emitted in fuel combustion. Studies have shown that ozone exposure is associated with reduced lung function, shortness of breath, chest pain, wheezing and coughing, asthma exacerbation, and poorer athletic performance (Thurston and Bates 2003). Emerging evidence suggests that ozone exposure may even increase the risk of developing asthma (McConnell et al. 2002). High ozone levels are a problem in nearly 500 counties in 31 states, according to the U.S. Environmental Protection Agency (EPA 2004). Ozone levels vary by season and time of day. Levels are typically higher in the summer and early fall and lower in the winter; levels are higher in the mid-to-late afternoon than in the morning and evening.

Particulate Matter

Particulate matter (PM), made up of tiny specks of dust, soot, or aerosol in the air, can come from vehicle tailpipes, factories, refineries, power plants, ships, locomotives, planes, forest fires, dust storms, and other sources. The tiniest of these particles, called ultrafine particles, typically result from the combustion of fuel. When inhaled, ultrafine particles can deposit in the lungs and, in animal studies, have been shown to get into the brain (Oberdorster et al. 2004). Particles may be dangerous in and of themselves, but they also have many harmful chemicals on their surfaces that can be carried into the body. Studies link particulate matter exposure to increased respiratory and cardiovascular illnesses and death, especially among the elderly and those with preexisting heart and lung disease (Pope et al. 2004) and diabetes (Bateson and Schwartz 2004).

Carbon Monoxide

Carbon monoxide (CO) comes from the combustion of fuel and is emitted by motor vehicles. Exposure to CO can alter the body's ability to supply oxygen to the organs, and at very high levels (such as from faulty venting of a gas heater) can result in sleepiness, unconsciousness, and death. CO levels are higher within 500 feet of busy roadways, according to studies done in communities with high traffic volumes (Zhu et al. 2002a, 2002b). Studies in Los Angeles, California, showed a relationship between CO levels (and other indicators of heavy traffic exposure) and both birth defects and low birth weight in babies of exposed mothers (Ritz and Yu 1999; Ritz et al. 2000).

Nitrogen Dioxide

Nitrogen dioxide (NO_2) results from chemical interactions in the air when nitric oxide (NO) is emitted by vehicles or through fuel combustion. NO_2 is a precursor of smog. NO_2 has been linked to a decrease in lung function growth and acute respiratory problems. It is unclear whether NO_2 causes these effects directly or whether it serves as a marker for other traffic-related pollutants. That is, there may be some other pollutant in traffic exhaust that is actually responsible for the health effects.

Sulfur Dioxide

Sulfur dioxide (SO_2) is emitted from industrial facilities such as power plants. Sulfur dioxide emissions are a problem particularly in Eastern and Midwestern states, where they have contributed to acid rain. Children with asthma may be especially sensitive even to low concentrations of SO_2 (ATSDR 1999).

Lead

Lead was a serious air pollution problem until its use in gasoline was finally phased out in the U.S. in the late 1970s. The average blood lead levels of children in the United States have dropped dramatically since that time—a public health success story. Today the main exposure sources for lead in the school environment are flaking lead-based paint, drinking water from systems with old leaded pipes, and contaminated soil. (See chapter 15 for more information on these sources and on the health effects of lead.) However, some communities may have smelters, metal scrap recycling operations, battery manufacturing plants or other factories that emit lead. These sources are of particular concern, as lead emissions can contaminate the air, soil, and workers' clothes; health problems can result in children whose homes or schools are nearby or whose parents work at the plant and bring their work clothes home.

Air Toxics

There are also hundreds of different air toxics—toxic chemicals released into the air from local air pollution sources such as neighborhood dry cleaning shops, refineries, or automobiles. Several hundred of these compounds are regulated by the Federal Clean Air Act. Air toxics are of concern because of their chronic (long-term) effects. In this chapter we discuss several air toxics that pose significant risk to children's health.

Health Effects of Selected Air Toxics

Diesel Exhaust

Diesel exhaust is emitted by diesel trucks, buses, cars, locomotives, ships, and a variety of off-road equipment. The health effects of diesel exhaust exposure include eye and respiratory irritation, asthma exacerbation, and increased cancer risk. Scientific studies also show that when people with allergies are exposed to diesel exhaust, they have increased allergic reactions, including allergic rhi-

nitis (hay fever–like symptoms), and that the genes of some people make them even more susceptible to diesel exhaust (Gilliland et al. 2004). In animal studies, researchers have shown that breathing diesel exhaust particles may be enough to induce acute asthma attacks (Hao et al. 2003).

Dioxins

Dioxin and dioxin-like chemicals are produced during incomplete combustion of chlorine-containing wastes like municipal solid waste, sewage sludge, and hospital and hazardous wastes. Studies of workers link dioxin exposure to increased risk of cancer and animal studies have demonstrated reproductive effects (EPA 2003). The proximity of schools to incinerators or hazardous waste sites is of concern.

Polycyclic Organic Compounds

Polycyclic organic matter (POM) is a class of chemicals comprising 100 different compounds, including polycyclic aromatic hydrocarbons (PAHs) such as benzo[a]pyrene. Most of these chemicals are attached to particulate matter. They arise from combustion processes such as forest fires, wood burning, agricultural burning, smoking of tobacco, and vehicle exhaust. Children may be exposed in the school environment, as POM can get indoors from the outdoor air, especially at schools near industrial or agricultural operations or freeways.

Acrolein

Acrolein is produced from the combustion of fossil fuels, tobacco, and forest fires. It is a by-product of atmospheric reactions involving 1,3-butadiene from vehicle exhaust and is also an ingredient in certain pesticides. Animal studies indicate that acrolein exacerbates asthma.

Cigarette Smoke

Both POM and acrolein are constituents of tobacco smoke. School administrators, nurses, and teachers might consider discussing the toxic chemicals in cigarette smoke in antismoking educational programs at their schools and include efforts to get parents to stop smoking as well.

Health Effects of Key Air Pollutants on Children

We have known for years that breathing high levels of air pollution (ozone, particles, and other pollutants) can cause acute changes in health, such as nasal congestion, irritated eyes, coughing, chest tightness or congestion, wheezing, and inability to breathe deeply. These short-term effects resolve when the person breathes cleaner air. Studies show the following:

- When ozone levels go up, the number of school absences due to acute respiratory illness increases (Gilliland 2001).
- When levels of ozone and particulate air pollution increase, children with asthma have more emergency room visits and hospital admissions (Peel et al. 2005)
- When air pollution levels decrease (e.g., during the Olympics in Atlanta, when traffic was reduced, and during a period in Utah when steel mill workers were on strike), children's health improves, with fewer hospital visits and admissions for respiratory problems (Friedman et al. 2001; Pope 1996).

Less is known about the chronic effects of air pollution. For the past 10 years, researchers at the University of Southern California have studied the chronic effects of air pollution on the health of school children in the Children's Health Study (CHS). They have followed thousands of children who attend schools in more than a dozen different communities with differing levels and types of air pollution. Some of their key findings (summarized in Kunzli et al. 2003) are:

- Lung function growth is slower in school children living in communities with higher pollution levels. In fact, by age 18 a higher percentage of children who grew up in polluted communities with high levels of particles and NO_2 have underdeveloped lungs compared to children in low air pollution communities (Gauderman et al. 2004).
- Lung function grows more rapidly when school children move away from more polluted communities to areas where particle levels are lower.
- Children with asthma have more bronchitis and persistent phlegm (mucous that makes them keep trying to clear their throats) when they live in more polluted communities.
- Children who play outdoor team sports and spend more time outside in high ozone communities have a higher incidence of newly diagnosed asthma. When the CHS looked at the students who exercised the most, those who played three or more sports and also lived in the communities with high ozone levels were found to have about a threefold increased risk of developing new asthma. By epidemiological standards, that is a very high risk (McConnell 2002).

Adults, especially the elderly and the ill, are also at risk of chronic health effects from air pollution. Studies show links between air pollution and lung cancer, and new concerns have also been raised about particle pollution and excess deaths from heart- or lung-related illnesses in older people and those who are ill.

Air Pollution and School Concerns

Health, economic, transportation, recreation, and urban planning concerns intersect around the issue of air pollution in the school environment.

School Absences

In the CHS, school absence rates increased as the levels of ozone increased. The study determined that nearly twice as many children are absent from school several days after the levels of ozone exceed state standards (Gilliland et al. 2001). This means that, as the air pollution gets worse, more children miss school. Further, when a young student misses school, someone typically misses work to take care of the sick child, meaning lost wages and lost productivity. An analysis of the CHS data calculated that reducing high levels of ozone could save approximately $67 million every year in Southern California alone in costs related to school absences, an average of $75 per year for every student. For many school districts, fewer school absences would also mean more money in the school budget, as daily student enrollment is often linked to state funding. More significant is the fact that a child who misses school regularly because of illness can easily get behind in schoolwork and may suffer academically.

Air Pollution on the Way to School

The mere act of being transported to school, whether in a school bus or car on a busy highway or freeway, can create some of the worst air pollution exposures during a child's day. A California Air Resources Board (CARB) study found that levels of pollutants in cars can be very high during the busiest commute time on freeways with high traffic volume (Rodes et al. 1998). A study on air pollution inside North Carolina state police vehicles also found that pollution was higher inside cars than outside (Riediker et al. 2003). Another CARB-funded study concluded that school children who ride in conventional diesel-fueled school buses are exposed to high levels of air pollutants from the school bus diesel exhaust seeping into the bus cabin, as well as from outside traffic (Fitz et al. 2003).

Diesel exhaust (see fig. 12.1) is a concern because it is linked to both cancer and asthma. The CARB bus study found air pollution levels two to five times higher inside regular diesel school buses than in diesel buses equipped with particulate traps or in compressed natural gas (CNG) buses. The two most significant scenarios for high exposure to pollutants on buses occurred when the bus windows were closed (pollutant levels were several times higher than when the windows were open) and when the windows were open and the bus was in traffic behind trucks or other buses (the pollutant levels inside the school bus were very high). Other children arriving at school and people at the school who were helping with loading and unloading the buses were exposed to diesel pollution as the buses arrived and departed. For the students commuting by bus, however, exposures inside the bus were much more significant than exposures that students experienced while getting on or off the bus or waiting to load.

Exhaust from gasoline-fueled cars and sport utility vehicles (SUVs) also contains hundreds of toxic chemicals that are harmful to health. Thus, school administrators should also be aware that the lineup of cars outside schoolyards during drop-off and pickup times can also create unusual amounts of air pollution. This is a particular concern in lower-income communities, where many of the cars are older and may not have appropriate pollution controls, or in more affluent communities, where many of the cars are SUVs that pollute more than regular cars and have fewer air pollution restrictions.

School Exercise and Outdoor Sports Practice

Regular exercise is critical for the health of school-aged children. In the face of high levels of community air pollution, however, school administrators are faced with difficult decisions about exercise, whether for recess, physical education, band or cheerleading practice, or team sports (see fig. 12.2). Precautions need to be taken because children breathe harder when they exercise. In fact, exercising heavily increases ventilation rates (how many breaths per minute someone takes), which

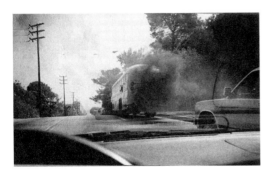

Figure 12.1. Diesel exhaust fumes from school buses can reach high levels both along the roadway and inside the school bus. (Photo by Andrea Hricko.)

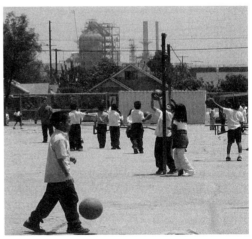

Figure 12.2. Children playing outside their school, near an industrial facility that may pollute the air. (Photo by Andrea Hricko.)

means breathing in a greater dose of airborne pollutants.

Air Pollution and School Siting

Only recently have scientists begun to consider what happens to the respiratory health of children who live or attend school near roads with heavy traffic. There is now compelling evidence that people whose homes or schools are close to busy roads have higher exposure to vehicle emissions than those who are farther away. For example, levels of ultrafine particles from vehicle emissions are 25 times higher right next to a busy freeway in Los Angeles than just 50 meters (165 feet) away (Zhu et al. 2002a, 2002b). Evidence also suggests that people in these situations may suffer adverse respiratory effects. In the Netherlands, studies of children who live near major roadways found decreased lung function and increased respiratory illness, particularly related to high volumes of diesel truck traffic (van Vliet et al. 1997). Dutch researchers also found that asthma is more often reported in children living within 100 meters of a freeway. Other scientific studies are now raising concerns about birth outcomes in mothers who live in high-traffic areas during their pregnancies, as an increase in premature births, certain birth defects, and even infant deaths has been observed (Kim 2004). The proximity of homes, daycare centers, schools, parks, and playing fields to busy freeways and roads is an emerging issue that school districts, residents, and local planning officials must consider, especially when siting new schools. In addition, it is not just air pollution that is an issue; noise from busy roads close to schools can also impact learning (see chapter 4).

Similarly, students and school staff may be at risk if a school is located close to a polluting factory. For example, chrome-plating plants next to homes and schools are coming under closer scrutiny, especially in low-income, minority neighborhoods. A chrome-plating facility next to a public school in downtown Los Angeles was the target of a 2004 lawsuit by the city attorney, who charged the facility with environmental contamination and cited environmental injustices. The chrome-plating factory, which was considered an inappropriate land use or zoning decision, was constructed after the school was built. In San Diego, California, a chrome-plating facility was shut down by the government after elevated levels of hexavalent chromium were found in adjacent homes. These actions were prompted by local residents, school staff, or parents of students who complained of respiratory and other illnesses. In each case, a community-based organization worked with the community to investigate the problem as an environmental justice issue, arguing that a polluting factory next to a home or school would not be allowed in a more affluent community (Environmental Health Coalition 2002).

Is There an Air Pollution Problem at the School?

To determine the types of outdoor air pollution problems a school may have, school administrators should be encouraged to form a committee to assess the problem. The committee would (1) investigate the levels of air pollution, the times of day during which the levels are highest, and nearby sources of pollution; (2) study students' transportation patterns; (3) conduct an inventory of the school bus fleet, and (4) determine what time of day outdoor practices are held for team sports, cheerleading, marching band, and other groups.

The regional air pollution district is a likely first stop in determining the levels of air pollution in the community. That agency's Internet site may allow a search for community air pollution levels to determine whether ozone is a problem there and whether there is a pattern of higher air pollution in the afternoon. Some communities also report area air pollution readings in the daily newspaper. At the national level, the EPA, through its AIRNow program, has maps showing current air quality and next-day forecasts for selected communities (see the list of resources at the end of this chapter).

Conducting an informal inventory of roads and businesses within one-quarter mile of the school, where exposures might be greatest, is another valuable tool to assess the potential risks a school might face. If the school has regular staff meetings, this process might be started by simply sharing the following information:

- distance to the closest busy roads (north, south, east, west)
- distance to other roads with a high volume of trucks or cars

- distance to the closest businesses, ports, rail yards, and factories
- information about the manufacturing (or otherwise polluting) processes at these sites.

At that point, if there are concerns, a committee could be formed to investigate further. For example, the local air pollution control authority may have information on emissions or violations from any of the identified facilities, and traffic counts may be available from the city's transportation department. High volumes of vehicles on nearby roads are of concern, especially when heavy-duty diesel trucks constitute a large percentage of the traffic. This information may be useful in determining routes that school bus drivers should avoid as air pollution inside buses can increase as a result of the outdoor traffic.

To identify industrial facilities that are large polluters, interested school personnel can turn to a number of databases. The EPA maintains the Toxics Release Inventory, which covers emissions of 650 toxic chemicals from facilities that emit significant amounts of the chemicals. The online U.S. EPA Envirofacts database (see the list of resources at the end of this chapter) allows Internet users to search for facilities and their emissions data by inputting the ZIP code of a school. Once the names of nearby facilities are obtained, the local air pollution control authority may be able to contribute additional information on emissions or violations. The Environmental Defense web site also has information on toxic releases (see resources). The Los Angeles Unified School District maintains a database of industrial facilities near schools (see resources). Finally, many states have their own databases that identify industrial facilities and their emissions of certain toxic chemicals, as does California with its Air Toxics Hotspots program (see resources). Once the school committee has identified these nearby fixed sources of pollutants, a qualified scientist should measure the levels of the pollutants of most concern at the school to better assess the impact of these emissions on the school's occupants.

Transportation services personnel may already have conducted an inventory of how students get to and from school. This is a useful assessment tool to determine how many students ride the bus, how many walk or bicycle, how many come in private cars, and whether any students take public or other forms of transportation. An important addition to this assessment is an analysis of bus routes and the length of time that students are on the bus. This information will help determine whether shorter bus routes are possible to reduce student exposure to diesel exhaust. Counting the number of students who come in private cars and taking photographs during morning drop-off and afternoon pickup times can help reveal problem areas. Alternative drop-off and pickup locations might be needed to reduce vehicle congestion and thereby decrease air pollution. School districts that are interested in encouraging more students to walk to school (after considering all of the safety implications) might consult the KidsWalk-to-School web site of the Centers for Disease Control and Prevention or consider a Walk to School Day to jumpstart their program (see resources and chapter 22).

A valuable part of the transportation assessment is an inventory of school buses to document their age and the type of fuel they use. From this information, school authorities can decide how to prioritize funding decisions on school bus replacements or retrofits, beginning with the oldest (and most polluting) buses.

Address Air Pollution at Schools

What to Do on Bad Air Days

School personnel have a responsibility to take appropriate actions at schools when the air quality is expected to reach unhealthy levels, which typically occurs in large urban areas every year between the beginning of May and the end of September.

If the regional air pollution control authority has a program to notify schools of bad air days or to inform them of the air quality index (AQI), the school should ask to be notified. (See chapter 28 for a full explanation of the AQI.) If the region does not have such a program, schools can try to work with the agency to develop one or establish a useful way to notify parents, students, teachers, coaches, school nurses, and other school personnel about air quality concerns (see box 12.2).

On days with bad air quality, one precaution is to keep the windows closed. Another is to ensure that the school's ventilation system is working effectively (see chapters 5 and 10). Ideally, schools in high-ozone or high-particle communities will have air-conditioning. In addition, schools can

▨ *12.2. Asthma-friendly flag program*

In 2004, the Merced/Mariposa County (California) Asthma Coalition developed an "Asthma-friendly Flag Program." The purpose of the program is to reduce or limit students' exposure to poor air quality, especially during outdoor sporting activities. The program is based on the U.S. EPA's AQI color code, with green flags denoting good air quality; yellow, moderate air quality; orange, unsafe for sensitive populations; and red, unhealthy for everyone. Each day schools raise the appropriate colored flag based upon the air pollution control district's air quality forecast, which is sent by e-mail to schools the day before (around 4 PM). Individual school districts determine who within the school receives the e-mail alert and ensures the appropriate flag is raised. For example, in one district this could be the safety control officer, and in another district it could be a vice principal, who then instructs maintenance or grounds personnel to raise the flag. Schools are responsible for having alternative activities in place on orange and red days, on which it is advisable to limit or forgo outdoor activities. (Because obesity is a countywide concern, schools are encouraged to have in place active indoor alternatives to sporting activities.) In 2004, Merced and Mariposa counties experienced 114 orange days and 7 red days. By early 2006, 95 schools in Merced County and three hospitals were displaying the flags, and the program had been replicated in numerous California counties, by school districts, chapters of the American Lung Association, and other asthma coalitions. The flag program has been recognized across the state, where more than 500 schools now use it, and it has been endorsed by the California Department of Health Services and the Environmental Protection Agency as a "best practice" for schools.

(Interviews with Alicia Bohlke, June 16, 2004, and Mary-Michal Rawling, January 10, 2006, staff of the Merced/Mariposa County, California, Asthma Coalition) ▨

schedule outdoor activities in the early morning to minimize ozone exposure. Coaches and teachers should pay special attention to students on bad air–quality days to detect early respiratory symptoms.

School Siting

New legislation in California addresses the issue of siting new schools along heavily traveled corridors. The legislation bans new school construction within 500 feet of busy roads and freeways, although it does not address the 200 California schools that have already been built within 500 feet of a freeway.

The California Office of Environmental Health Hazard Assessment (OEHHA) has suggested ways to reduce the exposure of students and staff at schools near dense traffic areas, including ensuring that recreational areas and playing fields are located as far as possible from busy roads; avoiding exercise during rush hour; installing and regularly maintaining air-conditioning systems; installing portable air-conditioning units; and using HEPA filters at

schools with the most serious exposures. The OEHHA plans to issue guidelines for better protection of students at schools near busy highways (see resources). As dense traffic often goes hand in hand with noise, school administrators should demand that sound walls be built to protect children from excessive traffic noise, which distracts students from their school work and interferes with student-teacher communication.

Retrofitting and Replacement of Diesel Buses

Some school districts have successfully retrofitted school buses with particulate traps to capture the particle pollution or replaced large numbers of old diesel buses with new or alternative fuel buses. An often-cited case study is a school district in Ardmore, Pennsylvania, that started to replace many of its diesel buses with CNG buses in 1995 (see box 12.3). By 2004, 75% of the school bus fleet in Ardmore consisted of CNG buses. The director of pupil transportation services reports that the state envi-

■ *12.3. Case study: Lower Merion School District and CNG school buses*

Ten years ago, neighbors were complaining about noise and pollution from diesel buses at the school district's bus yard, which was located in a residential neighborhood. The Lower Merion School District (LMSD) in Ardmore, Pennsylvania, decided to begin a replacement program of compressed natural gas (CNG) buses for older diesel buses, using state and other grants to buy them and build refueling stations. As of February 2004, the LMSD fleet contained 107 buses, 72 of which were operating on CNG. According to the head of pupil transportation services, the program has been well received, the complaints of residents have stopped, and the state environmental protection agency is pleased with the pollution reductions achieved.

(Natural Resources Defense Council 1998; Michael Andre, supervisor, Student Transportation Services, Lower Merion School District, Ardmore, Pennsylvania, personal communication, February 2004) ■

ronmental protection agency is pleased with the pollution reductions the school district is achieving and that the CNG buses have been well received by drivers, even though the buses have required somewhat more maintenance. He reports that one of the biggest challenges is finding the money to build the two refueling stations, which cost $350,000 each (Michael Andre, Ardmore, Pennsylvania, personal communication, February 2004). Interim steps in reducing diesel exhaust are to shorten bus routes to reduce commute time, use the cleanest buses for the longest commutes, decrease bus caravanning, and decrease idling time.

Idling Restrictions

Many school districts, cities, and states have regulations that limit idling time for school buses. The school district or state air pollution enforcement agency may already have an anti-idling rule. The California Air Resources Board has adopted a measure to eliminate the unnecessary idling of school buses at or near schools (see resources). These rules state that the bus driver must turn off the engine upon stopping at or within 100 feet of a school and must not turn the engine on more than 30 seconds before departing from a school or from within 100 feet of a school. In addition, the driver cannot idle the bus for more than 5 minutes at any location greater than 100 feet from a school. This regulation might be a starting point for a school district's discussions on idling restrictions.

Educational Campaigns

In the interim, several educational measures can be considered. In May 2002, the State of Maine Departments of Education and Environmental Protection sent a letter to public school superintendents statewide, warning them of the adverse health effects caused by exposure to diesel exhaust and rec-

■ *12.4. Protecting against exposure to diesel exhaust from school buses*

- Develop a priority schedule, replacing the oldest buses with new low-emission buses.
- Consider buses that use alternative fuels such as compressed natural gas.
- Retrofit older buses with particle traps.
- Study commuting routes and try to shorten commute time.
- Use the cleanest buses on the longest trips.
- When weather permits, keep the windows open on the buses.
- Limit or eliminate school bus idling.
- Invite bus drivers into the school in cold weather so they do not idle the buses to stay warm.
- Change bus schedules so buses do not caravan.
- Encourage drivers to maintain a good distance behind diesel trucks and buses.

(Adapted from U.S. EPA Clean School Bus USA at http://www.epa.gov/cleanschoolbus) ■

ommending diesel emission reduction strategies. The following month, a pledge card and magnet were given to school bus drivers as a reminder to turn off engines in the schoolyard and limit morning warm-up time whenever possible. (For more information on these programs, copies of the Maine letter, and the informational campaign materials, see the U.S. EPA Region 1 web site listed in the resources section.)

Air Conditioning

Chapter 10 addresses indoor air in schools, including good ventilation and filtration systems. However, because outdoor air finds its way inside, the following is a good frame of reference: If the air quality is good, open the windows unless noise levels are a problem. If the air quality is bad, keep the windows closed. Air conditioning definitely reduces the levels of ozone in the air and is recommended for schools in communities with high levels of air pollution.

Checklist for School Administrators

To address outdoor air pollution, school administrators can take the following steps:

- Limit outdoor activities on high ozone days. Keep students indoors for recess and practices. Ideally, cancel late afternoon practices or switch them to the morning.
- Protect students from nearby industrial facilities, busy roads, and ports by at least ensuring that school recreational facilities are located on the school grounds as far as possible from these sources of pollutants.
- Contact the air pollution control authority with any concerns about sources of pollution very close to the school, and discuss the record of the polluting facility. If there are violations, voice your concerns.
- Demand sound walls and other mitigation measures (such as soundproofing and double-pane windows) to protect against excessive noise from nearby airports, roads, or businesses.
- Consider switching to nondiesel school buses or retrofitting existing buses.
- Work with bus drivers to shorten bus routes,

use the cleanest buses for the longest commutes, decrease bus caravanning, and develop other ideas for limiting exposure to diesel exhaust.
- Enforce idling restrictions for cars and buses in front of schools.
- Consider air-conditioning at schools where air pollution levels are high, especially those that conduct summer sessions.

Acknowledgments

This research was supported by grant 5 P30 ES07048 from the National Institute of Environmental Health Sciences (NIEHS); grant 5 P01 ES09581 from NIEHS; and grant RD 83186101 from the U.S. Environmental Protection Agency.

Resources

- A Breath of Air: What Air Pollution Is Doing to Our Children. Educational video about air pollution's health impacts on children, summarizing the results of the Children's Health Study (28 minutes). Produced by the Southern California Environmental Health Sciences Center and the Annenberg School for Communications, University of Southern California. 2003. Available in Spanish and English versions. Free. http://www.arb.ca.gov/research/health/school/chs-vpform.htm.
- California Air Resources Board site on school bus idling regulations http://www.arb.ca.gov/regact/sbidling/revfro.doc.
- California Air Resources Board site on Air Toxics Hotspots Program http://www.arb.ca.gov/ab2588/ab2588.htm.
- California legislation on school siting: See fact sheet titled Air Pollution from Nearby Traffic and Children's Health: Information for Schools. http://www.oehha.ca.gov/public_info/facts/pdf/Factsheetschools.pdf.
- California Office of Environmental Health Hazard Assessment. Forthcoming guidelines on reducing exposure to air pollution for students and staff at schools near busy roads http://www.oehha.ca.gov/.

- Centers for Disease Control and Prevention KidsWalk-to-School http://www.cdc.gov/nccdphp/dnpa/kidswalk/.
- Environmental Defense web site on toxic chemicals in your community's air http://www.scorecard.org
- U.S. EPA AIRNow program with air quality forecasts http://www.epa.gov/airnow/.
- U.S. EPA Clean School Bus USA web site http://www.epa.gov/cleanschoolbus.
- U.S. EPA Envirofacts web site, including information on accessing the Toxic Release Inventory database http://www.epa.gov/enviro/html/tris/tris_query .html.
- U.S. EPA Region 1 web site on retrofitting diesel school buses http://www.epa.gov/ne/eco/diesel/school _buses.html#sarsbi.
- Los Angeles Unified School District. Industrial facilities near LAUSD schools http://www.lausd-oehs.org/industrial.asp
- Natural Resources Defense Council web site with report on alternatives to diesel fuel http://www.nrdc.org/air/transportation/ebd/ chap6.asp.
- Office of Environmental Health Hazard Assessment (information on selected air toxics and their effects on children) http://www.oehha.ca.gov/public_info/facts/ airkids.html.
- Walk to School Day http://www.walktoschool-usa.org/.
- With Every Breath: Health Effects of Smog. Educational video produced by the California Air Resources Board (20 minutes). 2004. Available in Spanish and English versions. Free. http://www.arb.ca.gov/research/health/school/ school.htm.

References

Agency for Toxic Substances and Disease Registry. 1999. ATSDR ToxFAQs for Sulfur Dioxide. Atlanta, Georgia: ATSDR. Available: http://www .atsdr.cdc.gov/tfacts116.html.

Bateson TF, Schwartz J. 2004. Who is sensitive to the effects of particulate air pollution on mortality? A case-crossover analysis of effect modifiers. Epidemiology 15:143–149.

Environmental Health Coalition. 2002. No more waiting: People power stops chrome plating. ToxInformer 21(2). Available: http://www .environmentalhealth.org/ ToxieApr2002ChromeEng.htm [accessed 11 January 2006].

Fitz D, Winer A, Colome S. 2003. Characterizing the range of children's pollutant exposure during school bus commutes: California Air Resources Board. Available: http://www.arb.ca.gov/research/ schoolbus/schoolbus.htm [accessed 11 January 2006].

Friedman MS, Powell KE, Hutwagner L, 2001. Impact of changes in transportation and commuting behaviors during the 1996 Summer Olympic games in Atlanta on air quality and childhood asthma. J Am Med Assoc 285:897–905.

Gauderman WJ, Avol E, Gilliland F, Vora H, Thomas D, Berhane K, et al. 2004. The effect of air pollution on lung development from 10 to 18 years of age. N Engl J Med 351(11):1057–1067.

Gilliland FD, Berhane K, Rappaport EB, Thomas DC, Avol E, Gauderman WJ, London SJ, Margolis HG, McConnell R, Islam KT, Peters JM. 2001. The effects of ambient air pollution on school absenteeism due to respiratory illnesses. Epidemiology 12(1):43–54.

Gilliland FD, Li Y-F, Saxon A, Diaz-Sanchez D. 2004. Glutathione-S-transferase M1 and P1 genotypes protect against xenobiotic enhancement of allergic responses. Lancet 363:119–125.

Hao M, Comier S, Wang M, Lee JJ, Nel A. 2003. Diesel exhaust particles exert acute effects on airway inflammation and function in murine allergen provocation models. J Allergy Clin Immunol. 112(5):905–914.

Hricko A, Preston K, Witt H, Peters J. 1999. Air pollution and children's health. In *Health atlas of Southern California* (Sommer H, Dear MJ, eds.). Los Angeles: University of Southern California, Southern California Studies Center. Available: http://hydra .usc.edu/scehsc/coep/coep_atlaschap.asp [accessed 21 December 2004].

Kim JJ. American Academy of Pediatrics Committee on Environmental Health. 2004. Ambient air pollution: health hazards to children. Pediatrics 114(6): 1699–707.

Kunzli N, McConnell R, Bates D, Bastain T, Hricko A, Lurmann F, Avol E, Gilliland F, and Peters J. 2003. Breathless in Los Angeles: The exhausting search for clean air. Am J Public Health 93:1494–1499.

McConnell R, Berhane K, Gilliland F, London SJ, Islam T, Gauderman WJ, Avol E, Margolis HG, Peters JM. 2002. Asthma in exercising children exposed to ozone: A cohort study. Lancet 359(9304): 386–391. [Erratum in Lancet 359(9309):896].

Natural Resources Defense Council, Coalition for Clean Air. 1998. Exhausted by diesel: How America's dependence on diesel engines threatens our health. Available: http://www.nrdc.org/air/transportation/ebd/ebdinx.asp [accessed 11 January 2006].

Oberdorster G, Sharp Z, Atudorei V, Elder A, Gelein R, Kreyling W, Cox C. 2004. Translocation of inhaled ultrafine particles to the brain. Inhal Toxicol 16(6-7):437–445

Peel JL, Tolbert PE, Klein M, Metzger KB, Flanders WD, Todd K, Mulholland JA, Ryan PB, Frumkin H. 2005. Ambient air pollution and respiratory emergency department visits. Epidemiology 16(2):164–174.

Pope CA III. 1989. Respiratory disease associated with community air pollution and a steel mill, Utah Valley. Am J Public Health 79(5):623–628.

Pope CA III, Burnett RT, Thurston GD, Thun MJ, Calle EE, Krewski D, et al. 2004. Cardiovascular mortality and long-term exposure to particulate air pollution: Epidemiological evidence of general pathophysiological pathways of disease. Circulation 109:71–77.

Riediker M, Williams R, Devlin R, Griggs T, Bromberg P. 2003. Exposure to particulate matter, volatile organic compounds, and other air pollutants inside patrol cars. Environ Sci Technol 37:2084–2093.

Ritz B, Yu F. 1999. The effect of ambient carbon monoxide on low birth weight among children born in southern California between 1989 and 1993. Environ Health Perspect 107:17–25.

Ritz B, Yu F, Chapa G, Fruin S. 2000. Effect of air pollution on preterm birth among children born in Southern California between 1989 and 1993. Epidemiology 11:502–511.

Rodes C, Sheldon L, Whitaker D, Clayton A, Fitzgerald K, Flanagan J. 1998. Measuring concentrations of selected air pollutants inside California vehicles. Available: http://www.arb.ca.gov/research/indoor/in-vehsm.htm [accessed 21 December 2004].

Schwartz J. 2004. Air pollution and children's health. Pediatrics 113:1037–1043.

Thurston GD, Bates DV. 2003. Air pollution as an underappreciated cause of asthma symptoms. J Am Med Assoc 290:1915–1917.

U.S. Environmental Protection Agency. 2003. Questions and answers about dioxins. Available: http://www.epa.gov/ncea/dioxinqa.htm [accessed 10 January 2006].

U.S. Environmental Protection Agency. 2004. Eight-hour ground-level ozone designations. Available: http://www.epa.gov/ozonedesignations/index.htm [accessed 21 December 2004].

van Vliet P, Knape M, de Hartog J, Janssen N, Harssema H, Brunekreef B. 1997. Motor vehicle exhaust and chronic respiratory symptoms in children living near freeways. Environ Res 74:122–132.

Zhu Y, Hinds WC, Kim S, Shen S, Sioutas C. 2002a. Study of ultrafine particles near a major highway with heavy-duty diesel traffic. Atmos Environ 36: 4323–4335.

Zhu Y, Hinds WC, Kim S, Sioutas C. 2002b. Concentration and size distribution of ultrafine particles near a major highway. J Air Waste Manag Assoc 52:1032–1042.

Toxic Hazards
in Schools

Troy A. Pierce and Robert J. Geller

Pest Control

■ *Summary*

- Insects, rodents, and other animals frequently cohabit indoor and outdoor human settings. They become pests when they put human health or property at risk.
- Pest control is important in minimizing the negative impact on human health and property, but the strategies by which it is achieved need to balance the risks presented by pest control against those presented by the pests themselves.
- Integrated pest management (IPM) aims to control pests by exclusion and changes in the indoor environment and by reserving pesticides for use only when these steps prove inadequate. IPM is the recommended strategy to control pests.
- Insecticides and rodenticides can be used with a high degree of safety if used in keeping with currently recommended practices. These agents should be used only as part of a coordinated program of pest control and should not be left to individual discretion. ■

Many creatures, including mosquitoes, bees, spiders, and rodents, are considered pests when found in human environments. People have always coexisted with these species, many of which serve important ecological functions. However, pests can cause discomfort, disease, and damage to property, so programs to control them are often necessary.

In the past, pest control consisted of little more than spraying pesticides routinely. This approach has major disadvantages: It is expensive, wasteful, and potentially dangerous. The modern approach to pest control is exemplified by integrated pest management (IPM), which is based on information on the life cycles of pests, how they interact with the environment, and what they need to survive. It emphasizes nonchemical means of control, such as creating inhospitable environments, removing sources of food, blocking entry into buildings, and placing traps. Pesticides are also used in IPM programs but in a judicious, targeted way. Pest control is a special challenge for schools for several reasons.

First, children may be especially sensitive to pesticides (National Research Council 1993), so it makes sense to use the least toxic pesticides possible and to use them sparingly. Second, children's habits, such as leaving food around, may inadvertently encourage the proliferation of pests. Third, human sensitivity to pesticides and to pests themselves varies considerably. For example, some children are highly allergic to bee stings. As a result, those who plan pest control programs in schools must minimize both the presence of pests and the use of pesticides—a delicate balance.

In this chapter we provide an overview of the various pests found in school environments and their effects on the health of students and staff. Next we review the health effects of pesticides. Finally, we discuss the concept of IPM and explain how it can be implemented in schools. The resource list at the end of the chapter offers additional sources of information.

The Pests

Cockroaches

Flies and cockroaches may spread foodborne pathogens such as salmonella, staphylococcus, streptococcus, and *Escherichia coli*. It has also been shown that cockroaches can harbor the polio virus, as well as the parasite that causes toxoplasmosis (Baumholtz et al. 1997). Many studies have shown that airborne cockroach body parts and excrement can cause allergic reactions and asthma attacks in children and adults who are sensitive. In fact, children who live in urban environments with high concentrations of cockroaches have significantly higher levels of asthma compared with other children (Rosenstreich et al. 1997; Custovic et al. 2002; DeVera et al. 2003).

Wasps and Bees

The various species of wasps and bees provide enormous benefits to the environment, including pollination and control of certain insect pests. It has been said that if all pollinators, such as wasps and bees, were to die, life on Earth would probably end as well. Wasps in and around schools, however, can have serious effects on children's health. While most people react to bee or wasp stings with only local pain and swelling, some people are allergic (i.e., they have IgE antibodies, which are involved in producing allergic reactions, to certain insect venoms) and can potentially have more serious reactions, such as difficulty breathing, low blood pressure, and even death. Yellow jackets can be especially aggressive and, like many wasps, deliver a painful sting that can be life threatening to allergic people. Social wasps like yellow jackets account for most of the insect stings to people. Bees, on the other hand, are usually nonaggressive unless directly agitated, although bees and wasps will defend their nesting sites aggressively.

Venom-specific IgE antibody can be detected for bees in 6–17% of the general population and for wasps in 12–21%, but many people with these antibodies do not demonstrate allergic responses after being stung (Annila 2000; Antonicelli et al. 2002). Sting reactions that extend beyond the site of the sting occur in only 0.3–7.5% of the general population, although only some of these stings pose the risk of a life-threatening reaction (Annila 2000).

It is important to remember that many commonly seen bees cannot sting. Carpenter bee males, for instance, are very aggressive at protecting their nest site but cannot sting, and a large increase in bumblebees often means the stingless males (drones) have hatched. The more we know about bees and wasps, the better we will be able to safely control them if they become pests.

Mosquitoes

Mosquitoes are principally found outdoors in warm, humid weather. They feed on the blood of several species of animals including humans. To feed, they inject minute amounts of a substance that permits the blood to flow without clotting. These substances may result in local itching or swelling or in allergic symptoms.

In the process of feeding, mosquitoes may acquire infectious agents from one victim and spread them to another host. In suitable climates, mosquitoes are a principal vector in the spread of malaria, West Nile virus, and other human diseases (Gratz 2004).

Spiders

Spiders may inflict painful bites, and some may pose a health risk (e.g., allergies, pain, skin destruction, secondary infection of bite site), especially in the case of the brown recluse and black widow. Most spiders hide and either ambush their prey or catch it in a web. Spiders are much more likely to scare people than to bite them. They can usually be captured in a cup with a lid and placed outdoors. Where large numbers of spiders are present, there is a strong likelihood that other pests that serve as food for them are in even greater numbers. Most spider bites occur when spiders hide in clothing or other materials that come into direct contact with humans. Some of the best ways to prevent spider bites include keeping rooms uncluttered and cleaning all areas of the classrooms regularly. Always shake out shoes that have not been worn in several days.

Rodents

Through chewing, excrement, dander, and secondary parasites, mice and rats may contaminate food and cause disease. In addition, rodents can trigger asthma attacks and cause structural damage to buildings. Yet another significant reason for keeping rodents from entering school buildings is the potential for damage to the electrical system or fire from chewing and nest building. It is well known that rodents can spread diseases such as bubonic plague, hantavirus, and salmonella. Less well known is the fact that rodents are very valuable to our outdoor environment. Many animals rely on abundant rodent populations for food, and rodents can bury plant seeds or deposit seeds through feces. Despite these benefits to the outdoor environment, rodents must be excluded from the school building for health and safety reasons.

Ants

Ants, and fire ants in particular, can pose challenges in school buildings and on school grounds. Ants that forage in schools can spread staphylococcal and streptococcal bacteria. The pharaoh ant is a familiar ant pest in homes and schools and specifically targets buildings for its nests. Several species of ants can bite or sting. In ant infestations, populations can easily number several thousand, and one colony of fire ants can consist of more than 100,000 individuals (Winn, 2000). Fire ants are a serious threat to children and the elderly, who cannot always prevent and defend themselves against attack. Because fire ants are very aggressive and will readily sting people, schools with fire ant concerns must have an effective prevention program to ensure the safety of students and personnel.

Termites

Structural damage to schools from termites can be a serious issue for financially struggling school districts. The costs of preventive treatment, annual inspection, and early detection are usually much lower than replacing walls and floors that have been compromised by termite activity. Termites themselves do not pose a disease risk, but their presence often indicates wet conditions that may be conducive to mold growth. Schools should always have at least yearly termite inspections and targeted treatment when termites are found to be actively feeding on the school structure. Termite prevention is also essential and can often be as simple as eliminating wood-to-ground contact and removing excess moisture through proper drainage and dehumidification. State government agencies (usually departments of agriculture) will usually inspect a school upon request to ensure the foundation of the school has been properly treated to help prevent termites.

Fruit Flies

Fruit flies are a problem very different from house flies. Fruit flies can infest a school cafeteria or other food-related area (such as a concession stand) quite easily. They need only very small pieces of ripened fruit, fermenting spills under a cabinet, or food residue in sink drains to breed and infest an area. Like larger flies, fruit flies can spread bacteria. Proper housekeeping, with particular attention to sink drains and disposals, is the best way to prevent fruit fly infestation.

Pesticides

The use of pesticides in schools dates back to the beginnings of formal education and pesticide development. Before the development of mass-market pesticides, teachers, headmasters, and monks brought in plants and various home remedies thought to repel insects and rodents. More recently, attitudes about how and when pesticides should be used in schools have changed. Increased concern about their effects on children and highly susceptible people has fueled the desire to find better options for pest control. Alternatives to traditional pesticide use in and around schools include IPM strategies that use better building technology and disrupt pest pressure with hormonal, genetic, and natural means that pose a lower risk to people and pets.

In addition to multiple brand names and a variety of packaging systems, pesticides present a number of possible health concerns. Companies submit data on the potential health effects of pesticides to the U.S. Environmental Protection Agency (EPA), which registers all pesticides for use in the United States. Many pesticides were approved for use decades ago, but the science and our understanding of acceptable risk factors have changed since the time of initial registration with the federal government. Pesticides registered by the EPA before November 1, 1984, are undergoing a reregistration process to make sure they do not present unreasonable risks to human health or the environment when used in accordance with approved label directions and precautions. Additionally, the Food Quality Protection Act, passed in 1996, established a new safety standard for pesticide residues in food, with an emphasis on protecting the health of infants and children. As a result of reregistration, many pesticides have new requirements for use, and some of them are no longer offered in the marketplace.

All pesticides registered for use in the United States should have an EPA registration number listed on the bottom of the pesticide label on the container.

The pesticide label (commonly called directions) should be followed exactly, and all the recommended precautions (e.g., wearing gloves, using eye protection) must be taken to ensure that the risk of being poisoned or otherwise affected by the pesticide is minimized. All pesticides should be in the original sealed container and stored in a location where children have no access. Moreover, because many pesticides degrade over time and temperature extremes can affect their usefulness and safety, the label directions for storing them must be followed.

Several large classes of pesticides are discussed here. More information on less commonly used agents may be obtained from the resources listed at the end of the chapter.

Organophosphate and Carbamate Insecticides

Organophosphate and carbamate insecticides (such as malathion, diazinon, and chlorpyrifos) have been used extensively for more than 50 years. Excessive human exposure to these agents may result in clinically evident toxic effects. Some people are more sensitive to these agents than others—young children may be more vulnerable to these agents' neurologic effects, for example. In addition, clinical effects may be difficult to distinguish from other illnesses.

Carbamates and organophosphates are cholinesterase inhibitors that kill insects by interfering with the proper functioning of their central nervous system. Cholinesterases are enzymes that are required to "turn off" signals once they are transmitted from one neuron to another within the nervous system. Preventing these enzymes from acting leaves the neuron that is receiving the message locked in the "on" position. Most animals have a reserve amount of more cholinesterase function than is needed to maintain normal function. Symptoms occur only when the amount of cholinesterase inhibition substantially exceeds the amount needed to maintain function. Insects are more sensitive to these agents than most people, which explains why insects can be killed while the people nearby are not adversely affected.

Cholinesterase inhibition can also occur in humans. The effects commonly noted after poisoning by these agents include a combination of nausea, vomiting, stomach cramps, diarrhea, excessive drooling and tearing, muscular weakness, and muscle tremors. Young children, however, may display sedation and other behavioral effects instead of these typical cholinesterase symptoms. Lingering effects have also been described, particularly after intense exposures.

Pesticide applicators who use these types of pesticides should be tested on a regular basis for cholinesterase inhibition and should have baseline blood work performed before any regular use of carbamates and organophosphates.

Pyrethroids

Pyrethroids belong to another class of insecticides in common use. The agents in this class, such as

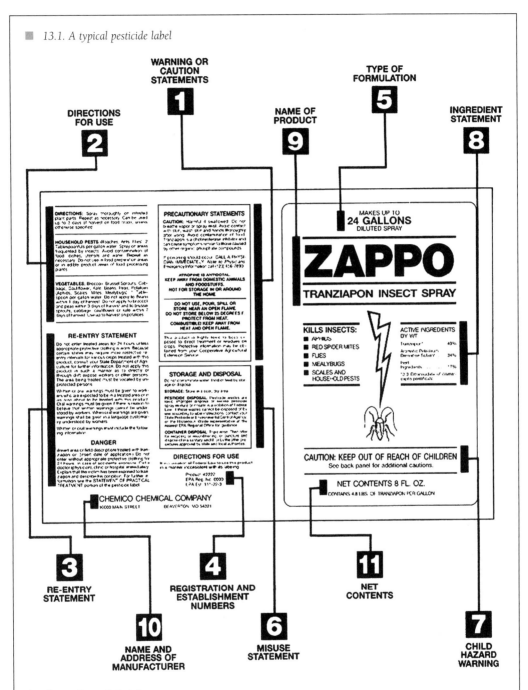

Reading a Pesticide Label

One of the more important tools for the safe and effective use of pesticides is the information on the product label. As legal documents, labels are required to contain directions on how to properly mix, apply, store, and dispose of a pesticide product. The numbers are keyed to the numbers used in fig. 13.1.

1. Warning or Caution Statements

Statement of practical treatment. The label must indicate how to avoid the hazards the product

(continued)

poses. Within the precautionary statement or elsewhere on the label, emergency first-aid measures must be stated. The label must also state what types of exposure require medical attention. Precautionary statements:

- Hazards to humans and domestic animals. This section indicates the ways in which the product may be poisonous. It also explains how to avoid poisoning, such as using appropriate protective clothing or ventilation. If the pesticide is classified as "highly toxic," this section must inform physicians of the proper treatment for poisoning.
- Physical and chemical hazards. This section indicates whether the pesticide may pose fire, explosion, or chemical hazards.
- Environmental hazards. If used improperly, pesticides or pesticide residues may contaminate water supplies, accumulate to dangerous levels in the environment, or harm birds, fish, or wildlife. To avoid these problems, the label may contain environmental precautions that apply to air, water, soil, or wildlife.
- Endangered species. If the pesticide has potential for harming an endangered species or its habitat, use restriction statements will indicate where the pesticide may not be used.

2. Directions for Use
The instructions on the label must explain how to use the product properly within its legal requirements to achieve the best results. The directions will state the following:

- the pests the product is registered to control
- the crops, animals, or other items on which the product can be used
- in what form the product should be applied
- how to apply the product
- how much to use
- where it should be applied
- when it should be applied
- how frequently it should be applied
- if applied to a crop, how soon the crop may be used or eaten after the product is applied.

3. Reentry Statement
This statement indicates how much time must pass before people can reenter a treated area without appropriate protective clothing and equipment. If no reentry statement appears, then all unprotected workers must wait until the sprays have dried or dusts have settled before reentering. If the reentry period is in effect and early reentry is required, the protective clothing that must be worn will be indicated.

4. Registration and Establishment Numbers
Every pesticide on the market must be registered with the U.S. Environmental Protection Agency. The registration number must be on the front panel of the label and is written as "EPA Registration No. XXXX." The establishment number, a code of the factory that made the chemical, must also be on every pesticide container. It usually appears underneath the registration number.

5. Type of Formulation
A pesticide may be available in more than one type of formulation (e.g., liquids, powders, concentrates, dusts). Different formulations require different methods of handling. The label will say what formulation the package contains and how to use it properly.

6. Misuse Statement
Chemical companies are required by law to do extensive testing on a product before it may be placed on the market. They must meet all of the labeling requirements and prove that the labeling information is correct. To use a pesticide product in any manner that is inconsistent with its labeling is a violation of federal law. The misuse statement reiterates this stipulation.

■ *13.1. (Continued)*

7. Child Hazard Warning

Every pesticide container must bear the statement "Keep Out of Reach of Children" on the front label.

8. Ingredient Statement

Every pesticide label must list what is in the product. It must show the name of each active ingredient, the percentage of each active ingredient, and the percentage of inert ingredients. The inert ingredients do not need to be named.

9. Name of the Product

Brand name: The name, brand, or trademark is plainly on the front panel of the product label. This is the name used in advertisements by the company that makes the product and is the most identifiable name for the product.

Common name: All chemicals have a scientific name. Many times a chemical with a complex scientific name is also given a simpler common name. The scientific and common names do not vary between companies. Brand names are different, depending on which company made the chemical.

10. Name and Address of the Manufacturer

The name and address of the company that made or distributed the product must be on the label so the purchaser knows who made or sold the product and can contact them if necessary.

11. Net Contents

The label must show how much of the product is in the container. This can be expressed in ounces, liters, pounds, or other similar units.

(Adapted from Michigan State University Extension Service Bulletin E-2182, Reading a Pesticide Product Label; http://web1.msue.msu.edu/msue/imp/mod02/01500584.html) ■

cypermethrin and resmethrin, are based on pyrethrin, which is isolated from the chrysanthemum flower. These agents interfere with nerve function in insects but generally have minimal, if any, effect on nerve function in mammals. Potential adverse effects in people are principally allergic in nature, or they may present as a local skin irritation that resolves rapidly without specific therapy. Pyrethroids are commonly mixed with piperonyl butoxide to enhance their effectiveness. This chemical is of low toxicity to mammals. Because of their greater safety, pyrethroids have become the main class of insecticides used in the United States.

Organochlorine Insecticides

Organochlorine insecticides, also called chlorinated hydrocarbon insecticides, were among the first insecticides used commercially. Agents such as DDT, kepone, chlordane, and lindane are members of this class. These agents have been recognized for their threat to human health and the environment. The toxic effects of these agents include seizures (after a large dose) and possible chronic effects such

as hormonal disruption and cancer. Their persistence in the environment, frequently for many years, has led to adverse ecological effects in animals and birds. Stringent restrictions have been imposed to limit further use of these agents.

The carcinogenicity of various pesticides has been investigated in studies carried out with animal models and agricultural workers. Although some studies have shown that these subjects had increased risks of cancer, it is unclear whether the increased cancer risk was related to exposure to several different pesticides over many years, to other occupational factors, or to a combination of factors. The organochlorine class of pesticides appears to pose the highest risk of carcinogenicity. Increased cancer risk in the children of parents who use insecticides in agricultural activities has also been explored (Flower et al. 2004). Current studies do not implicate pyrethroids or most of the organophosphate or carbamate agents.

Insect Repellants

Insect repellants for topical use have resulted from efforts to prevent the spread of mosquito-borne diseases and to reduce their undesirable interactions with people. DEET (*N,N*-diethyl-*m*-toluamide, also known as *N,N*-diethyl-3-methylbenzamide) has been shown to be the most effective chemical mosquito repellant to date (Fradin and Day 2002). DEET has a generally favorable safety record, although rare individuals have demonstrated sensitivity to this agent. Toxic effects, when they occur, generally follow dermal use of high doses for long periods of time or acute ingestions of large doses. Although rare, the most common toxic effects reported after the use of these agents are seizures or decreased level of consciousness.

The effectiveness of DEET as a mosquito repellant does not increase with concentrations greater than 50% (Koren et al. 2003). DEET should be used on limited areas of the body, in concentrations generally not exceeding 30% (Koren et al. 2003), and at intervals not exceeding the manufacturer's recommendations. DEET should not be applied to clothing or to the eyes, nose, or mouth. The use of DEET should be avoided by people who are sensitive to its adverse effects.

Although other insecticides and repellants exist, their use is much less common at this time. Further information about these agents can be obtained from regional poison centers (1-800-222-1222), the National Pesticide Information Center (1-800-858-7378), the EPA web site, and local county agricultural extension agencies.

Rodent Control

In the past, rodent control has been achieved by the widespread use of rodent-killing products. Some are highly toxic to humans, as well as rodents, and should not be used in home or school settings. The most commonly used product—because of its effectiveness and favorable safety profile with regard to people—is brodifacoum. This compound, which is the main ingredient in many products, is a long-lasting anticoagulant. When eaten in a single dose of an adequate amount, it will prevent an animal's blood from clotting for days to weeks. After even trivial injury, massive bleeding ensues, and the animal dies. The amount of this agent that is needed to cause human toxicity is much larger than that required to anticoagulate a rodent; thus this agent has achieved a favorable safety record.

Delivery and Safety

Pesticides can be delivered in many forms, including traditional sprays, powders, and baits. Some of these systems are much less likely to expose students and school staff to residues. Baits, such as bait stations and gels, are the preferred method for controlling ants and cockroaches (Stier et al. 2000) in schools. Pests are attracted to the bait stations and then feed on the bait. Many pests also take the bait back to the colony or nest and feed it to other members of the colony. Bait stations should be placed in areas that pests frequent, but not in any that are readily accessible to students.

Some pest control companies use gel baits, which are especially effective for ant problems. Gel baits are usually applied in areas where pests are active but out of the way of children. The gel is applied in small amounts (about an inch-long line) at wall and floor intersections and in cracks and voids. Gel baits can be valuable tools and, when used correctly, can provide targeted pest control with fairly low risk to students.

Baits and gels in schools are almost always preferred over other pesticide application methods. It is important to remember that the method of delivery and application of a pesticide relates directly to potential human exposure. The traditional method of spraying pesticides indoors can lead to pesticide residues in the air and on hard surfaces. Avoid spraying pesticides indoors. A school pesticide professional may spray pesticides indoors as an extreme measure when very severe pest pressure warrants such use, but, even then, the sprayed material should be carefully targeted. Pesticide sprays are always a last resort. Except for the management of Formosan termites (EPA 2002), using pesticide fumigants, fogs, or bombs is never recommended for schools because of the residue that is left on exposed surfaces.

The persistence of pesticides indoors can be a significant problem, as is the off-target movement of pesticides. Many pesticide labels state that the killing power is maintained for a certain length of time; that is, the pesticide is designed to persist indoors at a level that will kill pests for at least the indicated time. Frequently the residue persists in homes and buildings even longer than the time indicated on the label. Some pesticides used indoors can persist for long periods of time after their original use (Landrigan et al. 1999). Therefore, people who are highly sensitive to an agent should be discouraged from contacting the pesticide-treated surface for as long as the pesticide is present at an active level.

Schools are often treated with pesticides on a routine basis, with the assumption that a qualified professional is applying the chemical. Additionally, school administrators and other officials may pressure pest control companies to treat the schools with pesticides. School officials may threaten to change pest control companies if the current company is unwilling to spray pesticides on schedule, whether or not pest pressures warrant treatment.

Reasons to avoid spraying pesticides routinely in schools are numerous: reduced exposure to residues; prevention of insect resistance to the overuse of pesticides; and cost savings realized by eliminating unneeded applications. Why use a chemical when there is no need to do so? Less-frequent use of pesticides correlates directly with a reduction in potential exposure.

Pesticide application records are frequently either nonexistent or difficult to obtain. Anyone who applies pesticides in a school, including school personnel (e.g., janitors and groundskeepers) and contractors, should be state certified and provide proof of certification to the school. Such certification helps to ensure that those who are using pesticides in schools have been trained and tested by the state on their safe use.

Recognizing Pest Control Problems

You may have a problem with pesticide use in your school if you are routinely using them in the buildings or on the grounds. Furthermore, you may have a problem if you frequently encounter sighting of pests, teachers bringing pesticides into the classroom, and coaches allowing students onto athletic fields too soon after pesticide treatment. Most pesticides should not be applied while students are present in the building. If in doubt, do not apply the pesticide, and check the label directions to ensure proper use and application.

Untrained staff, administrators, teachers, and janitors should not bring pesticides into schools and certainly should not be applying them in classrooms and offices. Pesticide application in schools should be done by highly trained staff or professionals. The days of teachers bringing pesticides from home to spray ants should be over. With a proper IPM plan in place, such rogue sources of pesticide use will be eliminated.

Occasionally school officials request that janitors and other maintenance staff apply pesticides. All school staff who apply pesticides must have proper training by the state and should be certified to apply pesticides. Training can be acquired by contacting the state cooperative extension service. The state agency for pesticides, usually the state Department of Agriculture, can provide testing and certification.

Pest problems in classrooms arise when food is left in drawers and cabinets. Water leaks are also of primary concern in classrooms, not only for mold issues but also during the warmer days of summer, when many animals and insects are looking for water to drink. Food and drinks should be kept only in designated areas of the classrooms where a regular cleaning regime is in place. Candy and snacks in students' desks present a definite problem, as does the forgotten candy bar taken from a student and placed in the teacher's desk.

A growing trend in some school districts is to allow students to purchase sodas and bring them into class. Such sugared soda is a strong attractant for bugs and rodents, and the soda machines themselves can harbor pests if housekeeping around the heavy machines is poor.

Because of the nature of school cafeterias and the unique combination of food, water, and waste, schools see most of their troubling pest problems arising from housekeeping and maintenance of the cafeteria. Drains, grease traps, mops, storage, and locations of trash containers are all cafeteria variables that must be controlled and monitored. Drains should be cleaned of debris every night. Grease traps should be on a regular maintenance schedule for cleaning. Food must be stored off the ground on uncluttered shelving. Trash containers should be washed regularly, tightly sealed, and emptied every day. Trash dumpsters and outdoor containers of used grease should be kept away from the building and not allowed to overflow. Tightly sealed containers are a must.

Improving Pest Control: Integrated Pest Management in Schools

The U.S. Environmental Protection Agency (2004) has said that "The goal of a school IPM program is to protect human health by suppressing pests that vector diseases, to reduce losses from pest damage, reduce environmental pollution, reduce human exposures to pesticides, particularly that of children, and to reduce costs of pest control" (p. 3–4). IPM in schools is a proactive method of significantly reducing pesticide use while simultaneously eliminating the presence of pests. School IPM addresses the control of three basic needs of pests: food, water, and shelter. The school should be as inhospitable an environment as possible for pests while maintaining a comfortable educational setting.

School IPM has simple components that are common among the strategies currently being implemented across the United States. They are described in greater detail in the EPA's school IPM manuals (2003, 2004):

- Develop an official policy statement on school IPM.
- Determine baseline levels of pests, sanitation, and school building deficiencies.
- Remedy baseline sanitation and building deficiencies.
- Determine your tolerance for pests.
- Set action levels of pests that trigger various steps in the hierarchy of treatment.
- If an action level is reached, use the lowest-risk treatment first.
- Evaluate treatment effectiveness and adjust as needed.
- Continue monitoring and treatment as required by the action level.

In this section of the chapter we explore each of these steps in detail and discuss a model approach to adopting school IPM, the Monroe IPM Model. Additional sources of practical advice include the EPA's online how-to manual (listed in the resources section of this chapter) and local cooperative extension agents, who can often assist schools in adopting IPM.

Develop an Official Policy on School IPM

An official policy ensures that school administrators and staff are truly committed to school IPM and to reducing the use of pesticides. Such a policy should include the following:

- pest management reasoning
- IPM procedures

- record-keeping requirements
- pesticide treatment notification
- proper storage of pesticides
- application of pesticides.

Sample policies are available from the EPA, the University of Florida, and Pennsylvania State University at the web sites provided in the resources section at the end of this chapter.

Determine Baseline Levels of Pests, Sanitation, and School Building Deficiencies

A trained professional can determine baseline pest levels. In many cases, the county extension agent or state school IPM specialist will be able to identify a professional pest control operator (PCO) who would be willing to work with the school in adopting an IPM program. In some areas, however, it may still be difficult to find a PCO who understands basic IPM principles as they apply to schools. In that event, the local cooperative extension service may be needed to train PCOs. All operators, including house staff, must be properly trained in IPM and certified in pesticide application. Depending on the pest, methods for determining pest levels might include the following:

- glue traps for rodents
- roach-monitoring stations
- visible signs of pest trails
- nesting
- snap traps.

Knowing the Potential Pests in the Area Facilitates the Assessment of Baseline Levels

Baseline sanitation remains one of the most important elements of a school IPM program. Identifying simple sanitation problems (e.g., a trash dumpster next to the school building is an invitation to pests to eat and stay a while) can reap big rewards in the fight to control pests. Indoor trash containers should be inspected for cleanliness and spills, and garbage must be removed daily. School lockers, teachers' desks, janitorial closets, storage areas, cafeterias, concession stands, and other likely locations must be free of the trash, debris, and clutter that attract pests. All appropriate places in the school should be inspected to accurately determine the condition of the school. It is not unusual to find sanitation problems that need simple, common-sense approaches.

Initially, uncovering building deficiencies can be daunting. In a baseline assessment, all major problem areas must be documented, beginning with obvious items:

- holes on the outside of the building where pests can enter freely
- seams in the building where wood joints come together or brick meets wood
- locations of air-conditioning condensation pipes
- vents
- access doors
- windows
- roof gables
- wood-to-ground contact areas.

Remedy Baseline Sanitation and Building Deficiencies

As soon as possible, the easy-to-accomplish items should be addressed: moving the garbage dumpsters away from the building, cleaning the grease traps, and getting food and stored items off the floor and neatly stacked onto shelves. Repair of the next-hardest deficiencies involves having the maintenance staff seal cracks and holes in the building and around windows and other seams. The roof should be repaired if necessary. If the school is operating on a limited budget, the PTA or even parents with needed construction skills may be able to help. The final task is attacking the biggest problems, such as removing water from crawl spaces under the school and providing adequate drainage to prevent water from infiltrating the school. Eliminating all excess moisture from the school environment can help prevent future problems. Often a school simply needs regular, thorough maintenance to prevent pest infestation.

Determine Tolerance for Pests

Tolerance for pests can vary from school to school, based on acceptance of aesthetic, economic, and medical impact. Communities may have different standards for acceptable levels of pests and the use of pesticides around their children. Putting these into written form guides intervention in keeping with local preferences and community, state, and local laws.

Set Action Levels That Trigger Various Steps in the Hierarchy of Treatment

Action levels for pests should be set to avoid reaching injury levels. For example, if a school is using sticky-trap monitoring stations to judge cockroach levels in the school, what number of cockroaches per sticky trap over a prescribed time period warrants action? What number of cockroaches in monitoring stations triggers the use of pesticide baits versus a targeted spray treatment for an infestation? These questions must be addressed not only to prevent an injury but also to make sure the appropriate lowest-risk treatment is used.

If Action Level Is Reached, Use the Lowest-Risk Treatment First

The lowest-risk treatment is often not a pesticide at all: Finding an ant trail, removing the food source, and caulking the crack in the wall where the ants are entering are examples. The exclusion and elimination of pests' basic necessities are always first-choice treatments and tend to be longer-lasting solutions compared with the use of pesticides. Pesticides are almost always a temporary fix for the bigger problems related to the food, water, and shelter that pests need to survive. Targeted baits should be used, if needed, and pesticides should be sprayed only as a last resort for very targeted control of infestations. Pesticide labels must be read and carefully followed. On school grounds and athletic fields, children should not be allowed to enter treated areas until the restricted entry time has passed. Pest-resistant turf and plants on school property offer a safe, proactive option.

Evaluate Treatment Effectiveness and Adjust as Needed

Certainly, a bit of art accompanies the science of pest control, especially when it comes to choosing a strategy based on the unique environment of the school and on the community's desires. The key question is, did the strategy that was used produce acceptable results? If not, further questions are in order: Was the bait placed in the best locations? Was the building sealed correctly? Is a pest becoming resistant to the pesticide that the school has used for many years? These questions can lead to answers that are specific to the school and its pest problem. It is the very action of continuously evaluating pest treatment effectiveness that will ultimately lead a school to more permanent solutions to pest control and prevention. Cooperative extension agents and other pest management experts can help in long-term evaluation.

Continued Monitoring and Treatment as Required by Action Level

Many pest problems can be permanently controlled through a sound school IPM monitoring and treatment program. A school or pest management professional will conduct pest monitoring for the life of the school if requested. Over time, action levels and treatments will be tweaked and increase in precision and accuracy. Schools that make long-term use of IPM will notice marked decreases in pests, use of pesticides, and anxiety over pest control issues. The school will be prepared for occasional minor pest problems by having a well-established monitoring and treatment plan. Monitoring gives the school the ability to detect pest problems early. Familiarity with treatment options offers a wide variety of tools for solving pest problems at the lowest risk to students and supports permanent solutions.

The Monroe Model: A Practical Approach to IPM

The Monroe Model, developed by Dr. Marc Lame at Indiana University and named for Monroe County, Indiana, where it was first used, is a widely used step-by-step process for implementing a successful school IPM program (Lame 2005). It starts with asking and answering three basic questions: What action must be taken? Who will take that action? And, do they have the resources to take the action? The Monroe IPM Model combines the process for answering these simple questions with the Rogers Innovation-Decision process (Rogers 1995). As such, it provides an effective approach to implementing IPM, first on a pilot basis in just a few schools and later across an entire district. In fact, it also offers a useful approach for a wide range of other school programs. Twenty-two steps from the

Monroe Model are presented here to facilitate a successful school IPM program:

1. Agree on the program goals.
2. Scout for the most promising school and/or district.
3. Contact interested change agents at the school and residing in the target area (such as entomologists or regulatory personnel).
4. Obtain a verbal commitment from a high-ranking school official (preferably the superintendent).
5. Cooperate with a school official with some responsibility for and understanding of facility management (e.g., sanitation, maintenance, groundskeeping) in designing a pilot program.
6. Sweeten the pot by providing resources such as personnel, educational materials, or recognition (e.g., awards, publicity).
7. Obtain a memorandum of understanding (MOU) between the school, local change agents (e.g., extension agents and regulatory personnel), onsite IPM coordinator, and the implementation team; this memo should specify the work plan and expectations.
8. Assess the school district both technically (e.g., pests, pest-conducive conditions, pest management) and administratively (the school leadership's assessment of the current policies and the cost of pest management).
9. Train the trainers, including the contracted pest control operator, technicians, local change agents (e.g., extension, regulatory, and local activists), and the designated onsite coordinator.
10. Train the school staff adopters, including custodial, kitchen, maintenance, and other staff members, and, if possible, the principal and faculty.
11. Monitor at least monthly for the presence of pests and pest-conducive conditions, using varied methods (e.g., traps, staff interviews, visual inspection)
12. Introduce IPM more broadly to teachers, administrators, parents, and students, using a mass media approach.
13. Institute an ongoing newsletter and establish Web communication within the school community.
14. Set up a midterm evaluation of pest problems

and pesticide use and compare the findings with preprogram conditions.

15. Schedule a midterm adjustment meeting to explain and implement the midterm evaluation recommendations.

16. Initiate handholding or nurturing to reinforce IPM adoption.

17. Integrate the pest control operator into the model and specific IPM standards (a process of professionalization).

18. Make a final evaluation, using a comparison of the baseline, midterm, and end-of-program data, looking at costs, pests, pest-conducive conditions, pesticide use and exposure, and the attitudes of the school community, and share the results with others in the school district.

19. Recommend district expansion based on a successful pilot program. A standard plan would include funding options, a strategy for expansion (larger districts usually need to implement incrementally), personnel requirements (those who are acting as professional pest managers), training requirements and options, and even a public relations campaign.

20. Reward the successful users of such techniques with plaques, certificates, letters of congratulation, and positive media exposure.

21. Suggest expansion to other school districts.

22. Make a final report.

Conclusions

Many chemicals that make pesticides effective in controlling pests can act on humans in a similar fashion. It is the potential to detrimentally affect people that should force us to remain vigilant and limit pesticide use whenever possible. Of particular concern when using pesticides in schools are children with asthma or allergies, those with high levels of hand-to-mouth activity, and those with a history of adverse responses to chemicals.

Some pests are commonly seen in the school environment. By going outside unprotected when mosquitoes are biting or allowing gaps to form around water pipes where mice and roaches can enter, for instance, we create most of the opportunities ourselves for animals to become pests. If we can create these situations, we should also be able to limit them. This chapter has presented pest con-

trol strategies that attempt to limit infestation by modification of the school environment. Pesticides should be used only by the safest application method that will achieve control of the infestation— and only after exclusion and housekeeping methods have failed. Even then, pesticides in school settings should be used only by certified pesticide applicators who follow an established IPM program.

Resources

- California School IPM
  http://www.cdpr.ca.gov/cfdocs/apps/schoolipm/main.cfm
- *Consumer Reports* magazine
  http://www.consumerreports.org/cro/home.htm
- ExToxNet
  http://ace.orst.edu/info/extoxnet/
- Healthy Schools Network
  http://www.healthyschools.org
- Integrated Pest Management in Schools: A How-to Manual. Produced by the U.S. Environmental Protection Agency, this manual contains practical IPM strategies for several specific pests. This chapter was based in large part on the manual.
  http://www.epa.gov/pesticides/ipm/schoolipm/index.html
- National Foundation for IPM Education
  http://www.ipm-education.org
- Pennsylvania State University
  http://paipm.cas.psu.edu/index.html
- Texas A&M University, Southwest Technical Resource Center for IPM
  http://schoolipm.tamu.edu/
- University of Florida School IPM
  http://schoolipm.ifas.ufl.edu/
- U.S. Environmental Protection Agency: IPM in Schools
  http://www.epa.gov/pesticides/ipm

References

Annila I. 2000. Bee venom allergy. Clin Exper Allergy 30(12):1682–1687.

Antonicelli L, Bilo MB, Bonfazi F. 2002. Epidemiology of Hymenoptera allergy. Curr Opin Allergy Clin Immunol 2(4):341–346.

Baumholtz MA, Parish LC, Witkowski JA, Nutting WB. 1997. The medical importance of cockroaches. Int J Dermatol 36(8):90–96.

Custovic A, Murray CS, Gore RB, Woodcock A. 2002. Controlling indoor allergens. Ann Allergy Asthma Immunol 88(5):432–441.

DeVera MJ, Drapkin S, Moy JN. 2003. Association of recurrent wheezing with sensitivity to cockroach allergen in inner-city children. Ann Allergy Asthma Immunol 91(5):455–459.

Flower KB, Hoppin JA, Lynch CF, Blair A, Knott C, Shore DL, et al. 2004. Cancer risk and parental pesticide application in children of Agricultural Health Study participants. Environ Health Perspect 112(5):631–635.

Fradin MS, Day JF. 2002. Comparative efficacy of insect repellents against mosquito bites. New Engl J Med 347(1):13–18.

Gratz NG. 2004. Critical review of the vector status of *Aedes albopictus*. Med Vet Entomol 18(3):215–217.

Koren G, Matsui D, Bailey B. 2003. DEET-based insect repellents: Safety implications for children and pregnant and lactating women. Can Med Assoc J 169(3):209–212.

Lame ML. 2005. A worm in the teacher's apple: Protecting America's school children from pests and pesticides. Bloomington, IN: AuthorHouse.

Landrigan PJ, Claudio L, Markowitz SB, Brenner BL, Romero H, Wetmur JG, et al. 1999. Pesticides and inner-city children: Exposures, risks, and prevention. Environ Health Perspect 107 Suppl. 3):431–437.

Michigan State University Extension Service. 1998. Reading a pesticide label. Publication 01500584. Available http://www.msue.msu.edu/msue/imp/mod02/01500584.html [accessed 26 December 2004].

National Research Council, Committee on Pesticides in the Diets of Infants and Children. 1993. *Pesticides in the diets of infants and children.* Washington, DC: National Academy Press.

Rogers EM. 1995. *Diffusion of innovations,* 4th ed. New York: Free Press.

Rosenstreich DL, Eggleston P, Kattan M, Baker D, Slavin RG, et al. 1997. The role of cockroach allergy and exposure to cockroach allergen in causing morbidity among inner-city children with asthma. N Engl J Med 336:1356–1363.

Stier JC, Delahaut K, Pellitteri P, Kandziora P. 2000. Wisconsin's school integrated pest management manual. Available: http://ipcm.wisc.edu/programs/school/ [accessed 06 April 2004].

U.S. Environmental Protection Agency. 2002. Structural fumigation using sulfuryl fluoride: Dow-Elanco's Vikane gas fumigant. Available: http://www.epa.gov/spdpublc/mbr/casestudies/volume2/sulfury2.html [accessed 6 April 2004].

U.S. Environmental Protection Agency. 2003. Pest control in the school environment: Adopting integrated pest management. Publication EPA-735-F-93-012. Available: http://www.epa.gov/pesticides/ipm/brochure [accessed 29 December 2005].

U.S. Environmental Protection Agency. 2004. Integrated pest management for schools: A how-to manual. Available: http://www.epa.gov/pesticides/ipm/schoolipm/index.html [accessed 29 December 2005].

Weiss B, Amler S, Amler RW. 2004. Pesticides. Pediatrics 113 (Suppl. 4):1030–1036.

Winn J, ed. 2000. Managing imported Fire Ants in urban areas. University of Georgia College of Agricultural and Environmental Sciences, Cooperative Extension Service. Available: http://pubs.caes.uga.edu/caespubs/pubcd/B1191.htm [accessed 06 January 2006].

14

Stephen Ashkin and Richard Ellis

Cleaning Materials and Methods

■ *Summary*

- Clean schools minimize safety hazards and provide an optimal setting for learning.
- Conventional cleaning methods may incur health and environmental costs.
- "Green cleaning" is designed to produce an effective cleaning process that prevents toxicity among exposed persons while protecting the environment.
- Direct economic benefits of a green cleaning program include reductions in chemical use and labor costs.
- Indirect benefits, although less easily documented, frequently include improved performance and decreased absenteeism. ■

Cleaning is an essential activity in schools. Clean schools help teachers teach and help students learn productively, protect health and safety, maintain high morale, and prolong the useful life of equipment and facilities (fig. 14.1).

"Green cleaning" is an approach to cleaning designed to meet three different goals: effective cleaning, preventing discomfort and toxicity among people exposed to the cleaning process, and protecting the environment. Green cleaning offers special op-portunities in schools in several ways. First, children are especially susceptible to toxic exposures. Second, more than 50 million children spend their days in school, together with large numbers of teachers and staff, so protection could offer significant public health benefits. Third, the nation has more than 120,000 schools with 6 billion square feet of school space, and the scale of cleaning every day is enormous. Approaches that protect the environment could offer substantial benefits across the nation. Finally, because schools are educational settings, green cleaning offers an opportunity to teach students about healthy and environmentally responsible practices.

Cleaning Schools: An Overview

Schools are heavily used buildings. Busy children fill the classrooms, halls, and other facilities, often giving little thought to cleanliness. Before and after school hours, programs for children often occupy the school facilities, and parent and community groups may be present in the evenings and on weekends. In fact, schools often function as community centers, with large numbers of people constantly coming and going. Dirt is tracked in from

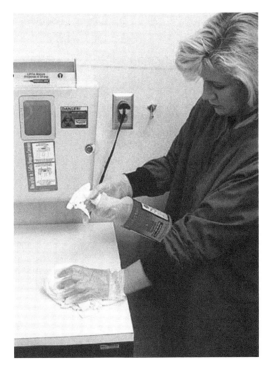

Figure 14.1. Disinfecting a school nurse's office. (Photo by Spartan Chemical Company.)

outside, paints are splashed, and food is spilled. Keeping schools clean is a formidable challenge, but it is essential.

Perhaps the two most important goals of cleaning are to provide an optimal setting for learning and to reduce hazards such as slippery surfaces. In addition, cleaning improves the school's appearance, extends the life of the building, and reduces the potential for transmission of infection. Some less obvious goals that are integral to green cleaning include minimizing the environmental impact of cleaning, keeping the school's waste stream to a minimum, and protecting the health of students and staff by using the least toxic materials possible.

Cleaning processes can be divided into three broad categories: mechanical cleaning, chemical cleaning, and surface-abrasion cleaning. *Mechanical cleaning* involves physically removing dirt and other particles. Two prime examples are sweeping and vacuuming. These processes can pose a problem if they increase exposure to particles. For example, a vacuum cleaner can dislodge dust from carpets and create clouds that students might breathe. *Chemical cleaning* involves the use of chemical agents, such as detergents or ammonia, that dissolve dirt or cre-

ate barriers (for example, stripping and waxing of floors) to protect surfaces. These processes can create a problem if students are exposed to harmful chemicals. Finally, *surface-abrasion cleaning* removes surfaces, usually with the use of machinery such as burnishers, which grind the floor finish from floors, and floor buffers, which both abrade floor surfaces and apply polish. These processes, like mechanical cleaning, can create clouds of airborne particles, some of which may be harmful.

Various degrees of cleanliness are required in different settings. Although there are no national standards, a five-tier system of expectations is emerging (National Center for Education Statistics 2003), each implying different staffing requirements.

- Level 1 entails very stringent cleaning that would be appropriate in operating rooms, for example, but rarely if ever needed in schools. Levels 2, 3, and 4 are often found in schools.
- Level 2 is the highest standard for most school cleaning and is generally reserved for restrooms and special education, kindergarten, and food service areas. A custodian can clean approximately 18,000–20,000 square feet to this standard in an 8-hour shift.
- Level 3 is the norm for most school facilities. It is acceptable to most stakeholders but may ignore some health issues. A custodian can clean approximately 28,000–31,000 square feet to this standard in 8 hours.
- Level 4 is not normally acceptable in a school environment. Classrooms are cleaned every other day, carpets vacuumed every third day, and dusting occurs once a month. At this level, a custodian can clean 45,000–50,000 square feet in 8 hours.

Custodians typically are responsible for a wide range of duties, such as

- cleaning throughout the school—classrooms and other instructional areas (floors, chalkboards); toilet areas (toilets, urinals, showers, sinks, locker rooms); administrative, support, and common areas (offices, lobbies, conference rooms)
- general floor cleaning (sweeping, vacuuming, mopping, polishing) of hallways, corridors, stairs, elevators, walkways, walkoff mats, other mats

■ *14.1. Johnny's story: An imaginary scenario*

6:00 AM   Another school day begins. Johnny's asthma is not a problem this morning as he wakes up. Across town, his third-grade teacher, Mrs. Hampton, is feeling rested after a good night's sleep. At the school, the buses are warming up, and the heating systems are starting their morning startup cycle with help from the morning custodian, Mr. Abbot.

7:00 AM   The school bus picks up Johnny, and he sits in his usual place, away from Dickie, the class bully, who taunts him when he has asthma attacks. Johnny has most of his asthma attacks at school lately. The bus arrives and discharges its 41 students in front, while other children arrive on foot, on their bikes, or in their parents' cars. A normal day.

8:15 AM   The day begins in Johnny's class with the flag salute, followed by spelling and math classes. The heating system rattles out its usual disruptive hum, while a first-grader down the hall throws up her breakfast and is taken to the sick room. Mr. Abbot arrives with his cleanup bucket and mop containing his old faithful cleaners. When he pours out the strong cleaners and disinfectants, one after the other, the first-grade room is overpowered by the smell. Mr. Abbot answers the ensuing complaints by reassuring everyone that if you can't smell the cleaners, they aren't strong enough to do the job. Down the hall, the odor in Johnny's room is a combination of human vomit mingled with strong bleach and ammonia mixed with something else that makes Johnny's eyes, nose, throat, and lungs begin to constrict. He needs to use his asthma medicine—again. Mrs. Hampton feels her head beginning to ache and throb, too.

10:00 AM   The air circulation slows down in the school as the temperature reaches its 72° set point. Meanwhile, Johnny and his classmates track in mud, sand, and sawdust from the playground. The air grows heavy and starts to smell like sweaty kids, vomit, cleaning solvents, and bleach. Fine dust and sawdust begin to settle visibly on the two computers in the room.

11:45 AM   As lunch recess begins, Mrs. Hampton's room is sweltering, and the lingering smell of the morning "accident" has hung around and kept her head pounding. Meanwhile, Mr. Abbot is vacuuming the lunchroom cafetorium carpet with his favorite "rug sucker" after generously applying some powdered cleaning chemicals to the six fresh, sticky milk, pop, and juice stains on the carpet. He dutifully presses the nozzle of his vacuum deep into the carpet so the worn-down bristles of the old beater bars can get at the stubborn stains. "Darn kids," he mutters. "They never learn." An invisible cloud of fine dust particles and germs follows the vacuum. They silently rise, enter the air plenum, and are sent quickly back to the classrooms, where the children, out of breath from running and playing during recess, are still inhaling deeply. The germs and fine particles enter their lungs without their noticing it. Quietly, the infection cycle at school continues.

2:45 PM   The final bell rings, and the other kids leave. Because he missed the morning quiz on Abraham Lincoln, Johnny stays behind with his teacher. As Mrs. Hampton reflects on the day's events, she sympathizes with Johnny. With her head still throbbing, she glances down at the computer and types in two unfamiliar words she just saw on one of the cleaners she has brought from home to clean her dusty computer. She enters the words "Green Seal" into the common search engine and gets 823 hits. Her eyes open wide, and during the next half hour, she surfs the Internet.

3:45 PM   Mrs. Hampton carries the printouts from the Green Seal search into the principal's office and points out the recommended ways of dealing with spills, handling chemicals, and improving the school environment. She is convinced that this will make a difference in student learning and attendance. Mrs. Hampton, driven by her pounding headache, is adamant, and the principal agrees to relate the ideas to the superintendent. The superintendent has been disturbed lately by the district's attendance figures, increased expenses for substitute teacher pay, and loss of revenues due to teachers' absences. In addition, he has concerns about meeting the district's learning objectives. ■

- cleaning of food service areas—kitchens, cafeterias, vending areas, break areas
- cleaning of vertical surfaces—walls, windows, mirrors, vents, blinds, partitions
- general dusting—horizontal surfaces, sills, counters, shelves
- removing trash
- coordinating recycling efforts
- replacing depleted supplies and controlling inventory of custodial supplies and equipment
- opening buildings at the beginning of the day and securing them at the end of the day
- performing minor maintenance—replacing light bulbs and air-conditioning filters, unclogging toilets, making small repairs, coordinating keys, repairing furniture, doing small paint jobs
- preparing for and cleaning up after events
- maintaining custodial equipment
- performing miscellaneous housekeeping duties
- coordinating safety and emergency responses
- maintaining material safety and data sheets
- initiating work orders
- maintaining the exterior of the buildings.

Health and Environmental Impacts of Cleaning

Conventional cleaning may impose significant health and environmental costs. Each year, the institutional cleaning industry uses 6 billion pounds of chemicals, many of which are known hazards. Consider the following statistics:

- The Janitorial Products Pollution Prevention Project, a U.S. EPA–funded effort in Santa Clara County and Richmond, California, found that the average janitor uses 23 gallons of chemicals per year, weighing 194 pounds, of which approximately 25% are hazardous ingredients (Barron et al. 1999).
- U.S. institutions, including schools and businesses, spend more than $75 million yearly on medical expenses and lost-time wages for janitors because of chemical-related injuries.
- Cleaning products are major sources of volatile organic compounds (VOCs), which can accumulate in buildings and contribute to

ozone formation. VOCs present a health threat, particularly in sensitized or compromised people.
- According to the Center for Building Science News, using safer cleaning products and better ventilation and cleaning could improve worker productivity nationwide by 0.5–5%, an annual productivity gain of $30–$150 billion (Fisk and Rosenfeld 1997).
- Cleaning substances were involved in more than 10% of exposures to potentially toxic compounds reported to U.S. Poison Centers in 2002. Fortunately, relatively few of these exposures resulted in severe illness (Watson et al. 2002).

These problems may be especially salient in schools for several reasons. First, modern schools often rely heavily on recirculated air. The venerable red brick schools of a few generations ago had large windows that opened, but in an effort to reduce energy costs, modern schools have much less circulation of outdoor air. Therefore, if any chemicals are introduced into the indoor air, they may circulate throughout the school and persist for a relatively long time.

Second, the timing of school cleaning may pose challenges in at least two respects. Bathroom cleaning, for example, is often performed throughout the day and sometimes even hourly, depending on the grade level and the need. Bathroom cleaning often entails the use of potential toxins such as acidic, caustic, or chlorinated cleaning agents. As a result, children confront regular opportunities for exposure. On the other hand, some cleaning is typically deferred until after school hours. At this time, the ventilation system is often turned down, so any fumes may be slow to dissipate.

Third, with increasing pressure on school funds, cleaning and maintenance budgets may be reduced. Neither custodians nor teachers are typically involved in budget decisions. Less-frequent cleaning may be a good thing if the cleaning process is hazardous, but not a desirable outcome if the school becomes dirtier. Moreover, accumulated dirt can be more difficult to clean, requiring more intensive use of cleaning agents. In fact, the level of school custodial staffing nationally is decreasing relative to increases in facility space. In K–12 schools, an average custodian is responsible for cleaning more than 23,000 square feet, about 10%

more than in 2001 (American School and University 2003). Such an increase is equivalent to adding an extra family home to a custodian's responsibilities in just 2 years and highlights the increasing pressure on those responsible for keeping schools clean.

Fourth, school custodians have a unique and challenging job. Unlike their counterparts in business and industry who have well-defined cleaning and custodial functions, K–12 custodians often find themselves doing maintenance, emergency work, groundskeeping tasks, and "other duties as assigned." Administrators, teachers, and students traditionally rely on several custodians to keep the entire physical plant running, walks swept and shoveled, flag in place, and restrooms, cafeteria, classrooms, windows, hallways, and floors clean. Custodians (fig. 14.2) and their supervisors may find it difficult to focus on the health and environmental aspects of cleaning.

Finally, many school systems are unaware that their approach to cleaning may impact people's health and the environment and thus may fail to take advantage of opportunities to improve the outcomes. Many health and environmental consequences of cleaning in schools relate to cleaning agents; some result from mechanical and abrasive procedures.

Schools typically use a wide range of cleaning agents. Although some of them pose little or no danger to people's health or the environment, others may be hazardous. These agents are shown in table 14.1.

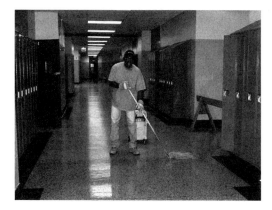

Figure 14.2. This custodian, in Chicago's Crane High School, is applying a low-odor, "green" floor finish acceptable for use while school is in session. (Photo by Stephen Ashkin.)

In addition, as mentioned earlier, mechanical and abrasive cleaning methods can pose health hazards. Schools use janitorial equipment, such as vacuum cleaners, floor buffers, and burnishers to maintain carpeting and hard flooring materials. Studies have shown that the soils removed by such equipment can be contaminated with toxic materials that include lead, pesticides, VOCs, mold spores, and other hazardous materials. These exposures are described more fully in chapter 15.

Some commonly used equipment can actually contribute to health hazards. Vacuum cleaners with poor-quality cloth bags may have no inner liners to adequately capture fine particles. Such vacuums can pull contaminants that would otherwise be trapped in a carpet and make them airborne. High-filtration bags should be used and replaced frequently and should not be allowed to get more than half full, as cleaning effectiveness is compromised when bags fill beyond this level. Custodians should check the bags frequently, at least once per hour.

High-speed burnishers without filter attachments grind the floor finish off the floor and send particles into the air to be inhaled or to resettle as dust on furnishings and elsewhere. Schools should specify and use burnishers and buffers with vacuum attachments and other janitorial equipment that captures and removes dust.

Green Cleaning

Green cleaning takes a systems approach to cleaning. It is based on careful assessment of cleaning needs; identification of healthy, environmentally sound, and cost-effective solutions; and evaluation of results, with adaptive program changes as needed. As with many of the programs discussed in this book, a team approach, with support from a range of stakeholders, is critical to success.

Improving cleaning practices can reduce hazardous exposures and improve the health and performance of students and staff. In the early 1990s, a study at the Frank Porter Graham Child Development Center in Chapel Hill, North Carolina, examined innovative cleaning procedures, including deep-cleaning methods, new equipment, and improved cleaning supplies. *Deep cleaning* includes a variety of techniques, such as pressure washing and high-efficiency vacuuming, that result in a significant reduction of pollutants and pollutant sources.

Table 14.1. Conventional cleaning agents and their risks

Product	Hazardous ingredients	Health or environmental concerns
Glass cleaners	2-Butoxyethanol (ethylene glycol monobutyl ether)	A commonly used solvent that can be absorbed through the skin and inhaled. Can damage the blood, kidney, and nervous system and possibly the liver and reproductive system.
	Methyl, ethyl, and isopropyl alcohol	Solvents used in glass cleaners because they remove greasy fingerprints and evaporate quickly. They are respiratory irritants, and methanol is a nervous system and optic nerve toxin. Some alcohols are poisonous if ingested and toxic to aquatic life once they enter the environment.
	Ammonia (ammonium hydroxide)	A rather old-fashioned cleaning ingredient that is a respiratory irritant and at high doses may damage the nervous, reproductive, and gastrointestinal systems. When inadvertently mixed with cleaning products containing chlorine, produces highly toxic chloramine gas.
Bleach	Sodium hypochlorite	Used commonly as a sanitizer and to remove mold and mildew stains. Bleach can irritate eyes, skin, and airways. It can damage carpets and other building finishes and, if inadvertently mixed with ammonia, will produce highly toxic chloramine gas.
Metal polish	Perchloroethylene (also called tetrachloroethylene)	A solvent "reasonably anticipated to be a human carcinogen" and a suspected reproductive and developmental toxin (Cal Prop 65, EPA SARA Title 3, ATSDR).
	Xylene	Considered a developmental, neurologic, reproductive, immune, and respiratory toxin.
All-purpose cleaner	Cocomide DEA (diethanol-amine)	One of the earliest naturally derived detergents. The DEA portion may form nitrosamines, which are carcinogenic.
	Alcohol ethoxylate	A common surfactant used in cleaning products. The ethoxylation process is typically contaminated with 1,4 dioxane, a known carcinogen with potential toxicity to blood, liver, kidneys, and nervous and immune systems.
Graffiti remover	Dichloromethane	Known carcinogen and potentially toxic to the reproductive, respiratory, cardiovascular, endocrine, gastrointestinal, kidney, and nervous systems.
	Perchloroethylene	See under "metal polish."
	Toluene	A known developmental toxicant that may affect the reproductive, respiratory, cardiovascular, endocrine, gastrointestinal, kidney, and nervous systems.
	Nonylphenol ethoxylates	Commonly used but older surfactant suspected to be an endocrine disrupter.
Carpet spot remover	2-Butoxyethanol	See under "glass cleaners."
	Methyl, ethyl, and isopropyl alcohol	See under "glass cleaners."
	Perchloroethylene	See under "metal polish."
Floor finish	Dibutyl phthalate	A commonly used plasticizer for floor finishes and a suspected developmental, endocrine, and reproductive toxicant.
	Tributoxyethyl phosphate	This ingredient hydrolyzes to 2-butoxyethanol, which is described above.
	Acrylic polymer	Traditional acrylic polymers use zinc, which can be a neurotoxin when it enters the environment after disposal (stripping floors).
	Diethylene glycol methyl ether	Suspected to be toxic to the developmental, endocrine, nervous, and gastrointestinal systems.

This approach reduced airborne dust levels by 52%, total VOC levels by 49%, total bacteria levels by 40%, and total fungi by 61% (Ashkin 2003).

In a daycare center for preschool-age children with Down syndrome, another study assessed a program of careful environmental cleaning and disinfection in addition to infection-control lectures, handouts, and posters. During a year of follow-up observation, decreases were reported in the monthly tallies of total illnesses per child (from 0.70 to 0.53), respiratory illnesses (from 0.67 to 0.42), physician visits (from 0.50 to 0.33), courses of antibiotics administered (from 0.33 to 0.28), and days of school missed as a result of respiratory illness (from 0.75 to 0.40). Although some of this benefit may have resulted from the educational portions of the program, cleaning was thought to account for part of the benefit (Krilov et al. 1996).

With regard to the effects of cleaning on school attendance, several researchers have documented improvements in attendance and the resulting financial benefits to the school district. For example, in the Syracuse, New York, public school district, attendance increased by 11.17% after an improved cleaning strategy that included high-efficiency backpack vacuums, high-efficiency vacuum filters, improvements in organization, and more efficient cleaning processes was implemented. The increased attendance resulted in approximately $2.5 million in additional state funding to the school district, or $25 million over 10 years—roughly the cost of a new elementary or middle school (Ashkin 2003).

How should a green cleaning program be established and operated? Six aspects deserve discussion:

- assessing needs
- building partnerships within the school or school system
- making the business case for green cleaning
- implementing green cleaning products and procedures
- managing personnel issues
- monitoring program success.

Assessing Needs

Before designing or implementing a green cleaning program, current practices must be evaluated and priorities for improvement identified. This is typically accomplished with a structured review, including a walk-through to evaluate issues such as water damage, dust, waste management, presence of clutter, overwatering of plants, and types of chemicals used; and an administrative review to evaluate issues such as the budget and workload for custodians.

One important factor to assess is the custodial workload, which is often measured in terms of how many square feet per hour custodians can clean. No official values for this are available, but 15,000–20,000 square feet per custodian for elementary schools and 17,500–22,500 for custodians in middle and high schools are reasonable benchmarks. The average allocation is larger than these values, and trends are moving in the wrong direction. According to the Maintenance and Operations Cost Study 2003, the latest in a series of annual reports published by *American School and University Magazine,* the number of square feet maintained per custodian has been increasing and reached 24,167 square feet in 2003 (from 23,985 square feet in 2002). This trend reflects declining budgets for school maintenance and raises concerns about the quality of maintenance.

Factors that impact custodial workload include the condition of the school, its size, the grades that are housed in it, the way it is equipped, the local site and climate, the age of the school, and building construction. Some schools are relatively easy to clean, whereas others are a custodian's nightmare. Smaller schools generally require more custodial labor per square foot than larger schools because the latter offer the custodian opportunities for greater efficiencies. Similarly, portable or modular buildings require additional custodial labor, mainly because of the time lost in moving from one building to another. Other uses of the school building may also play an important role. In particular, the extent of preschool, afterschool, and weekend use is directly related to the custodial staffing level needed. The emerging uses of schools as emergency shelters, homeland defense centers, and quarantine areas are important new issues that are beginning to play a significant role in many school districts. In some locations, schools also function as active community centers. Different cleaning approaches will also change the number of custodians. For example, "team cleaning" may not be possible in smaller schools, but it works well in many larger ones. The number of custodians needed also depends on the desired level of cleanliness.

The presence and use of potentially hazardous chemicals should also be assessed. Chemicals of concern include both cleaning materials and chemicals used for other purposes within and outside the classrooms (see chapter 15). To complete this assessment, the team should find, observe, and document every box, bottle, tube, and can containing cleaning materials, science room supplies, art and home economics materials, kitchen and custodial supplies, and any homemade or consumer products in storage areas, classrooms, and elsewhere. This assessment may be part of the housekeeping assessment if they are conducted together, or it may be documented separately as part of the school's chemical hygiene program (see chapter 15). The documentation should list each product, its location, the manufacturer, the hazardous ingredients, if any, and CAS (Chemical Abstracts Services) number, if applicable. Material safety data sheets, shipping manifests, and other documentation of transportation and disposal are also required in this assessment.

Schools should keep a log for all powered janitorial equipment, identifying the dates of purchase and documenting all repair and maintenance performed. Vendor technical bulletins for each piece of equipment in use should be kept with the logbook. These records are an important contribution to the initial assessment.

The housekeeping assessment should result in a written report, which is typically many pages long and may be organized into sections. One report format used widely in the field is shown in box 14.2. The report should be issued promptly after the assessment is completed, and the school should then prioritize its findings for action based on health and safety concerns, costs, and occupants' preferences and aesthetics (in that order).

Building Partnerships within the School or School System

Many members of the school community have reason to support green cleaning. Perhaps most important, custodians have a personal stake in adopting this approach, as they are primarily responsible for cleaning and are directly at risk from any hazardous chemicals in use. Teachers and students have an important stake as well—they spend their entire day at school and may benefit from safer, healthier cleaning methods. Parents and health care providers share an interest in safe and healthy cleaning practices. Environmental groups in the community favor decreased emissions, and the board of education appreciates the cost savings realized from green cleaning measures. It is important to reach out to each of these groups to build support for green cleaning and to implement it successfully.

Because the activities of each group impact the health and safety of other building occupants, each person in each group has a responsibility to help keep the building safe and healthy, a concept known as "the stewardship principle." Its application to green cleaning is shown in box 14.3.

An active stewardship role for teachers and students helps build a better understanding of the importance of cleaning in general (and of green cleaning in particular) and creates a sense of shared responsibility for green cleaning. An important benefit is enhanced awareness of good stewardship of our resources. In addition, the resources of the maintenance and custodial staff are multiplied without sacrificing time for learning.

Teachers and students can become involved in the stewardship role by picking up and preparing

---

■ *14.2. Elements of a needs assessment and ongoing evaluation of school cleaning*

- building usage, exterior site, and neighboring structures
- basements and crawl spaces
- garages, loading docks, and shop areas
- entryways and lobbies
- stairs and elevators
- classrooms
- offices, work spaces, and nurse's room
- specialty-use areas: pools, labs, gym
- kitchen and food preparation and eating areas
- washrooms, restrooms, showers, lockers, and bath areas
- mail, copy rooms, and computer rooms
- custodial closets and storage areas
- roof, mechanical, and overhead crawlspaces, HVAC areas, attics. ■

■ *14.3. Ten principles of stewardship for green cleaning*

1. Schools should celebrate and communicate their successes as part of their commitment to education, people, and better understanding.
2. Schools should establish a goal of cleaning to promote a safer, healthier learning environment. Improved appearance is a typical by-product of this goal.
3. Schools should make a decision to clean buildings as a whole, not as uncoordinated projects done with separate goals.
4. Schools should have written cleaning plans, schedule routine maintenance and cleaning activities, and document them upon completion.
5. Schools should develop response plans to deal with foreseeable incidents and accidents requiring the assistance of the custodial staff including spills, leaks, chemical contamination, smoke, and similar problems requiring fast action and coordination.
6. Schools should minimize human exposure to contaminants, provide adequate personal protection, and use the least hazardous materials for each activity and task in the building.
7. Schools should use cleaning practices that minimize chemical, particle, and moisture residues.
8. School should ensure that they have comprehensive health, safety, and risk management programs in place to protect all staff, students, and visitors.
9. Schools should focus on keeping contaminants out of the building as opposed to cleaning them up once they are inside. Entryways and air intake systems are two pollutant pathways that can be readily controlled.
10. Schools should dispose of waste in ways that encourage recycling, handle and dispose of garbage in a safe and environmentally sound manner, and minimize overall waste. ■

---

their areas before the custodians begin cleaning. This can be done at the end of the school day, with each student having an assigned responsibility such as stacking chairs on desks, picking up paper from the floor, cleaning the chalk boards and white boards, organizing recycling areas, and placing classroom, food, chemical, and other waste in appropriate containers. Another approach is to give a "Golden Trash Can Award" or "Green Cleaning Award" to the homeroom that is kept the cleanest during the week, with the winners earning a pizza party from the principal or maintenance department at the end of the month. Such efforts enable custodial resources to be spent in effective deep cleaning and sanitizing of critical areas.

Making the Business Case for Green Cleaning

The direct costs associated with cleaning the average school, including materials and labor, are approximately $1–$2 per square foot per year, depending on the district and the local labor market. Labor typically accounts for about 90% of the school's cleaning costs. Indirect costs can be considerable, although they are more difficult to calculate. For example, if cleaning is not carried out properly, indirect costs may include absenteeism or expenses for deferred problem solving such as mold remediation.

A careful business analysis can document the economic benefits of a program initiative such as green cleaning (see chapter 24). Savings may be readily available and easily documented (e.g., a metering system that mixes and dispenses cleaning chemicals can save personnel time and reduce the volume of chemicals used). Other benefits are evident as well, such as a reduction in employee exposure to chemicals and waste. Similarly, small adjustments in ventilation systems and cleaning materials can reduce the indoor concentration of contaminants. For teachers and students, a cleaner indoor environment often improves performance and reduces absenteeism. For a school district with escalating waste-disposal and tipping fees, recycling waste and purchasing durable and reusable materials can result in significant savings.

To illustrate the economic effect of green cleaning, consider school entryways. Cleaning industry estimates suggest that 85% of the dirt found in schools is tracked in, through entryways. Entrance mats that are properly sized and extend some distance into the school (typically 15 feet) can trap up to 80% of soil and moisture, reducing the need for vacuuming, dusting, washing, stripping, and recoating of floors (see box 14.4). Anecdotal experience suggests that effective use of mats can generate savings as high as 30–40% per year. In a facility with an average cleaning cost of $1.63 per square foot, the savings in dusting, vacuuming, mopping, waxing, and stripping floors could reach $0.41 per square foot. In a building of 100,000 square feet, this would represent $41,000 per year, roughly the amount needed to hire a custodian.

Implementing Green Cleaning Products and Procedures

The core components of green cleaning involve environmentally preferable purchasing (EPP) of supplies and equipment, the responsible use of these supplies and equipment, and responsible waste management practices.

EPP is a key element of a successful green cleaning program. As defined in Presidential Executive Order 13101 of 1998, Greening the Government through Waste Prevention, Recycling, and Federal Acquisition, EPP means buying "products or services that have a lesser or reduced effect on human health and the environment when compared with competing products or services that serve the same purpose. The product or service comparison may consider raw materials acquisition, production, manufacturing, packaging, distribution, reuse, operation, maintenance, or disposal." The following paragraphs provide specific information on EPP for equipment and cleaning products.

Vacuum cleaners should have high airflow (suction) for more effective soil removal and high-efficiency particulate air (HEPA) or a near-HEPA filter air-filtration system to prevent dust and other materials from passing through cloth bags and into the air. Unfortunately, some vacuum cleaners with HEPA filters are constructed so poorly that fine particles escape from the vacuum before being captured by the filter. Because filtration is the key element in school carpet soil removal, there is generally no need in most schools to use rotating brushes ("power heads") on vacuums. In fact, with modern institutional carpets, this can be counterproductive. The Carpet and Rug Institute, an in-

---

■ *14.4. Entrance mats: A simple preventive technology*

Entrance mats are a simple but effective way to reduce the amount of dirt and moisture tracked into a school. The mats must be wide enough to span the entire entrance way and should extend far enough—about 15 feet, the equivalent of five or six steps—to allow dirt to come off shoes and boots. It is important to consider mobility for students and staff who use wheelchairs or crutches; mats should not prevent the free use of this equipment (see chapter 26). Grit mats are designed to trap gritty or sandy types of soil. They have loops, bars, or ribs, feel hard to the touch, and are meant to scrape dirt off the bottom of shoes. Grit bars can also be incorporated into the entry as an inset in the floor. These mats are cleaned by taking them to a drainage area and using a hose.

Barrier mats are usually made of a synthetic carpet fiber, such as olefin or nylon, which is fused into a rubber or vinyl material. They come in a variety of lengths, widths, and colors and are meant to trap moisture. Olefin mats are economical and effective; nylon mats are more durable and have a higher absorbency rate.

Most people find that changing the mats is easier than continually cleaning the same one. In areas where moisture is high and tracking is constant, such as winter in the upper Midwest, barrier mats are rotated as often as twice a week. Otherwise, a rotation schedule of once every week or two is sufficient.

The most advantageous location for a mat is inside the access or entry areas of the building. Soil-control mats should not be placed on top of carpeting since that could discolor the carpet and also trap moisture. For maximum benefit and ease of maintenance, soil-control mats should be placed on hard surfaces. ■

dustry trade association, has developed a Green Label Program with guidelines that address air flow, particle capture, and other technical aspects of vacuum cleaner performance. The U.S. Green Building Council goes further, recommending that vacuum cleaners should exceed the minimum requirements of the Green Label Program in the following ways:

- greater ability to capture and contain fine respirable particles (capture 96% of particulates 0.3 microns in size as opposed to the usual high-level filtration number of 95%)
- more powerful air flow (> 90 CFM) and suction (static lift of > 80 inches) for enhanced cleaning performance
- durability to reduce the need for early replacement and disposal of old equipment (the manufacturer's warranty on parts and labor should run at least 2 years).

In addition to having the proper equipment, correct use is also important. Vacuuming should be performed on a regular schedule, usually daily, and disposable vacuum bags should be used and changed before they are half full to increase efficient particle capture.

Poorly designed floor buffers and burnishing equipment used to maintain hard flooring surfaces can actually cause unwanted exposures. For example, high-speed floor burnishers without vacuum attachments can generate airborne respirable dust. This equipment should have vacuum attachments.

Traditional string mops can be replaced with newer microfiber mops for cleaning and applying floor waxes, polishes, and other products. For ergonomic reasons and to prevent spills, shallow pans are preferable to buckets when working with microfiber floor applicators. Microfiber materials are also lighter and easier to use than traditional mops and buckets.

All powered equipment, including equipment used for both hard floor and carpet care, should be ergonomically designed to minimize vibration, noise, and user fatigue. Other ergonomic issues to consider include weight, ease of motion, and features of tools and accessories. Powered floor-maintenance equipment should have vacuums, guards, or other devices for capturing fine particulates and should operate with a sound level that is less than 70 dB.

Floor maintenance equipment should also have features to protect the environment. Propane-powered floor equipment should have high-efficiency, low-emission motors. Automated scrubbing machines should be equipped with variable-speed feed pumps to optimize the use of cleaning fluids. Battery-powered equipment should be equipped with environmentally preferable gel batteries, which reduce electricity costs up to 30%, are environmentally preferable to lead acid, and improve operational productivity through low to zero maintenance. Where appropriate, active microfiber technology should be used to reduce cleaning chemical consumption and prolong the life of disposable scrubbing pads. These round, microfiber cloth pads remove and hold dirt and other pollutants better than traditional fibers. Finally, janitorial equipment should have rubber bumpers to reduce potential damage to building surfaces.

Cleaning products are as important as equipment. In selecting cleaning products, several goals must be considered. Green cleaning can guide purchases of chemicals, paper products such as toilet tissue and hand towels, and other cleaning products. Careful selection can reduce toxicity and waste, protect health, and allow schools to model environmentally responsible practices for students to apply at home and in their future careers.

Cleaning products available on the market change frequently, and keeping up with the best ones requires some investment of time. Several sources can provide useful information. Green Seal is an independent, nonprofit organization that identifies and promotes green products and services and certifies them using standard criteria. Green Seal Standard 37 sets standards for three types of commercial cleaners: general-use cleaners, bathroom cleaners, and glass cleaners. Evaluation is based on characteristics such as the following:

- acute and chronic toxicity (eye and skin irritation, sensitization, reproductive toxicity, carcinogenicity)
- environmental impact (aquatic biodegradability, contributions to ozone formation and eutrophication)
- safety characteristics (combustibility, presence of fragrances, packaging and labeling).

Another useful source is the Standard Guide on Stewardship for Cleaning Commercial and Institutional Buildings published by the American Society of Testing and Materials (ASTM). Finally, the U.S.

■ *14.5. Criteria for selecting green cleaning products*

- low toxicity: (1) acute toxicity (e.g., skin or respiratory irritation); (2) chronic toxicity (e.g., liver damage, carcinogenicity)
- low environmental impact: (1) rapid biodegradation (the more rapidly a chemical breaks down, the less it persists in the school environment and the lower the exposure potential); (2) low bioconcentration factor (the lower the bioconcentration factor, the less likely the chemical is to accumulate in the food chain)
- favorable ingredient profile: (1) minimal volatile organic compounds (VOCs contribute to ozone formation and may be directly irritating to the airways); (2) made from ingredients derived from rapidly renewable natural ingredients and thus do not deplete finite resources, for example, surfactants (detergents); solvents made from natural oils such as citrus, coconut, and soy; vegetable derivatives such as cornstarch; (3) minimal cosmetic additives such as fragrances and dyes since some people cannot tolerate them
- favorable safety profile: nonflammable
- ability to minimize human exposure (the product dispensing method should include safety precautions designed to minimize exposure to the concentrated solution)
- animal testing not used in product development
- corporate environmental commitment by manufacturer. ■

General Services Administration has produced EPP purchasing "wizards." The resource list at the end of this chapter provides information on accessing each of these sources.

Cleaning Products

Described in this section are examples of recommended cleaning products that are readily available, are comparable in price to conventional products, and thhat have a neutral environmental and/or health impact. Each category has a limited number of health and environmental attributes that might differentiate one product from another. The product issues cover twenty individual products that represent the majority of janitorial requirements. This list is not intended to be complete but serves to identify some of the typical issues for each product type.

All-purpose cleaners. All-purpose cleaners consist of a broad array of possible formulations. Some of the specific issues to compare for this product category include

- pH: use those with a neutral pH (closer to 7) rather than those with an extreme pH (closer to 1 or 14)
- biodegradability: choose readily biodegradable products instead of those that are slower to degrade. Unfortunately, many older formula-

tions use ingredients that work quite well but cause serious environmental and health effects.

- dyes and fragrances: those with no dyes and fragrances (or very low levels of them) are preferable to products that are heavily dyed or scented. If dyes are necessary, they should be those approved for foods and cosmetics.
- VOCs: use those that have no or very few VOCs instead of alternatives with higher levels. Consider detergent-based products rather than those containing solvents.
- more preferable ingredients: surfactants containing terms such as lauryl, amides, and glycosides.
- less preferable ingredients: nonylphenol ethoxylates, NTA, EDTA, glycol ethers, sodium hydroxide, potassium hydroxide, sodium metasilicate, and phosphates.

Bathroom cleaners. Bathroom cleaners are often acids because of the need to remove mineral deposits from sinks, bowls, and urinals. They are often heavily dyed and strongly fragranced. Here are some of the specific issues to consider for this product category:

- pH: choose products with a more neutral pH over those with a very low pH (closer to 1). Green bathroom cleaners are more likely to have a pH of about 4 than are traditional products, which may have a pH below 1.

- dyes and fragrances: use those with no or low levels rather than heavily dyed or fragranced products. If dyes are necessary, those that are approved for foods and cosmetics are recommended.
- biodegradability: readily biodegradable products are preferable to those that are slower to degrade. Unfortunately, many older formulations use ingredients that perform well but have serious environmental and health effects.
- more preferable ingredients: surfactants containing terms such as lauryl, amides, glycosides, and citric or acetic acid.
- less preferable ingredients: nonylphenol ethoxylates, NTA, EDTA, hydrochloric acid, and phosphoric acid.

Bathroom disinfectants. Bathroom disinfectants are similar to general disinfectants but typically have an acidic pH (closer to 1) to remove hard-water deposits in sinks, bowls, and urinals. The selection issues include those listed previously under general disinfectants and bathroom cleaners. Care in selection and use is important. Here are some of the specific issues to consider (see bathroom cleaners for similar attributes):

- antimicrobial ingredients: choose products with antimicrobial ingredients that have a relatively low potential for persistence in the environment and accumulation in living tissue
- more preferable active ingredient: hydrogen peroxide
- less preferable active ingredients: sodium hypochlorite (chlorine bleach), quaternary ammonium compounds, alcohols, and phenolic compounds.

Carpet cleaners. See all-purpose cleaners (above). Select carpet cleaners that are not sticky or tacky when dry to minimize resoiling and extend the time between cleanings.

Chrome cleaners and polishes. Chrome cleaners and polishes frequently contain petroleum distillates, which are poisonous and derived from a nonrenewable resource. Consider the following for this product category:

- VOCs: choose those that have no or very few VOCs rather than alternatives with higher levels

- bio-based and renewable resources: use products that use oils derived from renewable resources
- more preferable ingredients: water-based emulsions
- less preferable ingredients: petroleum distillates, ammonia.

Drain maintainers. Drain maintainers and drain openers are typically strongly alkaline. They are extremely corrosive to skin and eyes, and can damage plumbing and may contain sodium hypochlorite (chlorine bleach) which is an eye, skin and respiratory irritant. Consider using mechanical snakes to remove clogs and nonpathogenic bacteria and enzyme-based products to maintain the drains and prevent clogs from forming. The following are some specific issues to consider in this category:

- pH: choose those with a more neutral pH instead of those with extreme pH
- more preferable ingredients: non-pathogenic bacteria and enzymes
- less preferable ingredients: sulfuric acid, sodium hydroxide, potassium hydroxide, sodium hypochlorite.

Floor finishes. Floor finishes must be durable and appropriate for the prescribed maintenance method; they typically contain heavy metals. Floor finishes must be compatible with the stripping solution. Specific issues to consider for this product category include the following:

- durability: choose finishes that are more durable (require less maintenance such as buffing, restoring, and recoating) rather than less durable finishes that require more frequent maintenance
- heavy metals: nonmetal cross-linked polymers are preferred over products containing heavy metals. Another significant benefit of nonmetal polymer formulas is that they can frequently be removed with less hazardous floor strippers.
- more preferable ingredients: metal-free polymers
- less preferable ingredients: metal cross-linked polymers.

Floor strippers. Floor strippers typically have an extreme pH value (closer to 14), solvents, and ammoniated compounds necessary to remove metal cross-linked floor finishes. Floor strippers must be compatible with the floor finish. Consider the following issues:

- pH: choose products with a pH closer to neutral (10–12) rather than those with an extreme pH (closer to 14)
- VOCs: use those that have no or very few VOCs compared with alternatives with higher levels
- bio-based and renewable resources: use products that contain naturally derived solvents rather than those containing nonrenewable derived solvents
- more preferable ingredients: d-limonene (citrus solvent) and methyl esters
- less preferable ingredients: ethylene glycol monobutyl ether (butyl cellusolve), 2-butoxyethanol, ammonia, and sodium hydroxide.

Furniture polishes. Furniture polishes frequently use petroleum distillates, which are poisonous and derived from a nonrenewable resource. Specific issues to consider are the following:

- VOCs: choose polishes with no or very few VOCs over alternatives with higher levels
- bio-based and renewable resources: use products with oils derived from renewable resources rather than oils from nonrenewable resources
- more preferable ingredients: citrus (lemon and orange) oils
- less preferable ingredients: petroleum distillates.

General degreasers. General degreasers are typically heavy-duty cleaners that include solvents for removing oil-based soils. Traditional solvents are usually derived from nonrenewable sources (e.g., petroleum), can be flammable, and have a high VOC level. As mentioned, VOCs can cause respiratory irritation and contribute to environmental pollution. Some also create severe health impacts. The following are some of the specific issues to consider for this product category (also see all-purpose cleaners, above):

- VOCs: use those with no or very few VOCs rather than alternatives with higher levels
- bio-based and renewable resources: choose

products containing oils derived from renewable resources rather than oils from nonrenewable resources

- flashpoint: choose products that have a high flashpoint rather those with a low flashpoint
- more preferable ingredients: d-limonene (derived from citrus fruits) and methyl esters from soy and corn
- less preferable ingredients: glycol ethers in general, ethylene glycol monobutyl ether (butyl cellusolve), and sodium hydroxide.

General disinfectants. General disinfectants are similar to bathroom disinfectants and cleaners (see all-purpose cleaners, above), with additional ingredients to kill bacteria and other unwanted organisms. Because disinfectants kill organisms, they are toxic by definition. Some are persistent in the environment and accumulate in living tissue. Care in selection and use is important. Consider the following issues for this product category (see bathroom disinfectants for similar attributes):

- antimicrobial ingredients: antimicrobial ingredients that have a lower potential for persistence in the environment and accumulation in living tissue are preferred over those with a greater potential
- more preferable active ingredient: hydrogen peroxide
- less preferable active ingredients: sodium hypochlorite (chlorine bleach), quaternary ammonium compounds, and phenolic compounds.

Glass cleaners. Glass cleaners have ingredients added to reduce streaking and to evaporate quickly. Traditional glass cleaners can contain alcohol and other solvents (typically glycol ethers) or ammonia. Specific issues to consider for this product category include the following:

- VOCs: choose those that have no or very few VOCs over alternatives with higher levels. Consider detergent-based products rather than those containing solvents.
- flashpoint: use products that have a high flashpoint rather than those with a low flashpoint
- pH: those with a neutral pH (closer to 7) are preferred over those with an extreme pH (closer to 1 or 14)

- biodegradability: use products that are readily biodegradable rather than those that are slower to degrade. Unfortunately, many older formulations use ingredients that work quite well but have serious environmental and health concerns.
- dyes and fragrances: the best products are those with no or very low levels of dyes and fragrances. If dyes are necessary, use those approved for foods and cosmetics.
- more preferable ingredients: surfactants containing terms such as lauryl, amides, and glycosides
- less preferable ingredients: ammonia, alcohols, propylene glycol, ethylene glycol, and other glycol ethers.

Graffiti removers. Before they were banned because of their environmental impact, graffiti removers were formulated with chlorinated solvents (e.g., methylene chloride). Many of them are packaged in aerosol containers that are full of highly flammable hydrocarbon propellants (e.g., propane, butane), which can contribute to indoor air quality problems.

- VOCs: choose products with no or very few VOCs. Consider detergent-based products rather than those containing solvents.
- flashpoint: use products that have a high flashpoint
- pH: products with a neutral pH (closer to 7) are preferable to those with an extreme pH (closer to 1 or 14)
- more preferable ingredients: n-methyl-2-pyrolidone, d-limonene
- less preferable ingredients: methylene chloride, petroleum distillates, propane, butane, isobutene, and sodium hydroxide.

Gum removers. Before they were banned because of their environmental impact, gum removers were formulated with chlorinated solvents (e.g., freon). Dry ice and carbon dioxide are preferable replacements. Degreasers can be used in some situations (see section on general degreasers).

- VOCs: choose those that have no or very few VOCs. Consider detergent-based products rather than those containing solvents.
- flashpoint: products with a high flashpoint are preferable to those with a low flashpoint

- pH: use those with a neutral pH (closer to 7) rather than those with extreme pH (closer to 1 or 14)
- more preferable ingredients: dry ice, carbon dioxide
- less preferable ingredients: freon, dichlorodifluoromethane, trichlorofluoromethane.

Lime and scale removers. Lime and scale removers are acids. They are used to remove mineral deposits from sinks, bowls, and urinals.

- pH: choose those with a more neutral pH instead of those with extreme pH (closer to 1). Environmentally preferable lime and scale removers may fall more in the range of pH 4, in contrast to traditional products, which may have a pH below 1.
- more preferable ingredients: citric or acetic acid
- less preferable ingredients: hydrochloric or phosphoric acid.

Solvent spot removers. Solvent spot removers are necessary for spot removal, particularly on carpets. Use detergent-based spotters if possible (they must be followed with extraction or other method to remove/absorb the detergent). (See all-purpose cleaners.) Look for these characteristics:

- VOCs: choose products that have no or very few VOCs
- flashpoint: products that have a high flashpoint are recommended
- more preferable ingredients: d-limonene (derived from citrus fruits) and methyl esters from soy and corn
- less preferable ingredients: mineral spirits, 2-butoxyethanol.

Urinal deodorizers. Urinal deodorizers are usually blocks placed in urinals to reduce odors. These deodorizers should be eliminated altogether, if possible, by more frequent cleaning and other methods of deodorizing. However, if deodorizers are still required, preference should be given to those with the safest ingredients.

- biodegradability: use detergents that are readily biodegradable. Unfortunately, many older formulations use ingredients that are very effective but have serious environmental and health concerns.

- more preferable ingredients: surfactants containing ingredients such as lauryl, amides, and glycosides
- less preferable ingredients: nonylphenol ethoxylates, paradichlorobenzene.

Wood and stone floor coatings. Wood and stone floor coatings have traditionally been solvent-based products. Although they are extremely durable and protect flooring materials that are expensive to replace, these coatings can be quite hazardous during the drying and curing period. The two primary issues to consider during product selection are the use of material with no or very few VOCs (to reduce indoor air quality concerns) and the product's durability, which is important in protecting the flooring and minimizing the cost of products and applications. Many janitorial firms lack specific expertise in the application of these types of finishes; for this reason, supplier support (e.g., training) is important.

- durability: choose durable finishes that require less maintenance (e.g., recoating)
- flashpoint: use products that have a high flashpoint
- more preferable ingredients: water-based or epoxy-based finishes
- less preferable ingredients: xylene, stoddard solvent.

Some custodians bring chemical "home recipes" to school or mix ingredients from the grocery or hardware store together at school—an unwise practice for several reasons. First, consumer products are not labeled to meet OSHA requirements and may create liability and training problems for schools. Second, home recipes are typically ready to use, which makes them more expensive than concentrated commercial products. Third, mixing chemicals may create health hazards. The classic example is mixing ammonia and bleach, which results in the release of chlorine gas which can be deadly. For these reasons, it is prudent to avoid using household cleaners at schools.

Reliable dispensing equipment systems are increasingly available for concentrated cleaners. Industry experience suggests that the use of dispensing equipment results in a 30–65%, reduction in chemical use, decreases environmental waste, controls costs, and reduces human exposure to chem-

icals. Systems for virtually every custodial product are available, and their use is encouraged.

Floor-coating products should be very durable in order to protect floor surfaces effectively, minimize the labor needed to maintain appearance and gloss, and reduce the frequency of reapplication. Products should be free of phthalates as well as metals such as zinc.

Because floor stripping is particularly hazardous for custodians, this process should be undertaken only when necessary and only when the school is unoccupied. Floor stripping and recoating are extremely labor intensive and should be performed only with the proper machinery and by those who have had proper training. This process can and should be minimized by using a floor-maintenance program.

A successful floor care program includes a solid foundation coating, followed by regular maintenance. An appropriate foundation is based on the durability of the finish and the number of coats (frequently 6–12 coats) used to make up the base. The maintenance program includes sweeping, dusting, vacuuming, mopping, and the use of walkoff mats to extend the life of the floor coating. Together these procedures maintain a superior appearance and reduce both labor and the amount of chemicals used and discharged into the environment. Some floor coatings are marketed on the basis of their high solids content. There is no evidence that the percentage of solid content is associated with a more durable product or a healthier building. The ingredients and manner in which the products are applied and maintained are the critical factors.

Hand care is an important component of school health. It is useful to provide proper products, dispensers, and facilities that encourage hand washing. Hand soaps that do not contain additional antimicrobial agents other than those needed as product preservatives are recommended, but health codes may require the use of such agents in food service areas and nurses' offices. Generally speaking, in bathrooms and classrooms with sinks, a liquid soap dispenser and 20 seconds of hand washing are very effective in preventing the spread of germs and will not introduce potentially toxic chemicals into the environment. Soaps made from ingredients that are derived from rapidly renewable natural ingredients and thus do not deplete finite resources are preferred, for example, soaps made from natural oils such as coconut and soy and from vegetable derivatives such as cornstarch.

Carpet care requires the use of proper cleaning chemicals. Green Seal, the Center for a New American Dream, the Carpet and Rug Institute, the carpet manufacturer, and other experts can provide useful information on the chemicals to use. School carpets should be extraction cleaned at least twice a year, usually before the school year starts and again during the winter break. The following precautions are recommended for extraction cleaning. Clean the carpet just before school opening, and completely dry it. If using a wet cleaning method, extract the moisture thoroughly. If possible, dry within 12 hours, but certainly within 24 hours. Indoor humidity greater than 60% is considered extremely high and can lead to mold growth. Consider using air movers or drying fans with wet cleaning methods. Follow the directions for mixing solutions carefully. Using a solution stronger than is recommended will not improve cleaning efficiency and may leave behind detergent residue that will accelerate carpet soiling. Limit access to the damp carpet until it is completely dry to avoid rapid resoiling. Various cleaning methods may be used separately or in combination for maintaining traffic areas and for overall cleaning. Always get the manufacturer's recommendations for preferred cleaning methods to prevent invalidation of applicable warranties.

Purchasing paper for schools is an opportunity to model leadership and environmental responsibility and at the same time to reduce expenses. Commercial and institutional use of paper towels, toilet tissue, and napkins accounts for billions of pounds of paper each year, the equivalent of millions of trees. Reducing paper waste and using paper made from recycled materials manufactured in a chlorine-free process decreases adverse environmental impacts significantly. Paper dispensed from large rolls reduces waste and packaging. To reduce the spread of infectious agents, the most effective dispenser is hands free and has no lever or cranks.

Disposable Paper and Plastic Bags

Selecting paper products is much easier than choosing cleaning products. The issues of concern for paper are focused primarily on the manufacturing stage of the product. Whereas cleaners may have more then a dozen ingredients that can vary significantly from category to category and even among different products within the same category, paper is relatively simple. It has fewer effects on health issues during the product's usage stage and fewer environmental impacts as a result of disposal.

The three basic concerns for paper usage include are total recovered material (recycled content), the postconsumer recycled content, and the bleaching process. Environmentally preferable paper products should meet the following standards for each of the product categories:

- bathroom tissue—minimum 20% postconsumer content
- facial tissue—minimum 10% postconsumer content
- toilet seat covers—minimum 40% postconsumer content
- paper towels and general-purpose industrial wipes—minimum 40% postconsumer content
- plastic trash bags—minimum 10% postconsumer content.

Two further recommendations for paper are no use of de-inking solvents containing chlorine or any other chemicals listed in the toxics-release inventory in the manufacture of paper products and no use of chlorine or chlorine derivatives in the bleaching processes for paper products. Paper dispensers—those used in restrooms to dispense paper hand towels, for example—should be touch free, which reduces the potential for cross-contamination of bacteria and other potentially harmful pathogens.

Janitorial Equipment

Finally, some considerations for equipment selection might include using vacuums with HEPA filtration capable of trapping 99.97% of all airborne particles collected by the vacuum. In addition, floor machines with guards and filters are preferable. Beater bars, an option for commercial vacuum cleaners, may be inadvisable, since institutional carpets usually have short pile; as a result, beater bars contribute little to cleaning, but may cause particles to become airborne and become a potential respiratory hazard. For all equipment purchases, select products that are durable, energy efficient, and quiet rather than less durable, less efficient, and noisier alternatives.

Choosing a Product Supplier

The final component in the selection of products is consideration of the supplier. The product supplier will play an important role as part of the Stewardship Task Force and may be intimately involved in training. Furthermore, the supplier's standard operating practices can impact inventory levels and the amount of materials, including hazardous items, that may be stored in the facility. Therefore, in addition to price and other traditional purchasing concerns, consider the suppliers' ability to train cleaning personnel and their expertise with green janitorial products and cleaning.

Managing Personnel Issues

In initiating a green cleaning approach and maintaining the program over time, custodial staff are critical to success. Custodians need to accept the principles of green cleaning and even become its champions. They should be trained in the rationale for green cleaning and involved in program implementation as much as possible. For example, if custodians play a role in product selection, they are more likely to buy into the program.

More broadly, successful school cleaning requires a well-run custodial program. Considerations for custodial management activities include the following:

- Does the personnel policy include maintenance and contracted staff?
- Do job descriptions reflect the identified needs of the organization?
- Do job descriptions outline the necessary qualifications to perform the work?
- Does the organizational chart accurately delineate reporting responsibilities?
- Are training opportunities available and relevant to the duties of the staff?
- Are all tradespeople and other outside contractors fully licensed for their work?
- Are industry guidelines used to determine custodial staffing needs?

Schools may consider supplementing in-house expertise with outside consultants. This is often unnecessary since resources such as the Healthy Schools Campaign's Quick & Easy Guide to Green Cleaning, Collaborative for High-Performance Schools (CHPS), the U.S. EPA's Tools for Schools,

and the Washington State School Indoor Air Quality Best Management Practices Manual provide free, expert advice. When a school decides to hire a consultant, the goal should be to create a high-quality cleaning program that will continue after the professional is gone. A prospective consultant should provide the school personnel with a current résumé and a list of completed school projects, including names and contact information for primary site contacts to verify the consultant's experience. It is useful to check for a professional's affiliation with major national organizations, including Green Seal; the U.S. Green Building Council (USGBC); Green Flag Schools; the Institute of Inspection, Cleaning, and Restoration Certification (IICRC); the International Sanitary Supply Association; the Center for a New American Dream; the National Environmental Health Association; the American Conference of Governmental Industrial Hygienists; and other reputable agencies and organizations with a track record of commitment to environmental health and safety in schools.

Monitoring Program Success

Program success is monitored with the use of standard outcome metrics. In an ongoing evaluation, baseline conditions are established, and trends are followed and reported on a regular basis. Some commonly used metrics are direct labor and material costs, administrative overhead, and claims paid. Employee and student absenteeism are also important to follow. In schools, academic performance is routinely followed through metrics such as standardized test scores, which can be correlated with changes in maintenance procedures. Employee satisfaction with the school environment can also be assessed. Custodial employees should be frequently consulted about the program, and their suggestions should be seriously considered. It is important to report the results of the program evaluation to all concerned parties.

Conclusion

Cleaning is an essential activity in schools. The emerging approach to cleaning schools known as green cleaning addresses each part of the "triple bottom line": environmental performance, cost, and human impact (including health, comfort, and performance). When implemented well, green cleaning also yields clean schools that provide positive settings in which students can learn and staff can work. Many green cleaning techniques are now well established and commercially available for schools to implement. Not only do they make good sense from the environmental, business, and health point of view, but they also provide an opportunity to educate students about optimal practices.

Resources

Green Cleaning Resources

- American Society of Testing and Materials, Standard Guide on Stewardship for Cleaning Commercial and Institutional Buildings (E-1971-98)
  http://www.astm.org
- Ashkin Group. Tips on green cleaning in schools
  http://www.AshkinGroup.com
- California Integrated Waste Management Board
  http://www.ciwmb.ca.gov/wpie/Purchasing
- Carpet and Rug Institute
  http://www.carpet-rug.com
- Center for a New American Dream. Environmentally Preferable Purchasing Program
  http://www.newdream.org; http://www.newdream.org/procure
- Center for Health, Environment, and Justice. Green Flag Schools
  http://www.greenflagschools.org
- Collaborative for High-Performance Schools, vol. 4
  http://www.chps.net/manual/index.htm
- Commonwealth of Massachusetts. Request for Response for Environmentally Preferable Cleaning Products (RFR #GR016). Awarded April 2003.
- Green Seal Standard 37 (GS-37) (www.greenseal.org). This private-sector resource provides guidelines for green purchasing. Specific information on cleaning supplies may be found at
  www.greenseal.org/standards/industrialcleaners.htm.
- Illinois Healthy Schools Campaign
  http://www.healthyschoolscampaign.org

- Leadership in Energy and Environmental Design (LEED) green building rating system for existing buildings
  https://www.usgbc.org/FileHandling/show_general_file.asp?DocumentID=913
- National Clearinghouse for Educational Facilities
  http://www.edfacilities.org/rl/cleaning.cfm
- Pennsylvania green building maintenance manual
  http://www.dgs.state.pa.us/dgs/lib/dgs/green_bldg/greenbuildingbook.pdf
- Presidential Executive Order 13101, Section 201: Greening the government
  http://www.ofee.gov/eo/13101.htm
- State of Washington K–12 health and safety guide
  http://www.k12.wa.us/SchFacilities/HealthSafetyGuide.aspx
- State of Washington school indoor air quality best management practices manual, 2d ed.
  http://www.doh.wa.gov/ehp/ts/IAQ/schooliaqbmp.pdf
- U.S. EPA. Environmentally Preferable Purchasing Program
  http://yosemite1.epa.gov/oppt/eppstand2.nsf
- U.S. EPA. Tools for Schools
  http://www.epa.gov/iaq/schools/tools4s2.html
- U.S. Green Building Council
  http://www.usgbc.org/

References

American School and University. 2003. Maintenance and operations cost study. Available: http://research.asumag.com/#MOCost [accessed 6 March 2004].

Ashkin S. The all-purpose solution. 2003. American School and University. Available: http://asumag.com/mag/university_allpurpose_solution [accessed 6 March 2004].

Barron T, Berg C, Bookman L. 1999. How to select and use safe janitorial chemicals. Project Completion Report. Janitorial Products Pollution Prevention Project. Available: http://www.wrppn.org/Janitorial/05%20Report.pdf [accessed 6 March 2004].

Fisk W, Rosenfeld A. Summer 1997. Improved productivity and health from better indoor environments. Center for Building Science News. Available: http://eetd.lbl.gov/newsletter/cbs_nl/nl15/productivity.html [accessed 6 March 2004].

Krilov LR, Barone SR, Mandel FS, Cusack TM, Gaber DJ, Rubino JR. 1996. Impact of an infection control program in a specialized preschool. Am J Infect Control 24(3):167–173.

National Center for Education Statistics. 2003. Planning guide for maintaining school facilities. Publication NCES 2003347. Washington, DC: Author. Available: http://nces.ed.gov/pubs2003/maintenance/ [accessed 16 January 2006].

Watson WA, Litovitz TL, Rodgers GC Jr., Klein-Schwartz W, Youniss J, Rose SR, et al. 2003. 2002 annual report of the American Association of Poison Control Centers toxic exposure surveillance system. Am J Emerg Med 21(5):353–421.

Jennifer Audi and Robert J. Geller

Chemical Exposures in and out of the Classroom

■ *Summary*

- Students and staff can be exposed to hazardous substances at school via inhalation, skin contact, or ingestion.
- Children may be more susceptible than adults to injury from toxic exposures.
- Outside the school, materials, including treated wood and roofing products, pose a hazard for toxic exposure. Contamination from landfills, groundwater, or well water can present additional toxic risk.
- Toxic exposure in the classroom can result from arts and crafts supplies or theater makeup, sets, and special-effects materials. Students and teachers in shop class are at risk for exposure from solvents and glue; paints, varnishes, and other finishes; metal reactions; and wood by-products.
- Exposure in the school building from asbestos, lead, insulation, and flooring is a concern, especially during periods of substantial renovation. Office equipment and supplies can cause respiratory and skin irritation in sensitive people. ■

On many occasions students, teachers, and staff may be exposed to hazardous substances. Pesticides are perhaps the best recognized of these materials (see chapter 13), and some cleaning materials are also hazardous (see chapter 14). Foods may contain various toxic substances or may cause allergic reactions in predisposed people. In this chapter we review some of the other toxic hazards that children might encounter in and around their schools. We discuss the ways in which a child might be exposed, as well as the possible effects of the exposures, and review strategies to reduce risks and manage the exposures if they do occur.

Toxic Exposures: An Overview

A toxin can be simply defined as any substance that can cause injury to an exposed person if the dose and time of exposure are sufficiently great.

Routes of Exposure

The most common routes of exposure to a toxin are inhalation, skin contact, and ingestion.

Inhalation

Inhaled substances in the form of airborne particles, spray mists, or gases may be toxic. Once inhaled, a toxic substance may irritate the lungs. Irritation of the lungs can cause coughing and shortness of breath and possibly worsen preexisting asthma or airway disease. After entering the lungs, the chemical may also be absorbed by the membranes of the lungs and possibly affect the rest of the body. Such an exposure can occur, for example, during renovation, painting, or installation of new furniture and carpets. Chemicals used in arts and crafts classes can also be inhaled.

Skin Contact

Particles, mists, and gases can be absorbed through the skin and result in toxicity. The eyes are particularly vulnerable to contact with airborne substances and irritating or toxic matter. Chemicals spilled on the skin can damage the skin, causing irritation, burns, or allergic reactions. Some chemicals absorbed through the skin have widespread effects throughout the body. The character and severity of such reactions are determined by the types of chemicals and the length of time they remain in contact with the skin.

Ingestion

Toxic exposures can occur from the ingestion of liquid or solid forms of potentially dangerous substances. When toxic substances are swallowed, they can irritate the mouth or the digestive system. If coughing or vomiting occurs during swallowing or while the substance is in the stomach, the chemical can be regurgitated into the lungs and cause damage at that site. As with skin contact, an ingested toxin can cause direct injury to the tissues it contacts, be absorbed into the body, and cause widespread effects.

Allergic Reaction or Toxicity?

Many people confuse an allergic reaction with illness caused by a toxic substance. A toxic substance is one that will have a deleterious effect on the body in most people exposed to a specific amount. An allergic reaction occurs when the body's immune system attempts to fight a substance that is not harmful in most people, and the body's defense

■ *15.1. Food allergies*

Some foods cause allergic reactions, and because many children eat as many as half of their weekly meals at school, it is not unlikely that they may experience such reactions during the school day. Peanuts, milk and dairy products, eggs, soy, corn, and wheat are the most likely food ingredients to cause allergic reactions in susceptible people. Some schools have addressed this issue by minimizing the potential for exposure to people already identified as sensitive to a specific food; other schools have altered their menus. Given the wide range of possible offending agents and the varying elements of food service, a single approach cannot be applied to all schools. ■

mechanism itself then becomes part of the problem. For example, a small percentage of the population is allergic to strawberries. When those people eat strawberries, they develop an allergic reaction that may include anything from a simple itchy rash to swelling of the lips and tongue and difficulty breathing. However, strawberries would not be classified as a poisonous or toxic fruit simply because some people have such a reaction (see box 15.1).

Children May Be More Susceptible

Children may be especially susceptible to injury from a toxic material for several reasons: Their bodies are typically smaller than adults, their organs are not fully mature, and they are still growing.

The dose–response relationship is an important concept. In general, when exposure to a toxin increases, the potential for toxicity in an individual also increases. When considering exposure to harmful substances, one must also consider the size of the person exposed. Because children typically are smaller than adults, the same dose of a particular toxin may be more harmful to a child than to an adult. The concept of dose per pound of body weight is important when evaluating the potential for harm from a particular exposure.

For many compounds, their distribution

throughout the body and their metabolism can be considerably different in children. Children have different ratios of body water and fat compared with adults, and this can affect the distribution of a particular substance. *Distribution* refers to the parts of the body to which the chemical spreads. In addition, certain metabolic processes (the mechanisms for breaking down certain chemicals or drugs) may not be fully developed in children. Where this occurs, the most common result is that the child is unable to convert a harmful substance into a nontoxic one as effectively as an adult. Moreover, the barrier between the blood compartment and the brain compartment is more permeable during the first few years of life. Children, especially those younger than 1–2 years of age, do not exclude some substances from their central nervous systems as well as adults and therefore may be more sensitive to particular chemicals.

Immature organs in children often have increased vulnerability to certain chemicals that injure cells only while the cells are growing. Once organs are mature, the toxins of this type are not hazardous. Liver, kidney, nervous tissue, heart, bone, and muscle all continue to grow well into childhood.

Environmental Factors

How children interact with their environments is also important to consider. Some toxic fumes and gases are heavier than ambient air and tend to settle closer to the ground. Children not only are generally shorter, but often spend a good deal of their play time sitting, crawling, and lying on the ground. While playing on the floor, children may also be exposed to pesticides, chemicals from the floor (both carpet and finished bare floor), and any particles that may have settled on the floor surface. Temperature and humidity also play a role in how people react to toxins in their environment. Some gases from flooring, treated-wood walls, and carpets are released more readily when the air in the room is warm.

Personal Safety

In some settings, products such as "pepper spray" or "tear gas," known by many trade names including Mace, may be carried as personal protection devices. Such agents pose the potential for irritation not only of both the intended recipient and the person activating the device, but bystanders as well. Pepper spray contains capsaicin, a potent irritant of the eyes, skin, nose, and throat with contact or inhalation. Tear gas contains one of several chemicals (lacrimators) that cause the eyes to water profusely.

Some people respond to irritants more than others, even at equal levels of exposure. If symptoms develop after exposure, the exposed area should be rinsed with large amounts of clean water. If symptoms persist or are severe, emergency medical help should be obtained.

Outside the School

Playgrounds

Playground safety is a broad topic encompassing injury prevention from falls and other mechanical issues, as well as enclosure maintenance. These topics are covered in chapters 8 and 18 of this book.

One area of toxic risk to children is the treated wood used in the construction of play structures. Some pressure-treated woods contain arsenic compounds, most commonly chromated copper arsenate, to prevent the deterioration of the wood from fungi and insects. Arsenic has been found to leach out of the wood and may be present in high levels in the surrounding soil. Arsenic compounds are not absorbed through intact skin but can be absorbed by the digestive tract if swallowed. In the United States, the production of pressure-treated outdoor wood with arsenic compounds has been eliminated recently in favor of ammonia-based compounds or other chromium-containing products. Because most of the leaching of arsenic and chromium occurs when the treated wood is first installed, older existing structures pose a lesser risk (Babich 1998; Gordon et al. 2002; Lesser and Weiss 1995; Schwar and Alexander 1988; Stadler et al. 1994; Stilwell and Gorny 1997; Tran et al. 2003).

Some lumber used in outdoor, exposed construction may also be treated with chlorinated phenols. This group of chemicals has been associated with human toxicity ranging from skin and respiratory irritation to the development of cancers. However, no data exist to link exposure to phenol-treated woods with human health effects. It is unclear whether there is sufficient phenol exposure from treated wood used in outdoor construction to cause toxicity (Daniels and Swan 1979).

Herbicides

Maintenance of school grounds often leads to the outdoor application of garden and lawn-care products (pesticide issues are discussed in chapter 13). Also worthy of consideration is the subject of herbicides. These weed-control products may come into contact with people during their storage or application or through contact with treated areas.

Commonly used herbicides include glyphosate (sold under trade names including Round-Up and Kleen-Up) and 2,4-D (2,4-diphenoxyacetic acid). Glyphosate is generally sold as a liquid and applied as a spray, while 2,4-D is frequently an ingredient of granular "weed and feed" products.

Glyphosate presents only a minimal toxic hazard to people, whether from direct contact or from contact with treated lawns and planting areas. Other ingredients are often added to the product to make the spray adhere better to the treated surfaces, and these ingredients may also pose a small risk of toxicity if they are swallowed or contact the skin extensively. Once the applied glyphosate product has dried on the treated area, it does not pose a risk of human toxicity from contact with the treated area. Cattle, sheep, and other ruminant animals should not be allowed to eat glyphosate-treated plants, as the glyphosate may prove harmful to them, particularly when eaten in large quantities.

In commonly available concentrations, 2,4-D is only a minimal toxic hazard to people. The herbicide used in the 1970s called Agent Orange contained 2,4-D as one of its ingredients, but the toxicity of Agent Orange is usually attributed to other ingredients of the mixture. Once the product has been applied and watered in as directed then allowed to dry, it does not pose a risk of human toxicity from contact with the treated area.

Roofing

Toxic chemicals in rainwater runoff from rooftops is an environmental consideration. Runoff can contaminate nearby groundwater and soil and may include particles of roof-top material or substances from the environment that have accumulated on the roof. Roofing materials include galvanized metals or asphalt shingles.

Runoff from roofs made of galvanized metals typically contains heavy metals such as zinc and cadmium. Other metals are often also present but in much smaller amounts. To date, there are no data proving a harmful effect on humans from rooftop runoff. However, in rural schools using well water, groundwater and well water should be tested periodically to ensure safety (Pickrell et al. 1983; van Faasen and Borm 1991).

Asphalt is used to coat roofing materials and road surfaces; because it is hot when applied, burns are a risk. As asphalt cools, it produces a characteristic and offensive odor and can give off toxic fumes containing hydrocarbons, methane, propane, hydrogen sulfide, and carbon monoxide. During ongoing roofing at school, children and staff should be kept away from the areas where there is active use of asphalt. Generally these types of construction activities occur outside, where there is natural ventilation. However, building air intakes located near asphalt activities can suck the odor and fumes into a building (Azizian et al. 2003; Farfel et al. 2003; Sullivan and Krieger 2001).

Proximity to cooling asphalt may result in difficulty in breathing, dizziness, or lightheadedness, as well as nausea from the hydrocarbons and carbon monoxide. Hydrogen sulfide has a strong odor, often reported as a "rotten-egg" smell, and most commonly causes irritation to the eyes, nose, and throat, as well as difficulty in breathing. At high enough concentrations, the gas can alter the ability of the blood to carry oxygen and thus cause fainting and possibly even life-threatening illness. People who exhibit symptoms after exposure to cooling asphalt should be removed from the area immediately into fresh air. Anyone who faints or has persistent symptoms should be evaluated by medical personnel.

In addition to the risks from close exposure to cooling asphalt, roadwork also has the potential to cause significant amounts of dust. People with underlying asthma or lung disease are likely to be more sensitive to dusts in the air and experience respiratory irritation and difficulty in breathing. Care should be taken to limit the amount of exposure in schools by moving classes away from areas of ongoing roadwork and supplying adequate fresh-air ventilation to classes that may be exposed to these dusts.

Contaminated Sites

Hazardous waste sites and landfills near schools are frequently topics of concern among parents and teachers. The U.S. EPA defines a "brownfield site" as a location that is complicated by the presence or potential presence of a hazardous substance, pollutant, or contaminant (http://www.epa.gov/brownfields). The toxin content in the runoff water (or leachate) from these sites raises the possibility of groundwater and soil contamination. The composition of these sites varies significantly, as they may contain myriad toxins in varying forms and levels. Contact the appropriate local, state, and federal officials if safety concerns arise in a school near such a site. The Agency for Toxic Substances and Disease Registry (ATSDR) has conducted a study of schools near brownfield sites in one region of the country and found no toxic hazards within the schools (ATSDR 2002; Greenberg 2003; Kaufman et al. 2003; Leung et al. 1993; Lockey and Wiese 1992).

Groundwater

When schools are located near a pond or lake, toxins may accumulate in the water; exposure may occur when children play in the water or when substances evaporate from the water. Compounds present in the groundwater under the school may also rise to the surface when environmental conditions are favorable, such as after heavy rain.

If concern develops about exposure to chemicals in this manner, testing of the suspect water may be appropriate. Care should be taken to make certain that testing is done by a qualified lab on a sample that has been carefully collected and stored (Azizian et al. 2003; Mushak and Crocetti 1990; Polkowska et al. 2002; Rudel et al. 2003).

Well Water

When a school's drinking water is supplied from a private well, periodic testing of the water is appropriate to ensure that it is free of bacterial or chemical contamination. Changes in the local water table or changes in land use may result in altered content at the well. The assistance of local water or health officials may be sought to collect water and have it tested appropriately.

Landfills

Schools are sometimes sited near sanitary landfills, and whether the landfill is closed or still operating, gases may be emitted from the area as its contents decompose. The gases that are emitted are usually methane and hydrogen sulfide. Methane is not toxic itself but may displace oxygen if it accumulates in a low-lying space. Hydrogen sulfide, with its characteristic rotten-egg smell, may displace oxygen and also interfere with the body's ability to use oxygen.

Air flow patterns fluctuate during the day and are altered by wind speed, wind direction, and weather. Where exposure to landfill emissions is of concern, the air should be monitored either continuously for several days or at various times of the day during differing weather conditions (Garcia de Cortazar et al. 2002; Isidori et al. 2003; James 1977; Stubblefield et al. 1989; Tarkowski et al. 2000; Van Metre and Mahler 2003).

In the Classrooms

In this section, we discuss hazards associated with specific types of classroom learning.

Arts and Crafts

Arts and crafts education encompasses a vast array of different activities that may pose health risks. Children participating in art classes must be supervised at all times. Students should use age-appropriate materials, and all materials should be nontoxic if possible. Donated art materials should be checked to determine whether they are nontoxic and safe before they are distributed and used. To limit the possible ingestion of materials, younger children should be given only small amounts of materials to work with at one time. To decrease the possibility of ingesting art materials, students should not be allowed to have food and drink in the classroom.

Good hygiene for both children and their work areas must be taught, encouraged, and enforced. Children who develop an adverse reaction to the materials they are working with should be removed from the area. Any spills onto their skin or clothes should be promptly cleaned off. If art materials come into contact with the eyes, the eyes should be flushed with large amounts of water. In addition, in the case of ingestion of art materials or contact with the eyes, contact the local poison center; the national poison center hotline number (1-800-222-1222) will reach the appropriate poison center for the caller's phone exchange anywhere in the United States. It is a good idea to keep the original containers of the materials for a quickly available list of the ingredients. Proper disposal of leftover art materials is also necessary to prevent future exposure.

The Art and Creative Materials Institute (ACMI; 2004) has developed labels for art supplies that designate their level of toxicity (table 15.1). The CP seal and the AP seal indicate that a product is nontoxic even if ingested. The CL seal indicates that a product contains toxic ingredients. Products labeled with the CL seal can be used safely but with caution. The HL seal indicates that a product contains one or more toxic components that are present in sufficient quantities to have an immediate or long-term effect on health. Products with CL seals (e.g., rubber cement containing n-hexane) should be used only by people who can read, understand, and follow the directions for safe use. These types of products should be avoided when working with young children. Products with HL seals are best avoided in the school setting (Babich 1998; City of Tucson n.d.; Tran et al. 2003; Watt et al. 2000).

Paint and Drawing Materials

Although numerous types of paint are available on the market, we discuss only the most commonly used media here. Watercolors and acrylics available in schools are generally nontoxic, but all labels should be carefully inspected. If a product is lacking a label indicating that it is nontoxic, the product

Table 15.1. ACMI art product labeling of possible toxicity

Label seal	Toxic risk
CP (Certified Product)	Nontoxic
AP (Approved Product)	Nontoxic
CL (Caution Label)	One or more toxic components; use with caution
HL (Health Label)	One or more toxic components; health effects possible even with appropriate use

should be used only with great caution and under direct faculty supervision until toxicity is determined, which may require contacting the manufacturer. Even though painting materials in schools should be nontoxic if swallowed, these products may cause respiratory irritation if their dust is inhaled.

Some products, such as oil-based paints, also contain substances that can be irritating to the skin of sensitive people. Oil paints are also used with turpentine and mineral spirits, which are toxic if swallowed and also absorb readily through the skin. With younger children, water-based latex paints should be substituted for oil-based paints unless there is a specific need for the oil-based product. Preteens and teens should be able to use oil-based products safely if good ventilation, appropriate supervision, and protective gloves and garments are provided. Ingestion of these compounds can cause sleepiness. If these products are swallowed and vomited, droplets can enter the lungs and cause inflammation and irritation. Children working with such chemicals must be closely monitored and given only small amounts to work with at one time. If exposure does occur, contact a poison center immediately for further instructions (1-800-222-1222).

Pastels, chalks, and charcoal dusts may cause irritation to the lungs, especially in people with underlying asthma. Some pastels may contain heavy metals such as lead, chromium, cadmium, and manganese in their pigments. These types of pastels should be avoided with younger children because the potential for ingestion and insufficient cleaning of work areas increases the risk of exposure. Felt-tip markers are generally nontoxic.

Glue

White glues that children use for construction projects are usually nontoxic. Many wood glues use the same technology as white glues but may also contain urea-resin technology or other adhesives. Rubber-based glues and rubber cements vary in their toxicity. Some may contain chemicals that can cause irritation and even burns with exposure to the skin. Other chemicals in rubber cement may be released into the air and cause respiratory symptoms, headache, nausea, and sleepiness. Rubber glues and cements that contain n-hexane should be avoided if possible.

Because urea-resin glues can release large amounts of formaldehyde fumes, they should be avoided where safer alternatives exist, unless excellent ventilation is maintained until the glue is fully dry. A person who develops symptoms should be removed immediately from the area and into fresh air; if symptoms persist, medical help should be promptly obtained. All labels should be inspected to ensure the least toxic product available is being used.

Ceramics and Sculpture

Ceramics and sculpture present a number of environmental risks. Dry clay dusts can cause difficulty breathing and worsen asthma symptoms. Ceramic colorants and glazes may contain heavy metals such as lead, barium, cobalt, and manganese. Each of these heavy metals can cause its own set of problems on exposure, which usually occurs through ingestion of the compounds (City of Tucson n.d.; Dorevitch and Babin 2001; Watt et al. 2000).

The following strategies can reduce the risks associated with ceramic glazes:

- The use of glazes that contain potentially toxic heavy metals such as lead, barium, cobalt, and manganese should be limited whenever possible.
- Proper cleaning of work areas and disposal of leftover materials significantly decrease risk.
- Only older children and adolescents with good work habits and the ability to understand and follow directions for safe use should be allowed to use glazes and colorants that contain toxic substances.
- Ceramic items intended for use as food-containing vessels should never be prepared with glazes containing these heavy metals.
- Only adult school personnel responsible for the class should execute kiln firing of ceramic pieces, as there is risk of fire, as well as carbon monoxide production, if the apparatus or area is not properly ventilated.
- Plaster of Paris heats as it dries and may cause a burn when applied directly to skin. Dusts from plaster of Paris and papier-mâché may be irritating.
- Sharp objects used for sculpting and clay work must be used only with direct supervision, especially with younger students.

Theater

Drama classes and theater productions offer another venue with potential for exposure to toxins. Scenery production on a large scale often involves painting, with the resulting hazards described previously. Construction of the set from wood or cardboard can result in respiratory irritation from particulate matter if these materials are cut. If particle board is used, formaldehyde may be released into the air and cause irritation of the breathing passages (Rice et al. 2002; Silbergeld 1997; Tran et al. 2003).

Smoke and Fog

Only adults who are supervising a theater production should use smoke-effect chemicals and other special effects. Several types of smoke and fog effects may be employed, the most common of which is dry-ice smoke. Dry ice is the solid form of carbon dioxide, which turns directly into a gas at room temperature. A fog forms when the cold gas reacts with moisture in the air. The dry ice itself must be handled with insulated gloves because it can cause cold burns to bare skin. Dry ice is one of the safest types of smoke effects. However, it must be used with adequate ventilation to prevent gas and fog accumulation, which would decrease the amount of oxygen in the air, especially closer to the ground. Actors who are lying or sitting on the set would be in the thickest part of the fog, with the lowest levels of oxygen. Low oxygen levels are dangerous and may cause fainting, cardiac arrest, and even death.

Other smoke-effect chemicals include oil-based and water-based fog fluids. These types of chemicals require special equipment to turn them into smoke and fog. All of them can cause skin, eye, mouth, throat, and respiratory irritation, and good ventilation is essential (Rice et al. 2002; Silbergeld 1997).

Any pyrotechnics that are necessary for a performance should be managed by someone who is qualified in this area, in consultation with local fire safety officials. The use of flame or flame-producing materials carries with it the risk of burns and the rapid spread of the fire to other areas of the set and scenery. In addition to carbon monoxide production during fires, materials that have been used to make the set may release other toxic fumes while burning.

Makeup

Stage makeup is generally nontoxic; the majority of adverse effects come from allergic reaction and contact irritation of the skin. Patch testing involves applying a small amount of the product to an area of skin (the inner forearm is usually recommended) and watching the area for 24 hours to determine whether the person is allergic or sensitive to the product. Patch testing is a prudent practice to adopt whenever new products are tried. Many manufacturers of cosmetics, stage makeup, and hair dyes recommend patch testing. Thorough cleansing of made-up areas after the performance is also important to minimize reactions. Any contact with the eyes should be avoided, and these products should not be swallowed (Tran et al. 2003).

Chemistry and Physics

Chemistry and physics classes are discussed in chapter 9. Please refer to that chapter for further information.

Shop Class

Shop, woodworking, and machining classes present numerous hazards. The majority of risks relate to the potential for physical injury, but several toxic exposures also exist and are addressed here. Ventilation of shops is important to reduce the inhalation of dusts and particles from wood and metal and to disperse any smoke and fumes from solvents and finishes in use (Babich 1998; Emerman and Cydulka 1998).

Solvents and Degreasers

Most solvents and degreasers contain hydrocarbons, a class of chemicals that can cause respiratory irritation if inhaled. After direct contact, they can also irritate and dry out unprotected skin and can be absorbed even through intact skin. After heavy exposure to hydrocarbons, liver or kidney damage may occur (Goldfrank et al. 2002; Tran et al. 2003; Sullivan and Krieger 2001).

Metal Reactions

Nickel allergy is a growing concern, and chromium can also cause reactions in certain sensitive people. If students are working with a metal that contains nickel, chromium, or both, they may have a reac-

---

■ *15.2. Huffing and other forms of solvent abuse*

Some teenagers use hydrocarbon solvent for the "high" feeling that results from inhalation. Several techniques may be involved. The solvent may be sniffed directly from the container. With a second method called "huffing," solvent is poured on a rag, the rag is held up to the mouth and nose, and the fumes are inhaled. The third and most dangerous method is called "bagging." The chemicals are placed in a bag, and the bag is then secured to the face to allow for continuous inhalation of the fumes.

Significantly dangerous and potentially fatal side effects are associated with solvent abuse. This type of drug abuse poses a high risk of suffocation, especially with the bagging method. This class of chemicals also causes the heart to become more sensitive to the body's own circulating epinephrine and other stress hormones. Hydrocarbon exposure is a common cause of abnormal heart rhythms in adolescents and young adults. Its abuse can cause cardiac arrest and death. ■

---

tion. Typically, this response is confined to a simple skin reaction, with an itchy allergic-type rash. If this occurs, the student should avoid working with all materials that contain the offending metal. Many alloys, including stainless steel, contain either nickel, cadmium, or both metals, and may cause reactions in nickel- or chromium-sensitive people.

Woodworking

Woodworking has several unique areas of interest. Sawdust, of course, may be irritating to the lungs and cause respiratory symptoms if inhaled. Particleboard and plywood, as discussed previously, are often treated with formaldehyde, which can also be irritating to the eyes, mouth, nose, throat, and lungs.

Treated Woods

Preservatives found in some woods can pose health hazards. Some woods may be treated with phenol chemicals, which can cause skin and respiratory symptoms. As discussed in the playground section, these woods may have been treated with antifungal and insecticide preservatives containing arsenic and copper. These heavy metals can cause multiple systemic effects if people are exposed to relatively large amounts all at once or if exposed to smaller, but still significant, amounts over a longer period of time. Adequate ventilation during woodworking is an important preventive measure against exposure to such preservatives.

Mechanisms to reduce exposures to sawdust, such as frequent cleaning of areas to reduce accumulation, automatic collection in a runoff container to reduce the spread of dust, and personal protective equipment, such as a mask and gloves, are effective. Any student or teacher who develops burning or irritation of the eyes, mouth, or throat, coughing, or difficulty breathing should immediately leave the area. The eyes should be rinsed immediately if chemicals or dust have been introduced. Washing of other exposed areas will decrease further exposure. Students who exhibit respiratory symptoms should go where they can breathe fresh, clean air and should seek medical care for persistent or severe effects.

Glue

Wood glues vary in their components and their toxicity, but white glues and similar glues have the best safety record among the various types. When resin-based glues, solvent-based adhesives, and other types of glues are preferred, these agents should be used carefully, and product instructions regarding ventilation and skin protection should be followed to minimize the risk of toxicity.

When using any kind of glue, use caution to prevent skin contact, exposure to eyes, and ingestion. If any of these problems occur, contact the local poison center, which can recommend treatment for the specific type of glue. It is especially important to keep the chemical in its original container and have the label information easily accessible.

Paints, Varnishes, Finishes, Stains, and Strippers

When using paints, varnishes, stains, and the like, excellent ventilation of the area is essential. Both paints and varnishes pose toxic risks. The individual containers and labels for all of these products should be retained, and directions for safe use specific to each product should be strictly followed. If an exposure does occur, contact the local poison center and relay the information from the container so that specific advice can be given.

Although each type of finish or remover will contain different chemicals, methylene chloride, which is found in paint strippers, is of particular concern. Methylene chloride is a solvent that, when inhaled, is converted to carbon monoxide. Carbon monoxide poisons the red blood cells, the oxygen-carrying cells of the body. The body is unable to utilize oxygen effectively, and the brain and tissues cannot get the oxygen they need to survive. The result of the exposure is determined by the amount of carbon monoxide in the blood and how quickly the person can be removed from the toxic atmosphere. Early signs and symptoms include headache, dizziness, nausea, and, with severe exposure, loss of consciousness. If symptoms develop and a carbon monoxide exposure is suspected, the victim must be moved as quickly as possible to fresh air. Immediate medical consultation should be obtained; further evaluation at a hospital may be required (Azizian et al. 2003; Goldfrank et al. 2002; Tran et al. 2003).

Toys

Phthalates are a class of chemicals widely used as softeners of plastics, components of perfumes and cosmetics, lubricants, and wood finishes. Because phthalates are so widely used, human exposure is common through food, water, and air. In the context of school environments, phthalates are of relevance because they are commonly found in soft plastic toys, food containers, and product packaging—items that may find their way into children's mouths. Children who mouth their toys, for example, can absorb a small amount of phthalate into their bodies.

Phthalates have been studied extensively in laboratory animals. Certain phthalates have been shown to be carcinogenic in some laboratory and animal studies, and some have been linked to animal fetal death and malformations (Shelby 2002). Some phthalates may be chemically similar to female sex hormones such as estradiol (Lorenz and Mignery 2000; McConnell 1994). However, it is unclear whether this corresponds to risk among young children and pregnant females (usually two of the most susceptible groups; Barr et al. 2003; Bouma and Schakel 2002; Kluwe 1982; Knight et al. 2000; Rossol and Hinkamp 2001; Shea 2003).

Although it is difficult to know how much of a problem phthalates pose to human health, the risk from this nonessential compound is best avoided. For that reason, regulations are in place in the United States that limit the amount of phthalates in toys made of soft plastic or polyvinyl chloride intended for children younger than 3 years of age to less than 1% by weight. Furthermore, the use of phthalates in infant bottle nipples, pacifiers, teethers, and infant toys intended for mouthing has been prohibited in the United States and Canada. Many countries in the European Union have banned the use of phthalates altogether or more extensively restricted their use, based on analysis of current data (Agency for Toxic Substances and Disease Registry 1996; Babich 1998; Blount et al. 2000; Kavlock et al. 2002a–g; Kluwe 1982; Knight et al. 2000; Lorenz and Mignery 2000; McConnell 1994; Rossol and Hinkamp 2001; Shea 2003).

In School Buildings

Building materials pose specific risks in terms of toxic exposures. When substantial renovation is ongoing within a school or classroom environment (such as removal of walls, stripping of paint or finishes, or replacement of windows), teaching activities should not be held in that particular area or classroom during the construction period. These areas should remain closed until the proper cleaning has been completed. The needed degree of isolation of the area will vary according to circumstances and from one phase of construction to another. Seek expert guidance when appropriate.

In this setting, the most likely route of toxicity is through inhalation of dust and particles; the most common health effects are respiratory irritation, development of asthma or airway disease, and worsening of respiratory conditions.

Asbestos

Renovation of older buildings raises the issue of asbestos exposure. Until the 1970s asbestos was used as an insulation material and pipe covering and in concrete flooring. It is composed of very fine fibers that, when disturbed, can circulate in the air for long periods of time. Once inhaled, these particles settle in the lungs. Because of the small size of the fibers, the lungs are unable to clear them

effectively and instead begin an inflammatory reaction around them. This process can lead to scarring and permanent lung damage. These particles can cause respiratory irritation, but the most serious health effects are delayed and include long-term lung disease and the potential development of cancer. These long-term effects are seen primarily in people who have worked with asbestos materials in industry or have been exposed during abatement work. Nonetheless, caution should be exercised to minimize any exposures during reconstruction and abatement (Agency for Toxic Substances and Disease Registry 2001; Babich 1998; Goldfrank et al. 2002; Mushak and Crocetti 1990; Norback et al. 2000).

Lead

For children, exposure to lead is an ongoing concern. Most states require the testing of blood lead levels in children at specific age intervals (usually about ages 1 and 2 years), with or without a history of exposure. The dangerous effects from lead vary according to how much lead the person has been exposed to, as well as the duration of exposure. Obviously higher levels and/or longer exposures are more dangerous (Agency for Toxic Substances and Disease Registry 1999; Costa et al. 1997; Flashinski et al. 1996; Goldfrank et al. 2002; Ryan et al. 2000; Sibbald 2002; Sullivan and Krieger 2001).

Many older homes and buildings still contain significant amounts of lead-based paint on walls, window frames, and woodwork. The manufacture of lead-based interior paint was discontinued in the United States in the late 1970s, but buildings and homes constructed and painted before 1980 may contain lead paint. When leaded paint flakes off from walls, children sometimes eat the chips. The dust from this paint can also be circulated through the air and inhaled or ingested, causing lead toxicity (Farfel et al. 2003; Leighton et al. 2003; Sanborn et al. 2002).

Among the many toxic effects of low-level, chronic exposure to lead are delays in learning and development. In general, even low levels of exposure may cause significant health effects. Typically, at low levels, children who appear to be asymptomatic may have subtle delays in neurological and cognitive development. Even low blood lead levels have been associated with decreased IQ, behavioral problems, decreased growth, hearing difficulties, and anemia. As blood lead levels increase, the severity of effects increases. Children with higher levels may have problems with nerve function and bone growth. Very high levels in children can result in abdominal pain, coma, or even death.

Older school buildings may contain water pipes with lead solder. Measures to eliminate these pipes are ongoing, but some schools in the United States may still have them. Soft water (low mineral content) and hot water are more likely to free up lead from the soldered joints of the pipes. Water standing in pipes will also increase the lead content of the water. In all schools, water should be tested regularly, in compliance with government regulations, and bottled potable water should be provided whenever high lead levels are found in the tap water until the situation can be remedied (Jirles et al. 1997; Langley et al. 2003; Lovekamp-Swan and Davis 2003; Moore 2000; Ward et al. 2002).

Lead may also be found in some ceramic glazes, which are discussed in the section on art materials.

All schools should minimize exposure by checking lead levels in water and eliminating the hazard of leaded paint from student-occupied buildings (Agency for Toxic Substances and Disease Registry 1999; Costa et al. 1997; Leighton et al. 2003; Murray 1991; Mushak and Crocetti 1990; Ryan et al. 2000; Sibbald 2002).

Flooring

Carpeting, especially recently installed carpeting, poses a unique set of health concerns. When first installed, many carpets release chemicals remaining from manufacture or introduced in the process of gluing or otherwise installing the carpets. These chemicals are included in a large group known as volatile organic compounds (VOCs; Agency for Toxic Substances and Disease Registry 2004; Costa et al. 1997; Dietert and Hedge 1996; Flanagan et al. 1990; Goldfrank et al. 2002; Morse et al. 1979; Stott et al. 1997). Some people are sensitive to these chemicals and develop respiratory complaints when they inhale them. However, data are lacking to prove any other significant or long-term adverse health effects from exposure to the compounds.

According to data from the Carpet and Rug Institute (2004), newer carpets emit far lower amounts of VOCs than older carpets, and the odors usually dissipate within 72 hours. Adequate ventilation provided to a heated room for 2–3 days (e.g.,

over a weekend) will hasten the process. The room should not be occupied until ventilation is complete. If children or school employees experience persistent problems, the process to air out the carpet should be repeated. Persistent respiratory conditions should be evaluated by a physician to rule out other illnesses. See chapter 10 for further information on indoor air quality (Dietert and Hedge 1996; Flanagan et al. 1990; Goldfrank et al. 20002; Morse et al. 1979; Smedje and Norback 2001a, 2001b; Taylor 1999).

Formaldehyde

Formaldehyde is used in the manufacture of resins, plastics, some textiles, wallboard, plywood, particle board, and certain types of insulation. The release of formaldehyde from these products into the air causes irritation of the mouth, throat, nose, and eyes and can worsen asthma symptoms. Formaldehyde has also been associated with headache and nausea. Although these symptoms can occur at very low levels of formaldehyde, effects are seen most frequently in industrial and occupational settings. In schools, only small amounts of formaldehyde are typically found in the air, unless new plywood or particle board or new furniture have been installed. Newly built portable classroom buildings pose a particular risk. As with chemicals released from new carpets, the majority of the release in portable classrooms occurs in the first few days after installation. To prevent adverse effects, these areas should be well ventilated prior to occupancy or avoided altogether for the first few days after new products are installed. If symptoms do occur, removing the affected person from the environment immediately and providing adequate ventilation of the space should alleviate the problem (Agency for Toxic Substances and Disease Registry 2004; Emerman and Cydulka 1998; Goldfrank et al. 2002; Harris et al. 1981; Koerner and Klopatek 2002; Morse et al. 1979; Sullivan and Krieger 2001).

Insulation Materials

As mentioned earlier, insulation materials no longer contain asbestos fibers, so the only potential for exposure to asbestos generally arises during abatement or reconstruction of an older portion of a building. Today, typical insulation materials are made of fiberglass. Fiberglass particles can cause irritation of the airways and the skin. Fiberglass belongs to a class known as synthetic vitreous fibers. Numerous investigations in the lab, in humans, and in large, long-term epidemiological studies have not provided firm evidence of long-term harmful effects to humans (Emerman and Cydulka 1998; Goldfrank et al. 2002; Hesterberg and Hart 2001; Litt and Burke 2002; Maas et al. 1994; Norback et al. 2000; Tepper et al. 1995).

Fiberglass fibers, unlike asbestos, are of a size that the lung is able to clear without persistent damage. However, because these fibers can still be irritating to the lungs (and may even trigger an asthma attack) and the skin, exposure should be prevented if possible. Areas where fiberglass insulation is being installed should be well ventilated and separated from occupied areas with tarps if the entire space cannot be closed off. Everyone within the installation area should have suitable masks and other personal protective equipment to minimize their exposure.

Office Equipment

Volatile compounds have been detected in the air around office electronic equipment. Printers and copiers may give off gases from the inks they use, and paper dust may also be irritating to some people. Allowing for good ventilation around this type of equipment is essential to protect sensitive people (Muller and Schaeffer 1996). Some people experience skin irritation and respiratory symptoms after handling carbonless copy paper. This is not a true toxic effect but rather an individual sensitivity to the compound. No long-term serious health effects have been found in office workers continuously exposed to this type of equipment in the workplace (Babich 1998; Calnan 1979; Emerman and Cydulka 1998; Furukawa et al. 2002; Kanerva et al. 1993; Koch et al. 2003; Koerner and Klopatek 2002; Tran et al. 2003; Adcox and Fast 2004; Wierniks 1996).

Conclusion

This chapter has provided a brief overview of some of the more commonly encountered hazards within the school environment. It is not meant to be all inclusive. The impetus for maintaining the safety of our schools is in the hands of our school officials,

---

> ■ *15.3. First aid for toxins at school*
>
> - If a student or school employee is having an adverse reaction of any kind from skin contact with a material or chemical, that person should immediately stop working with the substance and wash the area of contact to prevent ongoing exposure.
> - If students are having a reaction to something they are inhaling, they should move themselves or be removed from the area. Asthmatic symptoms should be treated appropriately, with medication and medical evaluation as needed.
> - Investigate all situations in which a substance has been swallowed. Unless the product is clearly indicated as nontoxic, contact a poison center for instructions, and seek medical care if necessary.
> - Any situations in which a substance gets into an eye should be handled by rinsing the eyes immediately with a large volume of clean water while contacting the poison center for further instructions and advice. ■

---

teachers, and parents. We must all be vigilant about recognizing potentially harmful substances in the school environment.

Resources

Arts and Crafts Information

- City of Tucson, Environmental Management Division
  http://www.ci.tucson.az.us/arthazards/home.html
- Western Washington University Wilson Library
  http://www.library.wwu.edu/ref/subjguides/art/arthazards.html

Environmental and Chemical Information

- Agency for Toxic Substances and Disease Registry
  http://www.atsdr.cdc.gov

- National Center for Environmental Health http://www.cdc.gov/nceh
- National Library of Medicine Hazardous Substances Database http://www.haz-map.com
- Poison Center Hotline: 1-800-222-1222
- U.S. Environmental Protection Agency http://www.epa.gov

References

Adcox R, Fast M. 2004. The Western Libraries' art hazards: Internet and library resources. Western Washington University Wilson Library. Available: http://www.library.wwu.edu/ref/subjguides/art/arthazards.html [accessed 10 October 2004].

Agency for Toxic Substances and Disease Registry. 1996. ToxFAQs for diethyl phthalate. Available: http://www.atsdr.cdc.gov [accessed 10 October 2004].

Agency for Toxic Substances and Disease Registry. 1999. ToxFAQs for lead. Available: http://www.atsdr.cdc.gov [accessed 10 October 2004].

Agency for Toxic Substances and Disease Registry. 2001. ToxFAQs for asbestos. Available: http://www.atsdr.cdc.gov [accessed 10 October 2004].

Agency for Toxic Substances and Disease Registry. 2002. Pilot exposure assessment of schools sited on or near hazardous waste sites in brownfields communities. Available: http://www.atsdr.cdc.gov/HEC/HSPH/v1n1-2part3.html, p. 3–4 [accessed 9 April 2006].

Agency for Toxic Substances and Disease Registry. 2004. Medical management guidelines: Formaldehyde. Available: http://www.atsdr.cdc.gov [accessed 10 October 2004].

Art and Creative Materials Institute. 2004. Safety: What you need to know. Available: http://www.acminet.org [accessed 10 October 2004].

Azizian MF, Nelson PO, Thayumanavan P, Williamson KJ. 2003. Environmental impact of highway construction and repair materials on surface and ground waters. Case study: Crumb rubber asphalt concrete. Waste Manag 23(8):719–728.

Babich MA. 1998. Risk assessment of low-level chemical exposures from consumer products under the U.S. Consumer Product Safety Commission chronic hazard guidelines. Environ Health Perspect 106 (suppl. 1):387–390.

Barr DB, Silva MJ, Kato K, Reidy JA, Malek NA, Hurtz D, et al. 2003. Assessing human exposure to phthalates using monoesters and their oxidized metabolites as biomarkers. Environ Health Perspect 111(9):1148–1151.

Blount BC, Silva MJ, Caudill SP, Needham LL, Pirkle JL, Sampson EJ, et al. 2000. Levels of seven urinary phthalate metabolites in a human reference population. Environ Health Perspect 108(10):979–982.

Bouma K, Schakel DJ. 2002. Migration of phthalates from PVC toys into saliva simulant by dynamic extraction. Food Addit Contam 19(6):602–610.

Calnan CD. 1979. Carbon and carbonless copy paper. Acta Derm Venereol Suppl (Stockholm) 59(85):27–32.

Carpet and Rug Institute. 2004. Carpet and VOC issues. Available: http://www.carpet-health.org/voc.asp [accessed 10 October 2004].

City of Tucson Environmental Management Division. N.d. Health and safety in the arts: A searchable database of health and safety information for artists. Available: http://www.ci.tucson.az.us/arthazards/home.html [accessed 10 October 2004].

Costa RA, Nuttall KL, Shaffer JB, Peterson DL, Ash KO. 1997. Suspected lead poisoning in a public school. Ann Clin Lab Sci 27(6):413–417.

Daniels CR, Swan EP. 1979. Determination of chlorinated phenols in surface-treated lumber by HPLC. J Chromatog Sci 17(11):628–630.

Dietert RR, Hedge A. 1996. Toxicological considerations in evaluating indoor air quality and human health: Impact of new carpet emissions. Crit Rev Toxicol 26(6):633–707.

Dorevitch S, Babin A. 2001. Health hazards of ceramic artists. Occup Med 16(4):563–575.

Emerman CL, Cydulka RK. 1998. Behavioral and environmental factors associated with acute exacerbation of asthma. Ann Allergy Asthma Immunol 81(3):239–242.

Farfel MR, Orlova AO, Lees PS, Rohde C, Ashley PJ, Chisolm JJ Jr. 2003. A study of urban housing demolitions as sources of lead in ambient dust: Demolition practices and exterior dust fall. Environ Health Perspect 111(9):1228–1234.

Flanagan RJ, Ruprah M, Meredith TJ, Ramsey JD. 1990. An introduction to the clinical toxicology of volatile substances. Drug Safety 5(5):359–383.

Flashinski RA, Taha T, Kanarek MS. 1996. Childhood lead paint poisoning: From past to present. Wis Med J 95(8):583–587.

Furukawa Y, Aizawa Y, Okada M, Watanabe M, Niitsuya M, Kotani M. 2002. Negative effect of photocopier toner on alveolar macrophages determined by in vitro magnetometric evaluation. Ind Health 40(2):214–221.

Garcia de Cortazar AL, Lantaron JH, Fernandez OM, Monzon IT, Lamia MF. 2002. Modeling for environmental assessment of municipal solid waste landfills, part 2: Biodegradation. Waste Manag Res 20(6):514–528.

Goldfrank LR, Flomenbaum NE, Lewin NA, Howland MA, Hoffman RS, Nelson LS, eds. 2002. *Goldfrank's toxicologic emergencies,* 7th ed. New York: McGraw-Hill.

Gordon T, Spanier J, Butala JH, Li P, Rossman TG. 2002. In vitro bioavailability of heavy metals in pressure-treated wood dust. Toxicol Sci 67(1):32–37.

Greenberg MR. 2003. Reversing urban decay: Brownfield redevelopment and environmental health. Environ Health Perspect 111(2):A74–A75.

Harris JC, Rumack BH, Aldrich FD. 1981. Toxicology of urea formaldehyde and polyurethane foam insulation. J Am Med Assoc 245(3):243.

Hesterberg TW, Hart GA. 2001. Synthetic vitreous fibers: A review of toxicology research and its impact on hazard classification. Crit Rev Toxicol 31(1):1–53.

Isidori M, Lavorgna M, Nardelli A, Parrella A. 2003. Toxicity identification evaluation of leachates from municipal solid waste landfills: A multispecies approach. Chemosphere 52(1):85–94.

James SC. 1977. Metals in municipal landfill leachate and their health effects. Am J Public Health 67(5): 429–432.

Jirles B, Thigpen J, Forsythe D. 1997. Lead in drinking water: A preventive solution. Environ Health Perspect 105(1):15.

Kanerva L, Estlander T, Jolanki R, Henriks-Eckerman ML. 1993. Occupational allergic contact dermatitis caused by diethylenetriamine in carbonless copy paper. Contact Derm 29(3):147–151.

Kaufman MM, Murray KS, Rogers DT. 2003. Surface and subsurface geologic risk factors to ground water affecting brownfield redevelopment potential. J Environ Qual 32(2):490–499.

Kavlock R, Boekelheide K, Chapin R, Cunningham M, Faustman E, Foster P, et al. 2002a. NTP Center for the Evaluation of Risks to Human Reproduction: Phthalates expert panel report on the reproductive and developmental toxicity of di-n-octyl phthalate. Reprod Toxicol 16(5):721–734.

Kavlock R, Boekelheide K, Chapin R, Cunningham M, Faustman E, Foster P, et al. 2002b. NTP Center for the Evaluation of Risks to Human Reproduction: Phthalates expert panel report on the reproductive and developmental toxicity of di-n-hexyl phthalate. Reprod Toxicol 16(5):709–719.

Kavlock R, Boekelheide K, Chapin R, Cunningham M, Faustman E, Foster P, et al. 2002c. NTP Center for the Evaluation of Risks to Human Reproduction: Phthalates expert panel report on the repro-

ductive and developmental toxicity of di-isononyl phthalate. Reprod Toxicol 16(5):679–708.

Kavlock R, Boekelheide K, Chapin R, Cunningham M, Faustman E, Foster P, et al. 2002d. NTP Center for the Evaluation of Risks to Human Reproduction: Phthalates expert panel report on the reproductive and developmental toxicity of di-isodecyl phthalate. Reprod Toxicol 16(5):655–678.

Kavlock R, Boekelheide K, Chapin R, Cunningham M, Faustman E, Foster P, et al. 2002e. NTP Center for the Evaluation of Risks to Human Reproduction: Phthalates expert panel report on the reproductive and developmental toxicity of di(2-ethylhexyl) phthalate. Reprod Toxicol 16(5):529–653.

Kavlock R, Boekelheide K, Chapin R, Cunningham M, Faustman E, Foster P, et al. 2002f. NTP Center for the Evaluation of Risks to Human Reproduction: Phthalates expert panel report on the reproductive and developmental toxicity of di-n-butyl phthalate. Reprod Toxicol 16(5):489–527.

Kavlock R, Boekelheide K, Chapin R, Cunningham M, Faustman E, Foster P, et al. 2002g. NTP Center for the Evaluation of Risks to Human Reproduction: Phthalates expert panel report on the reproductive and developmental toxicity of butyl benzyl phthalate. Reprod Toxicol 16(5):453–487.

Kluwe WM. 1982. Overview of phthalate ester pharmacokinetics in mammalian species. Environ Health Perspect 45:3–9.

Knight S, Junkins EP Jr., Lightfoot AC, Cazier CF, Olson LM. 2000. Injuries sustained by students in shop class. Pediatrics 106(1), part 1:10–13.

Koch HM, Drexler H, Angerer J. 2003. An estimation of the daily intake of di(2-ethylhexyl)phthalate (DEHP) and other phthalates in the general population. Int J Hyg Environ Health 206(2):77–83.

Koerner B, Klopatek J. 2002. Anthropogenic and natural CO_2 emission sources in an arid urban environment. Environ Pollut 116 (Suppl. 1):S45–S51.

Langley SJ, Goldthorpe S, Craven M, Morris J, Woodcock A, Custovic A. 2003. Exposure and sensitization to indoor allergens: Association with lung function, bronchial reactivity, and exhaled nitric oxide measures in asthma. J Allergy Clin Immunol 112(2):362–368.

Leighton J, Klitzman S, Sedlar S, Matte T, Cohen NL. 2003. The effect of lead-based paint hazard remediation on blood lead levels of lead-poisoned children in New York City. Environ Res 92(3):182–190.

Lesser SH, Weiss SJ. 1995. Art hazards. Am J Emerg Med 13(4):451–458.

Leung AK, Robson WL, Lim SH, Chopra S. 1993.

Playground safety. J R Soc Health 113(6):320–323.

Litt JS, Burke TA. 2002. Uncovering the historic environmental hazards of urban brownfields. J Urban Health 79(4):464–481.

Lockey JE, Wiese NK. 1992. Health effects of synthetic vitreous fibers. Clin Chest Med 13(2):329–339.

Lorenz J, Mignery T. 2000. Brownfield remediation. Occup Health Safety 69(11):77–78.

Lovekamp-Swan T, Davis BJ. 2003. Mechanisms of phthalate ester toxicity in the female reproductive system. Environ Health Perspect 111(2):139–145.

Maas RP, Patch SC, Gagnon AM. 1994. The dynamics of lead in drinking water in U.S. workplaces and schools. Am Ind Hyg Assoc J 55(9):829–832.

McConnell EE. 1994. Synthetic vitreous fibers: Inhalation studies. Regul Toxicol Pharmacol 20(3), part 2:S22–S34.

Moore NP. 2000. The oestrogenic potential of the phthalate esters. Reprod Toxicol 14(3):183–192.

Morse DL, Watson WN, Housworth J, Witherell LE, Landrigan PJ. 1979. Exposure of children to lead in drinking water. Am J Public Health 69(7):711–712.

Muller WJ, Schaeffer VH. 1996. A strategy for the evaluation of sensory and pulmonary irritation due to chemical emissions from indoor sources. J Air Waste Manag Assoc 46(9):808–812.

Murray R. 1991. Health aspects of carbonless copy paper. Contact Derm 24(5):321–333.

Mushak P, Crocetti AF. 1990. Methods for reducing lead exposure in young children and other risk groups: An integrated summary of a report to the U.S. Congress on childhood lead poisoning. Environ Health Perspect 89:125–135.

Norback D, Walinder R, Wieslander G, Smedje G, Erwall C, Venge P. 2000. Indoor air pollutants in schools: nasal patency and biomarkers in nasal lavage. Allergy 55(2): 163–70.

Pickrell JA, Hill JO, Carpenter RL, Hahn FF, Rebar AH. 1983. In vitro and in vivo response after exposure to man-made mineral and asbestos insulation fibers. Am Ind Hyg Assoc J 44(8):557–561.

Polkowska Z, Gorecki T, Namiesnik J. 2002. Quality of roof runoff waters from an urban region (Gdansk, Poland). Chemosphere 49(10):1275–1283.

Rice KC, Conko KM, Hornberger GM. 2002. Anthropogenic sources of arsenic and copper to sediments in a suburban lake, Northern Virginia. Environ Sci Technol 36(23):4962–4967.

Rossol M, Hinkamp D. 2001. Hazards in the theater. Occup Med 16(4):595–608.

Rudel RA, Camann DE, Spengler JD, Korn LR, Brody JG. 2003. Phthalates, alkylphenols, pesticides, polybrominated diphenyl ethers, and other endocrine-disrupting compounds in indoor air and dust. Environ Sci Technol 37(20):4543–4553.

Ryan PB, Huet N, MacIntosh DL. 2000. Longitudinal investigation of exposure to arsenic, cadmium, and lead in drinking water. Environ Health Perspect 108(8):731–735.

Sanborn MD, Abelsohn A, Campbell M, Weir E. 2002. Identifying and managing adverse environmental health effects: 3. Lead exposure. Can Med Assoc J 166(10):1287–1292.

Schwar MJ, Alexander DJ. 1988. Redecoration of external leaded paintwork and lead-in-dust concentrations in school playgrounds. Sci Total Environ 68:45–59.

Shea KM. 2003. American Academy of Pediatrics Committee on Environmental Health: Pediatric exposure and potential toxicity of phthalate plasticizers. Pediatrics 111(6), part 1:1467–1474.

Shelby MD. 2002. NTP center for the evaluation of risks to human reproduction phthalates expert panel reports. Reprod Toxicol 16(5):451.

Sibbald B. 2002. Arsenic and pressure-treated wood: The argument moves to the playground. Can Med Assoc J 166(1):79.

Silbergeld EK. 1997. Preventing lead poisoning in children. Annu Rev Public Health 18:187–210.

Smedje G, Norback D. 2001a. Incidence of asthma diagnosis and self-reported allergy in relation to the school environment: A four-year follow-up study in schoolchildren. Int J Tuberc Lung Dis 5(11): 1059–1066.

Smedje G, Norback D. 2001b. Irritants and allergens at school in relation to furnishings and cleaning. Indoor Air 11(2):127–133.

Stadler JC, Dudek BR, Kaempfe TA, Christoph GR, Hansen JF. 1994. Evaluation of a method used to test for potential toxicity of carpet emissions. Food Chem Toxicol 32(11):1073–1087.

Stilwell DE, Gorny KD. 1997. Contamination of soil with copper, chromium, and arsenic under decks built from pressure-treated wood. Bull Environ Contam Toxicol 58(1):22–29.

Stott WT, Beekman MJ, Johnson KA, Spencer PJ. 1997. Evaluation of a novel assay of potential toxicity/neurotoxicity of carpet emissions (VOCs) in mice. Food Chem Toxicol 35(2):241–254.

Stubblefield WA, McKee RH, Kapp RW Jr., Hinz JP. 1989. An evaluation of the acute toxic properties of liquids derived from oil sands. J Appl Toxicol 9(1):59–65.

Sullivan JB Jr., Krieger GR, eds. 2001. *Clinical environ-*

mental health and toxic exposures, 2d ed. Philadelphia: Lippincott Williams & Wilkins.

Tarkowski S, Jarup L, Laurent C. 2000. Biological monitoring in waste landfills studies. Int J Occup Med Environ Health 13(4):345–360.

Taylor D. 1999. Talking trash: The economic and environmental issues of landfills. Environ Health Perspect 107(8):A404–A409.

Tepper JS, Moser VC, Costa DL, Mason MA, Roache N, Guo Z, et al. 1995. Toxicological and chemical evaluation of emissions from carpet samples. Am Ind Hyg Assoc J 56(2):158–170.

Tran CL, Jones AD, Miller BG, Donaldson K. 2003. Modeling the retention and clearance of manmade vitreous fibers in the rat lung. Inhal Toxicol 15(6): 553–587.

van Faassen A, Borm PJ. 1991. Composition and health hazards of water-based construction paints: Results from a survey in the Netherlands. Environ Health Perspect 92:147–154.

Van Metre PC, Mahler BJ. 2003. The contribution of particles washed from rooftops to contaminant loading to urban streams. Chemosphere 52(10): 1727–1741.

Ward ML, Bitton G, Townsend T, Booth M. 2002. Determining toxicity of leachates from Florida municipal solid waste landfills using a battery-of-tests approach. Environ Toxicol 17(3):258–266.

Watt GC, Britton A, Gilmour HG, Moore MR, Murray GD, Robertson SJ. 2000. Public health implications of new guidelines for lead in drinking water: A case study in an area with historically high water lead levels. Food Chem Toxicol 38 (Suppl. 1): S73–S79.

Wieriks J. 1996. Photocopier toner dust and lung disease. Lancet 348(9040):1518–1519.

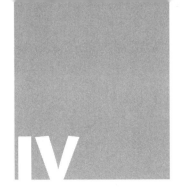

IV

Nutrition and Physical Activity

16

Jeannie Sneed

Food Safety

■ *Summary*

- Problems with food safety result from the presence of biological, chemical, or physical hazards in the food.
- Symptoms of foodborne illness may include nausea, vomiting, diarrhea, and, less frequently, fever or headache.
- Food consumed at school may be prepared by different people and served in multiple venues. Outside vendors may also prepare and serve school meals.
- Best practices for food safety in the school include food safety policy and procedures, adequate facilities to support food safety, proper food safety certification, implementation of an HACCP program, and food safety education for students. ■

Several children at an elementary school came down with diarrhea and vomiting, and foodborne illness was suspected. The health department was contacted to investigate the cause. Of 242 children who ate chicken sandwiches, 116 exhibited signs of illness—a far higher proportion than with any of the other foods served. Further investigation showed that the vehicle of transmission of the illness was the chicken sandwiches, specifically the bun. Norovirus was confirmed as the agent that caused the illness.

This scenario is dreaded by school administrators, school foodservice directors, and parents. In this situation, the source of the norovirus was identified, and the food vehicle was one that does not require cooking. The virus was likely spread by an employee who had not practiced good hygiene or through contact with an infected surface. Eliminating the spread of viruses requires frequent hand washing and surface sanitation. Another incident occurred when several children became ill after eating tacos in a school cafeteria. The ground beef used for the tacos was infected with *Escherichia coli* O157:H7 and was not cooked to an adequate temperature. Children became very ill, and some required hospitalization. Such situations emphasize the importance of sanitation and safety in the school environment.

Food safety is an important issue to parents. Parents want to ensure that every food item that their children eat is safe—whether that food is prepared at home, at a restaurant, or at school. This chapter introduces the field of food safety as it applies to schools. Chapter 17 introduces the field of nutrition in schools. Together these chapters present an overview of safe and healthy food in the educational environment.

What Is Food Safety?

Food safety is the appropriate handling of food as it travels from farm to table so that it is safe to consume. Problems related to food safety usually are unintentional and result from a biological, physical, or chemical hazard in the food. These hazards may result in foodborne illnesses, or illnesses caused by eating food.

Biological Hazards

Bacteria, viruses, parasites, and fungi are all biological hazards. Common bacterial causes of foodborne illness are *Salmonella, Listeria monocytogenes, Shigella, Staphylococcus aureus, Clostridium perfringens, Bacillus cereus,* and *Escherichia coli O157:H7.* In recent years, noroviruses (also called Norwalk and Norwalk-like viruses) have been the most common cause of foodborne illness. Other viral causes are hepatitis A and rotavirus. Parasites that can cause foodborne illness include *Trichinella spiralis, Anisakis simplex, Giardia duodenalis, Taxoplasma gondii, Cryptosporidium parvum,* and *Cyclospora cayetanensis.* Fungi include molds, yeasts, and mushrooms. Toxins produced by these organisms and by bacteria may also contaminate food and cause illness, even without causing infection.

Chemical Hazards

Cleaning chemicals, lubricants, and sanitizers that accidentally come in contact with food are examples of chemical hazards. Toxic metals, such as lead, copper, and brass, which are associated with equipment and utensils, may also present chemical hazards.

Physical Hazards

Foreign objects may create hazards in food. Some objects may be introduced to food during preparation—such as a staple from a food carton, a fingernail, or metal shavings from a can opener. Other physical hazards may be a natural part of the food itself, for example, a small bone from chicken that has been deboned and used for chicken and noodles.

> ### ■ 16.1. Food allergies
>
> Perhaps 1–3% of children are allergic to one or more specific food ingredients. For them, exposure to a food to which they are allergic may result in one or more of the following symptoms:
>
> - hives or other skin rashes
> - swelling of the face, tongue, or lips
> - wheezing or other difficulty breathing
> - nausea, vomiting, abdominal pain, or diarrhea
> - decreased blood pressure or other circulatory problems.
>
> These symptoms may occur almost immediately or may be delayed up to 2 hours after contact with the food. The degree of exposure that will result in symptoms varies. Usually, eating the food will cause the reaction; less commonly, skin contact or being near the food while it is being prepared or consumed may produce the allergic response. Most food allergies are triggered by a small number of foods:
>
> - milk
> - eggs
> - wheat
> - peanuts
> - soy
> - tuna or white fishes
> - shellfish
> - tree nuts (such as walnuts or pecans). ■

An important part of food safety programs involves analyzing these hazards and determining methods for preventing foodborne illness. Many food-handling practices can ensure that these hazards are prevented, eliminated, or reduced. Personal hygiene and time and temperature control are examples of two practices that can prevent a foodborne illness.

What Are the Symptoms of Foodborne Illnesses?

People with foodborne illness usually have nausea, abdominal pain, and diarrhea. Other symptoms, such as fever and headaches, vary with the type of illness. The onset of symptoms also varies. For example, *Clostridium perfringens* gastroenteritis is a common foodborne illness caused by products such as cooked meats, meat products, and gravy that have been stored at unsafe temperatures. The onset of this illness usually occurs within 10–12 hours of ingesting the bacteria. Symptoms include abdominal pain, nausea, diarrhea, and dehydration and rarely includes fever, headache, and vomiting. The onset of symptoms of staphylococcal gastroenteritis usually occurs within 1–7 hours, and the onset of symptoms from shigellosis usually occurs in 1–3 days.

Symptoms of foodborne illness are similar to those of other conditions; as a result, foodborne illnesses are not always diagnosed. When clusters of people have gastrointestinal illnesses, food is often the suspected cause. At that point, the health department is notified, and an exhaustive investigation is conducted to determine the cause of the illness.

Food Safety at School

Food is served in multiple venues in schools—in the cafeteria, in the classroom, from vending machines, from concession stands, and at school functions. Food consumed by children at school is prepared by many different people: foodservice workers who are certified in food safety; foodservice workers with limited training; teachers; support staff such as educational assistants; students; and parents or volunteers. Food may also be prepared and served by outside vendors such as restaurant companies.

More than 28 million children in the United States are served lunch daily, and more than 8 million of them are served breakfast daily at school as part of the federally funded National School Lunch and School Breakfast programs. The safety of those meals is of great importance because young children are vulnerable to foodborne illness. Food served in these programs generally is very safe. Millions more students are served a la carte items, purchase food from school stores and vending machines, and bring food from home. The U.S. Centers for Disease Control and Prevention has estimated that nearly 300 outbreaks affecting about 16,000 children in schools occurred between 1990

■ *16.2. Practical solutions for food safety*

Here are several practical solutions to minimize the possibilities for foodborne illness. They can be used both at school and at home:

- Wash hands with soap and water for 20 seconds (sing "Happy Birthday" two times), rinse, and dry with a single-use paper towel.
- Wash hands often—between tasks, after touching body and hair.
- Store foods at the appropriate temperature—dry storage between 50° and 70°F; refrigerators at 41°F or below; and freezers at 0°F or colder.
- Store foods in appropriate food-grade containers; label containers with contents and "use by" dates.
- Store foods off the floor.
- Cook all foods to the proper temperature and check the temperature with a thermometer. At home, ground beef should be cooked to 160°F, leftovers should be reheated to 165°F, and poultry should be cooked to 165°F.
- Keep foods out of the temperature danger zone (TDZ): 40°–135°F. Bacteria grow rapidly in the TDZ.
- Cool leftovers quickly. ■

---

and 1999 (Dyckman 2002). Dyckman has also noted that only 13 of the 20 largest school outbreaks were related to meals prepared and served by school foodservice personnel, and 3 of those were related to tainted burritos distributed to schools nationwide. Others were related to food prepared by others or brought from home.

Food handling in schools is generally very good. The U.S. Food and Drug Administration conducted an assessment of foodborne illness risk factors in hospitals, nursing homes, elementary schools, fast food and full-service restaurants, and retail food stores (including the deli, meat and poultry, produce, and seafood areas; U.S. FDA 2000). Schools had high compliance rates for the following risk factors: food from safe sources (94%); adequate cooking (94%); and protection from contamination (89%). The percent compliance with personal hygiene requirements (74%) and with proper holding times and temperatures (60%) indicated two areas in need of improvement. Compliance ratings in schools were higher than in many of the other operations, particularly restaurant and deli counters in grocery stores.

Section 111 of Public Law 108-265, the Child Nutrition and WIC Reauthorization Act of 2004, requires that school districts "implement a school food safety program in the preparation and service of each meal served to children, that complies with any hazard analysis and critical control point system established by the Secretary." Guidance was released by the U.S. Department of Agriculture in June 2005, with the requirement that school districts have a plan in place by July 2006. The new regulations require two inspections each year.

Is Food Safety a Problem in Your School?

Several important questions can help determine whether food safety is a problem in your school district. The following checklists can help identify areas that need attention.

School District
1. There is a school district policy on food safety that addresses the following:
   — foods served in the classroom
   — access to food production areas
   — use of the foodservice operation by people other than foodservice staff (e.g., groups such as parent-teacher-student organizations and others who are doing fundraising)
   — vending
   — concessions (such as food served at sporting events)
   — school foodservice program.
2. There is a school district policy on food security.
3. There is a policy, with appropriate procedures, on what to do in the case of a foodborne illness outbreak.
4. There are appropriate facilities to support food safety practices. For example, all of the restrooms are equipped with warm water,

soap, and single-use paper towels or a blow-dryer.

School Foodservice
1. There is an ongoing training program related to food safety for foodservice employees.
2. The foodservice director has food safety certification.
3. Foodservice workers have food safety certification.
4. Foodservice areas are adequately equipped to maximize safe food handling.
5. Foodservice operation has implemented a Hazard Analysis and Critical Control Point (HACCP) program, which is designed to identify high-risk activities and reduce their risk.
6. Foodservice has achieved the District of Excellence designation of the School Nutrition Association (SNA) through completion of the Keys of Excellence program evaluation.
7. Food safety education is provided to students through posters, menu messages, and so on.

Classroom and Curriculum
1. Teachers reinforce student hand-washing practices.

■ *16.3. Food for special events*

Food is often a part of class parties, school festivals, fundraising, sporting events, and other school activities. Some practical steps to ensure food safety:

- Obtain food from the school foodservice program if at all possible.
- Hire a school foodservice employee with food safety certification to work with outside groups during food preparation and service.
- If food is brought by individuals, use only items that have been purchased from approved vendors and that are still in their original wrappers.
- Distribute food-handling guidelines for teachers and parents. These guidelines should address hand-washing practices, potentially hazardous foods, and time and temperature guidelines. ■

■ *16.4. Lunches brought from home*

Sometimes children prefer to bring their lunches from home. These lunches require special consideration to ensure food safety. If refrigeration is available at school, many foods can be packed in lunches. Often, however, refrigeration is not available; thus, many potentially hazardous foods should not be packed. Potentially hazardous foods include milk and other dairy products, meat, poultry, fish, cheeses, rice, potatoes, and soy protein foods. These foods should not be packed unless there is a way to keep the food colder than 41°F or hotter than 135°F.

You may use insulated containers (such as Thermos or cold packs) to maintain temperature. Freezing food items ahead of time may also help with temperature maintenance. If you use one of these techniques, test it to make sure that the appropriate temperature is maintained. To do this, prepare a test meal and leave it sitting on the counter for the same length of time that your child would have it out at school. Take the temperature of potentially hazardous foods to make sure that they are outside the temperature danger zone (41°F–135°F). If they are within the temperature danger zone, do not send that lunch to school with your child. (Be sure to toss the test meal, too.).

From a nutritional standpoint, many prepackaged products marketed for lunches are high in sodium and fat. The school meal may be a better nutritional choice. ■

2. Food safety education is part of the curriculum at all grade levels.
3. School foodservice personnel serve as food safety resources for teachers.

An Approach to Ensuring Food Safety

Based on the foregoing determinations, the following best practices can help ensure food safety in the school environment. Some of these are policies that are implemented at the district level; others, such as providing hand-washing facilities, are implemented at the school level.

District Food Safety Policy

A food safety policy should be adopted by the school district to address food safety issues. This policy may be initiated by the district's foodservice director or the school superintendent and should be reviewed and approved by the school board. A sample food safety policy is presented in box 16.5.

Policy and Procedures for Foodborne Illness Outbreak

A districtwide policy and appropriate procedures should be in place in the event of a reported foodborne illness outbreak. These procedures specify who will take the report, who will communicate with the health department, who will communicate with the media, what information will be shared with the public, and so on.

Facilities to Support Food Safety

School administrators must provide adequate time and facilities to support student health behaviors related to food safety. For example, restrooms must be supplied with adequate warm water, soap, and paper towels or blow-dryers to encourage hand washing. Teachers can encourage hand washing, but it will not occur if there are not appropriate facilities and supplies. Water temperature is a big issue—often water is ice cold in restrooms, and that certainly does not encourage hand washing.

School Foodservice

The school's foodservice department plays a pivotal role in ensuring safe food, and the district's foodservice director must provide leadership for food safety programs and education. Best practices include the following five key areas:

1. food safety certification
2. adequately equipped foodservice areas
3. implementation of an HACCP program in the school district
4. recognition as an SNA District of Excellence
5. food safety education for students.

■ *16.5. Sample school district food safety policy*

Efforts will be made to ensure that all food served in the school district is safe for consumption by children and adults served by the district and that children will receive food safety education.

- Foods brought from home for consumption in the classroom must be purchased ready to eat and be wrapped in the original packaging.
- Vending companies that supply foods for vending machines must document that they follow a Hazard Analysis Critical Control Point (HACCP) program or Good Manufacturing Practices (GMPs).
- When groups operate concession stands or prepare and serve banquets or other meals, food must be purchased from approved sources and prepared under the supervision of someone with food safety certification.
- When external caterers are used, they must document that they follow an HACCP program.
- The foodservice program will be managed by someone who has a food safety certification, and foodservice employees will also be certified.
- The foodservice program will have an HACCP program.
- External groups that use the school kitchen must do so under the supervision of a food safety–certified foodservice employee designated by the district foodservice director.
- Food safety education will be provided to students in the classroom and in the school cafeteria. ■

Food Safety Certification

The foodservice director and foodservice staff must be certified in food safety. This certification indicates that foodservice staff have the requisite knowledge to use appropriate food-handling techniques to ensure the safety of the food they prepare. School district administrators must support food safety efforts by requiring food safety certification of staff and supporting ongoing food safety education.

There are several alternatives for certification, at both state and national levels. SNA certification covers professional competencies related to all areas of school foodservice operations and requires employees to complete a food safety training course. Courses such as Serving It Safe (provided by the SNA) meet the requirement. SNA certification does not require knowledge testing. Some states and municipalities require that foodservice managers and employees hold a nationally recognized food safety certification. Some national food safety training courses and certification programs require knowledge testing, such as the National Restaurant Association Educational Foundation's ServSafe, Experior's Certified Food Safety Professional or National Certified Food Manager, or the National Registry of Food Safety Professional's Certified Food Safety Manager.

Employees who have successfully passed the certification examination can use the designation offered by the certifying organization. In addition, some state health departments offer food-handling certification programs for foodservice workers in their state. To find out the requirements in your state, contact your state or local health department.

The school district's foodservice director should have, at a minimum, a bachelor's degree in dietetics, foodservice management, or family and consumer sciences to ensure the requisite knowledge and skills to provide leadership on food safety issues. The director should also have the School Food and Nutrition Specialist credential, which demonstrates knowledge of school foodservice programs. This credential is available through the SNA certification and credentialing program.

Adequately Equipped Foodservice Areas

Some school kitchens were built and equipped many years ago. Consequently, their equipment sometimes does not function properly or meet current needs. For example, as school districts either grow or decrease in size, food production is often centralized. Food that is produced in a central location is transported to other schools for service to students. Sometimes refrigeration for cooling foods is inadequate, or the transportation equipment cannot maintain safe food temperatures. Cooling of foods often does not meet the time and temperature recommendations of the U.S. FDA Food Code, a model offered for adoption by local, state, and federal governmental jurisdictions. "Blast chillers," although effective in eliminating many of these problems, may be prohibitively expensive. Often, however, inexpensive resources can be used in place of some of the more expensive equipment recommended in the code. For example, "chill sticks" can decrease the cooling time for soups and other liquid products, and color-coded cutting boards can decrease the possibility of cross-contamination. Equipment issues will surface with a comprehensive HACCP program, but resources must be available to ensure that equipment is adequate.

Implementation of an HACCP Program in the School District

An HACCP program helps ensure food safety in a school district because it is an integrated approach to managing food safety in a foodservice operation. The HACCP is a proactive program that focuses on food, identifying potential hazards and establishing mechanisms to control them. HACCP programs are not required in most states; however, implementation is a best practice that should be encouraged.

An HACCP program is based on seven directives:

1. Conduct a hazard analysis. Determine potential microbiological, physical, and chemical hazards and where and when they might occur.
2. Determine critical control points where intervention can prevent or eliminate hazards.
3. Establish critical limits or standards that should be met at each control point.
4. Establish a monitoring system to determine whether critical limits are met.
5. Establish corrective actions to be taken in the event that monitoring indicates that critical limits or standards have not been met.
6. Establish verification procedures to determine whether the HACCP program is working.
7. Establish documentation and record-keeping procedures.

Important prerequisite programs must be in place before an HACCP program can be implemented. Table 16.1 provides a checklist of these. HACCP programs are complex and often require implementation over 1 or 2 years, with continuous follow-up.

Recognition as an SNA District of Excellence

The SNA's Keys to Excellence in School Food and Nutrition program is a self-assessment tool that allows foodservice directors to evaluate their school food and nutrition program. The assessment covers four areas: administration, communication, nutrition and nutrition education, and operations. Food safety is an important component of the operations area. School districts that meet the criteria established by the SNA can be recognized as districts of excellence. Because of the importance of food safety in schools, districts of excellence must provide documentation that they have passed sanitation inspections for the past year with no critical violations and that they have implemented key components of an HACCP program. School districts should strive for this recognition because it demonstrates competence and can be used to promote a positive public image of the school district.

Food Safety Education for Students

The district foodservice director can provide leadership for food safety education for foodservice employees, teachers, support staff, students, and parent groups. The cafeteria should be a learning laboratory, and students should see appropriate food-handling practices demonstrated. For example, posters that illustrate the importance of hand

---

■ *16.6. Food safety fact*

In the early days of space exploration, NASA needed a system to ensure that astronauts would not become ill from the food they ate in flight. In the early 1960s, the Pillsbury Company—in cooperation with NASA and military research groups—developed the Hazard Analysis and Critical Control Point system. In the 1990s, HACCP was required in meat, poultry, and seafood processing by the U.S. Department of Agriculture (USDA) and FDA regulations. Although not required in most states, HACCP is used in many retail foodservice operations, such as schools, restaurants, and hospitals. ■

Table 16.1. Prerequisite program checklist

Prerequisite program	Yes	No	N/A
Supplier control			
Letter on file from all vendors stating that they have an HACCP program or follow good manufacturing practices			
Equipment installation and maintenance			
Equipment is installed properly			
Equipment maintenance schedules are in place and documented			
Calibration schedules are in place and documented			
Cleaning and sanitation			
Written procedures for cleaning and sanitizing equipment and facility are in place and documented			
Cleaning and sanitizing procedures are followed			
A master cleaning and sanitation schedule is in place			
Personal hygiene			
Written policy and procedures for personal hygiene for employees and all visitors (vendors, teachers, students, etc.) are in place and documented			
Personal hygiene policy and procedures are followed by everyone who enters the production or service area			
Training			
An orientation program on food safety for new employees is in place and documented			
An ongoing training program on food safety and HACCP is in place and documented			
Chemical control			
All chemicals are separated from food products (either in a separate storage area or in an area in storeroom well away from food)			
Written procedures to ensure separation of chemicals and foods are in place			
MSDS forms are available for each chemical stored			
Receiving, storing, and transporting			
All products are stored under sanitary conditions			
All products are stored in areas with appropriate temperature and humidity			
Traceability and recall			
All food products are dated when put into storage			
Pest control			
A pest control program is in place			
Pest control is done by a licensed pest control operator			
Documentation of pest control procedures is in place			
Food temperature control			
Food temperatures are monitored and maintained			
Potentially hazardous foods are monitored for time spent in temperature danger zone			

There should be standard operating procedures related to each of the prerequisite programs. The standard operating procedures should describe what tasks are to be done when the tasks will be done, who will complete the tasks, standards that must be met, and how the completion of the task will be documented. Documentation forms are needed to record actions and to identify corrective action taken if standards are not met.

washing can be placed in the cafeteria. Food safety messages can be printed on menus as an educational tool for both students and parents. Foodservice employees must demonstrate that they always follow good food-handling practices, such as taking temperatures of food and handling ready-to-eat foods with gloves.

Teachers can invite the foodservice director to provide lessons on food safety in the classroom. A number of activities can be used to reinforce safe

■ *16.7. Food security*

Food security is closely related to food safety and should be addressed in school districts.

What is food security? Food security and the related term *bioterrorism* have been added to our vocabulary in recent years. Food security relates to the prevention of intentional contamination of the food and water supply. Acts of bioterrorism are intended to make people ill and create panic.

While there have been no known incidents of bioterrorism or food tampering in foodservice, schools and other foodservice operations are encouraged to develop a plan for ensuring the security of their food supply. Many tools have been developed by private and government entities to assist foodservice operators. The USDA has published a biosecurity checklist for schools. This document will assist districts in developing action plans to support a policy that would include the following areas:

- communication
- handling a crisis
- choosing suppliers
- receiving deliveries
- storage areas, including appropriate storage of food and hazardous chemicals
- foodservice equipment
- foodservice personnel
- foodservice and food preparation areas
- water and ice supply
- personnel security
- operational security
- handling of mail
- training
- plan maintenance.

A short Food Security Checklist, based on the larger USDA checklist, addresses many of the related issues (see box 16.8). ■

■ *16.8. Food security checklist*

☐ Secure access points to the foodservice operation, using appropriate locks, alarms, cameras, and so on.
☐ Purchase food from reputable vendors.
☐ Have vendors establish delivery times and provide names of delivery personnel.
☐ Require that all food have tamper-proof seals.
☐ Inspect all food upon delivery to ensure that there has been no tampering.
☐ Store all food and chemicals in locked storage areas.
☐ Limit the number of people who have keys to storage and foodservice areas.
☐ Date all items upon delivery for traceability.
☐ Maintain a current inventory of all food and chemicals on hand.
☐ Limit access to the kitchen and loading dock to essential personnel.
☐ Visitors (pest control operators, health department personnel, salespeople, etc.) should be escorted.
☐ Make sure that at least one authorized foodservice employee is present when the kitchen is used (such as when outside groups use the facility).
☐ Provide employees with identification.
☐ Train employees on each job responsibility, emphasizing food safety and food security.
☐ Establish emergency notification procedures. ■

food-handling behaviors, for example, using an ultraviolet light with "glow germ" (cornstarch with a luminescent substance that glows under ultraviolet light) to demonstrate the effectiveness of hand washing.

Children of all ages benefit by learning about food safety. For young children, this knowledge can help minimize the spread of infections and reduce the possibilities of getting sick. As children age, they may become more involved in food preparation at home. Many high school students work in foodservice establishments and need to use good food-handling techniques when serving food to the public.

Another potential hazard in school foodservice involves the risk of tampering with the food supply. Security considerations are introduced in box 16.7, and box 16.8 provides a checklist for use in reviewing the school's food security preparedness.

Conclusion

Food safety is an important issue in schools and has implications for school district employees (administrators, teachers, and foodservice employees), parents, and students. Numerous resources are available to improve policies, practices, and educational programs for these people.

Resources

- *Bad Bug Book* provides additional information about foodborne illnesses.
  http://vm.cfsan.fda.gov/mow/intro.html
- Iowa State University provides a web site that offers HACCP resources for school foodservice, including downloadable self-assessment checklists, standard operating procedures, monitoring forms, a sample HACCP plan, and orientation and training materials. These resources can be modified to meet the needs of a specific school district.
  http://www.iowahaccp.iastate.edu/
- National Coalition for Food Safe Schools represents a collaborative effort between public and private organizations. The organization's web site serves as a gateway to Internet-based school food safety information and resources.
  http://www.foodsafeschools.org
- National Food Service Management Institute

(NFSMI) was established by Congress in 1990 to support nutrition programs for children. The goal of the institute is to provide professional resources that will assist in providing the nation's children with high-quality, nutritious, and cost-effective meals through the federally funded Child Nutrition Programs. The NFSMI provides the following food safety resources for both school foodservice and child-care environments:
- HACCP for Child Nutrition Programs: Building on the Basics, a train-the-trainer program on HACCP implementation
- Serving It Safe, a basic food safety training curriculum for employees
- Food Safety Mini Posters, a set of 14 laminated posters in English and Spanish with key food safety messages designed for use in school kitchens
- Ten-minute Lessons for School Food Service: Food Safety and Sanitation, a series of lessons that can be taught by foodservice managers in 10 minutes
  http://www.nfsmi.org

- School Nutrition Association (SNA) is the professional organization for people who are employed in school foodservice. It provides numerous member services, including a monthly magazine, *School Foodservice and Nutrition,* and a biannual research journal, *The Journal of Child Nutrition and Management.* The organization, along with the Child Nutrition Foundation, provides many educational programs and materials to support the continuing improvement of school foodservice programs. Important resources are available to support food safety in school districts:
- Keys to Excellence in School Food and Nutrition Programs, a self-assessment program, focuses on best practices for quality programs. Successful completion leads to recognition as a District of Excellence.
- The SNA food safety resources related to training and certification, regulations, consumer education, and updates on current topics.
  http://www.schoolnutrition.org

- U.S. Food and Drug Administration, Center for Food Safety and Nutrition
  http://www.fda.gov

References

Child Nutrition and WIC Reauthorization Act of 2004, 108th Congress.

Dyckman LJ. 2002. Food safety: Continued vigilance needed to ensure safety of school meals. GAO-02-669T. Washington, DC: U.S. General Accounting Office.

U.S. Department of Agriculture. 2003. A biosecurity checklist for school foodservice programs: Developing a biosecurity management plan. Available: http://schoolmeals.nal.usda.gov/Safety/biosecurity.pdf [accessed 23 March 2004]

U.S. Food and Drug Administration. 2000. Report of the FDA Retail Food Program database of food-borne illness risk factors. Available: http://www.cfsan.fda.gov/dms/retrsk2.html [accessed 23 March 2004].

U.S. Food and Drug Administration. 2004. FDA report on the occurrence of foodborne illness risk factors in selected institutional foodservice, restaurant, and retail food store facility types. Available: http://www.cfsan.fda.gov/~acrobat/retrsk2.pdf [accessed 23 March 2004].

U.S. General Accounting Office. 2003. School meal programs: Few instances of foodborne outbreaks reported, but opportunities exist to enhance outbreak data and food safety practices. GAO-03-530. Available: http://www.gao.gov/cgi-bin/getrpt?GAO-03-530 [accessed 23 March 2004].

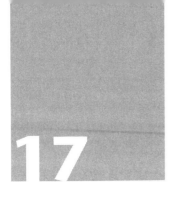

17

Nicole Larson and Mary Story

Nutrition at School: Creating a Healthy Food Environment

Summary

- The school food environment presents students with a range of food choices, from healthful foods to foods that are low in nutritional content and high in sugars, salts, and fats.
- A healthy school food environment can influence students to make healthful food choices, helping in turn to combat rising trends in overweight, obesity, diabetes, and related conditions among children.
- Obstacles to healthy school food environments include snack bars and vending machines, a la carte food programs, and easy access to fast foods. Many strategies are available to establish healthy food environments in schools, including School Nutrition Advisory Councils, school policies, educational interventions, and the provision of attractive, healthy food choices.

A school's food environment can have a significant impact on children's food choices and dietary quality because youth consume up to 40% of their total daily energy at school. Students today have many more food options at school than they did a decade ago.

Chapter 16 addressed the important topic of food safety and pointed out that food served at schools must be free of microbiological, chemical, and physical hazards. However, food must also be nutritious. With the ready availability of energy-dense (high-fat, high-sugar), low-nutrition foods and beverages in student stores, snack bars, vending machines, and a la carte cafeteria programs, there is growing concern about what students are eating. Establishing a school environment that fosters healthy eating behaviors can promote children's health and learning in the short term as well as reduce the risk of obesity and chronic diseases. This chapter describes nutritional concerns for youth, the impact of school nutrition programs, the current environment in schools, tools for assessing school nutrition environments, and model efforts to improve school nutrition. Table 17.1 provides a list of common terms and definitions related to school nutrition used in this chapter.

Nutritional Concerns for Youth

Diet is critical to both short-term and long-term health. During childhood and adolescence, good nutrition and dietary behaviors are important if

Table 17.1. Definitions of terms related to school nutrition

Term	Definition
National School Lunch Program (NSLP)	A program administered by the U.S. Department of Agriculture (USDA) in cooperation with state and local agencies. Subsidizes the cost of preparing and serving meals at participating schools. The program requires that lunches meet the Dietary Guidelines for Americans and provide one-third of the Recommended Daily Allowance for protein, vitamins A and C, iron, calcium, and energy.
National School Breakfast Program (NSBP)	A program that operates in the same manner as the NSLP. The NSBP requires that breakfasts provide one-fourth of the Recommended Daily Allowance for protein, vitamins A and C, calcium, and energy.
After-school Snack Program (AFSS)	A program available to after-school programs sponsored or operated by school districts running the NSLP. The AFSS reimburses schools for snacks that include at least two different components of the following four: a serving of fluid milk; a serving of meat or meat alternate; a serving of vegetables or fruits or 100% vegetable or fruit juice; a serving of whole-grain or enriched bread or cereal.
Free or reduced-price meal	Students are eligible for a free NSLP meal if their family income is 130% of the federal poverty level or below. Students are eligible for a reduced-price NSLP meal if their family income is between 130% and 185% of the federal poverty level. Students who do not meet the requirements for free or reduced-price lunches are allowed to purchase the NSLP meal at full price.
Universal Breakfast	A school program that offers breakfast at no charge to all regardless of income.
Competitive foods	Foods offered at school, other than meals served through USDA's school meal programs (e.g., school lunch, school breakfast, and after-school snack programs). Competitive foods are exempt from the dietary guidelines to which the NSLP meals must adhere.
Foods of minimal nutritional value (FMNV)	Competitive foods that, under current federal regulations, are not allowed to be sold in foodservice areas but may be sold anywhere else in the school at any time. FMNVs are defined as foods that provide less than 5% of recommended intakes for eight key nutrients. FMNVs include carbonated soda, gum, hard candies, and jelly beans. Other competitive foods may be sold at any time during the school day anywhere on the school campus, including the school foodservice areas. These foods include items that students purchase in addition to or in place of a reimbursable school meal, such as a la carte items and other foods and beverages purchased from school stores, snack bars, and vending machines.
A la carte	Foods sold individually and not as part of a complete NSLP meal. A la carte items are exempt from the dietary guidelines to which the NSLP meals must adhere and may include fast foods.
Fast foods	A wide variety of popular foods such as pizza and tacos, as well as cookies, chips, and pastries. Fast foods include branded and nonbranded items
Branded foods	Items sold under a recognized retail brand name such as Domino's Pizza or Taco Bell.
Foodservice area	Any area on school grounds where program meals are both served and eaten, as well as any areas in which program meals are either served or eaten.
Offer vs. serve (OVS)	Provision with the purpose of reducing food waste that authorizes schools to allow high school students to select as few as three of five meal components (fluid milk, meat/meat alternative, two vegetables and/or fruits, and grain/bread). Middle and elementary schools are given the option of implementing OVS.
Open campus	School environment where students are allowed to leave during break periods and lunch.
Closed campus	School environment where students are not allowed to leave during the school day.

Adapted from Craypo et al. (2002).

young people are to achieve their full growth potential and reduce their risk of chronic diseases in adulthood. Dietary practices affect young people's risk for a number of immediate health problems, including iron deficiency, obesity, eating disorders, undernutrition, and dental caries (U.S. Department of Health and Human Services 2000a). Long-term health is also of concern because certain dietary patterns developed in childhood and carried into adulthood can result in increased risk for chronic conditions such as heart disease, osteoporosis, cancer, and obesity.

Studies have frequently found that, as a group, children and adolescents have poor dietary habits that do not adhere to the Dietary Guidelines for Americans (U.S. Department of Health and Human Services, U.S. Department of Agriculture 2005). National surveys document that youth today consume excessive amounts of saturated fat, total fat, sodium, and soft drinks but inadequate amounts of fiber, fruits, vegetables, whole grains, and calcium-rich foods. Weight-related health problems are also of concern. The proportion of youth who are overweight has risen dramatically in recent years, and type 2 diabetes is increasing among children.

The School Nutrition Program: History and Impact

The oldest child nutrition program in the United States is the National School Lunch Program (NSLP), which Congress created in 1946 to respond to the high numbers of military recruits who showed signs of poor nutrition during World War II preenlistment physicals (Griffith et al. 2000). Congress passed the NSLP as a "measure of national security, to safeguard the health and well-being of the nation's children" (Griffith et al. 2000). The NSLP makes it possible for all school children in the United States to receive a nutritious lunch. School meals have become a primary resource for alleviating hunger in America's children (Griffith et al. 2000). In 2002 and 2003, 27.8 million children participated in the NSLP in more than 97,000 schools. More than half (57%) of NSLP participants received free or reduced-price lunches (Food Research and Action Center).

The School Breakfast Program (SBP) began as a pilot project in 1966 and was made permanent in 1975. The SBP operates in the same manner as the NSLP, and participating schools receive cash subsidies from the U.S. Department of Agriculture (USDA) for each meal they serve. In 2002 and 2003, 8.2 million children in more than 76,000 schools participated in the SBP. Of these children, 79% received a free or reduced-price breakfast (Food Research and Action Center). Since 1995, schools participating in the NSLP and the SBP have been required by the USDA to offer reimbursable meals that meet the Dietary Guidelines for Ameri-

cans. Schools are required to offer meals that provide no more than 30% of calories from fat and less than 10% from saturated fat. Regulations also require school lunches to provide one-third of the Recommended Dietary Allowances (RDA) for protein, vitamin A, vitamin C, iron, calcium, and calories and breakfasts to provide one-fourth of the RDA for these same nutrients.

Assessment of the national school meal programs indicates that participating children have higher intakes of most vitamins and minerals than nonparticipants. NSLP participants consume less added sugar and greater amounts of nutrients, including vitamins B_6, B_{12}, thiamin, and riboflavin, and minerals such as calcium, phosphorus, magnesium, and zinc (USDA 2001). Participants in the SBP had higher intakes of food energy, calcium, phosphorus, and vitamin C than did nonparticipants. One study found a reduced risk of overweight among girls (5–12 years of age) participating in the USDA Food Stamp Program, NSLP, and SBP compared with nonparticipants (Jones et al. 2003). Studies have also shown improvements in academic functioning among elementary school SBP participants (Griffith et al. 2000).

Although the NSLP and SBP offer numerous nutritional benefits, the high fat content of schools meals has been a concern. Recent findings show a significant trend toward lower levels of fat in school lunches (Fox et al. 2001). Despite these improvements, however, the average reimbursable lunch (not including a la carte items) served in schools provided about 33% of energy from fat, compared with the recommended goal of no more than 30% (Fox et al. 2001). Clearly, there is room for improvement.

The Current School Nutrition Environment

Just over a decade ago, the NSLP was the primary provider of food to children. Students today have multiple eating options in addition to those offered through the federally reimbursable national school lunch and breakfast programs. A variety of high-fat foods and high-calorie beverages is available for purchase from student stores, snack bars, vending machines, and a la carte programs, and the USDA nutrition standards for school meals do not apply to foods from such sources. Schools often sell food as part of fundraising programs. In addition, teachers may offer food as an incentive for good performance or behavior. Recent surveys indicate that the foods and beverages offered through these venues are less healthful. Federal regulations prohibit the sales of certain foods that offer minimal nutritional value (e.g., carbonated soft drinks, chewing gum, water ices, and hard candy) in the foodservice area during school meal periods. Although state and local authorities may enforce additional limits, federal regulations do not place any restrictions on the types of food offered for sale outside the foodservice area or within the foodservice area when school meals are not being served.

With increasing rates of child and adolescent obesity, the types of foods and beverages being offered in schools are a cause for concern. Schools are key settings of public health efforts to help prevent obesity and create healthier environments.

School Stores, Snack Bars, and Vending Machines

Stores, snack bars, and vending machines in schools provide regular access to high-calorie snacks and beverages of little nutritional value. Items available for purchase typically include soft drinks, sports drinks, fruit drinks that are not 100% fruit juice, salty snacks, cookies, and baked goods that are not low in fat (Wechsler et al. 2001). One recent survey of school stores in 24 San Diego County, California, public middle schools found that most (88%) of the snacks sold were high in fat and sugar, averaging 8.7 grams of fat and 23 grams of sugar (Wildey et al. 2000).

A recent national school survey found that almost all senior high schools (99%), 97% of middle and junior high schools, and 83% of elementary schools have stores, snack bars, or vending machines (U.S. General Accounting Office 2005). The majority of these schools allow students to purchase snacks and beverages at lunch (U.S. General Accounting Office 2005). In schools where purchases may not be made during lunch, students tend to purchase fewer soft drinks during the school week, but students still have access before classes in the morning or throughout the day when meals are not being served (Neumark-Sztainer et al. 2005). Students who stay for aftercare or after-school activities are also likely to have access to vended snacks and beverages at the end of the school day, when they are looking for a snack.

Although the majority of schools have made bottled water and 100% fruit juice available for purchase through vending machines or school stores, the opportunity to purchase healthful foods does not necessarily lead to their selection when popular, less healthful options are more widely available to students (U.S. General Accounting Office 2005). Soft drinks are particularly popular among school-age children and can often be purchased throughout the school day. A recent study in 20 urban Minnesota secondary schools found that 37% of soft drink vending machines were turned on at all hours (French et al. 2003). Consumption among students may further be promoted by contracts (made in nearly 50% of school districts) that give companies exclusive rights to sell soft drinks in the schools (U.S. General Accounting Office 2005). Often these contracts allow companies to advertise soft drinks in the school building, on school grounds, on playing fields, or on school buses. Each 12-ounce serving of soda contributes 9 teaspoons of added sugar to the diet (160 calories) but offers little else of nutritional value. National surveys indicate that, on average, young people consume more than 12 ounces of soda per day (French et al. 2003). Frequent consumption of soft drinks among children is related to the development of obesity and less consumption of nutritious beverages such as milk and 100% fruit juice (Harnack et al. 1999; Ludwig et al. 2001).

A la Carte Programs

A la carte programs offer students the opportunity to purchase individual components of a reimbursable meal or some items that are offered strictly for separate purchases (Fox et al. 2001). Although 39% of elementary schools, 8% of middle schools, and 6% of high schools have programs limited to milk, juice, and desserts intended to accompany meals brought from home, the majority of schools offer a greater variety of foods and beverages (Fox et al. 2001). A study in 19 junior and senior high schools in a large Midwestern metropolitan area found that, on average, 33 items were offered daily at each school (Harnack et al. 2000). Further analysis demonstrated that less than half (48%) of the items offered met the criteria for dietary fat (< 3 grams of fat per 100 grams), and students tended to purchase items higher in fat more frequently (Harnack et al. 2000). National surveys have also collected data confirming that, as a group, competitive foods are higher in fat than foods sold as part of the NSLP (Harnack et al. 1999). Access to a la carte programs is related to higher intakes of soft drinks, total fat, and saturated fat and lower intakes of key nutrients (e.g., calcium), fruits, vegetables, and milk among secondary school students (Cullen and Zakeri 2004; Kubik et al. 2003; Templeton et al. 2005).

Fast Food

Student consumption of fast foods, which tend to be high in fat and sodium, is another growing concern. Frequent fast-food consumption is related to higher intakes of soft drinks and fried foods and lower intakes of healthful foods such as milk, fruits, and vegetables (French et al. 2001). Fast-food restaurant patronage is increasing in the United States—most young people eat a fast-food meal an average of twice each week (Lin et al. 1999). Students have access to brand-name fast foods as part of reimbursable meal programs, on a la carte lines, and within the local neighborhood. A recent survey of high schools in California found that only 46% of districts that sell a la carte fast foods modified the traditional fast-food recipes to be low fat (no more than 30% of calories from fat) or to provide more fruits, vegetables, or fiber (Craypo, Samuels, & Purcell 2004). From 1994 to 2000, the percentage of middle and junior high schools and senior high schools offering brand-name fast foods increased from 17% to 25% (Wechsler et al. 2001). Although the majority (94%) of elementary schools, 89% of middle and junior high schools, and 73% of senior high schools implement closed-campus policies, many students have the option of traveling to a neighborhood fast-food restaurant or convenience store for their lunch (Wechsler et al. 2001). In one recent study of school food environments in Chicago, there were 3 to 4 times more fast-food restaurants near schools than would be expected had the locations been unrelated to school location, and the average distance to a fast-food restaurant allowed students to travel there in little more than 5 minutes of walking (Austin et al. 2005). Fast-food restaurants and convenience stores welcome young people and might also be frequented by students on the way home from school, when they are looking for a low-cost meal or a place to spend time with friends.

Food-related Fundraisers and Classroom Practices

Food is often sold within schools or the local community to support school-based organizations, and this may affect what students eat. In one national survey, 82% of schools reported that at least one organization had sold food or beverages during the preceding 12 months (Wechsler et al. 2001). The items most frequently sold included cookies, crackers, cakes, pastries, baked goods not low in fat, candy, soft drinks, sport drinks, and fruit drinks that were not 100% juice (Wechsler et al. 2001). Sales of healthful food items such as fruits, vegetables, and low-fat baked goods were less commonly reported. The predominantly high-fat, high-sugar foods that are sold likely contribute to excess energy consumption or replace more nutritious foods in students' diets. In one-third of schools, students are allowed to buy and sell fundraising items during the meal period in competition with the school lunch program (Wechsler et al. 2001).

In the classroom, students may also receive less healthful foods such as candy as a reward or incentive. Rewarding students with sweets and snack foods high in fat or sugar increases their preference for these foods (Baxter 1998). This practice is particularly common in elementary and middle schools, and it is prohibited in only 25% of the schools (Wechsler et al. 2001). One survey of 16 middle schools in the Midwest found that most teachers (73%) at least occasionally use candy as an incentive (Kubik et al. 2002). This practice in combination with other food practices related to the sale of food for school fundraisers and allowing food in the classroom have been related to school-wide prevalence of overweight (Kubik et al. 2005).

Concerns of the Current School Nutrition Environment

The wide availability of less healthful foods in student stores, snack bars, vending machines, a la carte programs, and local fast-food restaurants sends a mixed message to students about nutrition. Teaching students how to make nutritious food choices will not necessarily lead to healthy eating practices as long as the current environment in most schools provides ready access to many foods of limited nutritional value. In addition, the availability of these alternatives to the National School

Lunch and Breakfast programs threatens the continued viability of the programs and stigmatizes students who participate. Government-regulated meal programs, which adhere to established nutrition standards, have led to improvements in children's diets, but this progress may now be jeopardized by the many alternative food choices available. To ensure the development of healthy eating habits among students, local school systems must fully assess the nutrition environment they provide. School systems that participate in the federal school meal programs are further required to have wellness policies that focus on nutrition and physical activity in place by the 2006–2007 school year (see box 17.1).

Many opportunities exist for promoting healthy eating and reinforcing healthy eating messages within cafeterias and classrooms; however, educators, school personnel, students, parents, and the greater community must work together for optimal results. A self-assessment tool to help schools identify strengths and weaknesses of the current school nutrition environment and plan for improvements is shown in table 17.2.

Conducting a School Nutrition Environment Assessment

Create a School Nutrition Advisory Council

Establishing a school nutrition advisory council is one means of promoting healthier foods in schools. A diverse group of people (parents, teachers, students, school administrators, and health professionals) must be involved in assessing the school environment and developing recommendations. The involvement of partners helps foster a shared

---

■ *17.1. The 2004 Child Nutrition and WIC Reauthorization Act and local wellness policies*

On June 30, 2004, a reauthorization of the Child Nutrition and WIC Act was signed into law. Provisions of the act expand the availability of current programs and require improvements in the quality of food offered.

What changes were made to the NSLP and SBP? Among many improvements, new provisions provide for the following:

- expansion of the fresh fruit and vegetable pilot program
- resources that will allow five states to offer free school meals to families currently eligible for reduced-price meals
- automatic eligibility of migrant, homeless, and runaway children to have free school meals
- direct certification of food stamp households as eligible for free school meals
- a streamlined application process for low-income families to access reduced-price and free school meals (only one application per family per full school year is required)
- improvements in nutritional environments at school through local school wellness policies.

What is the local school wellness policy provision? All school districts that participate in the federal school meals programs must have a wellness policy by the first day of the 2006–2007 school year. It must include guidelines for school meals not to be less restrictive than current federal requirements.

What topics must be addressed by school wellness policies?

- goals for nutrition education, physical activity, and school-based wellness activities
- guidelines for the nutritional quality of all foods available at school
- plans for evaluation of policy implementation.

Who must be involved in the development of wellness policies?

The development process should involve school and community representatives (the school board, school administrators, school staff, students, parents, and the public).

Where can more information be obtained on the development of wellness policies and the reauthorization? More information can be obtained at www.frac.org or from local health departments. ■

Table 17.2. Creating a healthy school nutrition environment: A self-assessment tool

Complete the assessment tool for all five components of a healthy school environment. Add up the points for each column, based on the number of checks in each. Add the total points for each of the five components, and write that number underneath each section. If you need additional information before you can choose a response, put a check under the "Don't Know" column and investigate the item at a later time. When all components have been assessed, develop an action plan for creating a healthy school nutrition environment. Identify goals, who will work on the goals, when the goals will be achieved, and estimate the costs.

	Fully in place (3)	Partially in place (2)	Under development (1)	Not in place (0)	Don't know
School and community supports for healthy eating					
State & district health education curriculum standards/guidelines include nutrition. Nutrition is included in the daily education program from pre-K through grade 12.					
Administrators support the development of healthy lifestyles for students and establish and enforce policies that improve the school nutrition environment. They address issues such as the kinds of foods available on the school campus, mealtime schedules, and eating space and atmosphere.					
School staff, students, parents, and visitors are notified of policies, play a role in the policy-making process and support a healthy school nutrition environment.					
School food service staff is involved in making decisions and policies that affect the school nutrition environment.					
The school has a health council to address nutrition issues.					
Healthy eating is actively promoted to students, parents, teachers, administrators, and the community.					
Schools consider student needs in planning for a healthy school nutrition environment. They ask students for input and feedback and listen to what they have to say.					
Students receive positive, motivating messages about healthy eating throughout the school.					
Schools promote healthy food choices and do not allow advertising that promotes less-nutritious choices.					
Schools work with a variety of media to spread the word to the community about a healthy school nutrition environment.					
Point total: Possible points: 30					
Quality school meals					
Schools offer lunch, breakfast, and after-school snack programs, and students are encouraged to participate. Students are encouraged to choose healthy menu items including lean meats, fruits, vegetables, whole grains, and low-fat or nonfat milk.					
All school food service staff have appropriate training and regularly participate in professional development activities.					
Menus are planned with input from students and include local, cultural, and ethnic favorites of the students.					
Menus meet nutrition standards established by the USDA, conform to good menu-planning principles, and feature a variety of healthy choices that are tasty, attractive, of excellent quality, and are served at the proper temperature.					

	Fully in place (3)	Partially in place (2)	Under development (1)	Not in place (0)	Don't know

School food service staff use food-preparation techniques to provide meals that are lower in total fat, saturated fat, sodium, and sugar. They offer healthy food choices that include lean meats, fruits, vegetables, whole grains, and low-fat or nonfat milk.

Food safety is a key part of the school food service operation.

The school is prepared for food emergencies.

Point total: Possible points: 21

Policies and other healthy food options

All foods and beverages that are available at school contribute to meeting the dietary needs of students; that is, they are from the five major food groups of the Food Guide Pyramid.

School policies include nutrition standards for foods and beverages offered at parties, celebrations, and social events.

If foods are sold in competition with school meals, they include healthy food choices offered at prices children can afford.

If a la carte foods are available, they include a variety of choices of tasty, nutritious foods and beverages, such as fruits, vegetables, whole grains, and low-fat or nonfat dairy foods.

If foods and beverages are sold in competition with school meals, they are not marketed.

There are appropriate restrictions on students' access to vending machines, school stores, snack bars, and other outlets that sell foods and beverages, if these options are available (e.g., no access in elementary schools, no access until after the end of the school day for middle and junior high schools, and no access until after the end of the last lunch period in senior high schools).

School staff does not use food as a reward or punishment for students. For example, they do not give coupons for fast food as a reward for an "A" or withhold snacks as punishment for misbehaving.

The school encourages parents to provide a variety of nutritious foods if students bring lunches from home.

The school encourages organizations to raise funds by selling nonfood items.

Point total: Possible points: 27

(*continued*)

Table 17.2. (*Continued*)

	Fully in place (3)	Partially in place (2)	Under development (1)	Not in place (0)	Don't know

Pleasant Eating Experiences

Meal periods are scheduled at appropriate times; schools do not schedule other activities during meal times.

Meal periods are long enough for students to eat and socialize.

There are enough serving areas so that students do not have to spend too much time waiting in line.

Eating areas are attractive and have enough space for seating; tables and chairs are the right size for students.

Recess for elementary grades is scheduled before lunch so that children will come to lunch less distracted and ready to eat.

Schools encourage socializing among students and between students and adults. Adults supervise dining rooms and serve as role models to students.

Creative, innovative methods are used to keep noise levels appropriate (no "eat in silence").

Drinking fountains are available for students to get water at meals and throughout the day.

Schools use an accounting system that protects the identity of students who eat free and reduced-price school meals.

Facility design (including size and location of the eating/kitchen area, lighting, building materials, windows, open space, adequate food service equipment for food preparation and service, and food and staff safety) is given priority in renovations or new construction.

Hand-washing equipment and supplies are in a convenient place so that students can wash their hands before eating.

Point total: Possible points: 33

Nutrition Education

Students in pre-K through grade 12 receive nutrition education that is interactive and teaches the skills they need to adopt healthy eating behaviors.

Nutrition education is offered in the school cafeteria and classroom with coordination between school food service staff and teachers.

Students receive nutrition messages throughout school that are consistent and reinforce each other.

Nutrition is integrated into core curriculum areas such as math, science, and language arts.

The school conducts nutrition education activities and promotions that involve students, parents, and the community.

Point total: Possible points: 15
Overall Score:

Your score: _____
Total possible score: 126

	School & community supports for healthy eating	Quality school meals	Policies & other healthy food options	Pleasant eating experiences	Nutrition education
Your points:					
Total possible points:	30	21	27	33	15

Action plan

Goal #1: What needs to be done? Who will do this? When will it be accomplished? How much will it cost?

Goal #2: What needs to be done? Who will do this? When will it be accomplished? How much will it cost?

Adapted from Centers for Disease Control and Prevention (2000), USDA Food and Nutrition Service (2000).

understanding of how the current school environment may be promoting or discouraging healthy eating. A common vision is essential for developing and implementing necessary changes in policies and practices. For this reason, the USDA Food and Nutrition Service (2000) and the Centers for Disease Control and Prevention (2000) have developed tools to promote the establishment of school nutrition advisory councils and guide their work in schools.

Although the key people involved may vary from school to school, the Centers for Disease Control and Prevention School Health Index (SHI) recommends inviting a number of school and community representatives (box 17.2) or asking an existing health advisory council within the school to participate. To recruit members successfully, it may be necessary first to build support by meeting with administrators and others in the school community to explain the intent and proposed responsibilities of the council (Kubik et al. 2001). When a representative council has been recruited, the group should first spend some time to discuss and agree on the importance of creating an environment that fosters healthy eating habits. The SHI recommends that a minimum of two people from the council be asked to assess each of the following components of the school's nutrition environment:

- school policies and environment
- health education
- physical education
- school nutrition
- school health services
- school counseling, psychological, and social services

- health promotion for staff
- family and community involvement.

The entire council can then review the team's assessments to guide policy development and set priorities for creating a healthier school nutrition environment. Completing the adapted self-assessment tool (table 17.1) is a good first step that school advisory boards can take to assess the school's nutrition environment.

Develop School Policies

Council members who are delegated to assess strengths and weaknesses of the nutrition policies and environment need to consider the school's written policies, the community's awareness of them, administrative support of the policies, and schoolwide implementation. The policies should not only address the quality of school meals and food safety issues (see chapter 16) but also create an environment that supports healthy eating habits. Given their influence on food choices, environmental factors that include what foods are available, their prices and promotions, and the physical setting in which food is served and consumed should be covered by the policies (French et al. 2004; Neumark-Sztainer et al. 2005). Guidelines should restrict sales on school grounds of foods low in nutritional value and prohibit their use as rewards for student achievement. Similarly, guidelines for fundraising efforts should support healthy eating and recommend sales of nonfood items or healthful foods in place of items high in fat, sodium, and added sugar. When alternatives to the NSLP and SBP meals are available in the cafeteria or the

---

■ 17.2. *Key members of a school nutrition advisory council*

- School administrators
- Health and physical education teachers
- Other teachers
- Athletic staff
- School health personnel

- School nutrition personnel
- Parents
- Students
- Community health professionals

(Adapted from Centers for Disease Control and Prevention 2000) ■

---

greater school environment, these foods and beverages should be assessed to determine their influence on nutritional quality. Expert panels have developed standards for evaluating foods sold in competition with government-regulated school meals and recommended portion limits (tables 17.3 and 17.4).

Policies should ensure that the cafeteria environment is used to promote the selection of healthful foods, the cafeteria has an appealing atmosphere for student dining, and students have adequate time to consume their food. They should have a minimum of 10 minutes to eat breakfast and

20 minutes for lunch. Posters and other forms of advertising should not promote foods of limited nutritional value. Noise levels in the cafeteria should be controlled to promote a positive eating experience (see chapter 4). Nutrition services can make use of menus, displays, point-of-purchase advertising, and pricing structures to encourage the selection of healthful items.

Provide Education

To ensure that students gain the knowledge, attitudes, and skills to eat healthfully, the council

Table 17.3. Examples of model standards for competitive foods sold in schools

	Comprehensive school nutrition policy in Philadelphia schools[a]	Recommendations for competitive food standards in California schools[b]
Beverage standards	• Soft drinks will not be sold or served in school • Juice beverages must contain at least 25% real fruit juice • Water and flavored waters without added sugar, artificial sweeteners, or caffeine are allowed • Sports drinks are available during after-school hours in middle schools and high schools • Caffeine content of beverages is limited to 10 mg per serving	• Allow the sale of beverages that contain at least 50% fruit juice with no added sweeteners, water, low-fat milk, and nonfat milk • Eliminate sales of soft drinks, sports drinks, punch, iced tea, and other drinks containing less than 50% real fruit juice • Eliminate sales of beverages that contain caffeine (except chocolate milk)
Snack food standards	• Total fat content must not exceed 7 grams per serving • Saturated fat content must not exceed 2 grams per serving • Sodium content must not exceed 360 mg per serving • Sugar content must not exceed 15 grams per serving • Candy will not be sold or served during the school day	• Eliminate sales of snacks containing more than 30% of total calories from fat • Eliminate sales of snacks containing more than 10% of calories from saturated fat • Eliminate sales of snacks that are made with more than 35% sugar by weight

[a]Developed by the Philadelphia Comprehensive School Nutrition Task Force (2002).
[b]Developed by the California Center for Public Health Advocacy (2002).

Table 17.4. Recommended portion sizes

Item	Size (oz.)
Chips, crackers, popcorn, cereal, trail mix, nuts, seeds, dried fruit, jerky	1.25
Cookies, cereal bars	2
Bakery items (e.g., pastries, muffins)	3
Frozen desserts, ice cream	3
Yogurt	8
Beverages (no limit on water)	12

From the California Center for Public Health Advocacy (2002).

should carefully evaluate health and physical education curriculums. A school environment that provides nutritious foods and restricts access to foods of limited nutritional value can teach and support healthful eating behaviors, but children and adolescents must also receive nutrition information to balance the harmful messages about eating behaviors promoted in the commercial media. Students should receive education on using the guidelines for healthful eating, preparing nutritious foods safely, becoming critical consumers of nutrition information, and engaging in healthful weight management practices. These messages are transmitted most effectively when the curriculum is sequential, uses active learning strategies, and provides examples of concepts that are both culturally appropriate and personally relevant for students.

Provide Nutritious Food

The foods and beverages available in school cafeterias and other sites throughout school campuses impact the development of healthy eating habits. Council members should make sure that NSLP and SBP meals meet federal nutrition guidelines and are uniformly accessible to all students in a health-promoting context. Menus should include a variety of low-fat entrees, dairy foods, whole grains, fruits, and vegetables. Schools need to involve students and their families in planning menus, regularly evaluate whether the items served are acceptable to the majority of students, and offer a choice between at least two items in each food group daily. Nutrition service staff should purchase lower-fat foods and use food preparation methods that minimize fat content (e.g., baking or broiling instead of frying meat). When items are modified or new foods

added to the menu, students should be involved in taste testing to assess acceptance.

Involve Supportive School Services, Staff, Families, and the Community

To achieve a healthy school nutrition environment, school health-care providers, counselors, psychologists, and social services must be involved. The nutrition advisory council should promote collaboration among school administrators, teachers, nutrition services, and other support staff in creating and sustaining a healthy nutrition environment. A school staff that supports the physical, mental, and social health of the students plays an essential role in the identification of students with special needs or concerns related to eating (e.g., food allergies, weight issues, eating disorders, diabetes). Staff members should be skilled in working with teachers and parents to support students with eating challenges and making appropriate referrals to community services. Finally, all school staff and families are important role models for students. School-sponsored health promotion activities are effective ways to ensure that staff and families have opportunities to learn about nutrition. When assessing the school nutrition environment, council members should look for opportunities to expand staff health promotion, involve families in healthy eating programs, and collaborate with community programs.

Creating Changes That Support Healthy Eating in Schools

Change in the Schools: Research and Action

Promoting the consumption of fruits, vegetables, and lower-fat foods in schools using various approaches (table 17.5) can help young people eat more healthful diets. Success often requires a combination of several approaches. For example, Teens Eating for Energy and Nutrition at School (TEENS) is a school nutrition program developed for seventh- and eighth-grade students in Minnesota that made use of several techniques: peer-led classroom curricula, "parent packs" with newsletters and home activities, nutrition promotions in the

Table 17.5. School-based research on promoting consumption of fruits, vegetables, and lower-fat foods

Name	School level	Strategies	Results	Reference
The Lunch-power! Study	Elementary schools	• modification of recipes and food preparation practices • identification and selection of vendor products lower in fat and sodium • communication of healthy nutrition messages to students and parents via the school lunch menu	A review of school lunch menus demonstrated that energy from fat was reduced from 40% to an average of 28% without a change in student participation	Snyder et al. (1992)
Child and Adolescent Trial for Cardiovascular Health (CATCH), and Eat Smart School Nutrition Program	Elementary schools (third through fifth grades)	• classroom curricula • school meal program promotion • school meal food preparation guidelines • fat and sodium criteria for recipes, ingredients, and vendor-prepared products • home-based program activities	School lunch menus were modified to contain 11% less fat, 13% less saturated fat, and 13% less sodium than the original meals without compromising participation or the vitamin, mineral, and energy content	Nicklas et al. (1994)
Pricing Strategies to Promote Fruit & Vegetables	Senior high schools	• a la carte fruit, salads, and baby carrots were offered at half price • fruits and vegetables were promoted with signage and public address announcements	Fruit sales increased by fourfold, and carrot sales about twofold during the low-price period	French et al. (1997)
School-based Five-a-Day Research Initiatives	Elementary schools (fourth and fifth grades) and senior high schools	• classroom curricula • foodservice promotions and interventions to increase fruit and vegetable availability • parental involvement or home-based activities • community involvement (e.g., grocery store taste tests)	On average, the change in students' daily fruit and vegetable intake ranged from 0 to 0.6 additional servings	Perry et al. (1997)
Pathways	Elementary schools (third through fifth grades)	Development of • nutrient guidelines • skill-building behavioral guidelines • hands-on materials • twice-yearly trainings for foodservice staff to lower the amount of fat in school meals	A review of school lunch menus demonstrated energy from fat was reduced from 34%–40% to an average of 31%	Snyder et al. (1999)
Changing individuals' purchase of Snacks (CHIPS)	Middle and senior high schools	• low-fat snacks were added to vending machines and sold at the following four pricing levels: equal price, 10% reduction, 25% reduction, 50% reduction • snacks were sold without promotion, with a low-fat label, or with a low-fat label plus a promotional sign	Sales of low-fat snacks increased most with price reductions of 10%, 25%, and 50%. Promotional signage also increased sales of low-fat snacks but had less of an effect. Vending profits were not affected.	French et al. (2001)

Name	School Level	Strategies	Results	Reference
Food on the Run (FOR)	Senior high school	• trains high school students about healthful eating, physical activity, consumerism, advocacy, and the media • conducts classroom and campus- and community-related activities to advocate for healthful eating and physical activity options • integrates nutrition lessons into existing curricula that encourage students to eat healthfully, to keep moving, and to become smart shoppers and involved citizens.	Student advocates increased their knowledge of and positive attitudes toward nutrition as well as their healthy eating behaviors. Evaluation of the program found positive nutrition changes for students were related to the greater availability of healthful food options at school.	Agron et al. (2002)
Teens Eating for Energy and Nutrition at School (TEENS)	Middle and junior high schools (seventh and eighth grades)	• classroom curricula • family activities • school nutrition advisory councils (teachers, parents, and students)	Students reported increased consumption of fruits, vegetables, and lower-fat foods; students involved as peer leaders and/or in classroom curricula reported the largest increases in consumption	Birnbaum et al. (2002)
Middle School Physical Activity and Nutrition Study (M-SPAN)	Middle schools	• in-service education for child nutrition staff (CNS) • vendor fairs to let CNS view new lower-fat products and make connections with distributors • meetings to bring together key policy makers at each school (principals, nutrition staff, health teachers, students, parent-teacher association presidents, etc.) and select policy changes for implementation • taste testing with students and marketing low-fat foods at all school food sources (cafeteria breakfasts and lunches, vending machines, a la carte sources, school stores, and bag lunches) • parental education via school newsletters, posters, brochures, and presentations at meetings of the Parent Teacher Association	Students did not report reducing their consumption of fat, but CNS increased the availability of healthful, low-fat foods for reimbursable meals and a la carte.	Zive et al. (2002) Sallis et al. (2003)
Trying Alternative Cafeteria Options in Schools (TACOS)	Middle and senior high schools	• increased availability of lower-fat foods in school cafeteria a la carte areas • implemented student-based promotions targeting the lower-fat foods	Students purchased lower-fat foods more frequently	French et al. (in press)

cafeteria, and the development of policies and nutrition standards (see example in table 17.6) with a school nutrition advisory council (Birnbaum et al. 2002). Evaluation of the TEENS program found that students who were exposed to more program components consumed more healthful foods than students who were exposed to fewer components (Birnbaum et al. 2002).

Research-based guidelines for the promotion of healthy eating recommend integrating multiple methods, including classroom, family, environmental, policy, and community components. Current guidelines also emphasize the benefits of focusing on environmental change. Environmental approaches are often less costly and do not require sustained efforts to change eating behaviors. Box 17.3 highlights one example of a school that has translated these research guidelines into action and is using a combination of environmental techniques to help students develop healthier eating habits.

Challenges to Creating Change

The need for change is often clear, and examples of successful models are available, but schools face a

Table 17.6. Model standards for snacks and beverages sold in vending machines

Category of snack or beverage	Examples
Beverages to promote	100% fruit juice, bottled water, 1% or skim white milk, 1% or skim chocolate milk
Beverages to neither promote nor limit	Diet soda
Beverages to limit	Regular soda, fruit drinks, sport drinks, other sweetened drinks
Snacks to promote	Cereal, pretzels, rice cakes, real fruit snacks, low/lower-fat snacks (including chips, muffins, granola bars, popcorn, crackers, frozen desserts, and cookies)
Snacks to neither promote nor limit	Low-fat candy, low-fat pastries, nuts
Snacks to limit	Chips, cookies, crackers, granola bars, muffins, candy, frozen desserts, and popcorn (when not low in fat)

From Kubik et al. (2001), with permission of the American Dietetic Association.

number of barriers in creating healthy nutrition environments. Because school foodservice programs are generally required to operate on a break-even basis, financial demands and limited resources are among the greatest pressures they face. Efforts to make foods of limited nutritional value less available and provide healthier food choices are influenced by additional factors:

- competition with branded foods and established preferences among students for fast foods, sweetened beverages, and salty snacks
- the promise of substantial income or incentives tied to contracts that give corporations (e.g., soft drink companies) exclusive rights to sell their products in vending machines and at school events (among schools with contracts, 24% of elementary schools, 50% of middle and junior high schools, and 57% of senior high schools receive incentives such as cash awards or donations of equipment and supplies when receipts total a specified amount [Wechsler 2001]).
- inadequate facilities for efficient preparation and service of school meals (students are more likely to choose convenience foods from vending machines or other venues when dining facilities or the time available to eat is limited)
- reduced time in which to eat regular school meals as a consequence of efforts to foster academic performance by extending classroom time (when enrichment or extracurricular activities are only offered during meal periods, students may choose vended items more often or skip meals)

Schools and school foodservices have responded to these challenges with innovative efforts to promote nutritious food choices. In general, schools have found that students are more likely to make healthy food choices if a greater number and variety of options are provided. Many schools are making efforts to increase familiarity with and exposure to a variety of foods. A number of school foodservices allow students to try free samples of foods and complete an evaluation form to indicate how much they like or dislike the healthy items under consideration. Diverse schools that serve food to students of many cultures are incorporating nutritious, ethnic food items. In St. Paul, Minnesota, where almost one-third of the students are

▧ *17.3. Example of an environmental approach to the promotion of healthy food choices at school*

Eating Right at Central Middle School: A School Success Story from Whitefish, Montana

Principal Kim Anderson introduced the concept of a "healthy school nutrition environment" at Central Middle School after learning about the link between nutrition and learning at a Montana Team Nutrition conference. In his view, the key to success at Central was involving the whole school. Anderson believes that "eating right and being active are essential for school success." He has observed the benefits of providing healthy options firsthand and notes that "students who are nutritionally and physically fit have the energy, stamina, self-esteem, and brainpower to do well in the classroom and on the athletic field." The 700 students at Central now regularly enjoy healthy foods and beverages such as bagels, yogurt, fruit, low-fat sub sandwiches, water, and juice.

Change at Central
What changes were made to support healthy eating?

- involved parents, foodservice staff, and students in decision making and carrying out collaborative plans
- replaced the soft drinks in vending machines with bottled water and 100% juice
- replaced the candy in a la carte areas with homemade pretzels, bagels, salads, sandwiches, baked chips, and fresh fruit
- purchased a vending machine for the school foodservice program to sell milk, yogurt, pudding, string cheese, beef jerky, baked chips, and fruit
- increased efforts to promote the school breakfast program
- changed the school schedule so all students now have recess before lunch
- started a recycling program for the cafeteria

What changes did school administrators, teachers, and parents observe when healthy foods were made more available?

- increased net profits from vending and a la carte sales
- decreased lunchroom discipline problems
- improved student behavior and attentiveness during class periods immediately after lunch

What additional changes are planned for the future?

- development of a written nutrition policy to be included in student handbooks
- development of nutrition standards for vending and a la carte options
- purchase of additional vending machines for selling healthy foods as sales increase

(From Hayes D. 2003. Fit and healthy, anytime, anywhere: Healthy options at school. Deaconess Billings Clinic Nutrition News, September 10. Available: http://www.billingsclinic.com/AboutUs/NN_091003.htm.) ▧

Hmong, the district foodservice department has adapted students' family recipes for Hmong foods (Welbes 2003). To increase the appeal of healthful foods, schools have created packaging and brand names for school-made salads, reduced-fat pizzas, and sandwiches (U.S. General Accounting Office 2003). The addition of salad bars in California schools encouraged vegetable consumption when students were allowed to serve themselves as they would at a restaurant buffet (U.S. General Accounting Office 2003). A pilot program of the USDA that was implemented during the 2002–2003 school year also found that distributing free fruit and vegetables at times other than breakfast or lunch periods helped students make healthier nutrition choices (U.S. General Accounting Office 2002).

Faced with limits on finances, facilities, and time, other schools have implemented creative marketing strategies and formed new partnerships. Cafeterias with limited space and/or meal periods have been redesigned to resemble food courts with multiple serving lines so that students are able to spend less time waiting for food (U.S. General Accounting Office 2003). Each serving line features a unique theme and serves a different type of healthy food. One line features the standard school meal; other lines offer choices such as soup, salad, and low-fat submarine sandwiches. One school foodservice in California replaced high-fat snack bar and vended items (e.g., candy bars, potato chips) with healthier options such as fruit and low-fat baked goods and observed increases in sales and higher profits (U.S. General Accounting Office 2003). Schools in North Carolina, Florida, California, and Connecticut were able to address financial demands by implementing farm-to-school initiatives that involve cooperative buying agreements between schools and small, local farmers. Schools are able to provide students with fresh, tasty, nutritious produce with lower transportation costs, and farmers acquire new markets. These changes at the local school and district level have made important contributions to improving school nutrition environments, but policies and regulations are also needed to support good nutrition for students.

Identifying Successful Models: Key Legislation and Policy Initiatives

Although federal policies impose few restrictions on what foods and beverages are allowed in schools outside the federally reimbursable school meals, states, districts, and schools can implement additional guidelines to limit the types of products that are sold or the hours during which they are available. For example, Mississippi and Nebraska prohibit sales of competitive foods anywhere on school campuses during breakfast and lunch (USDA Food and Nutrition Service 2002). In California, the California Childhood Obesity Prevention Act (2003) addresses what beverages may be sold in schools. The bill limits sales of beverages to water, milk, 100% fruit juices, or fruit-based drinks with no less than 50% fruit juice and no added sweeteners from 30 minutes before school to 30 minutes after the end of the school day in elementary and middle and junior high schools.

At the district level, the Los Angeles Unified School District (2003) also adopted a resolution restricting beverage sales, and no sales of soft drinks are allowed in elementary, middle and junior high, or senior high schools. Governing boards or legislatures interested in adopting guidelines that encourage healthy eating can review these models, information at the USDA website about competitive food policies in other states (USDA Food and Nutrition Service 2002), or sample policies written by the National Association of State Boards of Education (NASBE). The NASBE advocates a comprehensive, environmental approach to encouraging healthy eating and has developed model policies (www.nasbe.org) to help schools create healthy nutrition environments and establish the following goals:

- a foodservice program that serves a variety of appealing and nutritious food choices
- a pleasant environment for eating unhurried meals
- a program of nutrition instruction that is sequential and integrated into the school health education curriculum
- an overall school environment that fosters healthy food choices
- a set of opportunities for staff to model good nutrition
- a program of services for students and staff with nutrition-related problems
- a set of strategies to involve students' families in nutrition programs.

Resources

For schools and communities considering changes in their nutrition environment, several resources and toolkits are available. Foodservice associations, health departments, and departments of education can often help schools find resources or connect with people who have expertise in nutrition and program planning. The USDA (www.usda.org), the Centers for Disease Control and Prevention (www.cdc.gov), the Center for Science in the Public Interest (www.cspinet.org), the Food Research and Action Center (www.frac.org), and many other organizations have online resources available.

References

Agron P, Takada, E, Purcel A. 2002. California Project LEAN's Food on the Run Program: An evaluation of a high school–based student advocacy nutrition and physical activity program. J Am Diet Assoc 102(3):S103–S105.

Austin SB, Melly SJ, Sanchez BN, Patel A, Buka S, Gortmaker SL. 2005. Clustering of fast-food restaurants around schools: A novel application of spatial statistics to the study of food environments. Am J Pub Health 95(9):1575–1581.

Baranowski T, Davis M, Resnicow J, Doyle C, Lin LS, Smyth M, et al. 2000. Gimme 5 fruit, juice, and vegetables for fun and health: Outcome evaluation. Health Educ Behav 27(1):96–111.

Baxter S. 1998. Are elementary schools teaching children to prefer candy but not vegetables? J Sch Health 68:111–113.

Birnbaum A, Lytle L, Story M, Perry C, Murray D. 2002. Are differences in exposure to a multicomponent school-based intervention associated with varying dietary outcomes in adolescents? Health Educ Behav 29:427–443.

California Center for Public Health Advocacy. 2002. National Consensus Panel on School Nutrition: Recommendations for competitive food standards in California schools. Davis, CA: Author. Available: http://www.publichealthadvocacy.org/center/center.htm.

Centers for Disease Control and Prevention. 2000. School health index for physical activity and healthy eating: A self-assessment and planning guide. Atlanta, GA. Available: http://apps.nccd.cdc.gov/shi/default.aspx. [accessed 26 December 2005].

Craypo L, Samuels SE, Purcell A. 2004. The 2003 California high school fast food survey. Oakland, CA: Public Health Institute. Available: http://www.phi.org/ [accessed 26 December 2005].

Craypo L, Purcell A, Samuels S, Agron P, Bell E, Takada E. 2002. Fast food sales on high school campuses: Results from the 2000 California high school fast food survey. J Sch Health 72:78–82.

Cullen K, Zakeri I. 2004. Fruits, vegetables, milk, and sweetened beverages consumption and access to a la carte/snack bar meals at school. Am J Pub Health 94(3):463–467.

Foerster SB, Gregson J, Beall DL. 1998. The California Children's 5-a-Day PowerPlay! Campaign: Evaluation of a large-scale social marketing initiative. Family Comm Health 21:46–64.

Food Research and Action Center. Federal Food Programs, Washington, D.C. Available: http://www.frac.org/html/federal_food_programs/federal_index.html [accessed 26 December 2005].

Fox M, Crepinsek M, Connor P, Battaglia M. 2001. School nutrition dietary assessment study 2: Final report. USDA Food and Nutrition Service, Office of Analysis, Nutrition, and Evaluation. Alexandria, VA: U.S. Department of Agriculture.

French SA, Jeffery RW, Story M, Breitlow KK, Baxter JS, Hannan P, et al. 2001. Pricing and promotion effects on low-fat vending snack purchases: The CHIPS Study. Am J Public Health 91(1):112–117.

French SA, Lin BH, Guthrie JF. 2003. National trends in soft drink consumption among children and adolescents age 6 to 17 years: prevalence, amounts, and sources, 1977/1978 to 1994/1998. J Am Diet Assoc 103(10):1326–1331.

French S, Story M, Fulkerson J, Gerlach A. 2003. Food environment in secondary schools: A la carte, vending machines, and food policies and practices. Am J Public Health 93:1161–1167.

French SA, Story M, Fulkerson J, Hannan P. 2004. An environmental intervention to promote lower-fat food choices in secondary schools: Outcomes of the TACOS study. Am J Public Health 94(9):1507–1512.

French SA, Story M, Jeffery RW. 1997. Pricing strategy to promote fruit and vegetable purchase in high school cafeterias. J Am Diet Assoc 97(9):1008–1010.

French S, Story M, Neumark-Sztainer D, Fulkerson J, Hannan P. 2001. Fast-food restaurant use among adolescents: Associations with nutrient intake, food choices, and behavioral and psychosocial variables. Int J Obes 25:1823–1833.

Griffith P, Sackin B, Bierbauer D. 2000. School meals: Benefits and challenges. Presented as a white paper at the National Nutrition Summit, Washington, DC, May 20.

Harnack L, Snyder P, Story M, Holliday P, Lytle L, Neumark-Sztainer D. 2000. Availability of a la carte food items in junior and senior high schools: A needs assessment. J Am Diet Assoc 100:701–703.

Harnack L, Stang J, Story M. 1999. Soft drink consumption among U.S. children and adolescents: Nutritional consequences. J Am Diet Assoc 99:436–441.

Jones SJ, Jahns L, Laraia BA, Haughton B. 2003. Lower risk of overweight in school-aged food insecure girls who participate in food assistance: Results from the panel study of income dynamics child development supplement. Arch Pediatr Adolesc Med 157:780–784.

Kubik M, Lytle L, Hannan P, Perry C, Story M. 2003. The association of the school food environment with dietary behaviors of young adolescents. Am J Public Health 93:1168–1173.

Kubik M, Lytle L, Hannan P, Story M, Perry C. 2002. Food-related beliefs, eating behavior, and classroom food practices of middle school teachers. J School Health 72:339–345.

Kubik M, Lytle L, Story M. 2001. A practical, theory-based approach to establishing school nutrition advisory councils. J Am Diet Assoc 101:223–228.

Kubik M, Lytle L, Story M. 2005. Schoolwide food practices are associated with body mass index in middle school students. 159:1111–1114.

Lin B-H, Guthrie J, Frazão E. 1999. Quality of children's diets at and away from home: 1994–1996. Food Rev 22:2–10.

Los Angeles Unified School District. 2003. Motion to promote healthy beverage sales on school campuses in the LAUSD. Bulletin no. Bul-26. Available: http://www.publichealthadvocacy.org/legislation/Healthy%20Beverage%20Resolution.pdf [accessed 14 April 2004].

Ludwig D, Peterson K, Gortmaker S. 2001. Relation between consumption of sugar-sweetened drinks and childhood obesity: A prospective, observational analysis. Lancet 357:505–508.

National Association of State Boards of Education. Fit, healthy, and ready to learn: A school health policy guide. Sample policies to encourage healthy eating. Available: http://www.nasbe.org/HealthySchools/Sample_Policies/healthy_eating.html [accessed 26 December 2005].

Neumark-Sztainer D, French SA, Hannan PJ, Story M, Fulkerson JA. School lunch and snacking patterns among high school students: Associations with school food environment and policies. Int J Behav Nutr Phys Act 2:14.

Nicklas TA, Johnson CC, Myers L. 1998. Outcomes of a high school program to increase fruit and vegetable consumption: Gimme 5—a fresh nutrition concept for students. J School Health 68:248–253.

Nicklas TA, Stone E, Montgomery D. 1994. Meeting the dietary goals for school meals by the year 2000: The CATCH Eat Smart School Nutrition Program. J Health Educ 25(5):299–307.

Philadelphia Comprehensive School Nutrition Policy Task Force. 2002. Comprehensive school nutrition policy. Philadelphia: Author.

Perry CL, Bishop DB, Taylor G, Murray DM, Mays RW, Dudovitz BS, et al. 1998. Changing fruit and vegetable consumption among children: The 5-a-Day Power Plus program in St. Paul, Minnesota. Am J Public Health 88(4):603–609.

Reynolds KD, Franklin FA, Binkley D. 2000. Increasing fruit and vegetable consumption among fourth-graders: Results from the High 5 Project. Prev Med 30:309–319.

Sallis JF, McKenzie TL, Conway TL. 2003. Environ-mental interventions for eating and physical activity: A randomized controlled trial in middle schools. Am J Prev Med 24(3):209–217.

Snyder MP, Anliker J, Cunningham-Sabo L, Dixon LB, Altaha J, Chamberlain A, et al. 1999. The Pathways Study: A model for lowering the fat in school meals. Am J Clin Nutr 69 (suppl. 4) (April):810S–815S.

Snyder MP, Story M, Trenkner LL. 1992. Reducing fat and sodium in school lunch programs: The LUNCHPOWER! Intervention Study. J Am Diet Assoc 92(9):1087–1091.

State of California. 2003. California Childhood Obesity Prevention Act. SB677.

Templeton SB, Marlette MA, Panemangalore M. 2005. Competitive foods increase the intake of energy and decrease the intake of certain nutrients by adolescents consuming school lunch. J Am Diet Assoc 105(2):215–220.

USDA Food and Nutrition Service. 2000. Team nutrition. Changing the scene: Improving the school nutrition environment. A guide to local action. U.S. Department of Agriculture. Available: http://www.fns.usda.gov/tn/resources/guide.pdf [accessed 15 April 2004].

USDA Food and Nutrition Service. 2001. Children's diets in the mid-1990s: Dietary intake and its relationship with school meal participation. Report No. CN-01-CD1. Office of Analysis, Nutrition, and Evaluation. Alexandria, VA: U.S. Department of Agriculture.

USDA Food and Nutrition Service. 2002. State competitive food policies: Food and nutrition service. Available: http://www.fns.usda.gov/cnd/lunch/competitivefoods/state_policies_2002.pdf [accessed 15 April 2004].

U.S. Department of Health and Human Services. 2000a. *Healthy people 2010: Understanding and improving health,* 2d ed. Washington, DC: U.S. Government Printing Office.

U.S. Department of Health and Human Services, U.S. Department of Agriculture. 2005. Dietary guidelines for Americans 2005. Available: http://www.health.gov/dietaryguidelines/ [accessed 26 December 2005].

U.S. General Accounting Office. 2002. *Fruits and vegetables: Enhanced federal efforts to increase consumption could yield health benefits for Americans.* Publication GAO-02-657. Washington, DC: Author.

U.S. General Accounting Office. 2003. *School lunch program: Efforts needed to improve nutrition and encourage healthy eating.* Publication GAO-03-506. Washington, DC: Author.

U.S. General Accounting Office. 2005. *School meal programs: Competitive foods are widely available and generate substantial revenues for schools*. Publication GAO-05-563. Washington, DC: Author.

Wechsler H, Brener N, Kuester S, Miller C. 2001. Foodservice and foods and beverages available at school: Results from the school health policies and programs study. J School Health 71:313–324.

Welbes J. 2003. *The world on a plate*. St. Paul, MN: St. Paul Pioneer Press.

Wildey M, Pampalone S, Pelletier R, Zive M, Elder J. 2000. Fat and sugar levels are high in snacks purchased from student stores in middle schools. J Am Diet Assoc 100:319–322.

Zive MM, Pelletier RL, Sallis JF, Elder JP. 2002. An environmental intervention to improve a la carte foods at middle schools. J Am Diet Assoc 102(3): S76–S78.

18

David Marshall

Safe and Healthy Sports Environments

■ *Summary*

- Athletic activities promote good health habits and provide many opportunities for developing social and leadership skills. Every year, millions of children in the United States participate in school- and community-sponsored sports.
- The inherent risks in outdoor sports participation can be mitigated by careful design and maintenance of playing fields, adequate lighting, and protective fencing. Indoor sports injuries can result from insufficient space allowances or inadequate equipment.
- Every school should have a general emergency plan that includes communication procedures, presence of an ambulance and emergency medical help at appropriate times, and proper medical equipment. Ideally, all coaches should be trained in CPR and the use of an automatic defibrillation device.
- Soccer, football, baseball, basketball, and gymnastics all present specific safety issues for participants and spectators.
- Environment-related conditions such as heat illness and dehydration are not uncommon in sports settings. Extreme cold and air quality are additional safety factors to be considered. ■

Each year in the United States more than 45 million children 16 years of age or younger participate in competitive sports programs. About half of these student athletes take part in school-sponsored athletics, and the others play in community-based programs. Regardless of where they play, the physical, emotional, and social benefits gained from athletic participation can carry over into all aspects of life (fig. 18.1).

The physical benefits of sports relate directly to fitness. In general, children who participate in sports are healthier than those who do not. As children learn the importance of caring for their bodies through proper nutrition and rest, they develop lifelong habits for good health. These habits are especially important for today's youth, given the alarming rise of pediatric obesity rates in recent years.

Participation in sports can also teach children to deal with success and failure in a positive way and thereby enhance their self-esteem. They learn to deal with adversity from losing a game or becoming injured, and they come to understand the

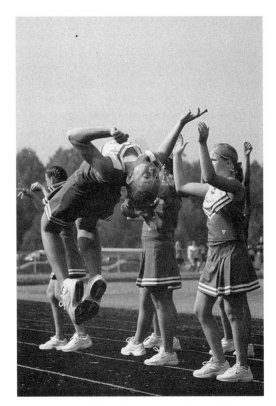

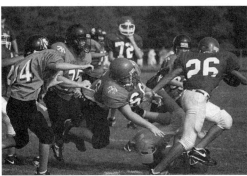

Figure 18.1. School athletic activities range from cheerleading to football, from basketball to volleyball. (Photo by Milestone Photography.)

importance of hard work, dedication, and patience to achieve their goals. Athletic activities can also present and encourage concepts such as time management, leadership, teamwork, controlling emotions, the importance of rules, and stress relief.

The greenspace available for the growing numbers of community-based programs such as club teams, travel teams, and Amateur Athletic Union–sanctioned teams is limited, so many of these community teams use fields already built and main-

tained by local school systems. In addition, millions of other children who are not involved in organized sports are participating in school physical education classes, which should encourage regular indoor and outdoor physical activity. Therefore, school athletic facilities are in use on a regular basis and, if not properly maintained and equipped, can increase the chance of injury.

Injury Patterns

Athletic participation at all levels carries an inherent risk of injury, both minor and life threatening, but we must not let the risk of sports injury outweigh the vast benefits:

- understanding the concepts of teamwork, sportsmanship, and fair play
- improvement in self-esteem
- development of physical skills
- creation of new friendships
- participation in daily exercise

According to data from the National Safe Kids Campaign and the American Academy of Pediatrics, each year approximately 3.5 million injuries occur in children 14 years of age and younger while playing sports or participating in recreational activities. This represents about one-third of all childhood injuries. The most common body parts injured are the knee and ankle; sprains and strains represent the most common type of injury. Most of these injuries result from falls, collisions, and overuse and occur most often during unorganized or informal activities. Of those injuries occurring during organized sports, 62% happen during practice (National Safe Kids Campaign 2004).

The National Youth Sports Safety Foundation and the National Safe Kids Campaign report the number of children ages 5–14 who are treated in hospital emergency rooms annually for sports injuries (table 18.1). Although baseball accounts for fewer injuries than bicycling, basketball, or football, it has the highest fatality rate among sports for children ages 5–14 and accounts for 3 or 4 deaths annually (National Safe Kids Campaign 2004.).

General Layout of Athletic Facilities

Athletic facilities should be constructed close to the school and be easily accessible to student athletes,

Table 18.1. Children ages 5–14 years who were treated in hospital ED for sports injuries in 2002

Sport	Number of children
Basketball	193,000
Baseball and softball	116,000
Bicycling	373,000
Football	187,800
Gymnastics	21,200
Ice skating	14,000
In-line and roller skating	85,600
Skateboarding	27,000
Sledding	23,500
Snow skiing	18,500
Snow boarding	19,000
Soccer	76,200
Trampolines	68,000

who should not have to cross roads or parking lots to gain access to the facility. Access should be away from heavy bus and automobile traffic areas where students are picked up. The fields should also be spaced and configured so that several teams can be practicing or competing simultaneously and not be in danger of being hit by batted balls, thrown discuses, and so on. The fields and facilities should be cared for and inspected on a regular basis, and repairs should be undertaken in a timely manner.

Because of the effects of weather and the high usage of outdoor fields, the conditions of the playing surface and turf can quickly deteriorate. When constructing new fields, the turf chosen must be compatible with the amount of anticipated usage, climate, and type of irrigation. A turf expert can provide guidance on soil conditions and turf types to find the best fit. Automatic irrigation systems are also strongly recommended to avoid turf damage due to drought. Through proper soil, irrigation, and turf management, turf may become stronger and reduce the incidence of knee and ankle injuries by stabilizing the root system and decreasing turf pull-up. Several schools in the Atlanta area are installing synthetic field turf of the type seen in many universities and professional stadiums. Although expensive, this artificial material is very durable and may prove cost effective in the long run.

Outdoor Fencing

Athletic fields should be fenced to limit access of nonschool personnel and activities. Allowing unlimited access puts the facility at risk for vandalism, theft, and animal waste and may increase the risk of injury to a student athlete from potholes, cans, bottles, sharp objects, and litter. However, for some communities, the athletic facilities, such as playground equipment and ball fields, may be the only facilities available for public recreational use and may therefore be accessible at all times. In this case, because the risk of vandalism, trash, and debris is higher and use may be greater, maintenance and supervision should be heightened.

Lighting and Parking Lots

Even if there are no plans for night contests, adequate lighting around the fields is essential for security purposes. Practices often continue until dusk, and student athletes leave the field and school in the dark. The gymnasium, as well as the parking lot used by spectators for outdoor contests, should be well lighted for security purposes. Students and parents are often excited about arriving at the sports venue and have a tendency to run between parked cars without looking both ways. Drivers are also frequently in a hurry and may drive too fast or without paying full attention while in the parking area. "Children at Play" signs or speed bumps throughout the parking area may help to decrease parking lot accidents. The parking lot should be designed for one-way flow for student drop-off and pickup. If curbside loading zones are not available, temporary signs can be posted to designate loading and unloading areas during high traffic times. These areas should be easily visible with reflective paint, signs, or speed bumps.

Locker Rooms

Locker rooms should be large enough to accommodate an entire team with adequate ventilation. Lockers must provide enough room to store school supplies and athletic gear and must be locked to avoid theft and vandalism. Floors should be nonslippery when wet and when students are walking with cleats. A windowed office in the locker room allows supervision by a coach until all student athletes have left.

General Emergency Action Plan

Each field or athletic venue should have an emergency action plan in case of serious injury or evacuation of the facility, and all of the coaches who will use the venue must be familiar with it. An emergency plan should include the following:

- access to the nearest working telephone (in case the coach does not carry a cellular phone or the battery is dead)
- predetermined directions for ambulance entry to the school and routing within the school grounds, including location of locked gates that may need to be opened for ambulance access
- location of shelters for evacuation of players and spectators in the event of lightning, tornadoes, or other severe weather conditions
- location of emergency medical equipment, if any (e.g., inhalers, EpiPens, spine board, airway and mask, automated external defibrillator)
- list of contact people and phone numbers and a protocol indicating when each person should be called (the list should be reviewed and updated periodically)
- emergency phone numbers and a list of relevant conditions for each student readily available

All coaches should be encouraged, if not required, to be trained and certified in CPR, which includes using an automated external defibrillator (AED).

Ambulances

In many jurisdictions, the presence of at least one ambulance and a paramedic crew is required for scheduled events. Having an ambulance immediately available at the scene reduces delay in transporting an injured person to the emergency department if needed. Where severe trauma or other life-threatening injury has occurred, eliminating even these few moments may reduce injury or prevent death.

Even if not required locally, having an ambulance and a paramedic crew available is preferable, particularly where transport time to the nearest emergency department would be prolonged by traffic, distance, weather, or other factors.

Automated External Defibrillator

Many life-threatening injuries or illnesses at sports events are cardiac in nature. Rhythm abnormalities may occur either as a result of decreased blood flow to the heart or, less commonly, as a result of blunt trauma to the chest wall. When these disturbances affect the ventricles (the pumping chambers of the heart), blood flow to the heart itself, as well as to the rest of the body, is impaired, often leading to cardiac arrest. The likelihood of a victim's surviving a cardiac arrest without permanent brain damage decreases with each additional minute required to restore circulation.

An AED can be used by staff with limited medical training. Once connected to the victim, the device will automatically analyze the heart rhythm. If appropriate, and only if appropriate, the device will deliver an electric shock to the victim's chest (defibrillate the heart) in an attempt to make the heart beat in an effective rhythm.

Every member of the coaching staff and school health personnel should be trained in the use of the AED. Although the device provides voice prompts to remind the user of the correct actions to take at each point in the setup sequence, this will not replace the initial training in the correct use of the device.

Activity-specific Issues

Pep Rallies

Many schools host pep rallies to boost school spirit and promote attendance at athletic events. These are often held after school or the evening before a contest and may take place indoors or outdoors. Indoor pep rallies pose risks that are different from those at outdoor rallies. Indoor events should be held only where emergency egress is maintained and where the safe capacity of the area is not exceeded. Adequate supervision should be provided to maintain crowd control at all times.

Bonfires have become popular events at evening outdoor pep rallies. The combination of a large number of spirited students and the will to build "a larger fire than last year" has obvious safety concerns. Bonfire risk can be reduced by following several precautions:

- Adequate adult supervision is essential.
- The fire should be located in a place far away from buildings, cars, or foliage and kept under strict control.
- Some type of nonflammable barrier must be used to keep students from getting too close to the flames.
- The local fire department should be informed of the event and, if possible, be present to monitor the size and control of the fire and to supervise the igniting and extinguishing of the flames. The presence of the fire department ensures their prompt response in the event of an emergency.

Football and Soccer

Soccer is one of the most popular sports worldwide, with more than 40 million players, and its popularity in the United States is growing each year. Currently more than 3 million U.S. players are registered in high school or youth soccer associations. As the number of these groups grows, fields for soccer use are in increasingly high demand. Community parks and fields designed for other sports are often converted and used for soccer. The U.S. Consumer Product Safety Commission has reported 24 deaths and hundreds of injuries since 1979 as a result of soccer goal accidents (U.S. Consumer Product Safety Commission 2005). Safety measures include the following:

- Before each contest or game, the field must be inspected for potholes, large rocks, glass, and other debris. This is especially important if the field has public access.
- The presence of drainage grates should also be noted and marked with visible orange cones.
- The corner boundaries should be marked with flexible or collapsible stakes to avoid injury to players.
- The yard line markers should also be made of padded material rather than wood.
- Soccer balls should be made of waterproof synthetic material rather than leather because

leather balls can become waterlogged and thus very heavy, making them dangerous.

- The goalposts for both soccer and football should be padded, and the end zone markers should be made of soft collapsible material or weighted with sand to allow them to stand up. Because soccer players do not wear head protection, the goalposts should be padded so that players do not sustain head injuries from direct contact with the goalpost.
- All soccer and football goals must be anchored to the ground. Even if they are properly built, soccer goals should be anchored to the ground from both the back and the base. Injuries are likely to occur when children climb on top of an unsecured goal (causing the crossbar to snap) or when the goal tips over onto another child.
- Soccer goals should be manufactured with heavy materials for the base and lighter materials for the crossbar and mouth. This will reduce the risk of the goal tipping over. High winds can also cause lighter, portable goals to tip over.
- The nets should be removed when not in use to prevent children from climbing on them. This will reduce the risk of injury from goal tipping or strangulation.
- When soccer goals are stored, they should be tipped over onto the mouth or locked together mouth to mouth. They can also be chained to a fence or fence post. A "Danger! No Climbing" sign may also serve as a deterrent.
- With the higher risk of head, neck, and spine injuries in football, the need for a well-planned and rehearsed emergency action plan cannot be overemphasized.

Lacrosse

Because lacrosse is gaining in popularity in high schools and middle schools, it should be mentioned.

- The facilities (field conditions, padding on goals) are similar to those for football and soccer, but, because of the speed of the ball when thrown toward the goal, the area behind the goal must be kept clear of spectators.
- If there is seating behind the goal, a safety net

should be installed to protect spectators (as with the net behind home plate at a baseball park).

Baseball and Softball

In the United States, nearly 6 million children 5–14 years of age participate in organized baseball and softball each year. Some of the related injuries requiring emergency department care may be preventable if certain measures are taken:

- Fields should be surveyed for hazards and debris before each use.
- The fencing around the field should be inspected for needed repairs, sharp edges, and stability.
- The top of the fence should be padded along the outfield and foul lines.
- A 6- to 8-foot warning track of dirt or crushed brick (rather than grass) should be installed in front of the outfield fence to warn players chasing a fly ball that they are approaching the fence.
- The dugouts, or player bench areas, should be protected with a fence to shield them from batted or thrown balls and thrown bats.
- The bullpen, or relief pitcher warm-up area, should be protected with a fence and provide an area for another player to sit to warn the players who are warming up of approaching balls.
- Similarly, the "on deck" (warm-up area for the next batter) should be beside or behind the dugout or eliminated completely to decrease the risk of players being struck by a wild pitch, foul ball, or thrown bat.
- The bases should be the breakaway type that detach when a player slides into them. These types of bases have been shown to decrease the risk of foot, ankle, and knee injuries caused by sliding.

Tennis

Tennis courts should be kept in good condition. Cracks, holes, and irregularities in the surface should be promptly repaired, and cranks for the nets should have safety locks.

Some schools may elect to keep the courts locked to prevent unauthorized use, whereas others may leave the courts accessible to the public. These courts should have signs prohibiting bicycles, skateboards, and rollerblades since they can damage the surface and pose an injury risk to tennis players.

Track and Field

The track should be inspected regularly for repair needs such as holes, defects, and debris. Rubberized surfaces are preferable to cinder or asphalt surfaces. They are more expensive than cinder or asphalt but decrease the risk of injuries to the lower extremities (e.g., knee pain, shin splints, stress fractures) from overuse.

Space must be adequate for field events such as the high jump, long jump, and pole vault to take place simultaneously. The landing pads should be inspected regularly.

The shot put and discus events must also be in a designated area where other athletes are not at risk of being struck. These events should not take place in the infield area, where unsuspecting athletes who are warming up might wander into the landing zone and be injured.

Cross-country

Because cross-country athletes often train off campus on public roads, certain safety issues warrant special attention. Runners should avoid running at dawn or dusk, when motorist visibility is poor. They should wear bright, reflective clothing to improve their visibility to motorists and run with a partner or in a group. The recommended direction for running is facing the traffic or on sidewalks, if available. Runners should wear well-padded running shoes and replace them at least every 350–400 miles.

Swimming

Schools with swimming and diving teams or those with a swimming pool on campus should follow certain safety guidelines:

- The pool should be locked when not in use to avoid unauthorized usage.
- A pool maintenance company or a school employee should be trained to provide daily chemical analysis of the water.

- Deep areas should be deep enough (at least 10 feet) to allow diving, and the ascent of the pool floor should be gradual enough to prevent neck and spine injuries to students diving.
- The depth of the water should be posted around the perimeter of the pool, and "No Diving" signs should be posted where appropriate.

Gymnasium Sports

Gymnasium sports include basketball, volleyball, gymnastics, cheerleading, and indoor rock climbing.

- The roof and floors should be inspected regularly for repair needs.
- Water fountains should be readily accessible but far enough from the playing floor so that splashes and spills do not pose a risk to players. For infection control, an individual water bottle for each player is desirable.
- Space from the boundary lines to the wall or bleachers should be sufficient for an athlete to slow down and stop (when saving a ball, for example). Many noncontact knee injuries, such as anterior cruciate ligament (ACL) tears and ankle sprains, occur when an athlete is suddenly decelerating to avoid hitting the wall or bleachers.
- The wall directly behind the baskets should be padded to prevent wrist, elbow, and head injuries in basketball players.
- Because of the increased popularity of rock climbing, some schools are installing rock-climbing walls for use in physical education classes. This equipment should be used only under close adult supervision and should be secured when adult supervision is not available. It should be installed and maintained as instructed by the manufacturer.
- Proper safety gear and harnesses should be used at all times.
- Gymnasts and cheerleaders need to have adequate padding under each apparatus, and the equipment should be inspected regularly. Because the sport of cheerleading now incorporates tumbling and stunts similar to those seen in gymnastics, cheerleaders also must

have adequate padding and mats during practice and competitions.
- Practicing jumps and tumbling on hard wood surfaces increases stress on the lower extremities, which may lead to overuse injuries. Cheerleaders, like gymnasts, should have access to padded, cushioned surfaces for tumbling, generally polyethylene foam athletic mats (such as Resilite or Ad-Mats).

Bleacher Seating

Bleachers must be kept in good condition. Wooden bleachers need to be inspected for rotten boards, sharp edges, nails, bolts, and so on. Aluminum bleachers must also be inspected periodically for abnormal wear. Rails should be installed on the ends of all rows. The gaps between the seats and between the seats and floorboards should be no more than 4 inches. Children have been seriously injured or killed because of falls through large gaps in bleachers. One solution is to place boards under all of the seats to reduce the gap to less than 4 inches. Another is to install safety netting under large gaps.

Heat Illness and Dehydration

Heat illness is one of the most common preventable and potentially catastrophic problems in sports. It accounts for 2–5 deaths each year among young athletes. The severity ranges from mild heat cramps to life-threatening heat stroke. Both athletes and coaches must be aware of the early signs of heat illness and, more important, know how to prevent it. The best prevention is adequate hydration, both before and during activity (fig. 18.2). Thirst is not always a good indicator of fluid needs, so fluid intake of prudent amounts should be encouraged, particularly in hot weather. On the other hand, excess fluid intake can lead to complications (including electrolyte disturbances such as hyponatremia and seizures) as well (Almond et al. 2005). The best type of beverage to use when encouraging fluid intake has been the subject of numerous studies, most (but not all) of which suggest that sodium-containing fluids reduce the risk of hyponatremia. These conflicting results may be explained in part by the small amount of sodium in many commer-

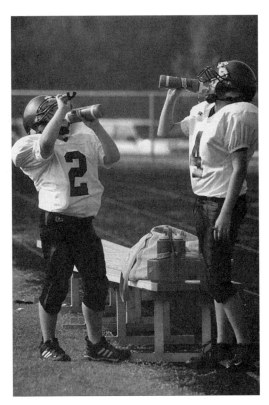

Figure 18.2. Adequate hydration is important for athletes, especially during warm weather. (Photo by Milestone Photography.)

cially available sports drinks, which may be too low to prevent hyponatremia (Maughan and Leiper 1999; Rehrer 2001; Speedy, Noakes, Schneider 2001; Tweronbold et al. 2003). Flavoring the beverage to make it more palatable may enhance its acceptance by the athletes and improve their fluid balance (Minehan et al. 2002).

Thermoregulation in young athletes is less efficient than in adults. Children generate more heat per pound of body weight than adults. They sweat later and less than adults, and they take longer to acclimate to heat and humidity than do adults. These factors place young athletes at increased risk of heat-related illness.

The following recommendations for young athletes may reduce or prevent heat-related illness:

- Before practice or games, drink at least enough to quench thirst, if not a bit more.
- Drink appropriate amounts of fluid every 15–20 minutes while exercising. For most school-aged children, 4–12 ounces every 15–20 minutes is probably reasonable.
- Water is usually sufficient if the activity lasts 1 hour or less and the fluid intake is less than 32 ounces. If the activity lasts more than an hour, a sports drink containing electrolytes (sodium and potassium) and carbohydrates is probably a good idea.
- Traditional advice has been to avoid salt tablets because of the danger of too much sodium intake, although this has not been well studied.
- Carbonated beverages offer little benefit beyond water; thus, electrolyte-containing solutions are probably preferable.

An athlete suffering a heat-related illness should be removed from activity immediately, allowed to rest in a cool, shaded place, and given fluids to drink. Measures to enhance cooling, such as removal of the outer layer of clothes, are often appropriate. Careful monitoring is essential. If the athlete becomes dizzy, disoriented, or confused or cannot drink, ice bags should be applied to the neck, armpits, and groin, and emergency medical help should be summoned.

Extreme Cold

Just as extreme heat can cause heat-related illness in athletes, exposure to extreme cold can cause cold-related disorders such as hypothermia and frostbite. These conditions are best prevented by being aware of the environmental conditions and the wind chill factor.

Hypothermia can occur with moderate temperatures as high as 65°F, and frostbite can occur when temperatures are 31°F and below. If the temperature is above freezing, hypothermia can occur with sweating and inadequate clothing, especially during rest breaks and windy conditions. During these times, dry clothing is essential to prevent excessive conductive heat loss through wet clothing. As the temperature drops below freezing, the risk of frostbite increases. Prevention measures include covering the exposed skin on the hands and face to minimize exposure. When the temperature drops to an extremely cold level (compared with the usual climate of the area), outdoor activities should be moved indoors or cancelled. Clothing for cold-

■ *18.1. The heat index*

The heat index incorporates both temperature and relative humidity. If the heat index is in zone 1, then general precautions with regard to outdoor exercise and hydration should be taken. If the heat index is in zone 2, outdoor activities should be shortened, regular hydration and rest breaks every 15 minutes should be mandatory, and unacclimated people should use extreme caution. If the heat index is in zone 3, administrators should consider moving events to cooler times of the day, unacclimated people should avoid strenuous activity, and all outdoor participants should use extreme caution.

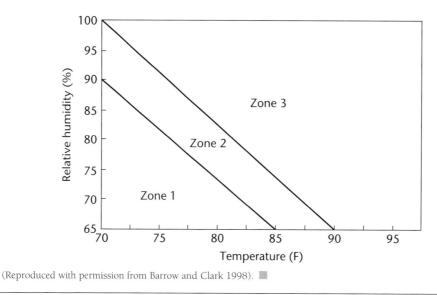

(Reproduced with permission from Barrow and Clark 1998). ■

environment activities should be made of a material designed to wick away moisture from the body and applied in layers for stepwise removal. A dry change of clothes should be available for excessive sweating.

Air Quality

If the air quality or pollution index is in the moderate range or above, people with acute or chronic lung disease such as asthma or cystic fibrosis should shorten their outdoor activities or remain indoors. Air quality is discussed more extensively in chapters 12 and 28.

Conclusion

As the number of school-age athletes in the United States grows, illness and injury related to sports, unfortunately, will also increase. When construct-

ing new athletic facilities or improving existing ones, we must be aware of the impact the design, layout, and materials will have on the health and well-being of the athletes. Points to consider include the following:

- the impact the playing surface may have on the development of injuries
- designation of someone to inspect and maintain the facilities and equipment
- implementation of an emergency action plan with CPR and AED training for all school personnel who work with student athletes
- implementation and maintenance of a campuswide communication system with the emergency management system
- programs to educate players, coaches, and administrators on the prevention and treatment of dehydration and heat-related illnesses
- the importance of the preparticipation physical examination.

References

Almond CSD, Shin AY, Fortescue EB, et al. 2005. Hyponatremia among runners in the Boston Marathon. N Engl J Med 352:1550–1556.

Barrow MW, Clark KA. 1998. Heat-related illness. Am Fam Physician 58:749–759.

Maughan RJ, Leiper JB. 1999. Limitations to fluid replacement during exercise. Can J Appl Physiol 24: 173–187.

Minehan MR, Riley MD, Burke LM. 2002. Effect of flavor and awareness of kilojoule content of drinks on preference and fluid balance in team sports. Int J Sports Nutr Exercise Metab 12:81–92.

National Safe Kids Campaign. 2004. Facts about childhood sports injuries. Washington, DC: National Safe Kids Campaign. Available: http://www.usa .safekids.org/content_documents/Sports_facts.pdf [accessed 11 October 2004].

Rehrer NJ. 2001. Fluid and electrolyte balance in ultra-endurance sport. Sports Med 31:701–715.

Speedy DB, Noakes TD, Schneider C. 2001. Exercise-associated hyponatremia: A review. Emerg Med 13: 17–27.

Twerenbold R, Knechtie B, Kakebeeke TH, et al. 2003. Effects of different sodium concentrations in replacement fluids during prolonged exercise in women. Br J Sports Med 37:300–303.

U.S. Consumer Product Safety Commission. 2005. Consumer product safety alert: Movable soccer goals can fall over on children. Washington, DC: Consumer Product Safety Commission, Document # 5118. Available: http://www.cpsc.gov/CPSCPUB/ PUBS/5118.pdf [accessed 11 January 2006].

V

Violence and
Disasters

19

Tod Schneider

Violence and Crime Prevention through Environmental Design

■ *Summary*

- Environmental changes can help protect schools from violence, crime, and other antisocial behavior.
- First-generation Crime Prevention through Environmental Design (CPTED) focuses on physical measures: improving natural surveillance, access control, and territoriality.
- Second-generation CPTED addresses the affective environment and promotes connectivity through a positive school climate and culture. Students feel connected to the school, the surrounding environment, the community, the teachers, and each other. ■

School Violence: Defining the Problem

In the school year that started in the fall of 1999, 32 students died violently at school-related events or facilities in the United States. Of those, 24 were murdered, and 8 took their own lives. These incidents were tragic, but they were rare. School-based crimes directly affected only 0.005%, or one in 20,000, of the 52 million children enrolled in school that year. During the same period 2124 juvenile homicides and 1922 suicides occurred away from schools (DeVoe et al. 2003). Schools are relatively safe havens from lethal violence.

In contrast, less-than-lethal violence and crime are not rare. In 2001 roughly 2900 children were kidnapped from schools by strangers, although available data do not specify the outcomes (Sedlak et al. 2002). The violent crime victimization rate has dropped dramatically over the past decade—from 48 violent crimes per thousand students in 1992 to 28 in 2001—but 451,000 students aged 12–18 years still suffered from nonfatal serious violence in 2001. In 1996 a serious assault occurred in 1 out of 10 public schools (Hevside et al. 1998). One in three high school students surveyed in 2003 reported having been in a physical fight during the previous 12 months, although only 12.8% reported having been in a fight on school property (Brener et al. 2004). More than 90% of secondary schools report at least some violence annually, and the incidence is generally higher in larger, poorer, urban schools (DeVoe et al. 2003). Offensive comments and graffiti that target race, religion, ethnicity, disability, gender, or sexual orientation are common. Thirty-six percent of students reported seeing hate-

■ *19.1. Risk to students*

Most of these 2001 statistics are good indicators of the present level of risk in the United States. In most cases, the rate of incidents is now significantly lower than during the previous decade:

- Students who saw hate-related graffiti at school: 36%
- Students who reported fighting either on or off school grounds: 33%
- Students who reported fighting on school property: 13%
- Ninth-graders who reported being threatened or injured with a weapon on school property: 13%
- Students ages 12–18 years who reported that someone at school used hate-related words (related to race, religion, ethnicity, disability, gender, or sexual orientation) against them: 12%
- Students who reported being threatened or injured with a weapon such as a gun, knife, or club on school property within the preceding 12 months: 7–9%
- Students ages 12–18 years who reported being bullied at school: 8%
- Students who reported being victims of crime at school: 6%
- Students who reported carrying a weapon to school within the past 30 days: 6%
- Twelfth-graders who reported being threatened or injured with a weapon on school property: 5%
- Students ages 12–18 years who reported avoiding one or more places at school: 5%
- Students in grades 9–12 who had at least one drink of alcohol on school property in the previous 30 days: 5%
- Students in grades 9–12 who smoked marijuana on school property in the previous 30 days: 5%
- Students who reported being victims of theft at school: 4%
- Students who reported being victims of violent crime at school: 2%
- Percentage of school-related juvenile homicides: 1%
- Percentage of school-related juvenile suicides: 0.4%
- Percentage of students who were victims of homicide or suicide: 0.00006%

(From Devoe et al. 2003) ■

related graffiti, and 12% heard hate-related comments; another 8% reported being bullied (DeVoe et al. 2003).

Bullying is a common problem, especially in the middle school years. Thirty percent of students report being either victims or perpetrators of bullying. Bullying generally correlates with other problems, including substance abuse and loneliness. In a 2001 North Carolina study, 10,000 middle school and high school students reported staying home at least once a week to avoid bullies, and more than one-third of students reported feeling unsafe at school (North Carolina Department of Juvenile Justice and Delinquency Prevention 2001).

■ *19.2. Risk to teachers*

Between 1997 and 2001, teachers in the United States were victims of 817,000 thefts and 473,000 violent crimes. During the 1999–2000 and 2001–2002 school years, 9% of all elementary and secondary school teachers were threatened with injury by a student, and 4% of all elementary and secondary school teachers were attacked by a student.

(From Devoe et al. 2003) ■

■ *19.3. Schoolwide risks*

The level of threat in U.S. schools may extend well beyond the relatively small number of students who are directly victimized. A violent incident can impact witnesses, bystanders, family members, and anyone else who even hears about it. With that in mind, consider the following data related to the 1999–2000 and 2001–2002 school years:

* Secondary schools that experienced a violent incident: 92%
* Schools with 1,000 or more students that experienced a violent incident: 89%
* Elementary, middle, and combined schools that experienced a violent incident: 61–87%
* Schools with fewer than 300 students that experienced a violent incident: 61%
* Schools that reported taking a serious disciplinary action: 54%
* Students in grades 9–12 who had at least one drink of alcohol in the previous 30 days: 47%
* Schools that reported property crimes: 46%
* Students in grades 9–12 who reported that someone had offered, sold, or given them an illegal drug on school property in the previous 12 months: 29%
* Schools that reported daily or weekly bullying: 29%
* Students in grades 9–12 who smoked marijuana in the previous 30 days: 24%
* All public schools that experienced one or more violent crimes: 20%
* Schools that reported student acts of disrespect for teachers: 19%
* Schools that reported student verbal abuse of teachers: 13%
* Public schools that took a serious disciplinary action for possession of a firearm or explosive: 4%
* Schools that reported occurrences of student racial tensions and widespread disorder: 3%
* Public schools that took a serious disciplinary action for the use of a firearm or an explosive device: 2%.

(From Devoe et al. 2003) ■

Although not nearly as commonplace as graffiti, harassment, or bullying, the wave of mass killings across the country in the 1990s riveted national attention on the issue of school safety. Schools across the nation scrambled to put security measures in place, even when such measures would not necessarily resolve the problems that inspired them. Locked gates after hours, for example, will not stop crime that occurs during school hours. Nighttime lighting will not prevent daytime incidents. Metal detectors at the front door will not deter students from bringing guns in through the rear entrance. Indoor security will not stop outdoor crime.

The approach known as Crime Prevention through Environmental Design (CPTED) addresses both physical and affective (emotional and behavioral) components of an environment. Together, these components can have a powerful effect on school safety.

Crime Prevention through Environmental Design

Crime Prevention through Environmental Design is the study and design of environments to promote desirable conduct while discouraging antisocial behavior. Conventional security measures can play important roles, but in isolation they can undermine the ambiance of an environment and give a school the feel of occupied territory. Security guards are unlikely to have much of an impact on verbal abuse or graffiti, and they certainly will not be able to turn around an otherwise poorly managed, academically uninspiring, or socially alienating school. Although CPTED incorporates conventional security measures as appropriate, it balances that approach with an emphasis on strengthening the primary function of an environment. Schools that are great places to teach and learn are less conducive to antisocial behavior.

■ *19.4. Inspired environments*

CPTED is truly a misnomer because, when it is applied well, the concepts focus not on crime prevention, but on building positive environments, motivating desirable attitudes and behaviors, and reinforcing primary intended functions. The focus is not on what should *not* happen, but on what *should* happen.

Community rehabilitation projects have successfully applied this concept in varied locales such as the South Bronx Banana Kelly neighborhood, Boston's Dudley Street, and Hope Community in Minneapolis. In each of these cases, slums were transformed into vibrant communities. The Hope for the Children project in Rantoul, Illinois, transformed a decommissioned U.S. Air Force base into a thriving model community of foster care to adoptive families and supportive seniors.

At their best, schools engage in similarly visionary work and grow safer not by becoming obsessed with crime, but by building safe, welcoming, and engaging environments that inspire teachers to teach and students to learn. Here are some encouraging examples:

- Reece Community High School in economically depressed Devenport, Tasmania, Australia, emphasizes connectivity, with a day-lit, welcoming layout that encourages small-group interaction, flexible use of technology, and project-based learning. Students in the upper grades have their own workstations.
- Island Wood School (K–12) on Bainbridge Island, Washington, is deeply embedded in the surrounding natural environment. Outdoor learning opportunities include shelters, bird blinds, and pedestrian trails. Solar panels, transparent building systems, and energy metering provide hands-on learning opportunities.
- West Metro Education Program in Minneapolis, Minnesota, emphasizes experiential learning and utilizes transparent technology and energy systems.
- Southridge High School, in Beaverton, Oregon, emphasizes lifelong learning, collaboration, and integration into the real world. Students spend half of their day at work sites. Halls become "streets," and "porches" mark the entry points to each "neighborhood."
- In Seattle, Washington, Whittier Elementary School, inspired by nearby ship locks, borrowed sea-related imagery to inspire the students. A whimsical sea serpent "swims" across their playground. ■

CPTED: A Historical Overview

The CPTED field emerged in the early 1970s with the publication of C. Ray Jeffery's *Crime Prevention through Environmental Design* (1971) and Oscar Newman's *Defensible Space* (1972). Newman's "broken windows" theory suggests that visual blight has an impact on neighborhood conditions, people's level of fear, and their subsequent behavior. The field evolved considerably in the following decades, and social ecologists examined the relationship between human behavior and the environment throughout this period (Moss and Insel 1974; Schalock 1989). Canadian academicians Pat and Paul Brantingham and consultants Greg Saville and Paul Wong made significant contributions from the 1980s on, while British criminologists Patricia Mayhew and Ronald Clark worked on situational crime prevention. Criminologist Tim Crowe's *Crime Prevention through Environmental Design: Applications of Architectural Design and Space Management Concepts* (1991) became a standard in the field. Stan and Sherry Carter, working in Florida, became CPTED leaders (Carter and Carter 2001), while Gerda Wekerle and Carolyn Whitzman, based in Toronto, applied CPTED to both urban design and women's safety. Chief Inspector Phil McCamley of the New South Wales Police in Australia built a CPTED risk assessment model that shows promise for use in urban areas. Greg Saville founded the International CPTED Association (ICA) in 1996. Australia-based educator Gerard Cleveland regularly teaches in partnership with Saville, promoting a second-generation CPTED approach incorporating affective issues.

Basic CPTED

Basic CPTED focuses on design features of the physical environment in three principal categories: natural surveillance, natural access control, and territoriality/maintenance.

Natural surveillance is the capacity to observe activity without having to take special measures to do so. Clear direct views, such as those provided by windows, provide opportunities for natural surveillance, which deters misbehavior. Students are less inclined to misbehave when they know they can be seen and thus are likely to be caught. In one study of five Midwestern high schools, of 166 violent incidents, none took place when adults were present, leading the researchers to conclude that the most effective deterrence to violence was the physical presence of teachers who were willing to intervene, together with a clear administrative policy on violence (Astor et al. 1999).

If responding to a call for help or a loud noise requires opening a solid door or stepping around a blind corner, natural surveillance is missing, and the response may be too little too late. In such situations school officials see the aftermath but do not know what initially occurred. Surveillance is further diminished if lighting is inadequate.

Natural access control is the capacity to limit entry to a facility. A school with dozens of unsecured exterior doors cannot hope to control comings and goings. Intruders have free rein, and schools must rely on other security measures. Without access control, a school must place much greater emphasis on surveillance, territoriality, security staffing, and a positive school climate to compensate.

Territoriality is the capacity to establish authority over an environment, making a statement about who is in charge, who belongs, and who is an outsider. Gangs use graffiti, for example, to establish their territory; schools take it back through repainting, following up with ongoing, vigilant maintenance. Signs that direct visitors to the office or spell out rules reinforce territoriality and influence behavior. In addition, if students wear uniforms, it is difficult for intruders to blend in.

The benefits of basic CPTED measures are fairly straightforward. With fewer access points and hidden areas,

- it becomes harder for intruders to enter the school undetected
- the need for teachers to serve as security guards decreases
- teachers can spend more of their time teaching
- the environment is more conducive to its primary functions of teaching and learning

Planning for CPTED

To determine whether a school has weaknesses that can be addressed through CPTED, it is useful to ask and answer eight key questions:

1. What risks and opportunities do students encounter between home and school?
2. What risks and opportunities do students encounter in areas directly adjoining school property?
3. Can office staff observe approaching visitors before they reach the school entry?
4. Can staff members physically stop visitors from entering?
5. How well can school employees see what is going on inside the school?
6. Do staff members have immediate lockdown capability in classrooms and other locations?
7. Are there identifiable or predictable trouble spots or high-risk locations?
8. Is the overall school climate prosocial; that is, does it reinforce respectful, responsible, mutually supportive attitudes and behaviors?

The following sections examine each of these questions at greater length. As an adjunct to this approach, audits of the school environment, typically conducted by consultants, can pinpoint areas of special concern (see box 19.5).

What Risks and Opportunities Do Students Encounter between Home and School?

Motor vehicle–related injuries are the most common cause of death for 5- to 19-year-olds (see chapter 21). But traffic is only one risk students confront between home and school. Gang conflicts,

---

◼ *19.5. CPTED audits*

In 2005, the National Clearinghouse for Educational Facilities, under the sponsorship of the U.S. Department of Education's Office of Safe and Drug Free Schools, integrated the nation's best school facility assessment measures into one comprehensive online source. Nationally recognized experts participated in the checklist's creation and oversee its maintenance and updating. The checklist was assembled by William Brenner and edited by Tod Schneider, with technical oversight by Michael Dorn, and peer reviewed by more than 24 specialists. The checklist is drawn from a half dozen primary sources, with additional contributions from 24 additional documents. This comprehensive checklist is now available, at no cost, at the clearinghouse web site (www.edfacilities.org).

The checklist can be customized to meet specific needs by selecting areas of interest on the setup page. Once selections have been entered, a customized checklist is generated. Be advised that the entire document may reach 40–50 pages in length, and require 4–10 hours of inspection time to complete.

The checklist is an exhaustive list of needed improvements, but it does not prescribe a holistic solution. Ideally, the information generated by using the checklist should be used in conjunction with an inspection and recommendations by a school design professional. ◼

---

war zones, drug dealers, predators, toxic exposure, barren landscapes, or isolating territory can also put them at risk.

Solutions

Make routes to school safer. Replace negative messages, such as demeaning advertising or graffiti, with inspirational artwork or student-generated posters. Encourage groups of students to walk or bicycle to school together, improving health while avoiding isolation. To reinforce territoriality and connection, work with the neighborhood to plant flowers and trees. By reducing students' anxiety,

these interventions may improve their school attendance, performance, and safety.

According to conventional security guidelines, bushes should be kept below 3 feet in height and lower tree limbs should be cleared to a height of 6 feet to maintain natural surveillance. Police, teachers, and students alike are in a better position to spot a threat if hidden areas are opened up. The Federal Emergency Management Agency (FEMA, 2003) expresses concern about thick ground cover, which, even at 4 inches in height, could hide an explosive device.

However, schools should apply these guidelines with care; clear-cutting school grounds and the surrounding neighborhood can be counterproductive. University of Illinois researchers found that inner-city girls who had a good view of greenery from their homes showed greater concentration, impulse control, and ability to delay gratification. Contact with nature was also associated with reduced aggression and violence in adults living in public housing (Kuo and Sullivan 2001) and with improved self-discipline in girls (but not in boys) (Taylor et al. 2002). If vigilant preparation for a remote possibility significantly undermines important daily activities, those measures may be inadvisable.

What Risks and Opportunities Do Students Encounter in Areas Directly Adjoining School Property?

Misbehaving students often gravitate to uncontrolled areas just off campus, where they are easy marks for offenders. They may annoy neighbors by littering or picking fights. Inadequate parking on campus can cause an overload off campus. Drug dealing or alcohol outlets near schools increase antisocial behavior related to substance abuse.

Solutions

Most cities impose enhanced penalties for crimes involving drugs, weapons, and other illegal activities near schools. As a condition of release, paroled sex offenders are usually barred from living near schools or children. Look into how aggressively these restrictions are enforced in your community.

Attend to conflicts that affect neighbors, and help design solutions. Ignoring off-campus problems is short sighted. If parking on campus is inadequate, make changes. Control parking with required stickers available only to residents and selected students. Open fields for overflow parking. Use incentives to encourage carpooling or mass transit.

Changes in fencing and landscaping can open up areas that are otherwise hidden from view. Replace solid wood with wrought iron fencing, and trim overgrown hedges. Remove visual obstructions from school windows. Encourage nearby businesses to clear their windows as well, allowing passers-by to observe crimes in progress and respond appropriately.

Reinforce connections with neighbors. Look for opportunities to put murals painted by students on otherwise blank walls. Display art or science projects in underutilized public spaces or storefronts. Offer after-school job and internship opportunities. Students who are recruited for neighborhood cleanups may mitigate immediate problems while building long-term goodwill. Positive interaction can build connectivity, which leads to mutual assistance when students or neighbors are in need of help.

Neighbors can serve as critical eyes and ears before and after school hours. No security service can provide greater vigilance, more affordable service, more continual presence, or greater commitment. Cultivate these neighbors as allies. Provide them with administrators' phone numbers, and entice them with binoculars, cell phones, or radios. Empower selected neighbors as quasi-official school caretakers, and reward them for calling in crimes in progress.

Consistent lighting throughout the site—including, in some situations, no lighting at all—is preferable to intermittent lighting, which creates dark pockets of shadow between well-lit locations. These pockets of shadow become magnets for undesirable behavior. Poorly angled lights can waste power by lighting the night sky or blind neighbors by shining in their windows.

Many schools have shifted toward darkened campuses at night, both to discourage loitering and to make intruders who carry flashlights more noticeable. The trend over the past few decades is clearly in this direction. Moreover, if there are no neighbors to watch over a site, excess lighting will be wasted.

Ultimately, lighting choices should be tailored to circumstances. If a well-lit campus is attracting misbehavior, shift to a darkened campus to see whether it helps. For example, Hillsborough County, Florida, switched to darkened campuses on September 1, 1995, in an effort to reduce utility costs. Arrests almost immediately went up, and property crimes went down. Flashlights and even burning cigarettes highlighted trespassers, making it easier for the police to capture them. On the other hand, if a darkened campus is providing locations for misbehavior, adding lighting may be productive. In high-security facilities where continual, active vigilance is necessary, night lighting is advisable (FEMA 2003). Bear in mind that whenever employees or students remain on site legitimately, they should have adequate lighting to reach their cars or buses and to see their surroundings en route. When uses and conditions change, responses must keep pace.

In cooperation with emergency personnel, assess neighboring facilities as emergency command posts or evacuation sites. If evacuation routes are predictable, watch for security weaknesses. Evacuation plans should include a scouting party that is activated immediately preceding a major evacuation to check for suspicious packages or people (see chapter 20).

Can Office Staff Observe Approaching Visitors before They Reach the School Entry?

Office workers should evaluate, direct, and control access by visitors. Many offices are located deep within schools, where they are ineffective guardians against unwelcome visitors. Even if the main office is located near exterior doorways, intruders may gain entry through secondary doors or windows.

School layout and signs often undermine territoriality, natural surveillance, and access control. Visitors may be instructed to check in at a distant office, but without clear directions this can be an invitation to prowl the halls while ostensibly searching for the destination. Even if the office is located at the main entry, it may lack well-placed windows. The assumption that office workers can deal with lethal threats that suddenly appear at the front desk is unrealistic. Ideally they should be able to see a threat before it arrives.

Can Staff Members Physically Stop Visitors from Entering?

Only about half of all public schools even claim to control access, and their level of success is not clear (Kaufman et al. 2001). Are the doors locked as a matter of course once school starts? How quickly and easily can staff members lock all of the entries, control visitors, or protect potential victims?

Solutions

To maximize control over visitors, reconsider office location and design. The following overview of seven levels of secure office design can serve as a guide:

1. The least useful location for an office is deep within the building, far from any primary entryway. The main office workers cannot see people who are approaching the building or prowling the halls, and they cannot control access.
2. A slight improvement puts the main office door flush with a main hallway, where it can be found more easily. However, because it is still distant from the main entrance, it provides no opportunity for natural surveillance of the area outside of the building. A small window facing into the hallway may provide a modest opportunity to view people passing by, but workers can neither anticipate nor control them.
3. Another advance in design would allow the office to protrude into the hall. With good layout and use of windows, school personnel would be able to look up and down the hallway.
4. A big step-up would position the office along the perimeter of the school, allowing natural surveillance to the outside. On the inside, the office should protrude into a main hallway, allowing natural surveillance up and down at least the main hallway and perhaps secondary hallways as well. This would allow extensive visual surveillance but would not establish control over visitors. Figure 19.1 shows an example.
5. A far superior design places the office directly adjacent to the main entry, protruding into the hallway and to the outside of the school. Visitors who approach the main entry are eas-

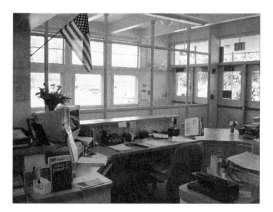

Figure 19.1. External surveillance from the office. This office offers good views of the school entrance, providing surveillance of arriving visitors. (Photo by Tod Schneider.)

ily seen and must pass close by to enter the building. Staff members have good visibility outside the main entry area and down the main hallway. Secondary entrances, if present, undermine the ability of the main office to observe or control unwanted visitors.
6. By securing all of the secondary entries, making them lock automatically upon closing, or by installing panic bars that convert secondary exits into emergency exits, schools can oblige all visitors to use the main entry. Only at this level of secure design, with well-placed windows and good internal layout, do employees achieve full natural surveillance over visitors. Electronic front door controls enable school authorities to enact lockdowns with the touch of a button.
7. At the highest level of security, an entry vestibule is added adjacent to the main office. Natural surveillance is then abundant in most directions. When visitors enter the vestibule, they cannot proceed until cleared by the office. In a high-security environment, this might include electronic screening for weapons and a pass-through window for suspicious packages. In this scenario, office workers are protected behind bullet-resistant glass.

How Well Can People See What Is Going on inside the School?

Blind corners and stairwells can hide inappropriate behavior. Some areas are especially difficult to

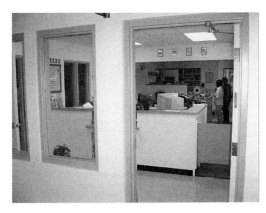

Figure 19.2. New windows improve surveillance. This office window looks out onto the main hallway, providing surveillance of activity within the school. (Photo by Tod Schneider.)

watch during times of peak usage—before and after classes—when most conflicts occur.

Solutions

The best solution is natural surveillance. Staff members should be readily able to see the source of a noise or observe activity. Windows add natural surveillance (fig. 19.2), while mirrors provide a secondary view. If neither of these is an option, cameras or staff patrols are alternatives. If objects such as posters or artwork on windows block natural surveillance, remove them. See-through backpacks and lockers can increase visibility. Because crowds can hide activity in otherwise open areas, mirrors, cameras, or observation posts can be useful in providing overhead views.

Do Staff Members Have Immediate Lockdown Capability in Classrooms and Other Locations?

Most schoolrooms would be difficult to secure at a moment's notice, and most of them do not have reliable communication devices readily available. Many rooms have outward-opening doors, which function well for emergency egress but not for other security purposes. In most cases, a teacher would have to insert a key from the hallway side to lock the door. That would mean stepping into the hallway, extracting a key ring, finding the correct key, and inserting it into the lock, possibly while shots are being fired. In a severe crisis, due to physiological changes that occur when the human fight-or-

flight response takes over, the teacher would probably lose the fine motor skills needed for inserting a key in a lock.

Entrapment is also a risk. If an intruder blocks a classroom door, students need secondary escape routes.

Solutions

Every schoolroom should be able to serve as a safe haven. The rooms should be easy to lock during a crisis without requiring someone to first move into a danger zone. The door should lock automatically or have a simple locking mechanism, such as a button to push in.

Each room should have a reliable communication device. Office staff should be able to tell everyone immediately to lock down, relocate, or evacuate.

Each room should be examined to determine where best to hide from shrapnel, bullets, or shards of glass. In general, dense, thick walls provide the best protection. In some cases, piled furniture may have to serve as a barricade.

Each location in the school will have strengths and weaknesses as a safe haven. Hallways, for example, may be too vulnerable to internal threats but can provide good shelter from external threats. Because of their thick furniture and piles of books, which offer added protection, libraries can serve well if securable. Gymnasiums do not always have communication devices or a quick method to secure doors. Safe havens can also become entrapment areas; escape routes must also be considered. If used as shelters during extreme incidents such as terrorist attacks or natural disasters, large shelter areas should have thick, poured-concrete walls, air-filtering systems, bathrooms, food, and emergency supplies that include plastic sheeting and duct tape.

Are There Identifiable or Predictable Trouble Spots or High-risk Locations?

In 1995, 9–15% of all students reported avoiding one or more places in school and feared being attacked at school or on the way to and from class (Kaufman et al. 2001). Parking lots, bus stops, stairwells, hallways, classrooms, offices, grounds, entry areas, breezeways, center courts, bathrooms, and cafeterias have all been sites of documented school violence (Kachur et al. 1996). Each of these locations merits individual attention.

Parking Lots and Bus Stops

Restrict parking to a compact, easy-to-patrol area, and investigate vehicles that circumvent this restriction. Require registration stickers for all student vehicles; record license plate and vehicle descriptions to make identification easier. Enclose the parking lots with fencing to control access, but leave escape routes for pedestrians to avoid entrapment. Taking present-day concerns about terrorist attacks into consideration, avoid building easy runways for launching car-bomb attacks on the school. Driveways should not lead directly toward the front door. Run driveways parallel to the school façade, with bollards, high curbs, or other obstacles to keep vehicles from running into the building. Such measures should protect students on adjacent sidewalks as well. Serpentine driveways or fairly sharp turns that force a reduction in speed are additional options.

As schools grow, new parking lots are often added. If not carefully situated, they can cause problems as well. Drivers will then use the closest doorway into the school, especially in inclement weather, creating a de facto new main entrance. If the main office remains on the north side of the building and the new parking lot is on the south side of the building, for example, there may be no guardian watching the new southside entrance. In this fashion, each new parking lot that is constructed generates a new main entry. Usually these new entries lack any natural or electronic surveillance or access control. Repairing this security breach requires new staffing, new office locations, new surveillance equipment, and/or new access controls. The following options should be considered:

- Move the main entry to the new location. If the old entry is still being used, however, access control will not improve.
- Designate a smaller parking lot for employees only, who can then be given proximity cards or similar devices to let themselves in through locked, unsupervised entries. Those doors can be monitored with video cameras.
- Install other staffed services at new entries. Workers who run these relocated services will provide natural surveillance and territoriality. The library, snack bar, custodian's office, school resource officer's office, or similar areas may be able to serve this function.
- Give all students proximity cards. This provides some degree of access control but does nothing to stop them from allowing intruders to enter with them.
- At all entrances, install security cameras that are linked to a central monitoring location (fig. 19.3).
- Hire security personnel to supervise all entries.
- Restrict secondary entry use to certain, supervised hours. Students who arrive at odd hours would be obliged to walk around to the supervised entry.
- Add emergency call buttons in parking lots. Video cameras in buses and radios or cell phones for drivers should also be considered. In the unlikely event of a hijacking, markings on bus rooftops will make them easier to identify from the air. Bus-tracking electronic devices are presently in the research stage.

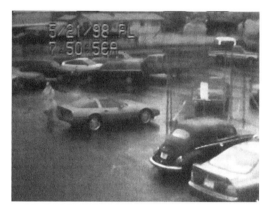

Figure 19.3. Kip Kinkle on security cameras. Security cameras may not guarantee anything more than evidence for prosecution after the fact. In May 1998, for instance, Kip Kinkle, a freshman at Thurston High School in Springfield, Oregon, killed two students and wounded seventeen others at his school, after murdering his mother and father in their home. As he approached the school, Kinkle was captured on tape, as shown on this photo, but to no avail. He was not identifiable, the weapons under his raincoat could not be seen, no one happened to be watching the monitor at the moment of his arrival, and, even if someone had been, it is unlikely that he could have been stopped. He reached the cafeteria by means of a back parking lot and an open breezeway. (Photo courtesy of Tod Schneider.)

Hallways

Hallways are a common setting for violent incidents for predictable reasons: large, noisy crowds; conflicting foot traffic; and little supervision. Spaces and unoccupied niches along the hallway often act as gathering spots. These spaces should be built out of the traffic flow to reduce unnecessary conflict. Spread lockers away from each other to reduce conflict between neighboring users. Avoid creating hidden locker areas, which can lend themselves to entrapment. Widen the hallway periodically, bringing the lockers out of the traffic flow without isolating them entirely from view.

Second-story internal balconies can provide internal views. Convex mirrors placed high up can improve surveillance over crowds and around corners. Where the architecture does not facilitate surveillance, cameras or human patrols may be additional options to consider. Improving natural surveillance by responsive teachers is probably the most effective solution.

Stairwells

The more open the stairway design, the better. Use slip-resistant surfaces and sturdy guardrails. Wherever solid walls block surveillance, look for ways to install openings or windows.

Grounds

Wrought-iron fencing is ideal for marking territory and controlling access because it is extremely vandal resistant and lacks enough surface space to attract much graffiti (see fig. 19.4).

Although it costs more than mesh fencing, wrought iron is a good long-term investment that enhances the school's image and climate, leaves natural surveillance intact, and controls access points. Heighten the definition of the enclosed area to enhance territoriality. Invite students, service clubs, and area residents to develop paths, gardens, sandboxes, wetlands, natural meadows, and amphitheaters as well as traditional sports fields. Group participation establishes a sense of stewardship. An in-residence caretaker is a good option to consider, especially for after-hours security. Attend to any hidden niches where misbehavior could occur. Open them up to view by installing mirrors or windows. Open other outdoor areas to view by lowering the height of visual obstacles such as walls

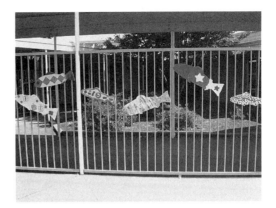

Figure 19.4. Wrought-iron fence with fish. One Springfield, Oregon, elementary school installed extensive wrought-iron fencing to establish access control but was determined not to end up looking like a prison. The solution was to have all of the students paint plywood fish, which were then mounted on the fence. Now the fish are more prominent visual features than the fence itself. Students proudly show off their artwork to friends and family. (Photo by Tod Schneider.)

or shrubs. In case of terrorist attacks, berms can be used to deflect explosions or vehicles.

Entry Areas

Upgrade front office design to provide surveillance over the exterior entry as well as the interior foyer and hallway. Avoid security measures that create bottlenecks. If students congregate outside while waiting to be frisked, they provide easy targets for mass victimization. Establish an adult presence wherever students congregate, and provide those adults with communication devices. Protect vulnerable locations with low walls or stanchions that can deflect bullets or out-of-control vehicles. At the same time, maintain natural lines of sight; do not build walls that block natural surveillance. Speed bumps can slow traffic near the main entry.

Breezeways

To control access, look for ways to enclose breezeways and connect buildings. Strengthen natural surveillance by installing windows in otherwise solid walls. Seal off secondary entry points, such as breezeway entries, with fire doors that close and lock automatically. Staff should have keys or proximity cards. Doors should be staffed when left open.

Bathrooms

Bathrooms should be located adjacent to supervised areas and within sight of school personnel. Maze entries should replace double-door entries for several reasons: Alarming sounds become more noticeable from the outside; offenders cannot count on the sound of the outer door opening to warn them that an authority figure is entering; and cigarette smoke is no longer masked (see fig. 19.5). As an added benefit, fewer un-sanitized hands have to share the same knob or doorplate. Regular maintenance is essential; bathrooms are often cited as scary places by students. If trash, graffiti, and vandalism gain a toehold here, the school appears to have ceded its authority over the bathrooms, which makes bullies and gang members feel right at home.

Locker Rooms

Locker rooms pose problems similar to those encountered in bathrooms and have long been notorious as sites for bullying and more serious assaults. The right to privacy should be balanced with protection from entrapment while students are undressing and vulnerable. Coaches have a responsibility to keep students who are in their charge safe. Locker room design weaknesses can be mitigated by using maze entries, lowering the level of lockers to allow more visibility over them, and stationing coaches' offices in the locker rooms to provide direct natural visual and auditory surveillance over students.

Cafeterias

Cafeterias are areas of concern because they are highly accessible gathering places where intruders can potentially enter and threaten large numbers of students. Other group gathering spaces, including gymnasiums and theaters, have similar vulnerabilities. The greater the accessibility, the more vigilance is required. It is critical to establish escape routes and provide communication devices to staff members. If screening occurs at some distance from the cafeteria, an offender is less likely to reach this destination undetected.

Technological Solutions

Ideally, the physical structure of a school should provide adequate natural surveillance, natural access control, and territoriality to minimize the need for technological fixes. Unfortunately, this ideal structure rarely exists. Improvements are usually necessary and may take the form of "Band-Aid fixes," major architectural remodeling, extra staffing, or electronic technology.

Because technology is constantly changing, investments in this area should always be carefully researched. New technology can sound dazzling. However, before committing funds, visit other schools to see the technology actually being used. Ask for references from satisfied customers. How finicky is the equipment? How difficult is it to arrange repairs or find parts?

Communication equipment is essential and can range from a public address system to CB radios, walkie-talkies, cell phones, and conventional phones throughout the site. On large campuses, schools should consider installing emergency call boxes in isolated locations. Students should be able to reach security personnel with the push of a button, and the location of the call box that is being used should be electronically identified at the receiving end.

Access control devices, such as pushbutton controls for entry doors or swipe cards for elec-

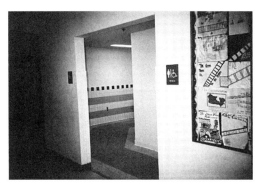

Figure 19.5. Bathroom vestibule, Shasta Middle School, Eugene, Oregon. Shasta Middle School had one troublesome bathroom that was hidden beside a pass-through vestibule between buildings. When the vestibule doors were closed, the vestibule completely muffled sound. The bathroom thus became a popular site for vandalism and other misbehavior. When anyone opened the door, vandals could hear them and hide their misbehavior until they were in the clear. The CPTED solution was to lock the vestibule doors in the open position. This cost-free solution immediately resolved the problem. (Photo by Tod Schneider.)

tronic entry points, permit greater access control with minimal staffing.

Although surveillance equipment is the most controversial security technology from a philosophical perspective, it is unquestionably a useful tool for identifying offenders after the fact. Cameras are of little value in preventing homicidal violence but effectively deter hallway fights and vandalism. Once offenders learn that misdeeds are being taped, their behavior improves. A successful instance of camera use at Berkeley High School in California is described in box 19.6.

Cameras are becoming both more affordable and more capable. A multiple camera system that records on a digital video recorder and is accessible through a modem or intranet hookup can provide officials with a remote view of live activity during a crisis, an invaluable tool for emergency personnel in a hostage situation. Expect to spend 10–15% of the initial cost for average annual maintenance, including replacement of parts as they wear out. Cameras that pan and tilt, for example, are likely to require more frequent maintenance than stationary cameras, and hard drives have an expected lifespan of about 5 years. Systems with similar capabilities are now frequently integrated into new school construction nationwide. (For an example, see the DVA CCTV surveillance system by Integral Technologies at www.integraltech.com.)

Terrorism

Terrorism-thwarting measures and technology can be extremely sophisticated and expensive and beyond the budgetary reach of most schools. However, a school that is particularly concerned about such attacks, such as one that is associated with the federal government or located near a likely terrorist target, may consider these measures. Options include the following:

- redundant utility sources (e.g., electricity, gas, phone, computer lines) that enter the building at different locations to provide backup sources if primary sources are sabotaged
- safe rooms capable of withstanding extremist attacks (such rooms might have 10-inch concrete walls poured on site)
- air-filtration systems
- chemical, biological, and radiological detection equipment
- protective gear and supplies

The Challenge of Large Schools

Large schools present greater security challenges. Multiple entry points will require an equivalent number of guardians. A labyrinth of add-ons often incorporates numerous blind corners and niches, creating hidden areas that are attractive for delinquent behavior. Individual at-risk students who may become lost in a crowd may not draw needed attention until too late. If the student body is large, staff and students alike may have trouble determining who belongs on campus and who does not.

Where enrollment limits are not feasible, a number of options can be considered. Converting secondary, unguarded doors into alarmed emergency exits, sealing off underutilized wings with metal accordion-style grates, recruiting volunteer hall monitors, and installing surveillance cameras are possibilities. Staggered schedules can reduce congestion. Large schools can be divided into smaller, specialized wings, houses, families, academies, or schools-within-schools. From a CPTED perspective, any arrangement that makes it easier for students to know each other and build bonds while enhancing staff surveillance and access con-

---

■ *19.6. Cameras in Berkeley and Biloxi*

Berkeley High School in Berkeley, California, is a sprawling inner-city campus of 17 acres serving 3,000 students with 150 teachers and 80 classified staff members. It also functions as the center of community activity 24 hours a day. In 2000, the school installed 80 cameras and noted an almost immediate decrease in misbehaviors, including starting fires in the hallways, setting off false fire alarms, and fighting. The school's next step was to close 11 of 14 entrances in order to improve access control.

Despite little history of student violence, the city of Biloxi, Mississippi, spent $2 million installing 800 cameras in schools. The cameras were credited with improving discipline and with apprehending a janitor who was stealing a television.

(From Dillon 2003). ■

trol is a step in the right direction. (For a discussion of school size, see chapter 2.)

School Safety Audits

Approaches to school safety audits vary according to budget, complexity, and primary concerns. A simple in-house survey, based on the eight questions posed at the beginning of this chapter, can provide a quick, solid start. At low to moderate cost, a consultant can bring a more practiced eye to the project, providing a CPTED "snapshot" and recommendations.

For more complicated environments or circumstances, such as high-crime schools, federal facilities, overseas academies, areas at great risk for natural disasters, or particularly well-funded projects, more thorough studies may include the following elements:

- crime mapping
- extensive surveys of students, teachers, parents, police, and neighbors
- crime, socioeconomic data, and risk evaluation
- review of crisis management plans
- in-depth research or literature reviews
- architectural design charettes (brainstorming by all involved parties) to discuss concerns (this may require hiring consultants with varied fields of expertise).

The clearer the goals of the survey, the more suitably it can be developed. Surveys funded by federal grants, for example, may require quantification of data, while a narrative description tailored to each site may be more useful at the local level.

When seeking grant funding or crafting bond measures, it is important to remember that, until a survey is conducted, the costs of remodeling cannot be accurately predicted. Core CPTED improvements can easily cost $100,000–$500,000 per school, although some schools have made dramatic improvements for as little as $20,000–$30,000.

Is the Overall School Climate Pro-social?

This chapter has emphasized physical characteristics of the environment. The other half of the social ecology equation is the affective environment—the social and emotional aspects of the school that influence behavior. An extremely secure physical design cannot compensate for a severely antisocial en-

vironment. If that were the case, prisons would be free of violence. Building a high-security school will be of little value if the anger of even one armed, disturbed student is allowed to fester. Design features may be able to restrict where the student erupts, but they cannot prevent the outburst from happening somewhere.

Reinforcing a secure physical facility with punitive behavioral controls may have its place in a prison environment but would be inappropriate for a public school in a democratic society. Zero-tolerance policies, although well intentioned, have drawn extensive criticism for inflexibility, over-zealousness, and a lack of common sense and may do more harm than good. Heavy-handed reactions rebuff students at one end of the spectrum who pose no threat, as well as those at the other end of the spectrum who most need help and represent the greatest risks to society. Mandatory sentencing approaches undermine respect for authorities and promote alienation rather than remediation. In those cases where involved students are indeed severely troubled, expulsions without attempts at reconciliation can exacerbate their rage and hopelessness and may increase the likelihood of violence rather than lowering it. A student who is banned from campus is no longer under supervision, and that student behavior is then harder to redirect or control.

Solutions

Basic school CPTED provides a physical framework in which to operate. Second-generation CPTED goes further, addressing these more important questions: Are the students receiving a quality education? How functional is the school itself, both academically and socially? Do the students feel as though they belong? Do they feel hopeful, effective, and successful? Do they see the value and relevance of what they are learning? Pay close attention to polarization, marginalization, bullying, or harassment. Invest proportionally more time and energy in reconnecting the most alienated individuals or groups. Look for the invisible students and the loners. Acknowledge them and help them develop their strengths.

Research over the past few decades has identified specific, overlapping risk factors for undesirable behaviors such as substance abuse, teen pregnancy, dropping out of school, delinquency, and violence (Posey et al. 2000). Across race and culture, the more risks a child faces, the greater the likelihood of a negative outcome. Established risk factors are often categorized into those that operate at school, in the community, and in the family.

School-centered risk factors include early and persistent antisocial behavior, early academic failure, early misbehavior, lack of commitment to school, hanging out with troublemakers, and alienation from school. Community risk factors include the availability of drugs or guns, media portrayals of violence, laws and norms that encourage misbehavior, fractured communities, poverty, and mobility. Family risk factors include family dysfunction, substance abuse, and violence.

Protective factors improve students' odds of overcoming these risks. These factors can be summarized in several ways. One simple approach identifies protective factors at three levels: the individual, the family, and society at large.

The Search Institute (www.search-institute .org) identifies 40 essential assets, which are broadly divided into two categories. External assets include support, empowerment, boundaries, expectations, and constructive use of time. Internal assets include commitment to learning, positive values, social competencies, and positive identity. Research has shown a strong association between the number of assets in a person's life and the likelihood of involvement in substance abuse, violence, or other antisocial behaviors. Students with fewer than 11 assets, for example, had a 61% probability of engaging in high-risk violent behavior, whereas students with more than 30 assets showed only a 7% involvement in violence (Scales and Leffert 1999).

A similar approach, called Communities That Care, focuses on five protective factors (Posey et al 2000): clear, healthy cultural standards; bonding; opportunities to succeed; skills; and recognition. Each of these corresponds to the concept of connectivity, a central focus of second-generation CPTED.

Many "strength-based" programs are designed to nurture these protective factors. The most successful ones are integrated throughout the school, and their concepts are reinforced by all of the staff members, the older students, and family members. Most of them combine academic training with development in social skills focused on empathy building, anger management, impulse control, and

similar goals. Examples of effective programs include the following:

- Second Step (Grossman et al. 1997): This is a violence-prevention curriculum for use in elementary schools. In a field study, physical aggression on playgrounds dropped by 29% among Second Step students, whereas it increased by 41% in a control group.
- The Good Behavior game (Kellam and Rebok 1992): Highly aggressive male first-graders who received this game-based intervention were found to be less aggressive in sixth grade than those who did not.
- The School Transitional Environment Project (Felner et al. 1993): This project focuses on multiple aspects of the school environment. Project students, who were low income, minority, or otherwise disadvantaged, dropped out at half the rate of the control group—21% instead of 43%—and achieved higher grades.

In addition to proactive, strength-based programs, schools should design comprehensive plans for problem solving, crisis management, and intervention. If all of the staff members know their responsibilities when misbehavior arises, problems are less likely to fall through the cracks or escalate into larger crises. Programs that include restorative justice approaches and reconnect troubled youth are far more productive than are punitive measures. Building networks and joint teams of police officers, social workers, teachers, and counselors will provide coordinated, consistent treatment for troubled students.

Learn the students' names and interests. Listen to them. Give them meaningful roles to play, such as service learning projects, surveys to conduct, projects to assist teachers, apprenticeships, or opportunities to help as grounds maintenance teams. Provide constructive after-school activities such as recreation programs, volunteer opportunities, internships, or homework clubs. Let them know you believe in them.

Measuring connectivity is a challenge. Surveys, onsite observations, and records of reprimands, visits to the school nurse, fights, or expulsions can provide some evidence. The physical environment can also yield clues (see the connectivity indicators in box 19.7). For example, elementary schools often reinforce students' strengths by displaying their

19.7. *Connectivity indicators and contraindicators*

Connectivity Indicators

1. Student-generated, prosocial messages (posters, announcements, extracurricular opportunities for building relationships)
2. Prosocial messages, nonstudent generated
3. Prominently displayed student artwork, accomplishments, awards across subjects (great writing, art, community volunteer work, sports)
4. Display cases, bulletin boards, display areas adjacent to related classes or work areas
5. Intimate spaces for student conversations, without blocking reasonable natural surveillance; separation of mobs into groups small enough for individual communication (i.e., small, round cafeteria tables, good separation of space)
6. Architectural elements enhancing connection: sense of belonging, ease of interaction (neighborhoods, blocks, halls, classrooms grouped in clusters, areas named or color coded, walls lend themselves to student displays and art, class ownership, wheelchair accessibility)
7. Classroom and work area layout and furniture enhance access to tools and communication and information devices/services
8. Evident community connection (community room, service activities, volunteers, field trips, visiting speaker, classes for area residents; parent info board near entry/pickup area).

Connectivity Contraindicators

9. Graffiti, vandalism, signs of disrepair
10. Dead walls (blank, windowless, messageless)
11. Divisive/polarizing messages from authority figures, others (negative statements toward minority groups or individuals; valuing of some groups to the exclusion of other groups)
12. Architectural elements alienating, fear reinforcing, demoralizing (such as a prison atmosphere).

Territoriality Indicators

13. Signs, name tags, dress codes, uniforms, or architecture defining access rights and directing visitors to office effectively
14. Clear border definition for school, wings, rooms, and other areas
15. Strong maintenance—all graffiti is immediately removed; locks, windows, doors, and so on, are in good repair.

artwork or awards in the hallways, but middle schools and high schools are less inclined to do so (fig. 19.6). When this public space goes unclaimed, an opportunity for reinforcing strengths is lost, and students may perceive an opportune venue for misbehavior. Studies show that teachers feel territorial in their classrooms but are reluctant to take responsibility in "undefined public space" (Behre et al. 2001). It was the students who advised the adults to reclaim their ownership of these areas.

The presence of adults does more than deter misbehavior; it also presents an opportunity to "catch children being good." Praising students for positive behavior reinforces bonding between stu-

dents, teachers, and, by extension, the school. Other indicators of connectivity (or the lack thereof) include underutilized display cases or a lack of intimate gathering spaces where students and teachers can converse in small groups. Provide benches in designated gathering areas, and encourage students to provide artwork or science projects for the display cases.

Conclusion

Basic CPTED is a key component of school safety planning. A site that is well protected with natural

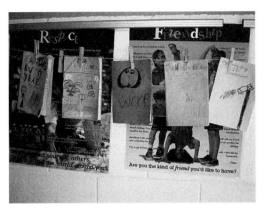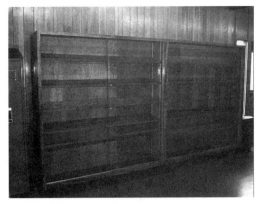

Figure 19.6. Student art (left) and empty display case (right). Creating a prosocial environment in schools is an important aspect of second-generation CPTED. Placing positive messages and student art in the halls helps achieve this goal, whereas empty display cases send a message of hopelessness. (Photos by Tod Schneider.)

surveillance, access control, and territoriality will require less staff time and energy to defend. This leaves the instructors more time to focus on teaching and students more time to focus on learning. Second-generation CPTED is equally important. Establishing an atmosphere of mutual support, respect, and connection between people and the environment should reduce the need for conventional security measures.

Resources

Several articles, monographs, and books provide useful background information on the causes of school violence and its prevention:

- California Department of Education. Safe schools: A planning guide for action. http://www.cde.ca.gov/ls/ss/
- Centers for Disease Control and Prevention. 2001. School health guidelines to prevent unintentional injuries and violence. Mortality and Morbidity Weekly Report, Recommendation Report 50(RR-22):1–74.
- Committee for Children. Seattle. Second step: A violence prevention curriculum. http://www.cfchildren.org/ssf/ssf/ssindex/
- Duke DL. 2001. *Creating safe schools for all children.* Boston: Allyn and Bacon.
- Gottfredson DC. 1997. School-based crime prevention. In *Preventing crime: What works, what doesn't, what's promising* (Sherman L, Gottfredson D, Mackenzie D, Eck J, Reuter P,

Bushway S, eds.). College Park: Department of Criminology and Criminal Justice, University of Maryland, 5.1–5.74.
- Schneider T, Walker H, Sprague J. 2000. *Safe school design: A handbook for educational leaders, applying the principles of crime prevention through environmental design.* Eugene, OR: ERIC Clearinghouse.
- Small M, Tetrick KD. 2001. School violence: An overview. Juvenile Justice 8(1):3–12.

Many organizations and agencies address the problem of school violence. Their web sites are useful sources of information, and many of them contain links to additional sources.

- Center for the Prevention of School Violence, Raleigh, North Carolina. This is a resource center for efforts that promote safer schools and foster positive youth development. It focuses on understanding school violence and developing solutions. The website provides a comprehensive list of violence prevention resources for specific areas of the school (e.g., gym, library) http://www.ncdjjdp.org/cpsv
- Channing Bete Company, Seattle, Washington. This source offers, among other items, a guide called Communities That Care Prevention Strategies: A Research Guide to What Works. It provides a comprehensive list of evaluated, successful programs, as well as assistance in selecting programs that best suit local needs.

http://www.channing-bete.com/positiveyouth/
pages/CTC/prevention_strategies.html

- Colorado Center for the Study and Prevention of Violence. This is an information source on evidence-based violence prevention programs.
http://www.colorado.edu/cspv

- Educators for Social Responsibility, Boston. ESR is a nonprofit organization that promotes the teaching of social responsibility in schools. Its Resolving Conflict Creatively Program, for grades K–8, teaches conflict resolution and intergroup relations based on character education and social and emotional development.
http://www.esrnational.org/home.htm

- Florida Department of Education. The Florida Department of Education website includes a useful set of Safe Schools guidelines.
http://www.firn.edu/doe/edfacil/safe_schools.htm

- Institute on Violence and Destructive Behavior, University of Oregon, College of Education, Eugene. This organization studies risk and protective factors related to violence, school failure, and other types of delinquency that affect adolescents.
http://darkwing.uoregon.edu/ivdb/index.html

- International CPTED Association. This is the umbrella organization for practitioners of Crime Prevention Through Environmental Design worldwide.
http://www.cpted.net

- National Clearinghouse for Educational Facilities. This organization maintains a voluminous web site and electronic library of articles and resources related to school design, as well as a free, customizable, downloadable safe school facilities checklist.
http://www.edfacilities.org

- National School Safety Center, Westlake Village, California. This center advocates for safe, secure, and peaceful schools worldwide.
http://www.nssc1.org

- Northwest Regional Educational Laboratory, Portland, Oregon. The NWREL provides online guidebooks that assist in developing strategies for safe learning environments.
http://www.nwrel.org/

- Safe Havens International. Home base for

Michael Dorn and associates, who provide consultation on all aspects of school emergency planning and policing.
www.safehavensinternational.org

- Search Institute, Minneapolis, Minnesota. The Search Institute is a nonprofit organization that promotes healthy children, young people, and communities through research, education, and the bringing together of community, state, and national leaders. The institute's work is built on the framework of 40 developmental assets that young people need to become healthy, caring, and responsible. Telephone: 800-888-7828. E-mail: si@search-institute.org.
http://www.search-institute.org)

- Transcending Violence, Eugene, Oregon. This is Tod Schneider's web site, a home base for a variety of safe school design and confrontation management-related services, including seminars and consulting.
http://www.transcendingviolence.com

- U.S. Department of Education Office of Safe and Drug-Free Schools. This is the national clearinghouse for all information nationally on related topics and publisher of the highly recommended report, *Practical Information on Crisis Planning* (May 2003). E-mail: edpubs@inet.ed.gov
http://www.ed.gov/emergency plan

References

Astor RA, Meyer HA, Behre WJ. 1999. Unowned places and times: Maps and interviews about violence in high schools. Am Educ Res J 36:3–42.

Behre WJ, Astor RA, Meyer HA. 2001. Elementary- and middle-school teachers' reasoning about intervening in school violence: An examination of violence-prone school subcontexts. J Moral Educ 30(2):131–153.

Brener N, Lowry R, Barrios L, Simon T, Eaton D. 2004. Violence-related behaviors among high school students: United States, 1991–2003. Mortal Morbid Weekly Rept 53(29):651–655.

Brown SL. 1994. Animals at play. National Geographic 186(6):2–34.

Carter S, Carter SP. 2001. Surrounded by safety: A crime prevention through environmental design (CPTED) handbook for youth. Miami, FL: Office of Juvenile Justice and Delinquency Prevention and Youth Crime Watch of America.

Crowe T. 1991. *Crime prevention through environmental design: Applications of architectural design and space management concepts.* Boston: Butterworth-Heinemann.

DeVoe JF, Peter K, Kaufman P, Ruddy SA, Miler AK, Planty M, et al. 2003. Indicators of school crime and safety: 2003. NCES 2004-004/NCJ 201257. Washington, DC: U.S. Departments of Education and Justice.

Dillon S. 2003. Cameras watching students, especially in Biloxi. *New York Times* (September 23), Section B, 9.

Federal Emergency Management Agency. 2003. Primer to design safe school projects in case of terrorist attacks. FEMA-428. Washington, DC: Author

Felner RD, Brand S, Adan AM, Mulhall PF, Flowers N, Sartain B, et al. 1993. Restructuring the ecology of the school as an approach to prevention during school transitions: Longitudinal follow-ups and extensions of the School Transitional Environment Project (STEP). Prev Hum Serv 10(2):103–136.

Grossman DC, Neckerman HJ, Koepsell TD, Liu PY, Asher KN, Beland K, et al. 1997. Effectiveness of a violence prevention curriculum among children in elementary school: A randomized controlled trial. J Am Med Assoc 277:1605–1611.

Hevside S, Rowland C, Williams C, Farris E, Burns S, McArthur E. 1998. Violence and discipline problems in U.S. public schools, 1996–1997. NCES 98-030. Washington, DC: U.S. Department of Education, Office of Educational Research and Improvement.

Jeffery CR. 1971. *Crime prevention through environmental design.* Beverly Hills, CA: Sage.

Kachur SP, Stennies GM, Powell KE, Modzeleski W, Stephens R, Murphy R, et al. 1996. School-associated violent deaths in the United States, 1992–1994. J Am Med Assoc 275:1729–1733.

Kaufman P, Chen X, Choy SP, Peter K, Ruddy SA, Miller AK, et al. 2001. Indicators of school crime and safety: 2001. NCES 2002-113/NCJ-190075.

Washington, DC: U.S. departments of Education and Justice.

Kellam SG, Rebok GW. 1992. Building developmental and etiological theory through epidemiologically based preventive intervention trials. In *Preventing antisocial behavior: Interventions from birth through adolescence* (McCord J, Tremblay RE, eds.). New York: Guilford, 162–195.

Kuo FE, Sullivan WC. 2001. Aggression and violence in the inner city: Effects of environment via mental fatigue. Environ Behav 33:543–571.

Moss R, Insel P. 1974. *Issues in social ecology: Human milieus.* Palo Alto, CA: National Press Books.

Newman O. *Defensible space: Crime prevention through urban design.* New York: Macmillan.

North Carolina Department of Juvenile Justice and Delinquency Prevention (NCDJJDP). 2001. Stats 2001: Selected school violence research findings from 2001 sources. Raleigh: NCDJJDP, Center for the Prevention of School Violence.

Posey R, Wong S, Catalano R, Hawkins D, Dusenbury L, Chappell P. 2000. Communities that care prevention strategies: A research guide to what works. Seattle: Developmental Research and Programs. Available: http://www.channing-bete.com/positiveyouth [accessed 22 December 2005].

Scales PC, Leffert N. 1999. *Developmental assets: A synthesis of the scientific research on adolescent development.* Minneapolis, MN: Search Institute.

Schalock RL. 1989. Person-environment analysis: Short- and long-term perspectives. In *Economics, industry, and the disabled: A look ahead* (Kiernan WE, Schalock RL, eds.). Baltimore, MD: Paul H. Brookes, 115–127.

Sedlak AJ, Finkelhor D, Hammer H, Schultz DJ. 2002. National estimates of missing children. Washington, DC: U.S. Department of Justice, Office of Juvenile Justice and Delinquency Prevention. Available: http://www.ncjrs.org/pdffiles1/ojjdp/196465.pdf [accessed 26 March 2005].

Taylor AF, Kuo FE, Sullivan WC. 2002. Views of nature and self-discipline: Evidence from inner-city children. J Environ Psychol 22(1–2):49–63.

20

Angelo J. Bellomo

Emergency Management

■ *Summary*

- Schools today must address a variety of health and safety risks. Preparation for school emergencies is a critical risk reduction measure.
- Adequate preparation for emergency events is a preventive strategy and improves the ability of school personnel to respond effectively to an incident and minimize harm.
- The Incident Command System used by fire and law enforcement personnel is easily adapted to the school environment. ■

Development of a comprehensive emergency response plan is key to ensuring a rapid and effective response to school emergencies.

During the past decade, the U.S. educational system has recognized the importance of maintaining a safe and healthy learning environment. Today, schools throughout the country are addressing a broad range of health and safety risks, many of which are addressed in the chapters of this book, such as the use of pesticides on campus, indoor and ambient air pollutants, unhealthy food choices, and emotional stress. These efforts are effective in reducing risk, but they advance on a relatively grad-

ual time frame. School officials, parents, and others who focus on these issues may overlook the importance of preparing for school emergencies as a risk reduction measure.

It is evident that when schools are adequately prepared to manage emergencies, the extent to which an incident causes harm is minimized. Though less apparent, the process of preparing for emergency incidents is often effective in reducing the potential for incidents to occur. As a result, emergency preparedness not only improves the ability of a school to respond to an incident but represents a preventive strategy as well.

Well-established principles of emergency preparedness can be applied specifically to the school environment. The Incident Command System (ICS) used by fire and law enforcement authorities throughout the country is easily adaptable to school use. This system can substantially improve the response capabilities of a school through the effective organization and management of personnel and provides a framework from which school staff are assigned to work on several defined emergency teams.

At the heart of preparing for school crises is the development of an emergency plan to deal with a range of scenarios likely to be encountered within the learning environment. Such situations might include natural disasters, traffic collisions, acts of violence, explosions, fires, and chemical emissions within the surrounding community. In view of regional differences, schools should identify other plausible incidents for inclusion in the plan. For each of the identified events, the emergency strategy defines a sequence of initial response actions and procedures.

The Changing Scope of School Emergencies

In recent years, the range of potential emergencies that schools must be prepared to manage has substantially expanded. School facilities have always been subject to fires, severe storms, flooding, earthquakes, and other natural disasters. But beyond these common risks, community development over time has placed industrial facilities, transportation corridors, and other elements of the built environment in proximity to schools, increasing the potential risks.

A growing immigrant population and severe overcrowding in many urban areas have increased multicultural tensions, contributing to an increased potential for violence in the learning environment. Finally, the current vulnerability of our nation's schools to potential acts of terrorism indicates that serious consideration should be given to this possibility in the development of emergency plans.

The range of emergencies encountered within the school environment is diverse and encompasses incidents due to both natural and manmade hazards (box 20.1).

The scenarios listed in box 20.1 are potential emergency situations in schools throughout the nation. The frequency of occurrence, however, varies among regions. For example, among "natural emergencies," earthquakes are more common in the western states, hurricanes occur with greater frequency in the southeastern states, and severe storms are especially common in the northeast. Schools in densely populated metropolitan areas are more likely to experience incidents involving violence or industrial explosions. As a result, planning for school emergencies in any given region should emphasize the scenarios that are most likely

20.1. Potential emergency situations in the school environment

- aircraft crash
- animal disturbance
- armed assault
- biological or chemical release
- bomb threat
- bus disaster
- disorderly conduct
- earthquake
- explosion or risk of explosion
- fire in surrounding area
- fire on school grounds
- flooding
- loss or failure of utilities
- motor vehicle crash
- psychological trauma
- suspected contamination of food or water
- threat of violence
- unlawful demonstration or walkout.

to occur. School staff should consider the scenarios listed in box 20.1 but modify the list as appropriate.

Framework for Managing School Emergencies

The effective management of school emergencies requires the development of adequate capabilities in both emergency preparedness and emergency response. These capabilities must be developed at individual school sites as well as within the central district organization.

Emergency preparedness is a term that is often misunderstood. Individuals and organizations strive to be "prepared" for emergencies, which often misidentifies emergency preparedness as an end point rather than a process. A basic level of preparedness can be achieved with the gathering of key supplies and equipment, as well as familiarization with standardized emergency procedures, yet this basic level of preparedness is absent in most households and government organizations.

An estimated 1 in 5 Americans, or 55 million children, teachers, and staff, spend their days in the nation's more than 120,000 schools. Given these numbers and the current range of potential risks encountered in school emergencies, it is prudent to establish a more advanced level of preparedness through comprehensive and detailed emergency planning. Preparedness within the school environment must be viewed not as an end point but as a planning process: to develop a broad range of contingencies and to define and communicate the roles and responsibilities of staff members. To be effective, this information needs to be documented in a school emergency plan that is periodically reviewed, evaluated, and revised.

Many basic improvements in the management of school emergencies can be identified during the process of preparedness. Other necessary improvements will be pinpointed during emergency drills and responses to actual emergencies. For this reason, school emergency plans should be reviewed and revised at regular intervals and after each drill and actual emergency incident. This process ensures continual improvements in both the level of preparedness and the capabilities for response.

Every school should formulate an emergency plan regardless of its physical size and number of students. Key elements include response procedures for a number of emergency scenarios, the assignment of school personnel to specific teams responsible for implementing the procedures, and an organizational framework for managing emergency response activities. The management framework presented in this chapter can be applied to any school, whether it is one of several schools in a small rural district or several hundred schools in a large urban district.

This chapter describes the changing scope of school emergencies and introduces a general framework for emergency management. "Organizing for School Emergencies" describes the general structure and presents an emergency management organization (EMO) appropriate for use in school emergencies. "Emergency Planning and Preparedness" addresses the preparation of a school emergency plan and the designation of emergency teams. "Initial Response to an Emergency" provides guidance for determining the nature and extent of a school emergency and a discussion of immediate response actions the school may employ. The final section, "Emergency Response Procedures," discusses the preparation of response procedures for emergencies typically encountered in a school setting.

Organizing for School Emergencies

Emergency Management at the School and District Levels

A well-coordinated response to school emergencies can ensure the protection of students and staff and minimize damage to school property. Schools can substantially improve their response to emergencies through the effective organization and management of personnel. The efficient use of employees and resources during an emergency can minimize the risk to students and staff and reduce the time required to recover and resume normal school operations.

The development and implementation of an EMO is critical to the success of emergency operations. An alternative organizational structure is appropriate because the operational functions and skills required during an emergency differ greatly from those used in normal school operations. Once an emergency is declared, the alternative management organization is activated to effectively manage the emergency operations.

Although school emergencies are common and often limited to a particular school, some emergencies are regional (e.g., earthquakes, hurricanes, wildfires) and involve multiple schools. For this reason, a separate EMO must be established for each school and for the school district as a whole.

Standard Emergency Management Organization

Several EMO models are available, most notably the ICS, which is universally recognized by police and fire authorities and is the system of choice for most governmental organizations throughout the country.

The ICS is designed to centralize and coordinate emergency response activities through the use of standardized terminology and processes. This approach facilitates the flow of information and resources among school personnel and among the multiple agencies involved in response to an emergency. The system also facilitates the coordination of efforts among the various participants and provides a common management organization that can be easily scaled up or down based on developments during the crisis.

All schools, regardless of size, should prepare

an emergency plan that includes specific response procedures to follow in an emergency, the assignment of school staff to carry them out, and a management framework for emergency response activities. Because the ICS is scaleable, it is appropriate for any school.

In the ICS model, school personnel are organized and assigned to five emergency response functions: (1) management, (2) planning, (3) operations, (4) logistics, and (5) finance. Following are brief descriptions of each of these functions.

Management

Under the management function, an incident commander, typically the school principal, is responsible for directing all emergency response actions. The incident commander constantly assesses the situation and develops and implements appropriate response strategies. The incident commander is responsible for monitoring and allocating resources, documenting response actions, and effectively communicating response strategies to others. A public information officer (PIO), safety coordinator, and agency liaison assist the principal in carrying out this function.

Planning

During an emergency, the planning function involves gathering information, evaluating the data and information for significance, and assessing school conditions as the crisis progresses. This function is vital to understanding the situation at hand and developing an appropriate response. A planning chief and/or two optional assignments, a documentation position and a situation analysis position, support the planning function.

Operations

All emergency response actions may be carried out under the operations function. This function is supported by staff members who perform first aid, crisis intervention, search and rescue, site security, damage assessment, evacuations, and the release of students to parents. These activities are assigned by the incident commander (principal) to one or more emergency teams:

- first aid/medical
- security and utilities
- assembly area
- psychological first aid

- supplies and equipment
- request gate
- reunion gate
- fire suppression and hazmat
- search and rescue.

Logistics

The logistics function supports emergency operations by identifying available personnel; assembling and deploying volunteer teams; providing supplies, equipment, and services; and facilitating communications among emergency responders. It is common for these activities to be performed by the security and utilities team and the supplies and equipment team, both of which report directly to the incident commander (or through a logistics chief, if assigned).

Finance

The finance function involves purchasing all necessary materials, tracking financial records, timekeeping for emergency responders, and recovering school records after a crisis. These activities may be performed by a "documentation" position that reports directly to the incident commander (unless a finance chief is assigned).

Figure 20.1 presents an EMO chart that is consistent with the ICS and modeled after the Standardized Emergency Management System (SEMS), which was developed by the State of California and is directly applicable to schools.

Emergency Planning and Preparedness

Preparing a School Emergency Plan

Central to emergency planning and preparedness is the development of a school emergency plan, the objective of which is often misunderstood. It should not be prepared as a general reference document, but rather as a blueprint for how emergency scenarios will be handled. It is a document to be employed during a crisis to guide the implementation of response actions following a defined set of procedures.

The plan specifies the organizational structure to be used in managing an emergency as discussed in "Emergency Management Organization" (see fig. 20.1). It defines the roles and responsibilities of school staff and illustrates relationships and team

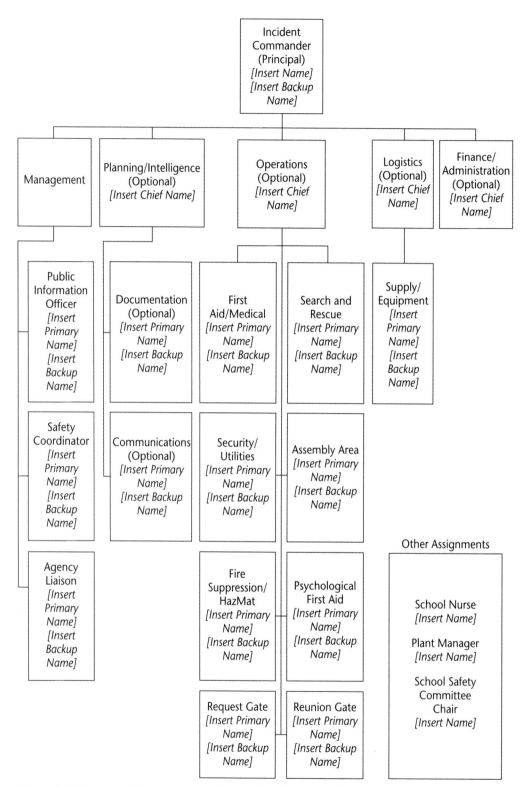

Figure 20.1. Emergency Management Organization Chart. This chart is based on the ICS and adapted for use by the Los Angeles Unified School District. School staff should use discretion in making further modifications to address the school's specific needs. The first name in each box represents the primary responsible person, and the second name denotes the designated backup.

assignments. In addition, the plan includes specific and detailed procedures to be implemented in response to a variety of emergency scenarios.

The process of preparing a school emergency plan should begin with a review of the organization and function of the ICS system by the school principal, which will serve as a reference base in building the school's EMO. Next, the principal should confer with the senior managers to review the five functions in the ICS and consider appointments to each of the positions identified in figure 20.1. The roles and responsibilities of these positions are defined in "Designating School Emergency Teams." After the senior managers of the EMO are assigned, they should collaborate in assigning other school employees to each of the emergency teams and any specialized positions the principal creates.

The EMO should identify a list of emergency scenarios to be covered in the school's plan. Although a list of scenarios is provided in box 20.1, school staff should identify those situations that are most likely to occur where the school is located. The last section of this chapter, "Emergency Response Procedures," includes general guidance for the 18 emergencies listed in box 20.1. The EMO should identify the appropriate scenarios and prepare a written procedure for each. Each of these procedures should then be prepared as a sequence of discrete steps to be taken for the given scenario. Each step should identify a specific action and the person who is responsible for taking the action (see box 20.2). The resulting emergency procedures constitute an essential part of the school emergency plan. For this reason, school personnel should carefully consider the challenges that each situation presents and the individual steps that will be taken to deal with them successfully.

Designating School Emergency Teams

The ICS consists of five separate but integrated functions: (1) incident command, (2) planning, (3) operations, (4) logistics, and (5) finance. During an incident, response activities are carried out by several emergency teams, each of which is assigned to work under a particular ICS function (see fig. 20.1).

Building an effective EMO requires more than assigning school staff to serve on emergency teams within the ICS framework. All members of the EMO must be familiar with the ICS and the purpose of each of the emergency teams. In particular, the emergency plan should specify the roles and responsibilities of the various teams, team leaders, and individual team members. The following general guidelines may be used to define the roles and responsibilities of the 10 key teams involved in responding to school emergencies.

Incident Command Team

The incident command team, led by the school principal (incident commander), directs all of the school emergency response activities. The team may also include a PIO, a safety coordinator, and an agency liaison. The principal, with assistance from the other members of the incident command team, directs the activities of all other emergency teams assigned to the four ICS functions.

The incident commander directs the emergency operations and should remain within a designated location, or command post, to observe and direct all operations. In a school setting, the duties of the incident commander may include the following:

- frequently assessing the situation
- directing the work of all of the emergency teams
- determining the need for outside assistance
- communicating with the district superintendent and school board members as the crisis develops.

As the official spokesperson for the school, the PIO is responsible for delivering public announcements and communicating with the media. Duties of the PIO may include receiving updates and official statements from the incident commander; maintaining a log of PIO actions and communications; preparing statements for dissemination to the public; monitoring news broadcasts as necessary to identify and correct any misinformation.

The designated safety coordinator ensures that emergency activities are conducted as safely as possible. Specific duties of the safety coordinator may include periodically briefing the incident commander; monitoring emergency response activities; identifying safety hazards; and ensuring that team members involved in the response use appropriate safety equipment.

The incident commander should designate an agency liaison to coordinate the efforts and flow of information between the school district and outside agencies. Other responsibilities typically include briefing agency representatives on the current situation, school district priorities, and planned actions, as well as keeping the incident commander informed of agency priorities and planned actions.

First Aid/Medical Team

The first aid/medical team ensures that first aid supplies are available and properly administered during an emergency. The team leader directs the team's activities by periodically interacting with the incident commander to determine medical needs and planned actions. The team leader is also responsible for collecting injured and missing persons reports from the first aid/medical team members and making these reports readily available to the incident commander. Specific duties of the team leader may include the following:

- assigning first aid personnel
- assessing the available inventory of supplies and equipment
- setting up first aid treatment areas that are accessible to emergency vehicles
- determining the need for and requesting skilled medical assistance
- overseeing the care, treatment, and assessment of patients
- keeping the incident commander informed of overall status
- keeping a log of injured and missing persons, compiled from the reports submitted from the first aid/medical team.

The members of the first aid/medical team assess injuries and administer necessary first aid and medical treatment. Specific duties may include setting up areas for triage, first aid, and temporary morgue; keeping accurate records of care given to injured personnel; and reporting any deaths to the first aid/medical team leader.

Crisis Intervention Team

The crisis intervention team is responsible for the care and safety of all students on campus during an emergency. The team also provides counseling and related psychological first aid as needed, both during and immediately after a crisis. The team leader directs team activities and interacts with the incident commander to identify problems and report status. The team leader is also responsible for assigning personnel as needed.

Team members monitor the safety and well-being of the students and staff in the assembly area. The team should direct all external requests for information on the status of students to the PIO. Specific duties of team members may include administering minor first aid and counseling; providing support to the release gate team as needed; ensuring the care and feeding of students and staff; and reassuring students on the steps being taken to protect their health and welfare.

Search and Rescue Team

The search and rescue team prepares and performs search and rescue operations during an emergency. Typically, two or more such teams are present in an earthquake or other large-scale disaster.

The search and rescue team leader directs team activities and keeps the incident commander informed of overall status. Specific duties of the team leader may include conferring with the incident commander on the identification of injuries and other situations requiring response, assigning personnel to teams, and recording the exact locations of casualties and structural damage.

Members of the team perform search and rescue operations, which typically include the following:

- searching an assigned area and reporting to the team leader any gas leaks, fires, or structural damage
- shutting off gas or extinguishing fires
- providing periodic reports to the team leader on the location, number, and condition of injured people
- carrying out preestablished search and rescue patterns
- checking classrooms, offices, storage rooms, auditoriums, and other rooms
- sealing off and posting areas where hazardous conditions exist
- notifying the security and utilities team to secure the building from reentry after the search.

Security and Utilities Team

The security and utilities team is responsible for the security of the school site and its population during an emergency. The team works closely with the reunion gate team to reunite students safely with their parents or lawful guardians. They also initiate short-term repairs and other necessary actions during a crisis. The effective response of this team in shutting down air-handling systems and gas, power, and water supplies can be vital in minimizing damage to school facilities.

The security and utilities team leader directs the team's activities and collaborates with the incident commander to review the status of site security and the condition of the utilities. The team leader is also responsible for direct contact with water, electricity, gas, and sewer utilities.

The team is typically staffed by janitorial and cafeteria workers, who are responsible for securing rooms, buildings, and the school perimeter. Team members lead the effort to lock down the campus when that action is ordered by the incident commander. The team also surveys all of the utilities and takes appropriate actions to shut off gas, water, and electricity. Other specific duties may include the following:

- locking and unlocking external gates and doors as appropriate
- assigning one team member at the main entrance to the school to greet parents and direct emergency vehicles to areas of need
- keeping students and staff from reentering buildings that have been closed
- providing assistance at the reunion gate as appropriate
- assisting the first aid/medical team in comforting students as needed
- assessing damage to school facilities.

The team is also involved in preparing and distributing food, checking the emergency water supply and preparing it for distribution, setting up portable toilets and temporary sanitation areas, assisting in the administration of first aid, and providing support as needed at the temporary morgue.

Supplies and Equipment Team

The supplies and equipment team ensures the availability and delivery of supplies and equipment during the course of an emergency. The team leader directs their activities and keeps the incident commander informed of overall status. Specific duties of the team leader normally include reporting equipment and supply needs, estimating the number of people requiring shelter, and determining the length of time shelter will be needed. Team members assess the adequacy of available water, food, and other supplies and organize resources,

including water, food, power, radios, telephones, and sanitary supplies, for immediate distribution. Other duties include distributing emergency water and food supplies, establishing a list of everyone who has been taken to a shelter and determining any special needs to support them, and implementing controls to conserve food, water, and other consumables.

Assembly Area Team

The assembly area team is responsible for the safe evacuation, staging, and accounting for all students and staff members during an emergency. The team also reports missing persons to the incident commander. The team leader directs their activities, collects information on injured or missing persons, and confers with the incident commander to ensure the safety of evacuated personnel. Members of the assembly area team are responsible for the safe evacuation of students and staff to a designated on-site or off-site assembly area. Specific duties include accounting for all students and staff at the designated assembly area, collecting reports of missing students from teachers and other school staff, and assisting the reunion gate team as required.

Request Gate Team

The request gate team is responsible for processing parents' requests for the release of their children during an emergency. The leader directs the team's activities and confers with the incident commander to identify problems and report status. The team leader refers all outside requests for information to the PIO.

Request gate team members greet parents, guardians, or designees and provide them with tags or other identifications that authorize the holders to reunite with students at the reunion gate. Specific duties of the request gate team may include directing parents and guardians to counselors as appropriate; reassuring them; maintaining order; and directing confirmed parents and guardians to the reunion gate.

Reunion Gate Team

The reunion gate team reunites parents or guardians with students. This is often a highly sensitive role, as some parents will be informed that their children may be injured, missing, or dead.

The reunion gate team leader directs team activities and periodically interacts with the incident commander to identify problems and report status. The team leader should refer all parent requests for information to the PIO and is also responsible for transmitting to the incident commander a written record of those students who are released to parents or guardians by team members.

Members of the reunion gate team greet parents and guardians; verify the authenticity of tags or identifications presented; dispatch student runners to the assembly area to escort students to the reunion gate; confirm that students recognize their parent or guardian; and reunite students with them.

Fire Suppression and Hazmat Team

The fire suppression and Hazmat team is responsible for extinguishing fires, conducting assessments of damage to school property, and assessing the potential release and/or discharge of hazardous materials.

The team leader directs team activities; confers with the incident commander to review status and identify problems; and submits damage assessment report forms to the incident commander.

Members of the fire suppression and hazmat team are responsible for the following:

- locating and extinguishing fires
- evaluating the potential release of hazardous materials
- conducting physical inspections of school buildings and other areas of the campus
- logging and reporting property damage by radio to the command post
- checking the gas meter for leaks
- shutting down the gas supply as appropriate
- cordoning off damaged buildings or hazardous areas.

Optional Assignments

Two additional assignments may be made by the school principal and placed within the planning function (see fig. 20.1).

A document position may be assigned to maintain a log of emergency developments and response actions, including financial expenditures, timekeeping, and other necessary records. This position would communicate directly with the incident commander and carry out a variety of tasks:

- documenting all communications between external agencies and the incident commander or other members of the Emergency Operations Center (EOC)
- maintaining a record on the number of students, staff, and other personnel on campus
- reporting missing persons
- ensuring that accurate time and activity records are kept by emergency personnel
- documenting site damage and first aid needs, in collaboration with the incident commander
- maintaining all emergency documentation in a secured location.

A communications position may be assigned to analyze emergency information, identify potential changes in emergency conditions, and maintain a status board within the command post or EOC. Other duties may include updating site maps and reports, using an area-wide map to record information on major incidents, such as road closures and utility outages, and preparing situation reports for the incident command team.

Supplemental Sources of Support

General School Employees

Most school employees have specific, preassigned tasks to carry out during natural disasters or other emergencies. Even when this is not the case, school employees play a vital role in ensuring the health and safety of students, and state law often designates employees as "disaster service workers" during declared disasters. For example, the State of California Government Code (chapter 8, section 3100) designates all public employees as "disaster service workers subject to disaster service activities as may be assigned to them by their superiors or by law." School employees should be advised of any such requirement associated with their employment.

All school staff should be familiar with the school emergency plan, their assigned responsibilities, and response procedures to be employed under various incident scenarios. Teachers should be informed that their initial responsibility is to ensure the safety of students in their class. If evacuation is required, teachers should lead the class to the assembly area, where the class may be reassigned to another staff member. The teacher can then carry out any assigned team responsibilities.

Centralized District Support

Depending on the nature and extent of an emergency, schools may receive centralized district support, which is limited for minor incidents. However, major school incidents (e.g., large fire, shooting) or situations involving several schools (e.g., earthquake, regional flooding) typically result in the activation of centralized sources of support. For larger school districts, such support may include school police, facilities maintenance, busing or trucking operations, crisis intervention, environmental health, or central emergency services.

Although the focus of this chapter is on emergency planning at the school level, school districts typically prepare a district emergency plan for managing major or multischool emergencies requiring districtwide support.

Police and Fire Services

Police and fire services are normally identified as first responders. However, school emergencies within large urban school districts occur daily and in many cases are resolved without the assistance of police and fire. For major incidents, these agencies play a vital role, managing emergency operations in a manner consistent with the ICS. This arrangement facilitates the coordination of efforts among school officials and the participating police and fire agencies.

Nongovernmental Organizations

The contributions of the Red Cross in the area of disaster relief are well known, and school districts often assist this organization by offering schools as disaster assistance centers. This relationship can facilitate the assistance that the Red Cross provides to a local school in times of crisis, particularly those involving a multiday response.

School officials should confer with the local chapter of the Red Cross and other sources of community support in the development of school emergency plans. In this way, the services available from nongovernmental organizations during an emergency can be identified and will be prearranged. Such groups should be asked to participate with school staff during emergency drills and tabletop exercises.

Initial Response to an Emergency

In an emergency, school personnel must quickly decide what initial response actions are required to ensure the health and safety of school occupants. This is a three-step process: Identify the type of emergency; identify the level of emergency; and determine the immediate response actions required to protect school occupants.

Identifying the Type of Emergency

Box 20.1 identifies emergency scenarios that can significantly impact school operations. A detailed and specific response procedure should be developed for each type of situation. These procedures are typically provided in the school emergency plan, and once the type of emergency is identified, school personnel can respond using the applicable procedure.

Identifying the Level of Emergency

The second step is to determine the level of emergency. School crises can range from small fires to major earthquakes and may be classified using the following three-tier rating system:

- Level 1: a minor emergency that can be handled by school personnel without assistance from outside agencies (e.g., a temporary power outage, a minor earthquake, a minor injury on the playground).
- Level 2: a moderate emergency that requires assistance from outside agencies (e.g., a fire, a moderate earthquake, a suspected act of terrorism involving the dispersion of a potentially hazardous material ["unknown white powder"]).
- Level 3: a major emergency event that requires assistance from outside agencies (e.g., a major earthquake, a civil disturbance, a large-scale act of terrorism). For level 3 disasters, the response time of outside agencies may be seriously delayed if the agencies are called to respond to multiple sites at the same time.

Determining Immediate Response Actions

Concurrent with identifying the type and extent of the emergency, school personnel must quickly determine whether any immediate response actions are necessary to ensure the protection of the school's occupants. The most common immediate response actions they might then initiate would include:

- duck and cover
- shelter in place
- lockdown
- building evacuation
- off-site evacuation
- all clear.

School emergency plans should review each of these responses and define when and how they should be implemented.

Duck and Cover

The duck-and-cover action is taken to protect students and staff from flying or falling debris. It is normally implemented where there is a potential for people to be injured by these objects. Such emergencies include earthquakes, shootings, and explosions.

This action is normally conveyed by the school principal using a public address (PA) system or two-way radio or by sending messengers to deliver the instruction. School occupants who are indoors are directed to duck under desks or tables and cover their heads with their arms and hands. Outdoor occupants are instructed to drop to the ground, place their heads between their knees, and cover their heads with their arms and hands. Students and staff are also directed to move away from doorways and windows.

Shelter in Place

A shelter-in-place action is taken to keep students indoors and away from adverse conditions in the outdoor environment. Its objective is to isolate students and staff from airborne chemical contaminants and includes the shutdown of the heating, ventilation, and air-conditioning (HVAC) systems.

A decision to shelter in place is normally conveyed by the school principal using a PA system or two-way radio or by sending messengers to deliver the instruction. Students and staff are advised that, because of a potential airborne hazard in the community, it is necessary to remain indoors, with doors and windows closed to minimize exposure to outside air. At the same time, maintenance personnel shut down the facility's HVAC systems.

Outdoor occupants are directed to return to their classroom or building only if it is safe to do so. If not, students are directed into nearby classrooms or other school buildings. Teachers and staff should consider the location and proximity of the identified hazard and move to an alternative indoor location if necessary.

To provide maximum protection of the indoor environment, maintenance personnel assist teachers and office employees in closing and securing doors and windows, sealing gaps with wet towels or duct tape, turning off pilot lights and other sources of ignition, and covering vents with aluminum foil or plastic wrap, if available.

Lockdown

A lockdown is initiated in response to gunfire or some other threat of violence. Lockdown orders are normally given by the school principal but may also be ordered by law enforcement personnel. Often this action is deemed necessary to prevent a perpetrator from entering occupied areas. During lockdown, students are directed to remain in classrooms, and staff members are advised to lock doors and windows and not open doors until notified by a school administrator or law enforcement personnel.

The difference between shelter in place and lockdown is that the former involves shutting down the HVAC systems and allows for the free movement of students within a building. Lockdown does not allow movement within a building and is designed to keep students confined indoors and perpetrators from entering the campus or occupied classrooms and buildings.

Indoor occupants are instructed to lie on the floor and close any shades or blinds if it appears safe to do so. Outdoor occupants are directed to go to their classroom if it is safe to do so. If not, they are directed into nearby classrooms or other school buildings.

When lockdown is initiated, maintenance personnel also secure all school gates against entry, except by law enforcement or emergency personnel.

This scenario often presents a significant challenge to teachers with regard to managing the classroom and specifically calming the activity of the students. Under either lockdown or shelter in place, this challenge includes three basic requirements: (1) keeping students safe; (2) calming the students' anxiety and actions; and (3) providing temporary toilet facilities within the classroom.

For lockdown, the primary strategy for keeping students safe is to ensure they remain in the middle of a locked classroom, away from windows and doors. Students' fears and anxieties are best managed through group activities led by the teacher. Most teachers are prepared for rainy days, in which students remain indoors and participate in group activities including games and open dialogue. Such activities may need to be modified during lockdown but nevertheless provide a base for communicating with students and calming their fears.

Finally, temporary toilet facilities are an essential requirement during lockdown for extended periods. This need can be met with the use of a metal trash can lined with a plastic bag and located in a cupboard with closeable doors. In addition to lining the trash can, large plastic trash bags may be used for constructing temporary curtains for privacy. Other essential supplies include toilet paper, waterless hand sanitizer, air freshener, a solidifying agent for collected urine, and duct tape for fastening trash bags used as privacy curtains.

Building Evacuation

A school building should be evacuated when it is determined that the occupants may be exposed to unsafe conditions inside. Such conditions may exist during a fire or after an earthquake or explosion. The decision to evacuate is normally made by the school principal but may also be made by law enforcement or fire personnel. This instruction is communicated by the school principal using a PA system or two-way radio or by sending messengers to inform teachers and students.

Personnel are directed to relocate students to a designated assembly area using evacuation routes identified in the school emergency plan. Teachers lead students to the assembly area, take attendance once the class is reassembled, and remain until further instructions are given.

Off-site Evacuation

An off-site evacuation is ordered when a determination is made that it is unsafe to remain on school grounds and that evacuation to an off-site assembly area is required. The school principal initiates this action by making an announcement on the PA system or two-way radio or by sending messengers to deliver the instruction.

The principal will typically consider the available evacuation methods (e.g., walking, school bus) and determine the safest one to use. Teachers are advised to accompany the students to the off-site assembly area and take roll once the class is reassembled. Students and teachers are also advised to remain there until they receive further instructions.

All Clear

The all-clear action notifies school occupants that normal operations are to resume. Following the signal that the danger has passed, teachers may be asked to initiate discussion and activities to address students' fears, anxieties, and other concerns about the incident.

Emergency Response Procedures

As mentioned earlier, an essential component of the school's emergency plan is a set of procedures to be implemented in response to various emergency scenarios. Each procedure should be written as a sequence of steps (each of which identifies a specific action) and identify the person responsible for taking the action. Box 20.2 shows a sample emergency response procedure template that may be used in preparing these procedures.

Aircraft Crash

An airplane or helicopter may crash into or near school property. Immediate response actions may include duck and cover, shelter in place, building evacuation, or off-site evacuation. If evacuation is required, staff and students should exit the buildings using prescribed routes or other safe routes to a designated assembly area. Once assembled, teachers should account for their students and notify the principal of anyone who is missing.

If the crash occurs on school property, the security and utilities team should secure the area to prevent unauthorized access. If the crash results in a fuel or chemical spill or an interruption in utilities, it will be necessary to implement procedures for these scenarios as well.

The school principal should direct the fire suppression and hazmat team to initiate fire suppression activities until the fire department arrives. The first aid/medical team should check for injuries and administer first aid, and the psychological first aid

■ *20.2. Sample emergency response procedure template*

This template is a sample response procedure written to spell out necessary actions after an aircraft crash on or adjacent to school property. It may be used in preparing a response procedure for any specific emergency scenario. Response procedures should be written as a sequence of steps, each one of which identifies a specific action and the person responsible for taking the action. The response procedures for any reasonable emergency scenario should be included in the school's emergency plan.

Response Procedure No. ____: Aircraft Crash

This procedure applies to situations involving an aircraft crash on or near school property. If the crash has resulted in a fuel or chemical spill on school property, also refer to section ____, response procedure no. ____, "Biological or Chemical Release." If a crash results in a utility interruption, refer to section ____, "Loss or Failure of Utilities."

School administrators must exercise caution in implementing any standardized procedure and consider modifications as necessary to ensure everyone's health and safety. In the following procedure, "school principal" means the school principal or a designee.

1. After an aircraft crash that potentially affects the school, the school principal will initiate an immediate response, which may include DUCK AND COVER, SHELTER IN PLACE, EVACUATE BUILDING, or OFF-SITE EVACUATION, as described in section ____ [refers to the appropriate section of the school's emergency plan detailing immediate response actions].
2. If the school principal issues the EVACUATE BUILDING action, staff and students will evacuate the building using prescribed routes or other safe paths to the assembly area.
3. In the event of an evacuation, teachers will bring their student roster and take attendance at the assembly area to account for students. Teachers will notify the assembly area team of missing students.
4. The school principal will call 911 and inform the operator of the nature of the emergency and its exact location, if known.
5. If on school property, the security and utilities team will secure the crash area to prevent unauthorized access. If the crash results in a fuel or chemical spill on school property, refer to section ____. If the crash results in a utility interruption, refer to section ____. [Indicate appropriate section in the school's emergency plan.]
6. The school administrator will direct the fire suppression and hazmat team to suppress any fires until the fire department arrives.
7. The first aid/medical team will check for injuries and provide appropriate first aid.
8. The school principal will notify the district superintendent of the incident and relay the status of the response activities.
9. Affected areas will not be reopened until the [specify the appropriate fire, police, or other regulatory agency] provides clearance and the school principal issues authorization to do so.
10. The crisis intervention team will convene on-site and begin the process of counseling and recovery as appropriate.
11. If it is unsafe to remain on campus, the school principal will initiate an OFF-SITE EVACUATION, as described in section ____. [Off-site evacuation may be warranted by changes in site conditions.] ■

team should convene to begin the process of counseling and recovery.

Animal Disturbance

The presence of a coyote, bear, mountain lion, or any other wild animal on school grounds potentially threatens the safety of students and staff. (Further details are provided in chapter 7.) Immediate response actions may include lockdown or building evacuation. The key to managing this scenario effectively is to isolate students and staff from the animal, and, for larger or more dangerous animals, this is normally accomplished by moving the exposed people into a secure building. At the same time, assistance may be requested from the local police or the animal control authority.

Injured students or staff should be moved to a secure area where they can receive first aid from the school nurse or other member of the first aid team. Rarely, if the animal cannot be quickly isolated or controlled, it may be necessary to initiate an off-site evacuation.

Armed Assault on Campus

Today, conceivable school emergencies include an armed assault on campus in which one or more people attempt to take hostages or cause physical harm to students and staff. Such an incident may involve individuals or groups who possess guns, knives, or other harmful devices.

In the past, such incidents in schools have been rare and typically limited to acts of violence by an individual student or small groups. These situations have less frequently involved armed adult perpetrators entering a campus with intent to inflict harm. However, more recent acts of terrorism have occurred within the school environment, redefining the scope and potential devastation of an armed assault on campus.

Whether the incident involves the actions of a single student with a gun or knife or a well-coordinated terrorist attack, the actions taken by school staff before the arrival of law enforcement can greatly influence the safety of the school's occupants and the ultimate outcome. The key strategy is twofold: Attempt to quickly isolate the school's occupants from the perpetrators, and care for the physical and emotional needs of students and staff during and immediately following the incident. The

course of this type of situation can change radically in a few minutes. As a result, staff members must be prepared to exercise discretion in responding to changing conditions.

At the first indication of an armed assault, the school principal should be notified. The principal should in turn inform the local police of the nature and extent of the incident. If possible, the notification should include the location of the perpetrators and any students and staff who are believed to be at risk. If it is safe to do so, someone should be designated to remain in communication with the police. Immediate response actions may include shelter in place, lockdown, building evacuation, or off-site evacuation. If it is safe to do so, the security and utilities team should secure all points of entry to the school, and teachers and staff should take steps to calm and control the students, maintaining separation between them and the perpetrators, if possible. Staff members should remain with the students and await the arrival of the police.

After the perpetrators have been neutralized, a head count of students and staff should be made, and the police should be notified of anyone who is missing. The first aid/medical team should identify casualties and work with the local authorities to ensure they receive medical attention. The principal should prepare a list of casualties and the locations to which they were transported.

After the incident, the school principal should debrief the staff and confer with the crisis intervention team to ensure the necessary care for school occupants and notification of parents, guardians, or other family members. The principal should also confer with the designated PIO and confirm the process for handling inquiries from the media.

Biological or Chemical Release

The potential release of a chemical or biological substance within or adjoining a school campus can present a substantial risk to school occupants. The discharged substance may be in a solid, liquid, or gaseous state. Although unlikely, such incidents could potentially involve radioactive materials. More common incidents in this category include the spillage of acid or some other chemical reagent in a school science laboratory, an explosion at a nearby oil refinery, or an overturned tanker truck or railcar in proximity to a school. Under any of these scenarios, the school's occupants may be exposed to the harmful substance via direct contact or inhalation of contaminated air.

Some incidents in this category may be readily apparent, whereas others may go undetected until school occupants begin to develop symptoms. Initial indicators of an exposure may be multiple occupants suffering from watery eyes, twitching, choking, loss of coordination, or labored breathing. It is helpful to plan for such situations by using alternative incident scenarios.

Scenario 1

A chemical substance is released inside a room or building. If students may be directly exposed, a likely immediate response is to evacuate the room or building. Staff members should use designated routes or other alternative safe routes to an assigned assembly area located upwind of the affected area.

Depending on the quantity and volatility of the substance released, a call should be made to 911, and the operator should be informed of the nature and exact location of the discharge. The security and utilities team should isolate or restrict access to the affected area, turn off local fans there, close the windows and doors, and shut down the building's air-handling system. These steps will limit the migration of the substance and minimize the potential exposure of the school's occupants.

Anyone who comes into direct contact with the substance should have the affected areas washed with soap and water, and any contaminated clothing should be immediately removed. Those who are contaminated topically by a liquid should be segregated from those who are not, although isolation is not required for widespread airborne releases. A list should be maintained of those who have been in direct contact with the substance or who may have otherwise been exposed.

The affected area should not be released for reoccupancy until authorized by local authorities or the school principal.

Scenario 2

A hazardous or unknown substance is released outdoors on campus grounds and localized. In this situation, the immediate response is remove outdoor students from the affected area to an assembly area upwind. It is important to consider the potential for the substance to drift into occupied buildings; if this is probable, the occupants of these buildings should also be evacuated to an upwind assembly area. The security and utilities team should turn off local fans in the area of the release, close the windows and doors, and shut down the air-handling systems of potentially affected buildings.

A safe perimeter should be established around the affected area to ensure that personnel do not reenter. As explained in scenario 1, those who come into direct contact with the substance should have the affected areas washed with soap and water, and any contaminated clothing should be immediately removed. Those who are contaminated topically by a liquid should be segregated from those that are not, although isolation is not required for widespread airborne releases. A list should be maintained of those who have been in direct contact with the substance or who may have otherwise been exposed.

Scenario 3

A hazardous or unknown substance is released in the surrounding community. For instance, if a chemical has been released from a nearby chemical plant or an overturned railcar or tanker truck, the security and utilities team should initiate shelter in place:

- Close and lock doors and windows
- Shut down air-handling systems in all buildings
- Seal gaps under doors and windows with wet towels or duct tape
- Seal vents with aluminum foil or plastic wrap, if available
- Turn off sources of ignition, such as pilot lights.

If outdoors, staff and students should immediately go to nearby classrooms or buildings (e.g., auditorium, library, cafeteria, gymnasium). A call to 911 should be made, noting the nature of the incident. The school should continue to enforce shelter in place until clearance is provided by local authorities.

Bomb Threat

The response to a bomb threat is typically initiated upon the receipt of a threatening phone call or discovery of a suspicious package on campus grounds. If via phone call, the person receiving the call should try to keep the caller on the phone as long as possible because this may provide important information on the nature and seriousness of the threat. At the same time, the person receiving the call should alert someone else to call 911. The person answering the threatening phone call should ask the standard questions:

- When is the bomb going to explode?
- Where is it?
- What will cause it to explode?
- What kind of bomb is it?
- Who are you?
- Why are you doing this?
- What can we do for you to prevent the bomb from exploding?
- How can you be contacted if we lose this connection?

The caller's answers to these questions should be recorded and passed along to the school principal and police.

At the principal's discretion, the search and rescue team should begin to search the campus for suspicious packages, boxes, or unfamiliar objects. It is important during such an incident that all cell phones, beepers, and hand-held radios be turned off since many modern explosive devices can be triggered by radio waves. If a suspicious package or object is identified, the room, building, or area should be secured. Once the search is completed, the principal should determine the need for lockdown, building evacuation, or off-site evacuation.

School Bus Emergency

Students often take field trips by bus and are frequently transported to and from school via bus. A school bus emergency can occur if students are in transit at the time of a severe storm, an earthquake, or a traffic collision. It is helpful to plan for such crises under alternative incident scenarios. An appropriate response procedure applicable to school bus emergencies should be prepared using the template provided in box 20.2 and placed within the emergency packet of each school bus.

It is important that bus drivers understand their responsibility to account for all of the students and accompanying staff throughout the emergency. Drivers should also understand that, although direction may be provided by the dispatcher or another school administrator, independent judgment is often required in these situations to ensure the protection of everyone who is in their care.

Scenario 1

Students are on the bus when an earthquake occurs. If the school bus is moving at the time, the driver should bring the bus to a safe stop, set the brake, turn off the ignition, and wait for the ground to stop shaking. It is important to stop the bus in a location away from power lines, overhanging trees, bridges, buildings, and other tall structures. Students should be checked for injuries and given first aid as appropriate. The driver should report the location and condition of the bus and any injured or missing students to the dispatcher or some other school administrator.

At the dispatcher's discretion, the driver should continue with the original route and destination but should not attempt to cross bridges, overpasses, or tunnels that may have been damaged. If the bus was originally en route to school, the driver should pick up the remaining students along the route and continue on to school. If it is not possible to reach the school, the driver should go to the nearest shelter indicated on the bus route map. At the shelter, the driver should notify the dispatcher or another school administrator of their arrival and remain with the students while waiting for further instructions. If the incident occurs when the bus is taking students home, the driver should continue, provided there is a parent or responsible adult at each bus stop. If not, the student should remain on the bus, and the driver should finish the route. At that time, any remaining students should be taken to the nearest shelter indicated on the bus route map, where the driver should also remain until further instruction is given by the dispatcher or school administrator.

Scenario 2

Students are on the school bus when a flood occurs. If flood conditions are encountered while en route, the driver should take alternative routes to a safe area and should never drive through flooded streets or roads. If the bus is disabled, the dispatcher should be notified of the location of the bus and the condition of the students, and the driver should stay in place until help arrives.

Scenario 3

Students are on a bus when a collision occurs. First, the driver should park the bus in a safe location, set the emergency brake, and turn off the ignition.

Obviously, the bus should be immediately evacuated if there is any indication of fire on the vehicle or within the engine compartment. When the students are in a safe area, they should be checked for injuries and given first aid if necessary. The driver should notify the dispatcher and 911 of the exact location of the bus and the students' condition and await the arrival of emergency responders.

Disorderly Conduct

Disorderly conduct on campus may involve either a student or staff member exhibiting threatening or irrational behavior. If the incident involves an armed perpetrator, the procedures in the section titled "Armed Assault on Campus" would be followed. Upon witnessing disorderly conduct, staff members should attempt to calm and control the situation and isolate the perpetrator from other students and staff, if it is safe to do so.

The principal or other school administrator should be notified as soon as possible. This person then determines whether it is necessary to initiate shelter in place, lockdown, or some other immediate response action.

Many incidents of disorderly behavior can be mitigated if the perpetrator is approached in a calm, nonconfrontational manner and requested to leave the campus. If the perpetrator is a student, contact with family members is advisable because they may have encountered similar behavior at home and be able to provide relevant information on how best to handle the current incident.

Earthquake

Earthquakes generally occur without warning and may cause minor to severe ground shaking, damage to buildings, and injuries. Even a mild tremor can create a potentially hazardous situation if panic ensues. For this reason, it is important that a detailed response procedure (using the template in box 20.2) be prepared and followed in response to all earthquakes, regardless of magnitude.

Upon the first indication of an earthquake, teachers should direct students to duck and cover. Everyone should move away from windows and overhead hazards to avoid glass and falling objects. When the shaking stops, all buildings should be evacuated along designated routes to the assembly area, where teachers will take attendance and report any missing students. Guards should be posted a safe distance away from building entrances to prevent access. School occupants should be notified of any fallen electrical wires and instructed to avoid touching them. In the assembly area, students and staff should be checked for injuries and administered first aid as appropriate.

The search and rescue team should make an initial inspection of school buildings to identify anyone who may have been injured or trapped. At the same time, the fire suppression and hazmat team should inspect the school buildings and maintain a log of its findings for review with the principal. The security and utilities team should notify the appropriate utility company of any damage to gas, power, and water or sewer lines. Affected buildings and areas should be secured to prevent access and not reopened until authorized by the principal or local fire authorities, if on-site.

Explosion or Risk of Explosion

For most urban school districts, three alternative scenarios involving explosions should be considered: explosion or risk of explosion on school property; explosion or risk of explosion in a surrounding area; and nuclear blast or explosion involving radioactive materials. Response procedures should be prepared for each of these scenarios using the sample response procedure template in box 20.2. School staff members should be familiar with the response procedure for each so that delays are minimized in an actual emergency. See the "Bomb Threats" section for additional information.

Scenario 1

There is an explosion (or risk of explosion) on school property. Under this scenario, the duck-and-cover response action should be implemented, and if an initial explosion on the campus has already occurred, staff should consider the possibility of another imminent blast. After the explosion, other immediate response actions may include shelter in place, building evacuation, or off-site evacuation. Typically, evacuation is warranted in some buildings, while others may continue to be used for sheltering in place. If evacuation is initiated, teachers should take their attendance roster and lead the students to the assembly area using the prescribed routes or alternates. Once gathered, teachers should take roll and notify the principal of anyone who is missing.

Staff members should attempt to suppress fires with extinguishers while the search and rescue and first aid/medical teams identify and care for the injured. First aid is also likely to be required for those who are in the assembly area. The affected buildings or areas should be secured to prevent access until inspected and cleared by local authorities. A perimeter should be established at a safe distance away from the building entrances to prevent people from entering. Employees should be prepared for further building evacuations or off-site evacuation that changes in site conditions may warrant.

Scenario 2

There is an explosion (or risk of explosion) in the surrounding area. If an explosion has already occurred or if the school receives a warning about an imminent explosion in the community, the school should initiate shelter in place. Depending on what is known about the timing and nature of the explosion or risk of explosion, other immediate response actions may be warranted (e.g., off-site evacuation). However, the school should continue to shelter until local authorities or the principal issue further instruction.

Scenario 3

There is a nuclear blast or an explosion involving radioactive materials. Today it is important that response procedures include contingencies for the possibility of a nuclear explosion. The magnitude of such an event would likely bring total devastation to the area immediately surrounding the blast. However, the health and safety of people in schools located farther away from the blast zone may be greatly influenced by the extent to which the school has planned for such an incident.

If a warning is given of a possible blast, the school should initiate shelter in place. A nuclear detonation is characterized by a sequence of intense light and heat, an air pressure wave, an expanding fireball, and subsequent radioactive fallout. For this reason, school occupants should try to establish adequate barriers or shielding (e.g., concrete walls, metal doors) between themselves and the source of the blast or explosion and avoid seeking shelter near exterior windows.

After the initial blast, it is advisable to remove students from damaged rooms and buildings, extinguish fires, and administer first aid to the injured. Students and staff on the upper floors of buildings should be relocated if possible. Members of the security and utilities team should shut down the school's main gas supply, turn off air-handling systems, and seal gaps under doors and windows with wet towels or duct tape. Vent grilles should also be sealed with aluminum foil or paper and tape, if available, and all pilot lights and other sources of ignition should be extinguished.

Local radio and television announcements should be monitored, and further actions initiated as appropriate. At the principal's discretion, employees should distribute emergency supplies including food and water. The school should continue to shelter until advised otherwise by local authorities.

Fire in the Surrounding Area

Fires in the vicinity of schools can potentially impact school operations and the health of school occupants. Many structure fires occur within industrial or commercial facilities that handle hazardous substances, which can release harmful vapors or particulates when consumed by fire, explode, or simply increase the intensity of the fire. Fires in the area surrounding a school may also be associated with railroad or roadway accidents that involve hazardous substances. Finally, wildfires often threaten to destroy schools in more remote or undeveloped areas with heavy accumulations of dry vegetative debris. Even these natural fires can release particulate matter into the air that is harmful when inhaled. Children with asthma, elderly people, and those with other respiratory problems are especially susceptible.

When a fire is identified in the area around a school, it is important to consider its location and size, its proximity to the school, and the prevailing wind direction before initiating a response. Response actions typically include shelter in place, building evacuation, or off-site evacuation. The effectiveness of each one may depend on the conditions already mentioned. For example, it would be inadvisable to shelter either within a school building that is close enough to a nearby fire to be threatened or in one that is downwind of the fire. If evacuation to an on-site assembly area or some other off-site location is initiated, care must be taken to ensure that the area is *upwind* of the fire.

If shelter in place is initiated, the security and utilities team should shut down the school building's HVAC systems and assist teachers and office personnel in closing and securing doors and windows, sealing gaps with wet towels or duct tape, covering vent grilles with aluminum foil or paper and tape, and turning off pilot lights and other sources of ignition. The key to effective sheltering is to isolate the occupants from harmful conditions outdoors and protect the quality of the indoor air.

Fire on the School Grounds

Most fires on school grounds involve ordinary combustibles and may be quickly extinguished by staff members who are familiar with the use of an extinguisher or a fire hose. Responding quickly to a simple fire will prevent its possible spread and avoid injuries and further property damage. It is important for school employees to report any fire, regardless of size, to the local fire department even if they manage to quickly extinguish it.

Immediately upon discovery of a fire, teachers should evacuate the affected room or building using prescribed routes to an assembly area. They should bring the student roster and take attendance at the assembly area, and members of the fire suppression and hazmat team should attempt to extinguish any remaining fires. First aid should be provided to injured people in the assembly area until the arrival of firefighters and paramedics.

The entrances to the affected buildings should be guarded to prevent reentry, and the school access road should be kept clear pending the arrival of emergency vehicles. No affected areas will be reopened until cleared by local authorities or authorized by the principal.

Flooding

The school emergency plan should include a procedure for natural flooding or situations in which water is threatening to inundate the school grounds or buildings. Although flooding often occurs as a result of prolonged periods of rainfall, it can also occur without warning, as in the case of damage to a water distribution system or the failure of a

nearby dam or levee. Immediate response actions include shelter in place, building evacuation, or off-site evacuation.

The local authorities should be contacted, and staff members should monitor local radio stations for current information as the situation develops. If evacuation is required, teachers should bring their student roster and take attendance in the assembly area to account for students. If conditions worsen, the principal should consider the need for off-site evacuation.

Loss or Failure of Utilities

The school emergency plan should include appropriate contingencies to address a possible loss of water, power, or other utility on school grounds. A loss of utilities includes the identification of a gas leak, an exposed electrical line, or a break in a sewer line since these would necessitate a discretionary shutdown of the respective utility. A response procedure should be developed for this scenario, using the template provided in box 20.2.

If a water or electrical line is broken, it is important to turn off the water or power source leading to the affected area. Staff members should contact the appropriate utility to determine the anticipated length of the interruption and the time that service is expected to resume. The response procedure for this scenario should include specific plans to supplement or make up for the loss of water, electricity, natural gas, or communications. A supplemental water plan should specify how temporary toilets will be provided in each classroom with materials that are available in the emergency supplies. The plan should also indicate how alternative drinking water will be distributed to students and staff. Finally, the plan should designate an alternative source of water for the purpose of extinguishing fires.

A supplemental electricity plan should specify how the school is to address the associated loss in ventilation and lighting. For example, natural ventilation may suffice for some schools and school buildings but may not be available for others. Emergency lighting is already a requirement in most public buildings, but the supplemental electricity plan should review the details of lighting that will be provided during a loss of power. The response procedure for this scenario should also include emergency plans for supplemental heating and communications.

Motor Vehicle Crash

Motor vehicle crashes are common in the vicinity of schools, and although most of them do not occur on school property, many involve injuries to students and are frequently witnessed by school occupants. Beyond the potential to seriously injure students, a vehicle crash in proximity to a school may also inflict psychological trauma to witnesses. For this reason, a response procedure should be developed for this scenario that takes into account the need for both physical and psychological treatment of affected students and staff. As with the other scenarios presented in this section, the effective response procedures may be prepared using the sample response procedure template in box 20.2.

Upon first indication of a collision that may affect school occupants, the staff should administer first aid to those in need, pending the arrival of fire rescue personnel. They should also attempt to secure the crash area to prevent direct access by students. Because motor vehicle crashes often involve the release of gasoline or cause damage to public utilities, it may be necessary to implement procedures in the school emergency plan addressing those situations. Conditions at the crash site may require school employees to initiate fire suppression activities until local firefighters arrive.

Psychological Trauma

Crisis management is a critical function that school personnel will need to implement both during and after any emergency that may have a psychological impact on students and staff. Such incidents may include an act of violence, the death of a student or staff member, an earthquake or other natural disaster, fears about potential exposure to toxic chemicals, and ethnic and racial tensions. These incidents usually produce one or more of the following conditions:

- temporary disruption of regular school functions and routines
- significant disruption of the ability of students and staff to focus on learning

- physical and/or psychological injury to students and staff
- concentrated attention from the community and news media

As a result, students and school personnel may exhibit a variety of psychological reactions, both short-term (Koopman et al. 1995) and long-term (Winje and Ulvik 1998; Yule et al. 2000). As soon as the physical safety of those involved has been ensured, attention must turn to meeting the emotional and psychological needs of students and staff, pursuant to the applicable response procedure in the school emergency plan. Members of the crisis intervention team are primarily responsible for providing emotional support to those in need during and immediately after the incident, including efforts to limit exposure to scenes of trauma, injury, and death. Team members should be familiar with the principles of postdisaster psychological support (Norwood et al., 2000; Chemtob et al. 2002a, 2002b; Pfefferbaum 2002; Stein et al. 2003).

Team members provide direct intervention during the emergency and assess the need for subsequent intervention services in the days after the crisis. The team also assists school administrators in restoring regular school activities as soon as possible.

Suspected Contamination of Food or Water

The school emergency plan should include measures to address situations in which evidence of tampering with food packaging is found, suspicious people have been observed in proximity to food or water supplies, or local health authorities have notified the school of possible food or water contamination. Indicators of contaminated food or water may include unusual odor, color, or taste or multiple employees who have unexplained nausea, vomiting, or other illnesses.

When contamination is suspected, the materials or area in question should be quarantined, and local health authorities notified. A list of all potentially affected students and staff should be compiled, including their symptoms, the nature and quantities of the items they consumed, time of symptom onset, and any other relevant information. The first aid/medical team should examine the affected victims, assess their need for medical attention, and provide first aid as appropriate (see chapter 16 for more information).

Threat of Violence

School personnel often learn of a threat directed to a targeted individual or group on campus. Such threats may be received in person or by written note, e-mail communication, or phone call. The principal should ensure that all threats are properly assessed in accordance with established policy. Additionally, a response procedure for this scenario should be prepared using the template in box 20.2 and included in the school's emergency plan.

The principal or designee should attempt to determine the source of the threat and conduct a threat assessment with school security and local police in accordance with established school policy and procedure. It is important that the threat be thoroughly assessed, including the identification of any warning signs, risk factors, stabilizing factors, and potential precipitating events.

The Los Angeles Police Department has established five risk categories for the purpose of assessing a threat of violence:

- Category 1: high violence potential that qualifies for arrest or hospitalization
- Category 2: high violence potential that does not qualify for arrest or hospitalization
- Category 3: insufficient evidence to establish violence potential, but sufficient confirmation of the repetitive and/or intentional infliction of emotional distress upon others
- Category 4: insufficient proof to establish violence potential, but sufficient evidence for the unintentional infliction of emotional distress upon others
- Category 5: insufficient evidence to establish violence potential and insufficient evidence for emotional distress upon others.

In categorizing the risk, school employees should attempt to answer two questions: Is the person moving on a path toward violent action? Is there evidence to suggest movement from thought to action? After this assessment, staff members should confer with the principal on a recommended course of action, which may include crisis intervention for those who are affected by the incident.

Unlawful Demonstration or Walkout

An unauthorized assemblage of staff or students for the purpose of protest or demonstration can present a significant risk of injury to school occupants and members of the adjoining community and should be managed like other emergency incidents. Such demonstrations can take place on-site or off campus. Because permits are issued for lawful protests, school staff and local authorities are able to review potential impacts and plan ahead to ensure the safety of both participants and nonparticipants in the event. It is common for unlawful protests to occur with little or no advance warning. For this reason, this type of incident must be considered in the preparation of the school's emergency plan.

At the first indication that an unlawful demonstration or walkout is about to begin, personnel should immediately notify the principal, who will normally inform school security and law enforcement authorities. The request gate team should set up at the main gate to control student ingress and egress. Although unlawful walkouts should be aggressively discouraged, it is usually inadvisable to attempt a lock-in of students once the walkout has begun. For this reason, the main gate should not be locked because a locked gate may create a serious hazard for students leaving or attempting to reenter the campus. However, all those who enter or leave the campus should be required to sign their name and indicate a home address, telephone number, and entry or departure time.

If students leave the campus, the request gate team, in consultation with the principal, should designate appropriate staff members to accompany them. The designated members should attempt to guide and control the actions of the students while off-site. Students who are not participating in the demonstration or walkout should be kept in their classrooms until further notice by the principal. Teachers should close and lock the classroom doors, and window blinds or curtains should be closed to protect the students from flying glass in the event that windows are broken.

The principal should designate a staff member to keep an accurate record of the events, conversations, and actions, and all media inquiries should be referred to a designated PIO. The principal should confer with local law enforcement and senior administrators and exercise discretion in managing the impacts of the demonstration.

This scenario often presents a significant challenge to school employees. Although a distinction between lawful and unlawful demonstrations can typically be made, this is not always the case. Staff members must frequently balance the need for order and the right of free speech as it is often practiced in an educational setting. Accordingly, discretion is nearly always required. In the case of school-based demonstrations, such tact can be extremely important.

References

Chemtob CM, Nakashima JP, Carlson JG. 2002a. Brief treatment for elementary school children with disaster-related posttraumatic stress disorder: A field study. J Clin Psychol 58(1):99–112.

Chemtob CM, Nakashima JP, Hamada RS. 2002b. Psychosocial intervention for postdisaster trauma symptoms in elementary school children. Arch Pediatr Adolesc Med 156:211–216.

Koopman C, Classen C, Cardena E, Spiegel D. 1995. When disaster strikes, acute stress disorder may follow. J Trauma Stress 8(1):29–46.

Norwood AE, Ursano RJ, Fullerton CS. 2000. Disaster psychiatry: Principles and practice. Psychiatric Q 71:207–226.

Pfefferbaum B. 2002. Treating children exposed to disasters. Arch Pediatr Adolesc Med 156:208.

Stein BD, Jaycox LH, Kataoka SH, Wong M. 2003. A mental health intervention for schoolchildren exposed to violence: A randomized controlled trial. J Am Med Assoc 290:603–611.

Winje D, Ulvik A. 1998. Long-term outcome of trauma in children: The psychological consequences of a bus accident. J Child Psychol Psychiatr 39:635–642.

Yule W, Bolton D, Udwin O, Boyle S, O'Ryan D, Nurrish J. 2000. The long-term psychological effects of a disaster experienced in adolescence. Part 1: The incidence and course of PTSD. J Child Psychol Psychiatr 41:503–511.

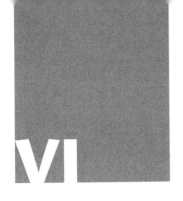

VI

Transportation to and from School

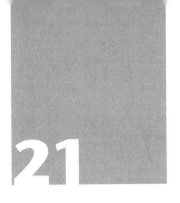

21

H. Douglas Robertson and Jeffrey C. Tsai

Safe School Travel

■ *Summary*

- School travel, although not risk free, is safer than most other types of travel.
- Modes of school travel are determined at school, at home, and individually, and the role of safety may be secondary to cost, convenience, and flexibility factors.
- Overall, the traditional school bus is the safest mode of school travel. Other modes include mass transit, private vehicles, walking, and biking.
- The safety of school travel can be markedly affected by shifting from one mode to another and by the immediate surroundings of the school.
- Checklists included in this chapter provide a means for assessing and reducing risk factors in school travel. ■

The trip to school is very much a part of the school environment. Two aspects of this trip bear directly on children's health and safety: the risk of injuries during the journey and the opportunity for health promotion through physically active travel such as walking and bicycling. This chapter addresses the first set of concerns, and the next chapter addresses the second.

How safe are children as they travel to and from school? Relative to most other types of trips, the answer is "very safe." However, school travel is not risk free, and mishaps (commonly called "accidents" and called "crashes" in the safety world) do occur, sometimes with injuries and occasionally with fatalities. This chapter briefly describes the risks of school travel and offers suggestions for reducing or minimizing them. The emphasis is on "getting it right" by those who are involved. Several checklists are offered for consideration of the types of actions that might reduce the risks associated with the most common means of school travel.

Much of the information in this chapter is drawn from a report published by the Transportation Research Board (TRB) of the National Research Council, titled *The Relative Risks of School Travel: A National Perspective and Guidance for Local Community Risk Assessment* (TRB 2002).

Background

Decisions about how a child travels to and from school are made at the school, at home, and individually. Safety is only one of several considerations in making those decisions, and it may take a back seat to cost, convenience, and flexibility. However, the safety of children traveling to and from school is a sensitive and high profile issue, especially when mishaps occur. In today's fast-paced environment, school travel is a complex topic affected by many factors, and no two school situations are exactly alike. Therefore, each state, community, school district, and school must assess its own circumstances. As characteristics and risk factors of school travel differ from school to school, so do the applicable treatments.

Children travel to and from school by a variety of means. The yellow school bus offers the most familiar image of school transportation, but other common modes include walking, biking, private automobiles, and mass transit. Each one carries some risk, a factor not well understood by parents or school-age children. As a result, these risks usually do not play a significant role in school travel choices. However, the shift from one mode to another can have a marked impact on the overall safety of school travel. In addition, a school's immediate surroundings can have a dramatic effect on the relative safety of the various modes of travel. Thus, the inclination to shift children to the overall safest mode—school buses—is not necessarily the right answer for every school situation.

Quantifying the Risks

To quantify and compare the risks of various modes of school travel, we need to calculate the rate of injuries or deaths per unit of travel. This ratio is an occurrence rate that can then be used to compare the risks of different modes of travel. The numerator data (injuries or deaths) come from national motor vehicle crash data collected in police reports (Fatality Analysis Reporting System 1991–1999; General Estimates System 1991–1999). The denominator data (amount of travel) come from the National Personal Transportation Survey (now called the National Household Travel Survey), the leading national data source on personal travel patterns (NHTSA 1995). Travel data can be expressed as the distance traveled, the time traveled, or the number of trips. In this chapter, for simplicity's sake, we place the number of student trips in the denominator. The rates calculated by trips and by

miles are similar when compared across modes. Both kinds of calculations are presented in the full Transportation Research Board report (TRB 2002).

Exposure to Risk

Of all modes of school travel, the school bus has received the most attention over the years with respect to safety, although school buses account for only 25% of student trips. Passenger vehicles account for 59% of student trips. The remaining trips are made by walking or biking or on public transportation and other types of buses. Table 21.1 depicts the exposure to risk across these modes in terms of student trips. Passenger vehicle data are distributed between adult and teen drivers, with teens driving about one in three student trips. Although walking accounts for 12% of the trips, it accounts for only 1% of the total miles traveled by students. These differences are important in understanding risk and are examined in more detail in later sections (TRB 2002).

Injuries and Fatalities

According to the TRB report, approximately 800 school-age children are killed each year in motor vehicle crashes during school travel hours. These fatalities represent about one in seven of the 5,600 child deaths that occur on U.S. roads each year and 2% of the more than 40,000 motor vehicle deaths in the nation each year. Of these 800 deaths, about 20 (2%)—5 school bus passengers and 15 pedestrians—are related to school buses. The other 98% of deaths among school-age children occur in passenger vehicles or to pedestrians, bicyclists, or other bus passengers. A majority of the passenger vehicle–related deaths (approximately 450 of the 800 deaths, or 55%) occur when a teenager is driving.

Injuries show a similar pattern. Approximately 152,000 school-age children are injured during school travel hours each year. More than 80% (about 130,000) of these nonfatal injuries occur in passenger vehicles; only 4% (about 6,000) are associated with school buses (about 5,500 school bus passengers and 500 school bus pedestrians), 11% (about 16,500) occur to pedestrians and bicyclists, and fewer than 1% (500) involve passengers in other buses (table 21.1; TRB 2002).

Table 21.1. Estimated annual trips and average annual student injuries and fatalities by mode during normal school travel hours

Mode	Student trips (× 100 million)		Average injuries per year		Average fatalities[a] per year	
	Number	Percent	Number	Percent	Number	Percent
School bus	58	25	6,000	4	20	2
Other bus	5	2	550	<1	1	<1
Passenger vehicle, adult driver	105	45	51,000	33	169	20
Passenger vehicle, teen driver	34	14	78,200	51	448	55
Bicycle	5	2	7,700	5	46	6
Walking	28	12	8,800	6	131	16
Total	235	100	152,250	100	815	100

Data from NPTS (1995); GES (1991–1999); FARS (1991–1999).
[a]A traffic fatality is the result of a fatal injury sustained in a police-reported traffic crash where death occurs within 90 days.

Injury and Fatality Rates

As mentioned earlier, the data presented in table 21.1 are used to calculate rates that permit us to compare the relative safety of different travel modes. These rates, calculated on a per-trip basis, are shown in figures 21.1 and 21.2. The highest rate of student fatalities and injuries per trip occurs for passenger vehicles with teenage drivers, and the second highest occurs among student bicyclists. The fatality rate for passenger vehicles driven by teenagers is roughly eight times higher than the rate

for those driven by adults and 44 times higher than the rate for school buses. School buses and other buses have the lowest injury and fatality rates. An obvious observation is that the modes where control resides with adults (i.e., buses and passenger vehicles with adult drivers) are safer than the modes with children in control (i.e., teen-driven passenger vehicles, biking, and walking) (TRB 2002).

Although walking and biking are, at present, relative risky ways to travel, a properly implemented infrastructure and procedures can substan-

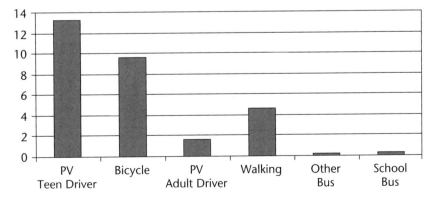

Fatalities per 100M student trips

Figure 21.1. Fatalities per 100 million student trips. PV = passenger vehicle. (Data from NPTS 1995 and FARS 1991–1999.)

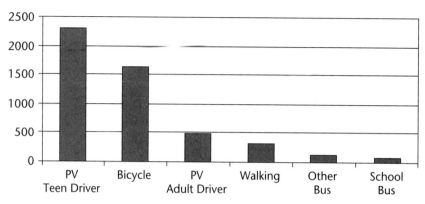

Figure 21.2. Injuries per 100 million student trips. PV = passenger vehicle. (Data from NPTS 1995 and NHTSA 1991–1999.)

tially improve their safety (see chapter 22) and yield the long-term health benefits of physical activity.

Non–School-Hour Travel

The data presented thus far have reflected mishaps during normal school travel hours. The risks faced by school-age children during non–school travel hours are worth noting. Across four age groupings, travel risks during non–school travel hours are approximately twice what they are during normal school travel hours on a per-trip basis. On a per-mile basis, the risks are approximately 20% higher during non–school travel hours and vary slightly across different age categories (TRB 2002).

Risk Factors

The risks of school travel are affected not only by the mode of travel but also by a range of other factors. The following discussion focuses on five categories of these factors:

- human
- vehicular
- operational
- infrastructure/environmental
- societal.

The material in the remainder of this section is largely drawn directly or paraphrased from chapter 4 of the TRB report, where further detail can be found (TRB 2002).

Human Factors

Pedestrians, passengers, and drivers all have attributes that can affect safety. Some human factors, such as age, gender, personality, and cognitive ability, cannot be directly changed. Others, such as experience levels, training, substance use, compliance, and peer pressure, can be modified.

Children must acquire numerous skills to become safe pedestrians. Children who are walking must be able to interpret the dangers represented by other modes that they may have to interact with during their travel. Critical behaviors such as crossing the street require the ability to judge vehicular speed and distance and safe gaps. Effective training programs, a well-designed pedestrian infrastructure, and adult supervision are needed to provide for the safety of children who walk or ride to and from school, bus stops, and the like.

In children, motor, cognitive, and behavioral skills develop chronologically and sequentially. Thus, age is a major risk factor in school travel, particularly for those younger than age 10 years who have not yet internalized the principles of safe travel and therefore may not exercise those principles during travel. Even with training, elementary school-age children may not make consistent, safe travel decisions, regardless of the modes they use. Between the ages of 9 and 12 years, children typically reach the maturity needed for safe behavior (Sandels 1975), although not every child will display or exercise it to the same degree.

Personality traits related to risk-taking and

sensation-seeking behavior appear to peak between 16 and 19 years of age, then decrease with age (Dewar 2002). These traits are also related to crash involvement. In addition, a relationship has been established between sensation seeking and risky driving (defined as excessive speed, increased frequency of speeding, less seat belt usage, and increased frequency of drinking and driving).

Higher risks of involvement in crashes or incidents are associated with age for both the young and the elderly and can be affected by numerous factors:

- driving experience
- training
- temperament and physical condition: visual acuity, reaction time, information-processing ability, stamina, alcohol impairment level.

Driver risk is higher for younger than for older drivers and higher for less-experienced than for more-experienced drivers, other conditions being equal. Teen drivers have substantially higher crash risks than adult drivers. Even within the teen years, the effects of inexperience and immaturity are evident: According to the Insurance Institute for Highway Safety (2004), 16-year-olds have almost three times the risk of a collision, per mile driven, as 18- to 19-year-olds.

Peer pressure and at times just the presence of peers are other important factors that influence children's behavior. Studies have shown that if the driver is wearing a safety belt, the passenger is more likely to do so. Other findings show that the risk of death for young drivers rises significantly with an increase in the number of passengers, regardless of time of day and gender of the driver (Williams 2001).

Vehicular Factors

Some vehicles are subject to numerous safety standards. Others, such as bicycles, are subject to a few; and still others, such as skateboards and scooters, are subject to virtually none. Motorized vehicles are regulated by Federal Motor Vehicle Safety Standards (FMVSS). These standards are performance standards, not design standards. In other words, they focus on what is to be accomplished, not how. There are 52 standards that apply to motor vehicles used to transport school-age children, and school buses are subject to 36 of these.

In addition to vehicle mass, the good safety record of school buses may also be attributed to several unique design features: their universally recognized bright yellow color and additional enhancements such as flashing red lights, stop arms, and (in at least 20 states and many more school districts) crossing control arms. Routinely enforced laws and regulations also afford school bus passengers special treatment during their boarding and alighting and at street crossings.

Unlike school buses, passenger vehicles used for school travel are not required to be a distinctive color or have special lighting, nor must they meet the same safety standards for occupant protection, joint strength of body panels, roof rollover protection, and so on. In addition, passenger vehicles do not have the capacity to transport as many students as school and other buses, nor do they have the same or comparable mass, crashworthiness, conspicuity, or maintenance and inspection requirements.

Bicycles are not subject to FMVSS and lack mass, stability, speed, and conspicuity (except for the bright-colored clothing worn by some bicycle riders). They have minimal crashworthiness characteristics, no restraints, and no maintenance or inspection requirements.

Operational Factors

In terms of operational characteristics, state and local school districts have established extensive policies and programs to ensure the safety of school travelers. Much of the guidance for these actions comes from Highway Safety Program Guideline 17. This guideline, which was originally a standard, "establishes minimum recommendations for a state highway safety program for pupil transportation safety including the identification, operation, and maintenance of buses used for carrying students; training passengers, pedestrians, and bicycle riders; and administration" (NHTSA 2000a).

School buses serve all types of areas (urban, suburban, and rural), all ages of children (prekindergarten through high school), and children with disabilities and special needs. They usually operate according to fixed routes with designated stops, although for children with special needs, they may provide door-to-door service according to a fixed schedule.

Because school bus drivers are responsible for

the safety and well-being of their passengers, they must sometimes discipline disorderly students. Unlike drivers of other forms of public transportation, school bus drivers cannot order an unruly student passenger off the bus. The driver can, however, ask system officials to suspend the student, pending correction of the misbehavior. School bus drivers also have more responsibility for the safety of students while they are pedestrians, particularly because the drivers must provide regular safety instruction to student riders and participate proactively when they cross in front of the bus. On undivided roadways, drivers are not to discharge students until other vehicles traveling in both directions have stopped in response to the bus driver's engagement of flashing lights and stop arms. Some states also require riders to wait for the bus driver's signal to cross the roadway. All school bus passengers ride seated. In fact, typical transit practices, in which passengers begin to walk toward the door as the vehicle approaches their stop, are prohibited on school buses.

The design goals and operating objectives of school and other buses reflect different needs. Other buses must accommodate a broader range of passengers (including school children), different destinations (including schools), different duty cycles and operating environments (some of which are similar to those of student transportation), and special user groups (elderly people and passengers with disabilities). However, the peak-hour nature of the majority of transit trips and the uneven distribution of passengers within these peaks lead to overcrowding and other operational issues. These, in turn, must be addressed by vehicle and operating characteristics such as room for standees; vertical and horizontal stanchions; flat, unpadded, and side-facing seats; irregular positioning of modesty panels; and other amenities not optimized specifically for student riders. Further, because passengers board and alight at the same stops, which does not occur during school bus service, passenger movement, boarding, alighting, crossing, fare collection, securing wheelchairs, lift usage, and so on are considerably different on non–school buses. Most important, because passengers do not cross in front of the bus, driver attention is diverted to many places it would not be during school bus loading, unloading, or crossing.

Students riding in transit or other buses to and from school face a number of operational factors that differ from those they encounter on a school bus. First, they mingle with the general population. Second, they must generally cross the street behind the bus rather than in front of it, except when the bus is stopped at the near side of a signalized intersection and the signal instructs pedestrians to cross. They must cross with no help from equipment and limited, if any, help from the bus driver and fellow motorists. In addition, these buses do not have identifying marks and flashing lights to indicate that they are carrying student passengers or that students are boarding or alighting. Motorists are not required to stop for transit buses loading and unloading passengers. Third, these students often spend more time than school bus riders as pedestrians, walking to and from the bus stop and waiting for the bus.

A considerable statutory and regulatory structure exists for passenger vehicles (e.g., mandatory child safety seat laws in all states and seat belt laws in many states), including distinctions that reflect driver's age, such as graduated licensing programs. In contrast, the framework for travel by bicycle and walking is generally personal. Guidance is provided by parents, relatives, and friends, occasionally with a contribution by the school, or learned through observation and experience.

Students traveling in a passenger vehicle often leave directly from their home (or some other origin) and thus do not make another trip, using a different mode, to an indirect transfer point (e.g., a bus stop). As a consequence, the total trip length and trip time are generally shorter, and the routing is more direct than is the case for bus trips. Passenger vehicles also have the ability to pick up and drop off passengers directly at their originating point and destination without the need to cross roadways or walk to bus stops. Like other non–school bus modes, however, passenger vehicles have no means of controlling other traffic (e.g., stop signal arms or flashing red lights).

Bicyclists, although using a nonmotorized vehicle, are considered vehicle operators according to traffic laws. Research indicates that wearing helmets could significantly reduce bicycle-related injuries and fatalities. As of 2002, 20 states and 84 localities had bicycle helmet laws (Bicycle Helmet Safety Institute 2002). In general, these laws are poorly enforced, except by parents and guardians. Largely because of the travel speed, the attractiveness of bicycling diminishes with increasing trip distance. As a consequence, bicycle trips are generally shorter in distance than school bus and other bus trips and may be shorter than passenger vehicle trips.

For students who walk to school, trip distances are significantly shorter than for any of the other modes. Like bicycle trips, walking trips are generally more direct. The relative risks of walking encompass a broad spectrum of considerations:

- trip length
- roadway and infrastructure conditions
- supervision
- intersections and signalization
- traffic volumes
- laws and law enforcement.

Infrastructure and Environmental Factors

Infrastructure and environmental risk factors are the characteristics of the travel route to and from school and of the school surroundings. These factors, which affect every travel mode, can be organized into four categories: (1) roadway characteristics and traffic control devices; (2) traffic characteristics; (3) adjacent land use characteristics; and (4) school zone safety and site location characteristics.

Roadway characteristics include road type (e.g., lanes, width, shoulders), surface (e.g., composition), condition (e.g., quality, irregularities), topography (e.g., degree of slope, straightness), and road hazards (e.g., detours). Traffic control devices include signs, signals, and pavement markings. Traffic characteristics include traffic volume, speed, and density, as well as the mix of traffic competing for the same space. Adjacent land use characteristics include lighting and light conditions, the presence of sidewalks and bike paths, and weather and atmospheric conditions. School zone safety and school site location factors include competing modes in and around the school zone, school-related traffic impacts on local roadway traffic, ingress and egress at the school, traffic-flow pattern at the school, and school site location and impact on modal choice.

Bicycles generally share the roadways with other vehicles (except when ridden on exclusive bike paths and sidewalks or other terrain). For bicycles, infrastructure and environmental features, especially if they are substandard or hazardous, will likely have a more direct impact on the likelihood of collisions than is the case for other vehicles.

Depending upon local conditions, numerous infrastructure features may contribute to or mitigate school travel risks (Ragland et al. 1992):

- presence or absence and condition of sidewalks
- number of street crossings students must negotiate to reach the school
- presence or absence of marked crosswalks and crossing guards
- signalization
- pedestrian-exclusive walkways and overpasses
- bike paths
- volume, density, and speed of vehicular traffic.

Such factors should be considered when selecting a particular mode if alternative modes are available, as well as when selecting potential school sites.

Societal Factors

Societal factors reflect the values of the community and its institutions and thus influence decisions and choices, including those related to travel. With respect to school travel, some of the more salient factors include the following:

- health and fitness
- security
- quality of life
- public spending and investment
- politics
- freedom of choice
- liability.

One example of how these concerns affect school travel decisions is the value placed on health improvement as a result of increased physical fitness. As chapter 22 points out, walking and biking offer important long-term health benefits if safety is ensured by proper infrastructure and procedures.

Other factors in this category, such as perceptions about security and safety, influence modal choices and may not be consistent with other factors related to the relative safety of the various modes. For example, many people believe that children are more secure in a passenger vehicle than on a bus. Likewise, a child who is assaulted on a bus may be statistically less likely than users of other modes to be killed in a vehicular crash, but that child's personal feeling of safety has been violated. In other cases, modal choices may be based purely on lifestyle factors, such as a teenager's preference for driving or riding in a peer's car rather than traveling by transit or school bus.

In every modern society, the notion of safety—the protection of human life and property—exists alongside the concept of holding individuals and organizations accountable for providing and ensuring safety. This latter notion is termed *liability*. But safety and liability are not merely related; they are inextricably intertwined. While laws, regulations, and practices establish safety criteria, verdicts and settlements often set standards that can diverge significantly from those criteria.

Under the U.S. legal system, an attempt is made to define the following:

- the elements and degrees of responsibility for safety (through statutes, regulations, and standards)
- nuances specific to each exercise of responsibility
- the responsible parties
- the parties entitled to relief when responsibilities are not met.

When a party violates prohibitions or fails to meet prescribed or generally accepted standards of care, that party is said to be *negligent*. Negligence consists of either things done wrong (errors of commission) or things not done that should have been (errors of omission). The U.S. legal system empowers the courts to assess monetary damages against parties who have violated various safety standards and practices. Although designed to compensate victims and deter both types of errors, these assessments have increasingly raised transportation costs, consumed human resources, and often complicated the provision of goods and services. On the positive side, the notion of liability has provided an additional incentive for parties to improve safety in an effort to avoid burdensome judgments or damage awards.

Another societal factor, the funding of school transportation, has become a major concern in recent years. Budgetary reductions in some school districts have resulted in competition for funding between transportation and classroom activities. These and other dynamics have led some states to consider alternatives for transporting students to and from school. For example, some smaller cities and rural areas have integrated a variety of student and social service transportation services with public transit services, thus mixing the school bus and other bus modes discussed in this study. However, federal law prohibits public transit agencies from providing exclusive school bus service (either separately or as part of their contracted provision of transit service) unless private operators are not available for the purpose. This prohibition was designed to ensure that transit agencies subsidized by public funds would not compete with private school bus operators. However, public transit can accommodate school children through regular transit service, including routes designed primarily for school travel, as long as that service is open to the general public as well.

Factor Summary

Certain factors in each of the five risk categories can be controlled by policies at the local, state, and federal levels. For example, safety education, bicycle helmet laws, and the availability of crosswalks can be changed through direct policy choices made by decision makers. Infrastructure that supports school travel must be designed, constructed, and operated to accommodate both the safety and mobility needs of children. Other factors, such as age and gender, cannot be changed but must be considered when making policy decisions.

Solutions and Applications

Combinations of factors from each of the foregoing five risk categories affect the safety of a school travel mode. The relative risk or net impact of these factors differs across modes, locations, and students. Communities are confronted with limited resources, multiple objectives, and conflicting priorities that nearly always prevent a school district from taking a safety-only perspective. Although steps can be taken to improve the safety of every mode, communities must balance safety with other goals. The actual cost of implementing a specific safety measure and the expected benefit are seldom known; thus decision makers must exercise informed judgment to select from known "best practices."

Managing Risk

A successful school transportation safety education program must be developed at a level that corresponds to the cognitive abilities of the children who will be receiving the training. Parents, as well as schools and law enforcement personnel, can assist in this effort. Attention must also be paid to the environment and infrastructure to safeguard the child pedestrian. It is important to understand the abilities and limitations of school-age children as they relate to behavior in the roadway and in the school environment.

The TRB report (2002) emphasizes the importance of considering the entire transportation system in managing risk: "Any risk reduction measures must be undertaken with the understanding that a change in a risk factor associated with one mode can shift students from/to other modes and affect a school's overall risk in unexpected ways" (p. 133).

Informed judgment can make it possible to evaluate alternatives designed to reduce the risks associated with each mode and can enable a school district to provide a range of choices for school travel that meet a variety of needs, including safety. Checklists (adapted from TRB 2002) are provided here for each mode and can be used by decision makers in a given community (whether policy makers, local administrators, or parents) to enhance the safety of school travel. Many states and school districts may already have addressed many of the items on these checklists. For these districts, additional risk reduction could be expensive and difficult to attain. For others, however, the checklists, when combined with the national statistics highlighted earlier in this chapter, can serve as a valuable starting point for discussing and prioritizing risk mitigation options.

Note that several of the questions are common to two or more of the lists. The checklists are presented and discussed in three groups: buses (boxes 21.1 and 21.2), passenger cars (boxes 21.4 and 21.5), and walking and biking (box 21.6).

All motorized vehicles are subject to FMVSS. In 1977, NHTSA issued three new FMVSS and modified four others to enhance the safety of school bus transportation. Some school buses built before 1977 do not incorporate later changes and are still used to transport school-age children. The use of these older buses puts their passengers at greater risk.

Unlike drivers of passenger vehicles, bus drivers are generally required to possess a commercial driver's license (CDL) or similar permit and receive considerable training. Moreover, federal regulations require drug and alcohol testing of bus drivers (initial, random, on suspicion, and postcrash). All CDL drivers are required to have a biennial physical, and in many states school bus drivers must have an annual physical exam. Not all states, however, have parallel requirements, including criminal history checks and other screening procedures.

It is also important for students to receive training on proper school travel behavior and safety. This passenger training, a safety feature unique to this mode, includes appropriate behaviors and activities while waiting for and riding on the school bus (e.g., remaining in one's seat, not distracting the driver, proper boarding and alighting procedures, proper street crossing, emergency evacuation). Students who ride other buses typically do not receive such training, or if they do, it is usually provided by parents or through observation of other passengers.

The integration or coordination of different modes such as school bus and transit service raises new challenges and opportunities that must be addressed at several levels:

- operating level (e.g., both drivers and students may need different training)
- vehicle level (e.g., the features that such vehicles should have to accommodate roadway crossing)
- societal level (e.g., concerns for security and liability)
- human level (e.g., whether such hybrid services may be less safe for school children of certain ages)
- environmental level (e.g., changes in roads, signage, and other infrastructure to accommodate the services).

Such changes are often complex, reflecting decades of development and refinement aimed at optimizing safety and other aspects of these modes as traditionally operated. As the National Transportation Safety Board (NTSB, 2000) has pointed out with respect to the comparative safety of school bus and motor coach vehicles, the safety of a vehicle is largely reflective of the type of service for which it is designed and in which it is operated.

Because of the rates of injuries and fatalities for

■ *21.1. Checklist for school buses*

Questions	Yes	No
1. Do all school buses meet current required Federal Motor Vehicle Safety Standards, including FMVSS 111, 131, and 222?	____	____
2. Have all drivers been properly trained?	____	____
3. Do school-age passengers receive training in loading, alighting, proper behavior while on board, and emergency procedures?	____	____
4. Do the passengers on the bus behave properly to minimize driver distraction?	____	____
5. Are school bus passengers who weigh less than 60 pounds transported in child safety seats?	____	____
6. Are children with special medical needs properly secured? Are wheelchairs, when needed, properly secured?	____	____
7. Are students on buses required to wear seat belts, where available?	____	____
8. Is after-hours/late bus service provided?	____	____
9. Are routes and pickup/drop-off locations selected, designed, and checked periodically for safety?	____	____
10. Are school-age children required to cross roads with less than average traffic volume only to get to and from the bus stop?	____	____
11. Do driver-training programs meet the recommendations of National Highway Traffic Safety Administration Guideline 17?	____	____
12. Do all drivers comply with Federal Motor Carrier Safety Administration (FMCSA) hours-of-service requirements?	____	____
13. Are on-board monitors required for the transportation of pupils with special needs?	____	____
14. Are all passengers provided a safe seat?	____	____
15. Are crossing guards employed to assist school-age children who need to cross the street?	____	____
16. Are roadways around the school adequate, safely designed, and in good repair?	____	____
17. Are passenger loading/unloading zones adequate and safely designed and supervised?	____	____
18. Are traffic-flow patterns designed to avoid or minimize people-vehicle and vehicle-vehicle (e.g., bus and passenger vehicle) interactions and conflicts?	____	____
19. Are speed limits in school zones obeyed?	____	____
20. Are traffic control devices properly installed and maintained?	____	____
21. Are video cameras installed on the buses?	____	____

---

passenger vehicles with teen drivers, the use of this mode is discouraged. However, given the propensity for this mode to be used, a number of issues can be addressed to help decrease the risk. Safety belt use is a proven injury reducer for people in passenger vehicle crashes. Graduated driver licensing (GDL) programs (especially those with passenger limitations) also reduces the risks associated with this mode. A carefully designed GDL system introduces young drivers to driving in stages and provides practical experience for extended periods of time before unrestricted driving is permitted.

■ *21.2. Checklist for other buses*

Questions	Yes	No
1. Do all buses meet current required FMVSS?	——	——
2. Have all drivers been properly trained?	——	——
3. Do school-age passengers receive training in loading, alighting, proper behavior while on board, and emergency procedures?	——	——
4. Do the passengers on the bus behave properly to minimize driver distraction?	——	——
5. Do all drivers comply with FMCSA hours-of-service requirements?	——	——
6. Are all school-age passengers provided a safe seat?	——	——
7. Is after-hours/late bus service provided?	——	——
8. Are routes and pickup/drop-off locations periodically checked for safety?	——	——
9. Are school-age children required to cross roads to get to and from the bus stop?	——	——
10. Are crossing guards employed to assist school-age children who need to cross the street?	——	——
11. Are roadways around the school adequate and in good repair?	——	——
12. Are passenger-loading/unloading zones adequate and safely designed?	——	——
13. Are traffic-flow patterns designed to avoid or minimize people-vehicle and vehicle-vehicle (e.g., bus and passenger vehicle) interactions and conflicts?	——	——
14. Are speed limits properly set and obeyed?	——	——
15. Are traffic control devices properly installed and maintained?	——	——
16. Are video cameras installed on the buses?	——	——

■

■ *21.3. Safety belts on school buses*

The issue of lap belts on school buses was addressed in a TRB report (1989) that concluded that a compartmentalized interior design (one with high-backed, padded seats front and back) provided adequate protection given both the small number of lives that would potentially be saved by lap belts and the high cost of installation. Other issues weighing against lap belts included the difficulty of fitting the range of sizes needed and the inability to keep youngsters belted. An NTSB report (2000) later indicated that compartmentalization is an incomplete measure for lateral impact with vehicles of large mass and in rollover collisions. A more recent NHTSA report (2002) shows that a lap and shoulder belt restraint system is superior to compartmentalization and to lap belts used in conjunction with compartmentalization. As school buses are replaced, they should have the newest and safest occupant-protection system. California is the only state at present to have adopted lap and shoulder restraints for all school buses; these restraints were implemented in the 2004–2005 school year (California Vehicle Code, section 27316, chapter 581, statutes of 2001 (California DMV 2002). The ongoing NHTSA research program is also addressing side-impact protection. ■

■ *21.4. Checklist for passenger vehicle with driver younger than 19 years of age*

Questions	Yes	No
1. Is seat belt compliance high?	____	____
2. Is a graduated driver-licensing program being used?	____	____
3. Are drivers alcohol and drug free?	____	____
4. Has driver education been successfully completed?	____	____
5. Are the students required to remain on school grounds during school hours unless they are enrolled in a work-study program or have special circumstances (e.g., doctor appointment, sickness)?	____	____
6. Are roadways around the school adequate and in good repair?	____	____
7. Are traffic-flow patterns designed to avoid or minimize people–vehicle and vehicle–vehicle (e.g., bus and passenger vehicle) interactions and conflicts?	____	____
8. Are speed limits obeyed?	____	____
9. Do drivers show caution toward pedestrians on school grounds?	____	____
10. Are traffic control devices properly installed and maintained?	____	____

This approach reduces collisions by 20–25% in the first years of driving (Foss and Evenson 1999). Having a closed campus where unwarranted passenger vehicle use during school hours is controlled can also reduce the possibility of crashes and the resulting fatalities and injuries.

For drivers younger than 19 years, the human risk factors described earlier in this chapter must be taken into consideration. For example, previous studies of the driving behavior of young drivers have provided much useful information about the relationship between collisions and behaviors such as alcohol and substance use, risk taking, and sensation seeking. If compliance with speed limits, traffic signals, and similar regulations is low, the risk associated with these factors is higher.

Finally, the importance of traffic-flow patterns and separation of different modes (especially at the school), proper installation of traffic control devices, and adequate repair of roadways around the school applies to all of the modes. Careful consideration should be given to the school site, including ingress and egress areas, where drivers are likely to encounter pedestrians and bicyclists.

■ *21.5. Checklist for passenger vehicle with driver 19 years of age and older*

Questions	Yes	No
1. Is seat belt compliance high?	____	____
2. Are drivers alcohol and drug free?	____	____
3. Are roadways around the school adequate and in good repair?	____	____
4. Are traffic-flow patterns designed to avoid or minimize people–vehicle and vehicle–vehicle (e.g., bus and passenger vehicle) interactions and conflicts?	____	____
5. Are speed limits obeyed?	____	____
6. Do drivers show caution toward pedestrians on school grounds?	____	____
7. Are traffic control devices properly installed and maintained?	____	____

Students who ride in passenger vehicles must receive effective, easily understandable instruction from school staff on appropriate locations for school pickup and drop-off and on safe procedures for crossing parking lots or streets.

Many interventions or countermeasures can be implemented in these two modes to mitigate the risks to school-age children. In particular, the risk of fatality and injury to a child bicyclist could be significantly reduced if bicycle helmets were worn universally. Research from several countries indicates that bicycle helmets reduce the likelihood of bicyclist fatalities by 73%, head injury by 60%, and brain injury by 58% in crashes (Attewell et al. 2001).

Educational programs that are age appropriate and properly designed and evaluated should be a component of strategies to enhance the safety of children traveling to and from school by these modes. Operational improvements have been achieved through the installation of bicycle paths. Numerous resources for bicycle and pedestrian safety are available (Federal Highway Administration 2002; NHTSA 2002; Schieber and Vegega 2001, 2002), and the Pedestrian and Bicycle Information Center (2003a, 2003b) has published walkability and bikeability checklists. These community resources identify goals and actions that can miti-

gate the risks identified in this chapter for school-age children.

Reduced speeds (and traffic volumes) result in increased pedestrian safety. School speed zones are usually instituted where pedestrians must cross roadways to get to and from a school. In most instances, these reduced speed limits remain in effect for specific time periods on particular days. School zone speed limits are set in relation to the regular speed limit on the roadway and are generally 10 mph below the road's posted speed limit. Various types of signs are used to inform drivers of these limits. A study by the Institute of Transportation Engineers (1999) revealed that about half of the motor vehicles in the school zone were in compliance with the posted speed restrictions and that flashing-light school zone signs were effective in slowing vehicles. The use of well-trained crossing guards is also one of the most effective measures for promoting the safety of children walking to and from school (Zegeer and Zegeer 1988).

Finally, the risk of injuries and fatalities from bicycling and walking could be reduced if the interaction of different or mixed modes were minimized by reducing the number of times they come together. For example, an infrastructure that included sidewalks, bicycle paths, and dedicated school-site access and egress for passenger vehicles

---

■ *21.6. Checklist for bicycling and walking*

Questions	Yes	No
1. Is appropriate crossing protection provided at intersections (e.g., crossing guards, signals, special signage)?	——	——
2. Are students trained in safe bicycling and walking behaviors and practices?	——	——
3. Are young bicyclists and walkers supervised or accompanied en route?	——	——
4. Are bicycle helmets required and used? Is compliance enforced?	——	——
5. Are safe and secure bicycling and walking routes designated?	——	——
6. Are bicycle paths and sidewalks available and in good repair?	——	——
7. Are traffic-flow patterns designed to avoid or minimize people–vehicle and vehicle–vehicle (e.g., bus and passenger vehicle) interactions and conflicts?	——	——
8. Are students on bicycles required to dismount and walk their bicycles on school property?	——	——
9. Are minimum walking distances realistic, given the associated risks?	——	——
10. Are traffic control devices properly installed and maintained?	——	——

in one area and bicyclists in another would be likely to increase safety for bicyclists and pedestrians. In addition, once on campus, bicycles should be walked.

Schools should work with communities and traffic engineers to provide an environment that enhances the safety of school travel by all modes. Planning for the transportation needs of children should be an integral part of the design of new school sites. According to the National Conference on School Transportation (National Highway Traffic Safety Administration 2000b), school officials should provide the following:

- separate and adequate space for school bus loading zones
- clearly marked and controlled walkways through school bus zones
- traffic flow and parking patterns for the public and for students who do not ride a bus that are separate from the school bus loading zone
- a designated loading area for passengers with special needs, if required
- an organized schedule of loading areas, with clearly marked stops

- a loading and unloading site to eliminate the backing of transportation equipment
- a procedure for evaluating each school site plan annually.

Safety at the School Bus Stop

The most dangerous part of the school bus ride is getting on and off the school bus. An average of 15 school children are killed each year while getting on or off school buses. Five are struck by another vehicle, and 10 by the school bus itself. The principal point of impact is the front of the bus. Half of the pedestrian fatalities in school bus–related collisions are children between 5 and 7 years of age.

The concept of the school bus "danger zone" should be taught and retaught in the school. The danger zone is an area 10 feet in front of the bus, 10 feet on either side of the bus, and the area behind the bus (fig. 21.3).

Best Practices for Reducing School Bus Stop-Arm Violations

The act of illegally passing a stopped school bus with flashing red lights is commonly known as a "stop-arm violation"—a reference to the stop sign–

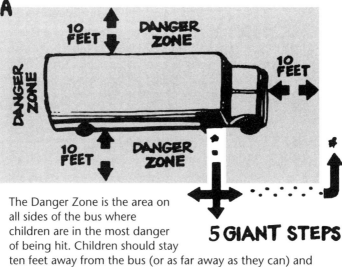

The Danger Zone is the area on all sides of the bus where children are in the most danger of being hit. Children should stay ten feet away from the bus (or as far away as they can) and never go behind it. They should take five giant steps in front of the bus before crossing, so they can be seen by the driver.

Figure 21.3. School bus danger zone. (From National Highway Traffic Safety Administration, US Department of Transportation.)

shaped arm that extends from the driver side of the bus when the red lights are activated. Every one of the 50 states has a law making it illegal to pass a school bus with its red lights flashing and stop arm extended that has stopped to load or unload students. However, some motorists simply choose to ignore the law.

Reducing the incidence of illegal passing of stopped school buses is easier said than done. The solution to this complex problem requires the involvement and cooperation of many groups (motorists, school bus drivers, law enforcement officers, prosecutors, and local judicial officials) to make sure the law is enforced. A successful comprehensive effort to reduce stop-arm violations requires a two-pronged approach involving education/awareness and enforcement.

The following steps are recommended for the education and awareness component:

- Teach bus drivers proper stopping procedures. In most states, bus drivers are trained to activate the amber warning light a few hundred feet before the red lights and stop arms are activated. The amber and red lights are the communication tools by which bus drivers alert motorists that the bus is ready to make a stop to load or unload school children. Consistency in using these warning devices is critical.
- Teach bus drivers the state's school bus stop-arm law. In most circumstances, a law enforcement officer must witness a violation of the law for a citation to be issued. Some states make an exception for the illegal passing of stopped school buses since such infractions are most often witnessed by school bus drivers and ordinary citizens. It is very important that school bus drivers understand the stop-arm law and be capable of making judgments on the validity of violations. School districts should involve local law enforcement and judicial officials in the training of school bus drivers for optimal results.
- Teach school bus passengers how to enter and exit the bus safely. Students must wait until the school bus comes to a complete stop, with the stop arm fully extended and all motorist traffic stopped, before crossing the road in an orderly fashion.

- Teach motorists the law. The consequences of not obeying the law (e.g., child death and injury, citations, fines, and points on the driver's license) should be emphasized. Remember that the ultimate aim is to influence behavior. Provide the information in a way that commands attention but does not offend motorists or make them unwilling to listen.

Increasing enforcement of the state's illegal passing law is a critical goal. How vigorously this objective can be pursued will depend on the commitment of law enforcement and on the community's resources. Studies have shown that, without the threat of enforcement and without the public actually seeing or hearing about the law being enforced (this includes prosecution and conviction), the program will have little, if any, impact.

Many communities have had positive experiences winning law enforcement commitment by videotaping stop-arm violations using a camera mounted outside of the bus (under the stop arm). Drawing media attention is an added bonus to the videotaping of these violations. It is also wise to consult your local judicial officials regarding the use of videotaping for this purpose.

Best Practices for Managing School Trip Carpools

Congestion in the carpool lane and the line of private vehicles waiting their turn to load and unload students may result in operational and safety concerns for pedestrians and drivers within and adjacent to the school campus. This congestion may be the result of, or at least be heavily dependent on, the economics of several public facilities associated with the carpool lane, including public roadway and street facilities, school buses, and school campuses.

School administrators who are facing carpool congestion problems may have the notion that the solution requires a reconstruction of internal and external traffic layout. In fact, most of these problems involve loading and unloading procedures. The actual loading and unloading of students in an efficiently managed loading area should take less than 10 seconds per vehicle. The complete process of a vehicle entering the loading area, loading or unloading passengers, then exiting the loading area can be completed in less than 45 seconds.

Traffic congestion on school campuses is more severe in the afternoon than in the morning. In the morning, vehicles arrive during a wider time window, so the line is often in motion. However, in the afternoon many of the parents are often already in line before the afternoon release time, so the later arrivals are often stacked outside of the designated loading area.

Solutions

The following recommendations and best practices offer practical solutions to the carpool congestion problem. Figure 21.4 shows a specific illustration and explanation of the best practices.

• Create short-term parking spaces past the student loading area and near the building en-

trance. These spaces can be identified by installing Visitor Parking signs at the designated spaces and should be used for parents who require an extended period of time to load or unload (location 1 in fig. 21.4).

• Clearly mark the loading area into separate bays for individual vehicles. There should be a maximum of 4–5 bays, and each one should be a minimum of 8 feet wide measured at the curb. The end bays should be a minimum length of 20 feet, and the middle bays should be a minimum length of 30 feet (location 3 in fig. 21.4).

• Limit options for parents, such as restricting access to certain parking areas and one-way traffic flow during the carpool hour, to reduce circumventions that may lead to vehicle-pedestrian and vehicle-vehicle collisions.

• If spillage onto adjacent roadways is a problem because of limited storage capacity, im-

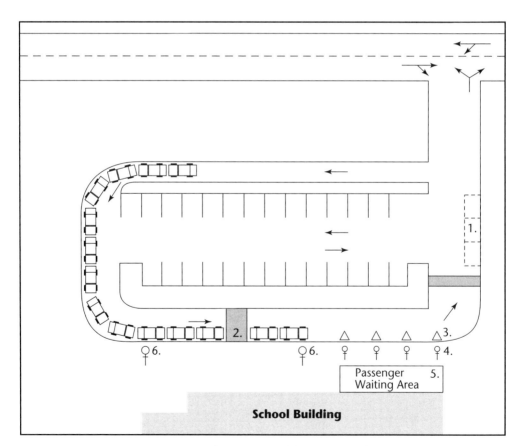

Figure 21.4. Best practices managing school campus carpool layout. See text for explanations of each numbered location.

plement a double lane for the carpool line at some point.

- Implement an advanced passenger identification system using numbers or name cards placed in the windshield of the vehicle waiting in the carpool. This will require at least two school staff members. The first one should stand five or six cars before the loading area and call out the names of the children over a walkie-talkie to the second staff member. The second staff member should be standing in the loading area itself, relaying the names or numbers with a speaker system and directing the students to the appropriate bay (location 6 in fig. 21.4).
- At the end of the school day, have the children wait in an organized fashion in the loading area or adjacent to it. Organization allows the children to pay attention and hear their name or number called and expedites the loading process by getting them to their vehicles more quickly (location 5 in fig. 21.4).
- Schools with large walking populations should stagger release times to separate walkers from carpool traffic. The walkers should be released first to provide them sufficient time to leave before the carpool process begins. Schools should also consider implementing programs such as the Walking School Bus (i.e., adult-supervised walking groups; see chapter 22) as a means to increase walking and thus reduce carpool traffic.
- Each loading bay should have its own safety assistant escorting children to their appropriate vehicles. The use of a safety assistant will expedite the loading and unloading process (location 4 in fig. 21.4).
- Crosswalks should be clearly marked. The first choice for location would be before the loading area, and the second choice would be after the loading area (location 2 in fig. 21.4).
- To prevent circumvention of the carpool, enforce No Parking and No Left Turn signs. This will avoid exposing pedestrians to risk during the pickup hour. Encouraging parents to enter the carpool lane and not circumvent the process will also minimize vehicle-to-vehicle conflicts in the lane and in the loading area.

Schools should also consider addressing private vehicle traffic congestion by encouraging mode shifts from passenger vehicles to the school bus and by promoting the health and physical fitness benefits of walking and biking. However safe walking and biking accommodations must be in place and carefully evaluated in order to support this alternative mode of school transportation (see chapter 22).

Chartered Buses for School Activity Travel

When charter motor coach services are used for school activity travel, it is important to understand some basics of the industry. If a vehicle is designed to transport more than 15 passengers including the driver, the motor carrier (that is, the charter motor coach company), the driver, the vehicle, and the motor carrier's agents are subject to the regulations of the Federal Motor Carrier Safety Administration (available at http://www.fmcsa.dot.gov/rulesregs/fmcsr/fmcsrguide.htm). Within these regulations are the requirements for controlled substance and alcohol testing, financial responsibility (minimum levels of insurance of $5,000,000), driver qualifications, driving rules, standards for parts and accessories for equipment, hours of service limitations for drivers, requirements for equipment maintenance, and hazardous material rules.

A carrier engaged in interstate commerce (that is, allowed to cross state lines) must be marked with the legal name or trade name of the carrier and must have the U.S. Department of Transportation number displayed on both sides of the vehicle.

A carrier must ensure that its drivers are qualified, as evidenced by a complete driver qualification file, and that they do not violate the hours of service limitations. The carrier must also maintain time records; 6 months of time records must always be on file. Drivers may not drive more than 10 hours without taking a break of 9 consecutive hours and may not drive after having been on duty 15 hours (part driving time, part nondriving time) without taking a break of 8 consecutive hours. Drivers cannot drive after having been on duty 60 hours in a 7-day period or 70 hours in an 8-day period, if operating vehicles every day of the week.

Nonprofit organizations are not required to comply with federal safety regulations if they carry only organization members or if passengers do not pay to ride.

Conclusion

In addition to the broad range of factors that must be considered in assessing the safety of various school travel modes, it is also important to keep in mind that the risks associated with each mode are partly generic (e.g., greater number of buses vs. automobiles or bicycles) and partly dependent on conditions at the local level (e.g., safety of bicycle path vs. road). The resources and values of the community must be taken into account as well.

The risk level of each mode can be affected positively or negatively by a variety of factors involved in its operation and in the local infrastructure and environment. In many cases, engineering, education, and enforcement interventions, whose effectiveness has already been proven by research, can have a highly beneficial impact.

The difficulty of evaluating the risks and making decisions accordingly is compounded by the fact that school trips often involve the use of more than one mode. Changes involving one mode used in the trip may adversely affect the risks associated with the other and in some cases may compound them. In addition, although students often go directly to school in the morning, they may take very different trips returning home in the afternoon, which complicates the application of treatments.

Finally, although the data presented in this chapter and elsewhere provide valuable insights regarding the relative safety of the various school travel modes, they are likely to be misleading if used to make policy changes at the local level without first considering the factors that affect the safety of school travel for a particular community. Although modes indeed have certain generic characteristics, it is also true that many of these features differ markedly from place to place. Local conditions that affect these characteristics must be considered in assessing the situation and implementing treatments.

Resources

- America Walks
  www.americawalks.org
- Institute for Transportation Research and Education School Transportation Group
  www.itre.ncsu.edu/STG/index.html
- National Center for Bicycling and Walking
  www.bikefed.org
- National Highway Traffic Safety Administration Traffic Safety Programs
  www.nhtsa.dot.gov/, then click on "Traffic Safety"
- National Safe Kids Campaign
  www.safekids.org
- Partnership for a Walkable America of the National Safety Council
  www.walkableamerica.org
- Pedestrian Bicycle Information Center
  www.pedbikeinfo.org and www.walkinginfo.org
- Street Design and Traffic Calming for Pedestrian and Bicycling Safety
  www.fhwa.dot.gov/environment/bikeped/index.htm
- U.S. Access Board
  www.access-board.gov

References

Attewell RG, Glase K, McFadden M. 2001. Bicycle helmet efficacy: A meta-analysis. Accid Anal Prev 33: 345–352.

Bicycle Helmet Safety Institute. 2002. Helmet laws for bicycle riders. Available: http://www.bhsi.org/mandator.htm [accessed 4 February 2005].

California Department of Motor Vehicles. 2002. Vehicle Code. Safety belts: Schoolbuses: Study. Section 27316. Available: http://www.dmv.ca.gov/pubs/vctop/d12/vc27316.htm.

Dewar RE. 2002. Individual differences. In *Human factors in traffic safety* (Dewar RE, Olson PL, eds.). Tucson, AZ: Lawyers and Judges Publishing, 111–141.

Fatality Analysis Reporting System (FARS). 1991–1999. Washington, DC: National Highway Traffic Safety Administration. Available: http://www-fars.nhtsa.dot.gov/.

Federal Highway Administration. 2002. Good practices guide for bicycle safety education. Washington, DC: Author. Available: http://www.bicyclinginfo.org/ee/fhwa.html [accessed 4 February 2005].

Foss RD, Evenson KR. 1999. Effectiveness of graduated driver licensing in reducing motor vehicle crashes. Am J Prev Med 16(Suppl. 1):47–56.

General Estimates System (GES). 1991–1999. National Highway Traffic Safety Administration. Available: http://www-nrd.nhtsa.dot.gov/departments/nrd-30/ncsa/ges.html.

Institute of Transportation Engineers. 1999. School zone speed limits. Washington, DC: Institute of Transportation Engineers.

Insurance Institute for Highway Safety, Highway Loss Data Institute. 2004. Fatality facts: Teenagers, 2002. Available: http://www.highwaysafety.org/ [accessed 23 March 2005].

National Highway Traffic Safety Administration. 1995. Nationwide Personal Transportation Survey (NPTS). Available: http://npts.ornl.gov/npts/1995/ Doc/publications.shtml [accessed 23 March 2005].

National Highway Traffic Safety Administration. 2000a. Highway safety program guideline no. 17: Pupil transportation safety. Available: http://www .nhtsa.dot.gov/nhtsa/whatsup/tea21/ tea21programs/402Guide.html.

National Highway Traffic Safety Administration. 2000b. National school transportation specifications and procedures. In *Proceedings of the 13th National Conference on School Transportation,* rev. ed. Warrensburg, MO: Central Missouri State University.

National Highway Traffic Safety Administration. 2001. National strategies for advancing bicycle safety. Available: http://www.nhtsa.dot.gov/people/injury/ pedbimot/bike/bicycle_safety/ [accessed 23 March 2005].

National Highway Traffic Safety Administration. 2002. School bus crashworthiness. Available: http://www -nrd.nhtsa.dot.gov/departments/nrd-11/schoolbus .html [accessed 5 February, 2005].

National Transportation Safety Board. 2000. Putting children first. Report No. NTSB/SR-00/02. Washington, DC: Author.

Pedestrian and Bicycle Information Center. 2003a. Bike-ability checklist. University of North Carolina–Chapel Hill, Highway Safety Research Center. Available: http://www.bicyclinginfo.org/cps/ checklist.htm [accessed 23 March 2005].

Pedestrian and Bicycle Information Center. 2003b.

Walkability checklist. University of North Carolina–Chapel Hill, Highway Safety Research Center. Available: http://www.walkinginfo.org/cps/ checklist.htm [accessed 23 March 2005].

Ragland DR, Hundenski RJ, Holman BL, Fisher JM. 1992. Traffic volumes and collisions involving transit and nontransit vehicles. Accid Anal Prev 24(5):547–558.

Sandels S. 1975. *Children in traffic.* London: Paul Elek.

Schieber RA, Vegega ME. 2001. National strategies for advancing child pedestrian safety. Atlanta: Centers for Disease Control and Prevention, National Center for Injury Prevention and Control. Available: http://www.cdc.gov/ncipc/pedestrian/newpedbk .pdf.

Schieber RA, Vegega ME. 2002. Reducing childhood pedestrian injuries: Proceedings of a multidisciplinary conference. Atlanta, Georgia: Centers for Disease Control and Prevention, National Center for Injury Prevention and Control. Available: http:// www.cdc.gov/ncipc/pedestrian/default.htm# proceedings.

Transportation Research Board (TRB). 1989. Special report 222: Improving school bus safety. Washington, DC: National Research Council.

Transportation Research Board (TRB). 2002. Special report 269: The relative risks of school travel: A national perspective and guidance for local community risk assessment. Washington, DC: National Research Council.

Williams AF. 2001. Teenage passengers in motor vehicle crashes: A summary of current research. Arlington, VA: Insurance Institute for Highway Safety. Available: http://www.hwysafety.org/ research/topics/pdf/teen_passengers.pdf [accessed 9 January 2006].

Zegeer CV, Zegeer SF. 1988. Pedestrians and traffic control measures: NCHRP synthesis of highway practice no. 139. Transportation Research Board, November.

22

Linda B. Crider and Amanda K. Hall

Healthy School Travel: Walking and Bicycling

■ *Summary*

- Walking and bicycling offer important health benefits to children, but the proportion of children who walk and bike to school has declined in recent years.
- Safe Routes to School is a set of strategies designed to promote walking and biking to class by providing safe, appealing pedestrian routes and encouraging their use. These strategies include engineering and environmental changes, enforcement of applicable laws, education of children, parents, and motorists, and encouragement (social marketing).
- Important elements of Safe Routes to Schools programs include team approach, surveys to assess needs before implementing the program, program evaluation once the program is in place. ■

If school is the child's workplace, then the daily trip to school is the child's commute. This trip may be taken in a car or bus, but if it is made on foot or by bicycle, it offers children an opportunity for regular physical activity—a vitally important benefit at a time when overweight and related disorders are increasingly common. Chapter 21 discussed the relative advantages of various travel modes in terms of safety. This chapter takes a complementary approach. Given the health benefits of walking and bicycling, how can these modes be encouraged as a safe and preferred alternative?

The Decline of Walking

Walking and bicycling to school have declined precipitously in recent years. In 1969, when the first National Personal Transportation Survey was conducted, 48% of students walked or biked to school (Environmental Protection Agency [EPA] 2003). By 2001, according to the National Household Travel Survey, that proportion had fallen to 15% (EPA, 2003). Riding has replaced walking; half of children are now driven to school in private vehicles, and one in three rides a bus (Dellinger and Staunton 2002). A study in Georgia revealed even less walking; in a statewide sample of more than 1600 children, 49% rode the bus, 47% were driven in a car by an adult, and only 4% walked to school most days (Bricker et al. 2002). And in a study of urban and suburban elementary schools in South Carolina, only 5% of children were observed arriving and leaving on foot or bicycle, irrespective of the level of urbanization, school size, socioeconomic status, weather, or temperature (Sirard et al. 2005).

There are several reasons for this decline. First, suburban sprawl over recent decades has reshaped many communities. Walkable neighborhoods with neighborhood schools have given way to vast residential developments whose schools are miles away (Beaumont and Pianca 2002; EPA 2003; Frumkin et al. 2004; McMahon 2000). In fact, policies in many states require building a new school whenever renovation costs would exceed 50% of new construction costs (Gurwitt 2004). In addition, standards in many states require schools to have generous allotments of land; for elementary schools, for example, a typical guideline is ten acres plus one acre for each 100 students (McMahon 2000) (although this requirement may be changing; see Council of Educational Facilities Planners International 2004). Lot size requirements on this scale are difficult to meet in existing residential neighborhoods. As a result, the new schools are typically built on a large parcel of land in a suburban or exurban location. Because these schools are distant from most students' homes and reachable only on busy roads that lack walking and biking infrastructure, students must be driven to school (EPA 2003). For the entire life of the school, students are effectively constrained from walking or biking to school.

Parents perceive these conditions as important barriers to allowing their children to walk to school. In a national survey in 1999, parents were asked about the factors that made it difficult for their children to walk to school. The most frequently cited barriers were distance (55%) and traffic danger (40%). Others included bad weather (24%), crime danger (18%), and school policies (7%; Dellinger and Staunton 2002). In the past, parents may have walked their young children to and from school, but with more two-career families, time pressures can preclude this morning ritual. And with children carrying heavy packs full of books and other school supplies, walking may be an impractical alternative (see chapter 6).

The Benefits of Walking

The decline of walking and bicycling is regrettable. Overweight and obesity have reached epidemic proportions among children in the United States (Ogden et al. 2002; Strauss and Pollack 2001). More than 15% of school-age children are now overweight, a threefold increase in less than 25 years, and the numbers continue to rise. This trend is evident in all ethnic and racial groups, but it is especially marked in black and Hispanic children; by the age of 12, nearly one in four of these children are overweight (Ogden et al. 2002). Overweight children suffer a number of health problems, including hypertension, high cholesterol levels, and impaired glucose tolerance, a precursor of diabetes (Dietz 1998). In addition, overweight children suffer low self-esteem and may be at increased risk of depression (Strauss et al. 2001). Overweight children are likely to become overweight adults (Serdula et al. 1993), with attendant risks of cardiovascular disease, cancer, and other ailments.

Why are more children becoming overweight? Part of the explanation is dietary; larger portions of calorie-rich foods are increasingly marketed to children and form a substantial part of some children's diets (see chapter 17). However, a decline in physical activity also plays a role. More "screen time" in front of computers and televisions, less freedom to roam and play in neighborhoods, and the elimination of physical education programs in schools all contribute. In this setting, walking or bicycling to school—sometimes called "active commuting"—could play a valuable part in keeping children physically active.

Walking and bicycling to school have other benefits as well: Children have an opportunity to explore the neighborhood, learn to find their own way, and develop confidence and independence (David and Weinstein 1987; Matthews 1992; Proshansky and Fabian 1987; Siegel et al. 1978). Children who are driven to school and other destinations not only miss the opportunity to exercise and develop a "cognitive map" of their surroundings but also forfeit the acquisition of vital traffic safety skills. When simply observing traffic from the back seat of a car, they may not develop the skills they will need as young drivers to operate safely in complex situations. Moreover, when children form the habit of car dependence early on, they are often more reluctant to walk or bicycle as teens and young adults (Bradshaw 2001).

Children who are driven to school and other important destinations forfeit important developmental opportunities. Walking and bicycling to school could play a valuable part in this aspect of a healthy childhood.

The Hazards of Walking

The unfortunate irony is that walking and biking, despite their health benefits, can also be hazardous ways to travel to school—the reason many parents cite for not allowing or encouraging their children to walk and bicycle. As chapter 21 explains, walking and bicycling pose a considerably higher risk of injury and death than being driven by an adult or riding on a bus. Per capita pedestrian fatality rates in children are falling (a pyrrhic victory since the major cause is that fewer children are walking), but they remain too high. Parents who keep their children from walking to school because of safety concerns have a basis for their belief.

Travel to school needs to be both safe and healthy. Parents will not want their children to walk or ride their bicycles until the route to school is safe. Fortunately, the risk factors for pedestrian injuries and fatalities among children are well known; they include wide streets, high-volume traffic, high-speed traffic, and the need to cross streets frequently (Macpherson et al. 1998; Malek et al. 1990; Rivara 1999; Roberts et al. 1995; Schieber and Thompson 1996). Based on this knowledge, safety interventions such as better street design and "traffic calming" can be implemented. And happily, when more and more people walk and bike, the pattern reverses, and walking and biking do become safer. In Holland and Germany, where far higher proportions of trips are taken on foot and bicycle than in the United States, pedestrians and cyclists are killed at far lower rates (Pucher and Dijkstra 2000, 2003). This presumably results from several factors: better pedestrian infrastructure, more effective traffic calming, drivers who are more aware and considerate of pedestrians, and safety in numbers, which is perhaps related to better visibility. Underlying these attributes is the political will to accommodate pedestrians and bicyclists and to design and build infrastructures accordingly.

The next part of this chapter describes a set of strategies often known as "safe routes to school." These initiatives have two explicit goals: preventing injuries and encouraging walking and bicycling.

Promoting Health and Ensuring Safety

"Safe Routes to School" is an international transportation and public health movement focused on the child's journey to school. To achieve twin goals—improving safety and promoting walking and bicycling—Safe Routes to School programs typically rely on the classic "three Es" of injury control—education, enforcement, and engineering—together with a fourth strategy, encouragement. Education focuses on both children and drivers, enforcement focuses on compliance with traffic laws near schools, and engineering aims to calm traffic and improve pedestrian and bicycle infrastructures. Encouragement refers to social marketing—promoting walking and bicycling through public campaigns and similar means.

Some of the first such programs arose in Denmark in the 1960s, when that country had Western Europe's highest rate of traffic-related fatalities among children. Copenhagen and Odense began traffic-calming procedures to reduce vehicle speeds and achieved substantial reductions in fatality rates (Appleyard 2003). Traffic safety programs oriented to children appeared in Great Britain, emphasizing government policy for road safety (U.K. Department of Transport 1990), and Australia, emphasizing safe routes to school during the 1980s.

In the United States, safety patrols and crossing guards became common in the 1960s and 1970s. There were attempts to teach pedestrian safety to children, such as the 1979 AAA brochure "The Safest Route to School." However, it was not until the 1990s that dedicated programs emerged in response to child pedestrian fatalities (e.g., the "Safe Routes Program" in Bronx, New York City). These programs addressed school travel, both to improve safety and to promote waking and biking. In 1997 Florida launched a pilot research project involving 10 schools called "Safe Ways to School." Concurrently, the Centers for Disease Control and Prevention (CDC) was developing a set of survey instruments on the subject. Within 2 years, the National Highway Traffic Safety Administration (NHTSA) had funded pilot programs in Arlington, Massachusetts, and Marin County, California. Participating public schools in the Marin County program, called "Safe Routes to School," reported increases in school trips made by walking (64%), biking (114%), and carpooling (91%) and a 39% decrease in trips by private vehicles carrying only one student (Staunton et al. 2003). These pilot programs inspired an upsurge of programs and legislation across the United States. In 2004, "Safe Routes to School" legislation had been passed in 14 states, and several more were considering it. Many of these initiatives are showcased on the NHTSA Safe Routes to School web site (http://www.nhtsa.dot .gov/people/injury/pedbimot/bike/Safe-Routes-2004 /index.html). NHTSA also coordinates a network of professional engineers, administrators, educators, law enforcement personnel, legislators, and activists who provide guidance and support for this growing movement. Important federal legislative initiatives included the Pedestrian and Cyclist Equity Act, proposed in 2003 but not passed, and the Safe Accountable, Flexible, and Efficient Transportation Equity Act of 2005 (SAFETEA), which allocated $612 million for "Safe Routes to School" projects.

Strategies to Encourage Walking and Biking to School

The Importance of a Team Approach

The old adage that "it takes a village to raise a child" is apt in the context of child mobility and safety. Successful programs typically benefit from both top-down support from superintendents, city managers, public works directors, school board members, and county and city council representatives and bottom-up involvement of parents, children, teachers, neighborhood residents, and local activists. The team approach is critical.

In identifying problems and suggesting and implementing solutions, parents and children need to be actively involved throughout the process.. There are several ways this can be achieved. A typical start is the formation of a school traffic safety team that consists of the principal, a traffic engineering representative, school crossing guards, a city council representative, a Department of Transportation designee, a physical education or health teacher, parents, and children. It is the task of the school traffic safety team to assess conditions at the school and in the surrounding neighborhood, identify existing and potential walk routes, survey parents and children for their concerns, identify existing fund-

ing sources, and create an action plan for improvements.

The Four Es: Engineering, Enforcement, Education, and Encouragement

Developing walking and bicycling routes to school can be modeled on the "Four Es" of injury control programs: engineering, enforcement, education, and encouragement.

Engineering

Engineering solutions involve changes in the physical environment, such as features of the roadway that reduce the risk of pedestrian injuries and improve infrastructure for those on foot or on bicycles. While each school is unique and needs to be individually assessed, some of the solutions are universal.

For example, reducing traffic speed is critical, both to prevent encounters between vehicles and pedestrians and to reduce the mortality resulting from such encounters when they do occur. In a British study, the risk of pedestrian death in crashes rose from 5% at 20 mph to 45% at 30 mph and 85% at 40 mph (Pucher and Dijkstra 2003). Accordingly, many engineering solutions attempt to reduce traffic speed.

In the immediate vicinity of schools, much of the traffic often consists of parents themselves, dropping children off and picking them up. Slowing the traffic is accomplished with traffic-calming techniques such as single-lane roundabouts, raised or colored crossings, speed humps, curb extensions (bulb-outs) at intersections, and pedestrian warning signs or flashing devices. Widened sidewalks, exclusive pedestrian signal phasing, pedestrian refuge islands, and increased intensity of roadway lighting are also in the "tool box" of infrastructure improvements that enhance the pedestrian and cycling environment (Retting et al. 2003). Children face a greater risk when trying to walk or bike across larger and more complex intersections. Therefore, measures that focus on improving pedestrian safety along heavily traveled roads and crossing major intersections are critical to improving safety. Box 22.1 shows additional engineering solutions, and box 22.2 provides broader principles of school traffic management.

Another important environmental solution is

▨ *22.1. Engineering measures to improve pedestrian safety and encourage walking and bicycling*

- Increase school zone beyond school property boundary to include major crossings adjacent to school.
- Install overhead and solar panel flashers for school zone designation at crossings.
- Use special emphasis markings at crosswalks (including yellow paint rather than white for crossing stripes in school zones); construct raised pedestrian crossings (stamped or real brick inlay).
- Establish staggered dismissal times to separate students who are walking from car traffic.
- Designate parent drop-off zones away from school site but adjacent to designated walk routes.
- Use bright yellow-green school zone and pedestrian-crossing signs to designate school zones.
- Paint pavement markings and build bulb-outs at corners to reduce crossing distance and tighten turning radii.
- Use traffic-calming techniques including vertical deflections such as speed bumps and rumble strips; horizontal deflections such as chicanes (a series of street narrowings on alternating sides of the street, forming S-shaped curves); road narrowings; and islands in streets, including pedestrian refuges
- Install "No Turn on Red" or exclusive pedestrian signaling. ▨

▨ *22.2. Principles of school traffic management*

- Keep all movements separate (i.e., pedestrian, bicycle, auto, bus).
- Keep all turning movements low speed.
- Reduce speed in school walk zones to 20 mph or lower.
- Provide well-identified (high-emphasis) crossings (i.e., "zebra" striping or brick).
- Give priority to pedestrians and bicyclists.
- Release walkers and bicyclists before auto pickup begins.
- Do not permit lining up in undesirable locations.
- Do not permit drivers to cross main pedestrian routes.
- Use school crossing guards and safety patrols for elementary students.
- No right turn on red, if signalized, in school zone crossings.
- Avoid multiple-lane highways at school entrances.
- Encourage access management techniques for ingress and egress.

(From Walkable Communities, Inc.) ▨

the provision of dedicated bicycle and pedestrian pathways that are separated from motor vehicle traffic. These may be built on utility corridors, abandoned railways, or storm water or pipeline easements. Connections utilizing parcels owned by neighborhood associations from the end of culs-de-sac to school grounds can also facilitate shorter, more direct routes for children. Florida has several examples (Duval and Sarasota counties) where storm water easements or neighborhood association parcels have been used to create shorter, connected trails.

The site selection of schools may also contribute to environmental solutions. Newly built schools in remote locations require students to travel by bus or car. If a school is located within a mile of a child's home and if the neighborhood is walkable, with features such as trees on the streets, short block lengths, and mixed land uses, then children are more likely to walk (McMillan 2003). An EPA study (2003) in Gainesville, Florida, has suggested that living closer to school and having plenty of sidewalks on the route to class predicts a higher level of walking. Therefore, siting schools in pedestrian-oriented residential neighborhoods appears to be an effective way of promoting walking and biking. This finding may factor into decisions about whether to renovate an existing neighborhood school or build a new structure. It may also influence decisions about where to site new schools.

Enforcement

Enforcement addresses parental and community concerns about two kinds of danger: automobile traffic and crimes against children. With regard to automobile traffic, enforcement focuses on visible, consistent application of speed limits and similar laws and the presence of crossing guards. Speed limits should be held to 20 mph or less during morning and afternoon walk times and strictly enforced. Many communities impose double fines for speeding in school zones. With regard to crime, abduction, and bullying, enforcement consists of highly visible and reassuring tactics such as the presence of police, crossing guards, and other adult eyes on the street (see chapter 19). Many of these enforcement strategies help address both kinds of safety concerns. Some of the enforcement techniques are listed below:

- site-based crossing guards (school teachers and parent volunteers) who receive four-hour training sessions for on-site guards in the school zones
- off-site crossing guards who are hired, trained, supervised, and strategically placed by the law enforcement agency
- sheriff's "citizen courtesy notices" as a type of community watch program
- speed trailers with variable message signs for speed control
- bike patrols and cadet bike patrols on duty in school zones during school start-up and dismissal times
- speed limits visibly posted and aggressively enforced
- neighborhood watch programs and similar "eyes on the street" programs.

Education

Education takes many forms, beginning with early pedestrian safety education for children, as well as education aimed toward parents and motorists in school zones. Pedestrian education targeted at school children has been shown to have mixed effectiveness; children's knowledge of safe crossing techniques and their crossing behaviors show some improvement, but this is inconsistent across studies (Rivara et al. 1991; Duperrex et al. 2002). However, in combination with other approaches, education may well improve safety.

Early and repeated instruction for children in the techniques and skills of pedestrian and bicycle safety can be delivered through physical education classes, videos, and presentations by safety officials. A curriculum on pedestrian and bicycle safety is ordinarily designed as a continuum, with age-appropriate materials for elementary through high school students (when it is incorporated into driver's education classes). One commonly used activity involves children and their parents mapping and walking their route to school, identifying the safest route as well as any hazards, and addressing ways to minimize the hazards (see fig. 22.1). This can be coordinated with an early fall PTA walk-to-school program when there are still plenty of daylight hours. Education for parents who drive their children to school focuses on raising their awareness of children walking and bicycling and reminding them not to speed away after dropping off their own children. School zone signage, overhead flashing lights, bright yellow and green pedestrian crossing signs, and speed radar trailers are techniques mentioned earlier under engineering or enforcement, but all of these serve to alert and educate motorists on roadways surrounding the school grounds. Other educational strategies include PTA programs with safety topics, student-produced materials asking parents to slow down and watch for children crossing, and student-created "Parents Be Safe" videos.

Safe Routes to School programs in Great Britain have also incorporated environmental education, extending the understanding of traffic impacts on air pollution, congestion, and resource use (Newson 1999).

Encouragement

Encouragement, the fourth E, corresponds to social marketing, in that both parents and children are persuaded that walking and bicycling are viable choices (fig. 22.2; Dewey-Kollen 2003).

International Walk to School Day is an annual event that promotes this concept (the web site is provided in the resource section). This event provides an opportunity for the parents to network and make plans to facilitate walking and bicycling to school and for the administration to demonstrate its support for such initiatives. While it is done only as a one-day event, the goal is to motivate walking and bicycling on an on-going basis. Social marketing efforts such as these can be used to promote

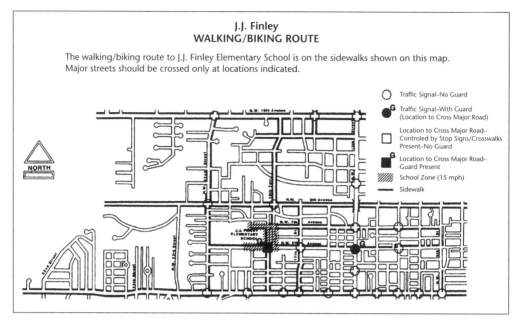

Figure 22.1. School walk map. (Courtesy of J. J. Finley Elementary School, Gainesville, Florida.)

the benefits of increased physical activity through walking and bicycling to parents and children.

An increasingly popular technique is the use of "walking school buses" or "bicycle trains." These are coordinated, scheduled group journeys to school on foot or by bicycle. In a typical program, a route to school and a schedule are established and announced. Each morning the "bus"—a group of children walking with a parent or other adult volunteer escort—departs from a fixed location and continues along a predetermined route. As the "walking bus" proceeds, children can join it for the walk to school. Some groups pull along a cart to carry heavy backpacks and musical instruments, and some use special flags or vests to alert motorists. This technique offers security, a friendly, social atmosphere, and the encouragement of peers who are also walking (fig. 22.3).

One good example of a walking school bus program is the one in Marin County, California. Since

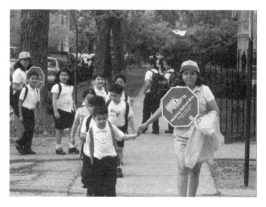

Figure 22.3. A walking school bus consists of children walking as a group, with adult supervision, according to a schedule. This picture was taken in Chicago at the beginning of the school year. (Photo by City of Chicago Police Department.)

Figure 22.2. Paw prints painted on sidewalk marking walking route to school. (Photo by Linda Crider.)

■ *22.3. Techniques to encourage walking and biking to school*

- children's "frequent rider" (bicycle or carpooler) miles certificates
- competitions among schools for the best innovations to promote walking and bicycling (e.g., the British "Safe and Sound Challenge" program, which offers cash prizes to winning schools)
- "Walk on Wednesdays" programs, providing small gifts, pizza lunch, or certificates for the class with the greatest number of walkers on that day
- footprints or "paw prints" (representative of a school mascot) imprinted or painted on the sidewalk along the designated safe path to school (see fig. 22.2)
- schoolwide safety week, poster contests, class prizes for highest percentage of walkers and bikers (pizza party, morning snacks)
- banners for street "reclaiming" or to celebrate "Walk a Child to School" week
- Bike Safety Festival Day
- "corner captains" (retirees reading the newspaper in their front yards as "eyes on the children")
- neighborhood safe watch programs
- "safe house" designations
- school "phone trees" for safe arrival
- "walking school bus." ■

its beginning in 2000, this program has supported more than 186 projects using federal, state, local, and private funding. The initial projects focused on neighborhood design changes, including the installation of sidewalks and curb ramps, the inclusion of pedestrian signals and crosswalks at signalized intersections, and the installation of traffic-calming measures, such as traffic circles and speed humps. A notable feature of this program was the careful evaluation that followed; at the end of the pilot phase, for example, participating schools experienced a 57% increase in the number of children walking and biking and a 29% decrease in the number of children arriving alone in a car (Anderson et al. 2002).

The walking school bus has become a significant part of the United Kingdom's "Transport 2000" program, through partnerships formed by a nonprofit organization, Sustrans, the Department of Health, and various county councils. An accompanying program, the "Safe and Sound Challenge," invites schools in England to bid for prizes of up to £6,000 with proposals for imaginative and practical ways of getting children to school without depending on private cars (Newson 1999). Additional examples of walking school bus plans can be found at the web site of the Pedestrian and Bicycle Information Center, www.walkingschoolbus.org.

Additional techniques for encouraging walking and bicycling to school are shown in box 22.3.

Survey Instruments and Needs Assessment Tools

Many Safe Routes to School or Safe Ways to School programs have developed survey instruments that identify barriers to walking and establish a baseline against which to evaluate subsequent changes. These include travel mode surveys, parent surveys, "walkability audits" for school and neighborhood walk routes, engineering studies, and Geographic Information Systems (GIS) crash data mapping.

Travel mode surveys identify how children get to school. These help determine opportunities for promoting walking and bicycling and provide a baseline against which to evaluate progress. The Florida Safe Ways to School "tool kit" includes a one-page student travel survey that can be administered in homeroom classes on the same morning at the beginning of the school year (see box 22.4). In this simple, ten-minute, teacher-administered questionnaire, children raise their hands to report the way they came to school. In order to track changes in the number of children walking and bicycling, results can be summarized for each school in a district and repeated on a regular basis. It can also be used to prioritize schools and neighborhoods for programs. For example, a neighborhood with a high proportion of children who live within walking distance but are still driven by car or school bus due to hazardous conditions may be a likely candidate for intervention.

Parent surveys are a means of assessing parents' concerns and building their involvement. Without their active participation, money can be spent with-

---

■ *22.4. Student travel survey*

Dear Teacher:

Your help is needed to assist with a schoolwide survey of how students travel to and from school each day. On the day that you receive this form, please record the number of children in your class that came to school by school bus, city bus, car, bicycle, or on foot and send the results back to the office on this form, along with your name, class grade, and number of students present today.

Please follow the script below to gather the information from your students. (The students should be raising their hands for only one mode of travel.)

Number of Students:

1. If you walked to school today, raise your hand: _____

2a. If you rode a bicycle to school today, raise your hand: _____

2b. If you used a bicycle helmet today, raise your hand: _____

3a. If you came in a car, with either your parents or someone else,
      raise your hand: _____

3b. If you used your seat belt in a car today, raise your hand   _____

4. If you came by day-care bus or van, raise your hand: A.M. P.M.   _____

5. If you came by school bus, raise your hand: _____

6. If you came by city bus, raise your hand: _____

Teacher's Name: _____   Grade: _____

Date: _____   # of Students in Class Today: _____

Please complete and return this form to the principal's office TODAY. This information will allow us to better plan ways for our children to get to and from school each day.

*Note to Principals: Please reproduce and distribute this form to all homeroom or first-period teachers at your school. It is important that **all classes be surveyed on the same day**. Please collect all survey forms and return to _____   by _____*

Thank you.

The Florida Traffic and Bicycle Safety Education Program—Safe Ways to School Tool Kit ■

---

out producing any change in the parents' behavior or willingness to allow their children to walk or bicycle. Too often issues of prime importance to parents, such as crime or morning darkness, are overlooked while focusing on engineering and infrastructure needs alone. By using both parent surveys and focus groups at schools (during PTA meetings or back-to-school nights), it is possible to identify parents' specific concerns and formulate acceptable solutions. Most of the Safe Routes to School programs use a parent survey instrument (examples are cited in the resource section at the end of this chapter). Successful questionnaires are no longer than one or two pages, easy to fill out, and convenient to return, using such methods as stamped return envelopes or homework assignments that students are expected to return the next day (with prizes for the class that brings back the most surveys).

Several instruments have been used to assess the walking and bicycling suitability of sidewalks and roads. NHTSA has developed a "walkability audit" and a "bikeability audit" that can be found on its web site. The Florida program recommends the assistance of a traffic engineer for completing the neighborhood site assessment instrument (downloadable from its web site, http://www.dcp.ufl.edu/centers/trafficsafetyed/safeways.htm). This assessment examines various conditions associated with roadways adjacent to walk routes (speed, amount of traffic), sidewalks (presence, completeness, surface condition, continuity), intersections and crossings (presence of crossing assistance such as guards or signals), and factors associated with security (crime activity, troublesome dogs, predator activity, etc.).

Potential Funding Sources

Many federal, state, and local funding sources can be tapped for safety projects related to walking and bicycling. Some state legislatures have appropriated special Safe Routes to School funds. Others utilize existing sources, with leverage given for school-related projects:

- federal funding through the Federal Surface Transportation Program (STP), Safe Routes to School federal earmark to states, Transportation Enhancement Activities (TEA 21), Congestion Mitigation and Air Quality program (CMAQ), and Statewide Transportation Improvement Program (STIP) (these sources must all be programmed through a regional transportation planning agency or local metropolitan planning organization [MPO] and approved by the state's Department of Transportation)
- federal discretionary and demonstration projects programmed through local members of Congress
- traffic safety grants (section 402) awarded through state offices of traffic safety
- county transportation sales tax measures or local-option gas or sales taxes funds
- local neighborhood traffic management and sidewalk program funds

- county health department funds
- local private organizations or companies such as SafeKids coalitions, AAA, 3M, Federal Express
- school capital improvement funds (state, district, or local level)
- private donations from charitable organizations or individuals.

Program Evaluation

There are two aspects of evaluation to be considered as part of a Safe Routes to School program. The first applies criteria that identify the greatest need for funds and staff resources. The second assesses progress toward established goals.

A community seeking funds for a Safe Routes to School program should develop a comprehensive plan, demonstrate an understanding of the process to assess its needs, follow through on proposed solutions, and provide evidence-based estimates of the impact of the proposed project for both risk reduction and health promotion (Local Government Commission n.d.). California's CalTrans Local Assistance Program has generated specific criteria for funding:

1. potential for reducing child injuries and fatalities
2. potential for increasing walking and bicycling among students
3. demonstrated need of the applicant
4. identification of safety hazards along existing walk and bike routes
5. support from school administration, local traffic engineering, PTA, local officials, and law enforcement officials
6. other population demographics and characteristics.

Florida has also added to this list of criteria the element of funding spent to bus children because of "hazardous walking conditions."

When projects are initiated, planners often set goals or benchmarks. For example, a school might aim for a 40% prevalence of walking at least twice each week, up from 25% at the inception of a program. Once projects are under way, it is important to monitor progress toward goals. This can be accomplished in several ways.

First, student travel patterns can be tracked. The Student Travel Survey not only assesses baseline travel patterns but can also monitor progress over time. Geographic Information System mapping and database programs have tremendous potential to store and track information relative to walk routes, student population demographics, location of residences, and pedestrian and bicycle crashes (U.S. Department of Transportation 2000).

A second basis for evaluation is improvements in walking infrastructure. Comparison of walkability and bikeability audits before and after projects can help track such improvements (Emery et al. 2003).

Traffic crash reports and trauma center data can assess changes in bicycle and pedestrian injuries and fatalities. However, because these incidents are usually rare at the level of a single school, even substantial improvements in safety may not lead to demonstrable changes in injuries and fatalities, at least over the short term.

Financial records of expenditures for "courtesy busing" for hazardous conditions paid for by state or local school districts provide another element for evaluation. A final benchmark is acceptance by school administrators, parents, children, and the community. This can be determined through follow-up surveys, school or community meetings, interviews, press stories, and observations.

Ultimately, successful programs create a virtuous cycle. As more children walk and bicycle to school, morning and afternoon traffic decreases. With less-congested roads and calmer neighborhoods and with more children walking, parents become more confident about their children's safety during the school trip, and more of them permit their children to walk or bicycle. The result is more livable communities and healthier, more active children.

Resources

National Safe Routes to School Web Sites

- Go for Green (Canada)
  http://www.goforgreen.ca
- Safe Routes to Schools Clearinghouse
  http://safety.fhwa.dot.gov/saferoutes/

- Sustrans (England)
  http://www.saferoutestoschools.org.uk

State and Local Safe Routes to School Web Sites

- Bronx Safe Routes to School Program
  http://www.transalt.org/campaigns/reclaiming/saferoutes.html
- California Safe Routes to School Initiative
  http://www.dhs.ca.gov/epic/sr2s/
- Florida Traffic and Bicycle Safety Education Program:
  http://www.dcp.ufl.edu/centers/trafficsafetyed/safeways.htm
- Marin County, California
  http://www.saferoutestoschools.org/
- Massachusetts Safe Routes to School Program
  http://www.walkboston.org/projects/safe_routes.htm

Events and Programs

- CDC, Kidswalk to Schoolhttp://www.cdc.gov/nccdphp/dnpa/kidswalk/pdf/kidswalk.pdf
- International Walk to School Week
  http://www.iwalktoschool.org
- Partnership for a Walkable America, National Walk to School Day
  http://www.walktoschool-usa.org

Related Agencies and Organizations

- Active Living by Design
  http://www.activelivingbydesign.org
- America WALKS
  http://www.americawalks.org
- Centers for Disease Control and Prevention. 2003. KidsWalk-to-School: Resource Materials: Fact Sheet. Available:
  http://www.cdc.gov/nccdphp/dnpa/kidswalk/fact_sheet.htm
- League of American Bicyclists
  http://www.bikeleague.org
- Local Government Commission
  http://www.lgc.org
- National Center for Bicycling and Walking
  http://www.bikewalk.org
- National Highway Traffic Safety Administration
  http://www.nhtsa.dot.gov

- National Safe Kids Campaign
  http://www.safekids.org
- Pedestrian and Bicycle Information Center
  http://www.pedbikeinfo.org
- Rails-to-Trails Conservancy
  http://www.railtrails.org
- Surface Transportation Policy Project
  http://www.transact.org/
- Walkable Communities, Inc.
  http://www.walkable.org

Other Sources

Savage JP Jr., Brix VC, MacLeod E, Reckord T, Boeck D. 1996. A guidebook for student pedestrian safety. Olympia: Washington Department of Transportation.
http://www.wsdot.wa.gov/Bike/PDF/PedSafetyGB
.pdf

References

Anderson C, Boarnet M, McMillan T, Alfonzo M, Day K. 2002. Walking and automobile traffic near schools: Data to support an evaluation of school pedestrian safety programs. Berkeley: University of California Transportation Center. Available: http://www.uctc.net/papers/557.pdf.

Appleyard BS. 2003. Planning safe routes to school. Planning 69(5):34–37.

Beaumont CE, Pianca EG. 2002. Why Johnny can't walk to school: Historic neighborhood schools in the age of sprawl, 2d ed. Washington, DC: National Trust for Historic Preservation. Available: http://www.nationaltrust.org/issues/schoolsRpt .pdf.

Bradshaw R. 2001. School children's travel: The journey to school. *Geography* 86:77–78.

Bricker SK, Kanny D, Mellinger-Birdsong A, Powell KE, Shisler JL. 2002. School transportation modes: Georgia, 2000. Mortal Morbid Weekly Rept 51(32):704–705.

Council of Educational Facilities Planners International. 2004. Schools for successful communities: An element of smart growth. Scottsdale, AZ: Author.

David TG, Weinstein CS. 1987. The built environment and children's development. In *Spaces for children: The built environment and child development* (Weinstein CS, David TG, eds.). New York: Plenum, 3–20.

Dellinger AM, Staunton CE. 2002. Barriers to children walking and bicycling to school: United States, 1999. Mortal Morbid Weekly Rept 51(32):701–704.

Dewey-Kollen J. 2003. Get kids in step. Traffic Safety 3(4):16–17.

Dietz WH. 1998. Health consequences of obesity in youth: Childhood predictors of adult disease. Pediatrics 101(3, Part 2):518–525.

Duperrex O, Bunn F, Roberts I. 2002. Safety education of pedestrians for injury prevention: A systematic review of randomized controlled trials. Br Med J 324:1129–1133.

Emery J, Crump C, Bors P. 2003. Reliability and validity of two instruments designed to assess the walking and bicycling suitability of sidewalks and roads. Am J Health Promot 18:38–46.

Environmental Protection Agency. 2003. Travel and environmental implications of school siting. EPA 231-R-03-004. Washington, DC: Author. Available: http://www.epa.gov/smartgrowth/pdf/school _travel.pdf.

Ewing R, Schieber RA, Zegeer CV. 2003. Urban sprawl as a risk factor in motor vehicle occupant and pedestrian fatalities. Am J Public Health 93:1541–1545.

Frumkin H, Frank L, Jackson R. 2004. Urban sprawl and public health: Designing, planning and building for healthy communities. Washington, DC: Island Press.

Gurwitt R. Edge-ucation. 2004. What compels communities to build schools in the middle of nowhere? Governing (March):22–26.

Hoehner CM, Brennan LK, Brownson RC, Handy SL, Killingworth R. 2003. Opportunities for integrating public health and urban planning approaches to promote active community environments. Am J Health Promot 18:14–20.

Huston SL, Evenson KR, Bors P, Gizlice Z. 2003. Neighborhood environment, access to places for activity, and leisure-time physical activity in a diverse North Carolina population. Am J Health Promot 18:58–69.

Jones SE, Brener ND, McManus T. 2003. Prevalence of school policies, programs, and facilities that promote a healthy physical school environment. Am J Public Health 93:1570–1575.

Killingsworth R, Lamming J. 2001. Development and public health: Could our development patterns be affecting our personal health? Urban Land (July): 12–17.

Local Government Commission. n.d. Transportation tools to improve children's health and mobility. Fact sheet. Available: http://www.lgc.org/freepub/

PDF/Land_Use/fact_sheets/sr2s_transportation
_tools.pdf.

Macpherson A, Roberts I, Pless IB. 1998. Children's
exposure to traffic and pedestrian injuries. Am J
Public Health 88:1840–1843.

Malek M, Guyer B, Lescohier I. 1990. The epidemiology and prevention of child pedestrian injuries.
Accident Anal Prev 22:301–313.

Matthews MH. 1992. *Making sense of place: Children's
understanding of large-scale environments.* Lanham,
MD: Barnes and Noble.

McMahon ET. School sprawl. 2000. Planning Com-
missioners Journal 39:16–18.

McMillan TE. 2003. Walking and urban form: Modeling and testing parental decisions about children's
travel. Ph.D. diss., University of California, Irvine.

Moudon AV, Lee C. 2003. Walking and bicycling: An
evaluation of environmental audit instruments.
Am J Health Promot 18:21–37.

National Highway Traffic Safety Administration. 2002.
Safe routes to school. Report #HS-809-497.
Washington, DC: Author.

Newson C. 1999. A safer journey to school: A guide to
school travel plans. London: Transport 2000
Trust. Available: http://www.dft.gov.uk/stellent/
groups/dft_susttravel/documents/page/dft_sust
travel_504076-06.hcsp.

Ogden CL, Flegal KM, Carroll MD, Johnson CL. 2002.
Prevalence and trends in overweight among U.S.
children and adolescents, 1999–2000. J Am Med
Assoc 288(14):1728–1732.

Proshansky HM, Fabian AK. 1987. The development
of place identity in the child. In *Spaces for children:
The built environment and child development* (Weinstein CS, David TG, eds.). New York: Plenum, 21–
40.

Pucher J, Dijkstra, L. 2000. Making walking and cycling safer: Lessons from Europe. Transport Q
54(3):25–51.

Pucher J, Dijkstra L. 2003. Promoting safe walking
and cycling to improve public health: Lessons
from the Netherlands and Germany. Am J Public
Health 93:1509–1516.

Retting R, Ferguson SA, McCartt AT. 2003. A review
of evidence-based traffic engineering measures designed to reduce pedestrian-motor vehicle crashes.
Am J Public Health 93:1456–1462.

Rivara FP. 1999. Pediatric injury control in 1999:
Where do we go from here? Pediatrics 103(4, Part
2):883–888.

Rivara FP, Booth CL, Bergman AB, Rogers LW, Weiss
J. 1991. Prevention of pedestrian injuries to chil-
dren: Effectiveness of a school training program.
Pediatrics 88:770–775.

Roberts I, Ashton T, Dunn R, Lee-Joe T. 1994. Preventing child pedestrian injury: Pedestrian education or traffic calming? Aust J Public Health 18(2):
209–212.

Roberts I, Norton R, Jackson R, Dunn R, Hassall I.
1995. Effect of environmental factors on risk of
injury of child pedestrians by motor vehicles: A
case-control study. Br Med J 310:91–94.

Saelens BE, Sallis JF, Black JB, Chen D. 2003.
Neighborhood-based differences in physical activity: An environmental scale evaluation. Am J Public Health 93:1552–1558.

Sallis J, Owen N. 1999. *Physical activity and behavioral
medicine.* Thousand Oaks, CA: Sage.

Schieber RA, Thompson NJ. 1996. Developmental risk
factors for childhood pedestrian injuries. Inj Prev
2(3):228–236.

Serdula MK, Ivery D, Coates RJ, Freedman DS, Williamson DF, Byers T. 1993. Do obese children become obese adults? A review of the literature. Prev
Med 22:167–177.

Siegel AW, Kirasic KC, Kail RV Jr. 1978. Stalking the
elusive cognitive map: The development of children's representations of geographic space. In
Children and the Environment. Vol. 3: *Human behavior and environment* (Altman I, Wohlwill JF,
eds.). New York: Plenum, 223–258.

Sirard JR, Ainsworth BE, McIver KL, Pate RR. 2005.
Prevalence of active commuting at urban and sub-
urban elementary schools in Columbia, SC. Am J
Public Health 95:236–237.

Sjolie AN, Thuen F. 2002. School journeys and leisure
activities in rural and urban adolescents in Norway. Health Promot Int 17(1):21–30.

Smith RC, Harkey DL, Harris B. 2001. Implementation of GIS-based highway safety analyses: Bridging the gap. Report # FHWA-RD-01-039. Washington, DC: Federal Highway Administration.

Staunton CE, Hubsith D, Kallis W. 2003. Promoting
safe walking and biking to school: The Marin
County success story. Am J Public Health 93:1431–
1434.

Strauss RS, Pollack HA. 2001. Epidemic increase in
childhood overweight, 1986–1998. J Am Med Assoc 286(22):2845–2848.

Strauss RS, Rodzilsky D, Burack G, Colin M. 2001. Psychosocial correlates of physical activity in healthy
children. Arch Pediat Adol Med 155(8):897–902.

Transportation Alternatives. 2002. The 2002 summary
of Safe Routes to School programs in the United
States. New York: Transportation Alternatives.
Available: http://www.transact.org/PDFs/sr_2002
.pdf.

Tutor-Locke C, Neff LJ, Ainsworth BE, Addy CL, Pop-
kin BM. 2002. Omission of active commuting to
school and the prevalence of children's health-

related physical activity levels: The Russian Longitudinal Monitoring Study. Child Care Hlth Dev 28(6):507–512.

U.K. Department of Transport. 1990. Children and roads: A safer way. London: Author.

U.S. Department of Transportation, Federal Highway Administration. 2000. GIS tools for improving pedestrian and bike safety. Washington, DC: Author. Available: http://www.walkinginfo.org/rd/safety.htm#gis

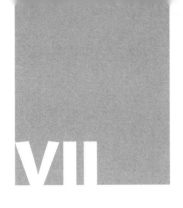

Managing for Safe and Healthy School Environments

23

Charles Eley

High-Performance School Buildings

■ *Summary*

- High-performance schools are designed to achieve a combination of goals: to be safe and healthy settings for students, teachers, and staff; to protect the environment; and to be economical to build and operate.
- High-performance schools achieve these goals through technical aspects of heating and air conditioning, lighting, and acoustics; explicit goal setting and integrated planning and operations, beginning early in the design process; commissioning, a quality assurance process that monitors the building function; and training and participation of building occupants.
- The benefits of high-performance schools include improved health and comfort for students, teachers, and staff; improved academic performance; protection of the environment; and cost savings. ■

What Is a High-Performance School?

The chapters of this book focus on many aspects of the school environment that affect the health and well-being of students, teachers, and staff—aspects such as lighting (chapter 3), noise (chapter 4), temperature and humidity (chapter 5), and indoor air quality (chapter 10). However, the importance of these factors extends beyond health and well-being; they also affect environmental performance and economics. This chapter reviews some material covered in the earlier chapters and introduces some new material, presenting it in the broad context of high-performance schools.

High-performance school buildings are designed to be efficient in their use of energy, water, and materials. They are intended to be not only adaptable and easy to operate and maintain but also comfortable, safe, secure, and healthy for teachers and students. "High performance" characterizes both the building and the people within it. Specifically, a high-performance school building is:

- Healthy. The significant amount of time that students and teachers spend inside schools during their educational career, combined with children's increased susceptibility to indoor pollutants, underscores the importance of good indoor air quality (IAQ).
- Thermally, visually, and acoustically comfortable. Thermal comfort means that teachers,

students, and administrators should be neither hot nor cold as they teach, learn, and work. Visual comfort means that quality lighting makes visual tasks, such as reading and following classroom presentations, easier. The lighting for each room is carefully considered. Acoustic comfort means teachers and students can hear one another easily. Noisy ventilation systems are eliminated, and the design minimizes the amount of disruptive outdoor and indoor noise.

- Energy efficient. Energy-efficient schools cost less to operate, which means that more money can be used for books, computers, teacher salaries, and other essential items. Energy-efficient schools also reduce emissions to the environment since energy use is related to emissions of chemicals that contribute to global warming and acid rain. Energy-efficient buildings take advantage of the sun's light energy year-round and of its heat energy in the winter. They also are designed to protect the building from unnecessary heat buildup in the summer.

- Materials efficient. To the maximum extent possible, the school incorporates building materials that have been recycled or produced in a way that conserves raw materials. These may be manufactured with a rapidly renewable resource or recycled content, are durable, can be recycled or reused, or are regionally produced. In addition, the school has been planned and built in a manner that reduces waste and keeps reusable or recyclable materials out of the landfill.

- Resource efficient. Even more than choosing materials wisely, a school can have a great environmental impact by choosing to reuse and adapt its existing resources, including buildings, furnishings, and equipment. Historic preservation and adaptation of turn-of-the-century schools may have many benefits for a community, ranging from enhancing its sense of identity and history, to taking advantage of higher quality materials and workmanship than would be affordable in a new building. Renovation is widely accepted as the first choice for sustainable development because of the much smaller resource load it entails.

- Water efficient. Preservation of natural water resources is a major issue. A high-performance school is designed to use water efficiently, saving money while reducing the depletion of aquifers and river systems and minimizing the use of sewage-treatment systems. The school uses as little off-site water as possible to meet their needs, controls and reduces water runoff from its site, and consumes fresh water as efficiently as possible.

- Easy to maintain and operate. Building systems are simple and easy to use and maintain. Teachers and administrators have good control over the temperature, airflow, acoustics, and lighting in the building and are trained in how to most effectively use the controls systems.

- Commissioned. The school operates the way it was designed and meets the district's needs. This happens through a formal commissioning process—a form of "systems check" for the facility. The process tests, verifies, and fine-tunes the performance of key building systems so that they perform at the highest levels of efficiency and comfort and then trains the staff to properly operate and maintain the systems.

- An environmentally responsive site. The site is recognized as an essential element of the school building's high-performance features. To the extent possible, the site conserves existing natural areas and restores damaged ones; minimizes storm water runoff and controls erosion; and incorporates products and techniques that do not introduce pollutants or degradation to the project site or at the site of extraction, harvest, or production.

- A teaching tool. By incorporating important concepts such as energy, water, and material efficiency, schools can become tools to illustrate a wide spectrum of scientific, mathematical, and social issues. Heating, ventilation, and air-conditioning (HVAC) systems; lighting equipment; and controls systems can be used to illustrate lessons on energy use and conservation, and daylighting systems can help students understand the daily and yearly movements of the sun.

- Safe and secure. High performance does not compromise safety. Students and teachers feel safe anywhere in the building and on the grounds. A secure environment is created primarily by design: Opportunities for natural surveillance are optimized; a sense of community is reinforced; and access is controlled.

- A community resource. The most successful schools have a high level of parent and community involvement. This participation can be enhanced if schools are designed for neighborhood meetings and other community functions.
- Architecturally stimulating. High-performance schools should invoke a sense of pride and be considered a genuine asset to the community.

Designing high-performance schools may seem prohibitively expensive and time consuming. Fortunately, this is not generally the case. The key lies in understanding the lifetime value of these schools, hiring skilled designers, and effectively managing priorities during the design and construction process. Building a high-performance school does not require buying and installing the latest, most expensive equipment. Rather, it requires a focus on student and teacher performance, a concern for the environment, and a commitment to cost effectiveness, all of which support a design philosophy focused on choices that improve the learning environment and that conserve resources. Some choices are essential and others are discretionary; it is important to keep the range of choices in perspective and to focus on the key design issues.

Benefits of High-Performance Schools

The quality of school facilities affects the city, town, or district on many levels. Perhaps most important, high-performance schools help educate students. Six primary benefits resonate from the individual classroom to the district office:

- improved academic performance, as reflected by indicators such as higher test scores
- increased average daily attendance
- reduced operating costs
- increased teacher satisfaction and retention
- reduced liability exposure
- reduced environmental impacts.

Academic Performance

It makes intuitive sense that students in quiet, well-lit, and properly ventilated classrooms with healthy air will learn better because they are more comfortable, are sick less often, can see and hear better, and are less distracted by extraneous noise. Poor lighting, poor acoustics, and poor indoor air quality are barriers to education. The evidence that documents these advantages is incomplete, but a growing number of studies support a relationship between a school's physical condition—especially its lighting, acoustics, and indoor air quality—and student performance. These studies are well reviewed in several publications (e.g., Schneider 2002; Mendell and Heath 2005).

Lighting has profound effects on humans, and research has linked daylight with student performance. One study was based in school districts in California, Washington, and Colorado; students in classrooms with the most daylighting progressed 20% faster on math tests and 26% faster on reading tests in a one-year period than their counterparts in classrooms with the least amount of daylight (Heschong Mahone Group 2003a, 2003b). Swedish researchers followed 90 eight-year-old students for a year and found that behavior, hormone levels, and health were significantly associated with daylight levels. They concluded that poorly lit rooms "may influence the children's ability to concentrate or cooperate, and also eventually have an impact on annual body growth and sick leave" (Kuller and Lindsten 1992). And in a study in North Carolina, children who moved to daylit schools showed up to a 14% improvement in standardized test scores (Nicklas and Bailey 1996).

Indoor air quality may also have a substantial effect on learning. Inadequate outside air ventilation may lead to the accumulation of carbon dioxide, volatile organic compounds, and other indoor pollutants, which can cause discomfort, headaches, difficulty concentrating, and other symptoms (fig. 23.1). Virtually no research has addressed the association between indoor air quality and student academic performance (Mendell and Heath 2005). However, a summary of nearly 150 field investigations of indoor air quality complaints in schools in California and other states found high levels of headaches, fatigue, memory problems, eye irritation, cough, and other symptoms in affected schools (Daisey and Agnell 1998). Similar symptoms in office buildings have been associated with reduced worker productivity (Mendell and Heath 2005), suggesting that school IAQ problems can be severe and persistent enough to affect students' learning.

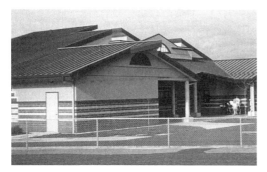

Figure 23.1. Natural ventilation. Despite the school's location in California's central valley, all of the instructional spaces in Roseville's 500-student Maidu Elementary School have completely natural ventilation. Classrooms have operable windows. The library and media center are surrounded by classrooms, limiting exterior exposure. Operable windows in these spaces create a chimney effect to draw air from the classrooms and exhaust it through clerestories, while spreading natural light throughout the space. In 1998 this school won a Coalition for Adequate School Housing/American Institute of Architects Award of Merit. (Photo courtesy of Stafford King Wiese Architects.)

Improved Attendance

The average daily attendance of students and staff is an important metric. Most children who miss school are not seriously ill, but missing school does indicate an illness severe enough to disrupt normal functioning and has implications for family members (such as parents who must miss work) as well (Weitzman 1986). Moreover, frequent absenteeism predicts lower academic performance and social problems (Rozelle 1968). Although many factors can influence whether a student comes to school, inadequate facilities can cause and exacerbate disorders that lead to absenteeism.

A key example is asthma, which is a leading cause of school absenteeism and accounts for more school absences than any other chronic disease (Parcel et al., 1979; Celano and Geller 1993; Mannino et al. 2002). Asthma exacerbations may be triggered by poor indoor air quality. Improved air quality in schools would be expected to reduce absenteeism, thereby improving learning and reducing costs (Rosen and Richardson 1999).

Reduced Operating Costs

High-performance schools are specifically designed—using life-cycle cost methods—to minimize the long-term costs of facility ownership (fig. 23.2). By using less energy and water than standard schools, they have lower overall operating costs—a notable advantage in times of rising and uncertain energy prices—and, with good operation and maintenance, will continue to do so for the life of the facility. School districts can save 20–40% on annual utility costs for new schools and 20–30% for renovated schools by applying high-performance design concepts (fig. 23.3). In a recent study of green schools, annual financial benefits exceed the costs of building "green" by more than 15-fold; of these benefits, about 25% represents reduced energy costs, and more than 50% represents increased future earnings for students related to their improved academic performance (Kats et al. 2005). These savings can be used to supplement other budgets, such as maintenance, computers, books, special education, additional classrooms, and salaries.

Increased Teacher Satisfaction and Retention

Many school districts face teacher shortages and high turnover rates. The educational and financial costs of recruiting and training teachers are significant. High-performance classrooms are designed to be pleasant, effective places to work. Visual and thermal comfort is high, acoustics are good, and the indoor air is fresh and clean. Such environments become positive factors in recruiting and retaining teachers and in improving their overall satisfaction with their work (Kats et al. 2005).

Reduced Liability Exposure

Because they emphasize health and superior indoor environmental quality, high-performance school buildings may reduce a district's exposure to health-related problems, lawsuits, and adverse publicity. Remediation expenses for schools with indoor environment problems often reach a quarter of a million dollars, and legal costs can be much higher. Consequently, proactive measures that prevent problems are sound investments.

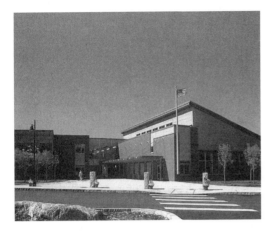

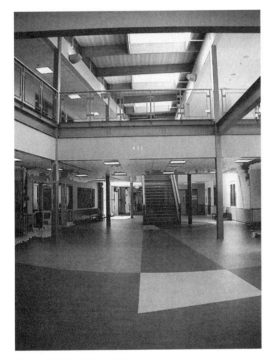

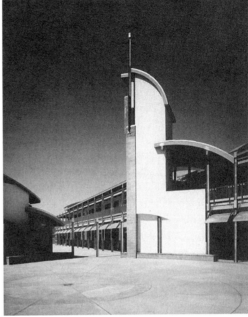

Figure 23.3. Energy efficiency in a school. At Wangenheim Middle School in San Diego, California, this 24-classroom addition is designed to optimize energy efficiency and indoor comfort using passive systems. The site and envelope design of the new one- and two-story buildings promote cross-ventilation and daylighting through the use of operable windows, clerestories, light shelves, and interior reflective surfaces. Appropriately sized shading devices protect the interiors from unwanted solar gain. Teacher response has been favorable. Comments include: "On bright days, we operate the classrooms frequently without any of the lights on." "We like the cross-ventilation. These classrooms are much more comfortable than the others. On hot days, the classrooms are at least ten degrees cooler than the portables." (Photo courtesy of Platt/Whitelaw Architects, Hewitt Garrison, photographer.)

Figure 23.2. High-performance school. The design approach of the Chickering School in Dover, Massachusetts, emphasizes the importance of the educational environment, focusing on natural light, indoor air quality, and acoustics. Standard unit ventilation was rejected in favor of a quieter, fully ducted, 100% outside air ventilation system. This system includes heat recovery of the exhaust air in order to reduce energy costs. Natural light is abundant, with all classrooms glazed from wall to wall. Interior public spaces surround a sky-lit commons, which also receives natural light from the two-story glazed walls at each end. (Photo courtesy of Flansburgh Associates.)

Reduced Environmental Impacts

High-performance school buildings are designed to have low environmental impact. They are energy and water efficient. They use durable, nontoxic materials high in recycled content, and the buildings themselves can be recycled. They preserve pristine natural areas on their sites and restore damaged ones. And they use nonpolluting, renewable energy to the greatest extent possible. As a consequence, these facilities are good environmental "citizens" and are designed to stay that way for their entire lifetime.

Achieving a High-Performance School

Building a school that encompasses all of these concepts requires an integrated, "whole building" team approach to the design process. From the beginning of the design process, key systems and technologies must be considered together and optimized based on their combined impact on the comfort and productivity of students and teachers. The 14 items listed in box 23.1 provide guidance for creating a high-performance school.

Set Design Goals Early and Use an Integrated Design

The typical design process for schools begins with programming and the selection of an architectural-engineering team. The sooner high-performance goals are considered in the design process, the easier and less costly they are to incorporate. The goals established during programming should be clearly stated in all aspects of project documentation—in the educational specifications, in the re-

quest for proposals to select the design team, in the instruction to bidders, and as part of the project summary.

Integrated design is the consideration and design of all building systems and components together. It unites the various disciplines involved in designing a building and reviews their recommendations as a whole. It recognizes that each discipline's recommendations have an impact on other aspects of the building project, allowing for optimization of both building performance and cost. Too often, for example, HVAC systems are designed independently of lighting systems, and lighting systems are designed without consideration of daylighting opportunities. The architect, mechanical engineer, electrical engineer, contractors, and other team members all have their scopes of work and often pursue them without adequate communication and interaction with other team members, resulting in oversized systems or systems that are optimized for atypical conditions.

For a high-performance school, team collaboration and integration of design choices should begin no later than the programming phase. The team may be more broadly defined than in the past and include energy analysts, materials consultants, cost consultants, lighting designers, and commissioning agents. Design activities may include charrettes, modeling, and simulations.

Consider Renovation Instead of New Construction

Some states now encourage renovation and reuse of existing facilities, an approach that is environmentally preferable from many standpoints. It takes advantage of existing infrastructure such as utility, water, and sewer services, it minimizes the conversion of "greenfield" land, it reduces resource use, and it often enables schools to be located in residential neighborhoods rather than in remote locations, permitting children to walk and bike to school (see chapter 22). Many states and school systems previously followed a guideline known as the "50% rule," under which a renovation projected to cost more than 50% of the equivalent new construction would not be approved. However, budget constraints and environmental concerns are spurring a growing preference for renovation.

▦ *23.1. Achieving a high-performance school*

1. Set district goals early and use an integrated design.
2. Consider renovation instead of new construction.
3. Choose and develop the site wisely.
4. Use sustainable construction practices.
5. Choose materials wisely.
6. Use high-performance HVAC strategies.
7. Protect the indoor air quality.
8 Use daylighting.
9. Install high-performance lighting and controls.
10. Optimize acoustics.
11. Minimize water use.
12. Do not forget the portables.
13. Train the staff and maintain the building.
14. Commission the school. ▦

Choose and Develop the Site Wisely

A school district faces many issues during site selection. Cost, student demographics, and environmental concerns all influence when sites are acquired and how the district uses them. As a crucial element in determining the overall sustainability of the school design, sites are sometimes purchased years in advance, and some options are thus out of the control of the districts and/or designers at the time the school is built. However, districts that are considering multiple sites can substantially lower the environmental impact of the school by wisely choosing their location, carefully orienting the buildings, protecting the ecosystems, and designing to control urban heat islands. Protecting student health is an essential consideration during site selection. Caution should be exercised when considering "brownfield" (former industrial) sites or locations near pollutant sources. Sites must not contain toxins, pollutants, or safety hazards that will impact student well-being. Of particular concern are:

- hazardous agents, including industrial, agricultural, and naturally occurring pollutants such as asbestos and heavy metals. Hazardous materials in existing buildings are also a concern.
- nearby facilities that might reasonably be anticipated to produce harmful air emissions or to handle hazardous or acutely hazardous materials
- other objects that are potentially harmful if located near a school, such as hazardous pipelines, heavily trafficked roads, high-voltage power-line easements, railroad tracks, high noise levels, and airports.

In addition to protecting student and staff health, districts should also consider ways to protect valuable land and open space. Options include:

- Channeling development to sites that are centrally located within the student population. Over the lifetime of the building, schools and parents invest significant amounts of time, energy, and money transporting students to and from class. Cars driven by parents, guardians, or the students themselves are the largest resource users and sources of transportation-related pollution. Centrally located sites allow more students to walk or bike to school, an important health goal (see chapter 22), and also to reduce the distance cars must travel.
- Entering joint use agreements in which parts of the school buildings, parks, or recreation space are shared with community organizations. Joint use is a growing trend across the country because it can have a variety of benefits, including increasing campus security, improving community integration, and reducing site acquisition and construction costs.
- Avoiding development on prime farmland, within flood zones, on habitat for threatened or endangered species, or public parkland
- Avoiding development on greenfields. Greenfields are defined as sites that have not been previously developed or have been restored to agricultural, forestry, or park use. Urban redevelopment reduces environmental impacts by utilizing established infrastructure and preserving the open space of undeveloped lands.
- Promoting alternative transportation. The energy use and pollution associated with transportation often dwarf the total lifetime energy used by the school itself. Locating the site close to public transportation, creating bike facilities and safe access, and offering bus service all reduce the automobile-related pollution.

The orientation of the buildings on the site is also important because optimal orientation can greatly reduce energy consumption related to heating and cooling. When site conditions permit, buildings should be oriented with their major windows facing either north or south (except in the far northern latitudes). Position classrooms so that light and air can be introduced from two sides. Utilize the potential contributions of the sun, topography, and existing vegetation for increased energy efficiency by maximizing heat gain (or minimizing heat loss) in winter and minimizing heat gain in summer. In the case of existing buildings, the arrangement of interior spaces, strategic landscaping, and modifications to the building envelope can mitigate an unfavorable orientation.

The orientation can also help with noise control. Reduce the impact of exterior noise sources by locating noise-sensitive areas such as classrooms, away from noise sources such as roadways and train tracks.

A high-performance school is designed for ecosystem protection. As much as possible, the school incorporates products and techniques that do not introduce pollutants or otherwise degrade the project site. Designers should take steps to preserve natural features and restore damaged areas whenever possible.

Storm water runoff is precipitation that flows over surfaces on the site and enters either the sewage system or receiving waters. Storm water carries sediment and pollutants from the site into the sewage system and/or local bodies of water. In addition, the cumulative runoff throughout the local area requires significant investments in municipal infrastructure to handle peak runoff loads. Reducing the amount of runoff is the most effective way to minimize its negative impacts. Strategies include (1) significantly reducing impervious surfaces, maximizing on-site storm water infiltration, and retaining pervious and vegetated areas, and (2) capturing rainwater from impervious areas of the building for groundwater recharge or reuse within the building.

Heat islands are caused when surfaces such as parking lots and rooftops absorb the sun's energy, warm up, and radiate heat. On the school site, rising temperatures make the air conditioners work harder, increasing discomfort and energy costs. Across an entire metropolitan area, the heat island effect substantially increases the amount of energy used for air-conditioning and exacerbates urban smog problems. Providing shade is the best way to reduce the heat island effect. Where possible, shade dark surfaces such as parking lots and walkways or replace them with vegetation. Alternatively, use materials with a high reflectance. Cool roofs reflect most of the sun's energy instead of absorbing and radiating it into the interior spaces below.

Use Sustainable Construction Practices

During the construction of new buildings and the renovation of existing ones, general and trade contractors play a significant role in making efficient use of materials, preventing future indoor air quality problems, and protecting the site from degradation. These responsibilities take several forms.

Effective job-site waste management reduces the amount of construction and demolition waste generated and diverts materials from disposal to reuse (salvage) and recycling. Some waste reduction can be designed into the building project, such as standardized dimensioning, the use of modular or panelized building units, reduced corners and angles in the structural footprint, and the layout of openings. A feasible goal is to recycle, compost, and/or salvage 50–75% (by weight) of construction, demolition, and land-clearing waste. The materials included in this effort include corrugated cardboard, metals, concrete brick, asphalt, land-clearing debris, beverage containers, clean dimensional wood, plastic, glass, gypsum board, and carpet.

In general, construction and demolition waste reduction should reduce overall construction costs, especially as this becomes standard operating procedure and the construction and demolition recycling and reuse infrastructure matures. If revenues from waste reduction, reuse, salvage, and recycling are allocated to the contractor, it gives the contractor both the responsibility and an incentive for waste reduction. Most contractors report that having a good waste reduction program in place results in a cleaner, safer site.

Indoor air quality should be protected during construction through planning and preventive job-site practices.

It is also important to protect the site during construction by paying attention to soil disturbances, erosion, and sedimentation in receiving waterways. An effective site protection plan includes construction practices that eliminate unnecessary site disturbance, minimize impact on the site's natural (soil and water) functions, and eliminate water pollution and water quality degradation. To achieve these goals, the protection plan should include protocols for operating and parking construction equipment, protecting and reusing topsoil and vegetation, managing hazardous materials, and installing and maintaining erosion control and storm water management measures.

Contractors can play a key role in effective commissioning by providing timely documentation, understanding the importance of thorough testing and tuning, paying attention to detail when correcting problems, and in general being responsive to the commissioning agent's recommendations and requests.

Choose Materials Wisely

Embedded within all materials are the resources, energy, chemicals, and environmental impacts of their entire life cycle, from the time they are produced and installed until they are ultimately recycled or buried in a landfill, possibly in your own community. Interior surfaces and furnishings provide an excellent opportunity to highlight the high-performance approach. Environmentally preferable choices of materials simultaneously protect the health of students, staff, and the larger natural environment. On its Environmentally Preferable Purchasing web site, the U.S. Environmental Protection Agency states that "environmentally preferable" refers to "products or services that have a lesser or reduced effect on human health and the environment when compared with competing products or services that serve the same purpose" (http://www.epa.gov/opptintr/epp/).

In a high-performance school, materials are selected for their efficiency and effect on indoor environmental quality. These criteria go beyond the traditional issues of performance, price, availability, and aesthetics. Box 23.2 outlines the basics of material selection. Other important concepts include:

- designing an area within the building dedicated to separating, collecting, storing, and transporting materials for recycling, including paper, glass, plastics, and metals
- reducing the amount of construction waste

■ *23.2. Guidelines for environmentally responsible material choices*

Designers should look for materials that are:

- Durable. These types of materials have been shown to offer a longer service life than other options in a given product category.
- Readily available. Designing with common, modular dimensions and specifying building systems that precisely fit the module promotes materials conservation. Using preconstructed building elements can also reduce waste. Materials should also be marketed in an environmentally responsible manner (e.g., sold with minimal packaging).
- Salvaged or reused. This includes materials that are refurbished and used for a similar purpose; they have not been processed or remanufactured for another use.
- Sustainably produced. This means they are extracted, harvested, or manufactured in an environmentally friendly manner. This includes materials that are grown or cultivated and can be replaced in a relatively time (i.e., rapidly renewable materials). One example is certified wood products, which are produced from trees grown and harvested from forests that are certified and sustainably managed by the Forest Stewardship Council (FSC). The FSC is the accrediting agency for organizations such as the Smart Wood program of the Rainforest Alliance and the Forest Conservation program of Scientific Certification Systems, which in turn oversee forestry practices and certify their sustainability.
- Made with recycled content, which includes materials that have been recovered or otherwise diverted from the solid waste stream, after-consumer use (postconsumer), or the manufacturing process (preconsumer). Always maximize the amount of postconsumer material. Specify products with higher postconsumer recycled content because this is waste that would have gone into landfills. High amounts of secondary or preconsumer content may perpetuate inefficient manufacturing processes. The use of recycled materials helps address problems of solid waste disposal, energy used during manufacture, and the consumption of natural, virgin resources. Related materials are those made with industrial byproducts (fly ash, for example) and include material that is created as a result of an industrial process.
- Recyclable. These materials can be collected, separated, or otherwise recovered from the solid waste stream for reuse or from the manufacture or assembly of another package or product. ■

that goes to landfills with a management plan for sorting and recycling it. Consider a goal of recycling or salvaging 75% (by weight) of total construction, demolition, or land-clearing waste.

- maximizing materials efficiency through the use of standard dimensions that reduce waste during construction. For example, modular systems such as carpet tile instead of carpet greatly minimize this particular construction waste stream. Additional building techniques for minimizing waste include reducing unnecessary corners and angles in the structural footprint and utilizing preconstructed elements, such as modular wall panels.

Use High-Performance HVAC Strategies

A school's HVAC strategy brings together many important characteristics of high-performance design, including energy efficiency, thermal and acoustic comfort, and indoor air quality. When designed, installed, and maintained correctly, HVAC systems are rarely noticed and quietly deliver the benefits of clean, comfortable air. However, if problems arise, HVAC systems can quickly become the largest source of service calls and comfort complaints. Chose an HVAC strategy that optimizes performance over the lifetime of the building, is easy to control, and meets the needs (and maintenance skills) of the district.

Energy efficiency is a key consideration, as the HVAC system is one of the largest energy consumers in a school. Even modest improvements in efficiency can yield relatively large savings to a school's operating budget. With the highly efficient systems available today—and the sophisticated analysis tools that can be used to select and size them—there is no reason why every school HVAC system cannot be designed to the highest levels of performance.

Always consider life cycle costs of operation and maintenance when choosing an HVAC strategy. To ensure peak operating efficiency, the HVAC system in a high-performance school should:

- Use high-efficiency equipment. When possible, model the energy use of the entire facility with energy modeling software. The U.S. Department of Energy's guidebook *School Operations and Maintenance: Best Practices for Con-*

trolling Energy Costs (2004) and the U.S. EPA Energy Star program (www.energystar.gov) are two places to start when looking for high-efficiency equipment. Consider recovery systems that preheat or precool incoming ventilation air and "economizer cycles" for small, packaged systems. In hot, dry climates, consider evaporative cooling.

- Be sized correctly for the estimated demands of the facility. Select systems that operate well under partial-load conditions, and consider standard HVAC sizing safety factors as upper limits. Apply any safety factors to a reasonable base condition for the building, not the hottest or coldest day of the year with maximum attendance and not the most temperate day of the year with the school half full.
- Include controls that boost system performance. Provide individual HVAC controls for each classroom. Consider integrated building management systems that control HVAC, lighting, outside air ventilation, water heating, and building security.

The key to optimizing HVAC system performance is an integrated design approach that considers the building as an interactive whole rather than as an assembly of individual components. For example, the benefits of an energy-efficient building may be negated if the HVAC equipment is not sized to take advantage of it. Oversized systems, based on rule-of-thumb sizing calculations, will not only cost more but will also be too large ever to run at peak efficiency and will waste energy every time they turn on. An integrated approach, based on an accurate estimate of the impact of the high-efficiency building, will allow the HVAC system to be sized for optimum performance. The resulting system will cost less to purchase, use less energy, and run more efficiently over time.

High-performance HVAC systems also promote thermal comfort, which is primarily a function of the temperature and relative humidity in a room, but air speed and the temperature of the surrounding surfaces also affect it. A high-performance school should ensure that rooms and HVAC systems are designed to allow temperature and humidity levels to remain within the "comfort zone" at all points in an occupied space. Thermal comfort guidelines, listed below, are discussed further in chapter 5:

- Design in accordance with the standards of the American Society of Heating, Refrigerating and Air Conditioning Engineers (ASHRAE). Standard 55-1992 (with 1995 addenda) defines thermal comfort standards. When a design incorporates natural ventilation (e.g., operable windows to provide direct outdoor air during temperate weather), consider adjusting the requirements of ASHRAE Standard 55-1992 to account for the impact.
- Install controls and monitor system performance. Provide controls in each classroom to give teachers direct control over thermal comfort. Evaluate the potential impact of such controls on the overall efficiency of the HVAC system. Consider temperature and humidity monitoring as part of the building's overall energy management system to ensure optimal thermal comfort performance.
- Analyze room configurations and HVAC distribution layouts to ensure that all parts of a room are receiving adequate ventilation and that heat gains from windows and skylights are properly controlled.

Thermal comfort is strongly influenced by the way in which a specific room is designed (for example, the amount of heat its walls and roof gain or lose, the amount of sunlight its windows let in, whether the windows can be opened) and by how effectively the HVAC system can meet the specific needs of that room. Balancing these two factors—room design and HVAC system design—is a back-and-forth process that continues throughout all of the stages of developing a new facility. In a high-performance school, the process ends with an optimal blend of both components: rooms configured for high student and teacher productivity and served by an energy-efficient HVAC system that is designed, sized, and controlled to maintain thermal comfort under all conditions.

Protect Indoor Air Quality

The need for excellent air quality in schools is discussed in chapter 10. A high-performance school should provide superior indoor air quality by eliminating and controlling the sources of contamination, providing adequate ventilation, commissioning the building, and implementing effective operations and maintenance procedures.

Adequate ventilation is the cornerstone of good indoor air quality and is critical to removing indoor pollutants from the classroom. Many schools do not meet the recommended ventilation levels specified in ASHRAE Standard 62.1-2004). A 1995 California Energy Commission (CEC) report (Lagus Applied Technologies 1995) found that schools consistently had substandard ventilation rates and that one in three classrooms was ventilated at less than half the legal minimum. Even when a room has sufficient ventilation, the air may not be distributed effectively to all its occupants. Of particular concern are portable classrooms with loud HVAC systems. Teachers are commonly forced into the unacceptable compromise of turning off noisy air conditioners (and sacrificing ventilation) in order to communicate with their students. Districts and designers must ensure that the proper amount of air is reaching all students and staff.

Maintenance practices are crucial to preventing indoor air quality problems. Mold and microbial growth are the largest potential problems (see chapter 11). Any moisture intrusions or spills must be cleaned up thoroughly and immediately to prevent mold from growing. Once mold is established, it can be very difficult to effectively remove; accordingly, prevention is essential. All of the teachers and staff members should be trained on how to identify and prevent mold.

HVAC systems must be regularly inspected and maintained to ensure adequate ventilation rates. Filters should be regularly replaced to ensure their effectiveness.

Maintenance practices themselves can introduce and/or remove pollutants. Regular carpet and floor cleanings minimize surface dust. Many cleaning solutions emit volatile organic compounds and other chemicals that can remain in the classrooms and cause indoor air quality problems. Districts should consider using interior surfaces that require less frequent or less toxic maintenance practices. They should also evaluate their cleaning and landscape management products and consider less toxic alternatives (see chapter 14). Because herbicides and pesticides are of particular concern, districts should employ integrated pest management techniques to minimize the use of potentially toxic pesticides (see chapter 13).

Material selection may play an important role in avoiding IAQ problems. Architects may be required to specify materials that resist the growth of molds and mildews and that minimize emissions. Some school designers require manufacturers to perform chamber testing of their materials prior to installing them in schools. The testing is capable of identifying hundreds of potentially harmful chemicals and their rates of emission. This information may be combined with information on the surface area of the material, the volume of the room, and the ventilation rate to determine whether the material is safe. At its web site (www.chps.net), the Collaborative for High-performance Schools (CHPS) provides a list of materials that have been tested to be safe in schools. Tests are in accordance with the California Department of Health Services Standard Practice.

Use Daylighting

Daylighting is central to sustainable, high-performance school design. A high-performance school should provide a rich visual environment—one that enhances, rather than hinders, learning and teaching—by carefully integrating natural and electric lighting strategies; by balancing the quantity and quality of light in each room; and by controlling or eliminating glare.

Principles for designing daylit schools are shown in box 23.3. In implementing these principles, it is important to use integrated design principles, to communicate daylighting goals clearly with the design team, and—at the conclusion of the project—to educate the buildings' occupants about how the systems work. Lighting options range from no-cost and low-cost choices to sophisticated state-of-the-art systems, so solutions are available for widely differing budgets.

Install High-Performance Lighting and Controls

Electric lighting is one of the major energy uses in schools. Enormous savings are possible through the use of efficient equipment, effective controls, and careful design. Using less electric lighting reduces a major source of heat gain, thus reducing air-conditioning demand, increasing the potential for natural ventilation, and reducing the space's radiant temperature (improving thermal comfort). Electric lighting design also strongly affects visual performance and visual comfort by maintaining adequate, appropriate illumination and controlling reflec-

tance and glare. Finally, visual, accessible light and power meters can educate students and faculty about how lighting systems and energy controls work. Box 23.4 provides guidelines for electric lighting design.

Optimize Acoustics

The detrimental effects of excessive noise in schools are discussed in chapter 4. Recognition of the widespread acoustic problems in U.S. schools spurred the development in 2002 of ANSI Standard S12.60-2002, the American National Standard Acoustical Performance Criteria, Design Requirements, and Guidelines for Schools. The information and tools needed to design classrooms for high acoustical performance are readily available and can be used to ensure that any newly constructed classroom provides an acoustic environment that enhances the learning experience for both students and teachers. To ensure a superior acoustical environment, designers should:

- reduce sound reverberation time inside the classroom
- limit the transmission of noise from outside the classroom. Standard building construction and glazing do not easily control exterior noise intrusion from traffic and/or aircraft.
- minimize background noise from the building's HVAC system. Teachers must sometimes resort to shutting off ventilation systems that are too loud, which can have the unfortunate side effects of reducing indoor air quality and thermal comfort. Typical, low first-cost heating and ventilating systems often cannot meet the recommended levels for background noise. Unit ventilators, "through-the-wall" systems, and window-mounted air conditioners are the worst performers.

These issues are discussed in more detail in chapter 4.

Minimize Water Use

A high-performance school should control and reduce water runoff from its site, consume fresh water as efficiently as possible, and recover and reuse gray water to the extent feasible. Basic water efficiency measures can often reduce a school's water use by 30% or more. These reductions help the local and

---

■ *23.3. Six principles for designing schools with daylighting*

The following six principles provide fundamental guidance in designing schools that utilize daylighting:

1. Prevent direct sunlight penetration in classrooms. Direct-beam sunlight is an extremely strong source of light. It is so bright and hot that it can create great visual and thermal discomfort, although it may also provide a comfortable, warm, sunny spot for reading or activities for small children in the winter months especially. Daylight, on the other hand, which comes from the blue sky, from clouds, or from diffused or reflected sunlight, is more gentle and can efficiently provide excellent illumination without the negative impacts of direct sunlight.

2. Provide gentle, uniform illumination. Daylight is most successful when it gives gentle, even illumination throughout a space. Evenly diffused daylight will provide the most energy savings and the best visual quality. Daylight designers achieve this balanced diffuse daylighting by using techniques such as clerestories (structures that extend above roofs and whose walls contain windows for lighting the interior) and luminaires (fixtures that contain a light source together with components to position the lamps and distribute the light). The arrangement of reflective surfaces that help distribute the light are just as important as the arrangement of daylight openings for providing gentle, uniform illumination.

3. Avoid glare. Excessively high contrast causes glare. Direct glare is the presence of a bright surface (for example, a bright, diffusing glazing or direct view of the sun) in the field of view that causes discomfort or diminished visual performance.

4. Provide control of daylight. Because it is highly variable throughout the day and the year, daylight requires careful design to provide adequate illumination for the maximum number of hours while contributing as little as possible to the cooling load. Teachers should have easy access to controls for shades or blinds to adjust light levels as needed throughout the day. These systems should be reliable, easy to operate, and economical to clean and repair.

5. Integrate with electric lighting design. The daylight and the electric light systems should be designed together so they complement each other to create high-quality lighting. This requires an understanding of how both systems deliver light to a space. The electric lighting should be circuited and controlled to coincide with the patterns of daylight in the space, so that the lights can be turned off in areas where daylight is abundant and left on where it is deficient.

6. Plan the layout of the interior spaces. Successful daylighting designs must include a careful consideration of the interior space planning. Since daylighting illuminance can vary considerably within a space, especially with side lighting, it is important to locate work areas that have appropriate daylighting. ■

---

regional environment while decreasing operating expenses. While current cost savings may be modest (since water is relatively inexpensive in most areas of the country), there is a strong potential that savings will rise over time, especially in areas where water is scarce and becoming more expensive.

Design landscaping to use water efficiently by reducing water use and specifying hardy, native vegetation. Consider using an irrigation system for athletic fields only, not for plantings near buildings or in parking lots. Where irrigation is used, use high-efficiency irrigation technology (e.g., drip ir-

rigation in lieu of sprinklers). If the local climate allows, use captured rain or recycled site water for irrigation, and utilize cisterns for capturing rainwater.

Set water use goals for the school. A good initial target is 20% less than the water use calculated for the building after meeting the fixture performance requirements of the Energy Policy Act of 1992. This can be reached with a combination of water-conserving fixtures and equipment such as low-flow or waterless toilets and urinals, automatic lavatory faucet shut-off controls, low-flow show-

■ *23.4. Principles of electric lighting design*

The principles of electric lighting design are discussed in chapter 3 and are covered only briefly here.

Horizontal Illumination

Longstanding customs and antiquated standards, on which many school lighting systems were based, often result in excessively high horizontal light levels. The Illuminating Engineering Society of North America (IESNA) now recommends a horizontal illuminance level of 30 foot-candles for most classroom and office reading tasks, although some classroom tasks may justify up to 50 foot-candles (IESNA 2000); lighting in this range is a good choice.

Vertical Illumination

Adequate vertical illumination is key. Most visual tasks other than desktop reading are heads-up activities that require proper vertical illuminance. Adequate vertical illuminance also creates a sense of lighting quality, supports social communication, and, at night, promotes facial recognition to enhance a sense of safety and security.

Glare Control

Light sources that are too bright create uncomfortable glare. In extreme cases, direct or reflected glare can also impair visual performance by reducing task visibility. Glare causes eye fatigue by forcing the eyes to work much harder. All sources of light, including daylight, must be carefully controlled to avoid causing discomfort or a disabling glare. Common problems in classrooms include uncomfortable direct glare from overhead sources, reflected glare from computer screens and whiteboards, and direct glare from uncontrolled windows or skylights.

Lighting Uniformity

For the most part, illuminate school-building spaces as uniformly as possible and avoid shadows or sharp patterns of light and dark. Uniformity can be achieved by avoiding traditional recessed or surface-mounted parabolic fixtures, restricting very bright sources to high spaces such as gyms, using cove lighting and indirect luminaires in ordinary classrooms and other spaces, using light-colored surface materials, and illuminating vertical surfaces and ceilings.

Lighting Control Flexibility

Lighting controls should be user friendly and flexible, with multiple-level switching or separate circuiting of light fixtures. This permits teachers to adjust the lighting according to changing needs or daylight levels and helps save energy. Teachers should be able to override automatic dimming and/or occupancy sensor controls so that they can switch lights off when necessary.

Integration with Daylight

Integrating electric light with daylight is one of the more challenging aspects of school lighting design. Luminaires should be circuited to match the way daylight enters a space. Those closest to windows or skylights should be circuited separately from the other lights to allow them to be turned off during the day. Dimmers permit additional flexibility in balancing electric lights with daylight. ■

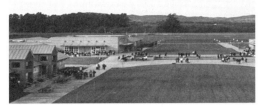

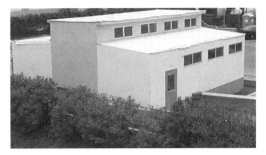

Figure 23.4. Reclaimed water. The grounds at Windsor High School in Windsor, California, are irrigated with reclaimed water from the local water municipality. The municipality waived the hookup costs, and the school saves money every month by not using potable water for irrigation. (Photo courtesy of Quattrocchi Kwok Architects.)

erheads, and high-efficiency dishwashers and laundry appliances.

Use reclaimed water. Reclaimed water is treated, nonpotable water and is an excellent resource for irrigation or flushing toilets. Reclaimed water is available in many areas at low and sometimes no cost (fig. 23.4).

Don't Forget the Portables

Portable (or "relocatable") classrooms have been a feature of U.S. schools for years. From a school district's perspective, the two advantages of relocatable classrooms are low initial cost and short time between specification and occupancy. They are intended to provide flexibility to school districts because they enable quick response to demographic changes and can be moved from one school to another as demographics change (fig. 23.5). However, relocatable classrooms often become permanent fixtures of the school.

The effects of poor indoor air quality in relocatable classrooms are no different from those in permanent classrooms. School buildings generally use similar construction and furnishing materials, so the types of chemicals present in indoor air are not likely to be different for relocatable versus permanent classrooms. However, pressed-wood products (often with high concentrations of formaldehyde) are used more in the factory-built relocatable units than in buildings constructed on-site. As result, levels of airborne chemicals may be higher in new relocatable classrooms, especially if ventilation is reduced (Shendell et al. 2004).

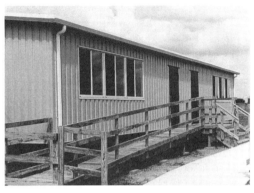

Figure 23.5. Rethinking the portable classroom. Typical modular classrooms (bottom) can pose problems with crowding, noise, lighting, and indoor air quality. Recognizing that relocatable classrooms are often used as permanent structures, Southern California Edison created its Rethinking the Portable Classroom program to redesign the standard relocatable building. The project, which involved numerous parties with an interest in relocatable classrooms, led to the development of a prototype (top) designed to be a cost-effective alternative to site-built projects. This model is constructed of metal with little or no use of wood other than the plywood sheeting used for flooring. (Photo courtesy of Parkline, Inc.)

The most common problems with relocatable classrooms include:

- poorly functioning HVAC systems that provide minimal ventilation of outside air
- poor acoustics as a result of loud ventilation systems
- chemical off-gassing from pressed wood and other high-emission materials, compounded by quick occupation after construction or installation of carpets
- site pollution from nearby parking lots or loading areas.

The solutions to these problems are the same as the recommendations for improving indoor air quality in permanent structures. Relocatables also range in quality. Care should be taken to ensure that money and student health are not compromised by low-quality designs.

Train the Staff and Maintain the Building

Effective maintenance and operations procedures are fundamentally important to sustaining the performance of all of the building systems. Student and staff health and productivity can be affected when these systems fail to operate as designed. Substandard maintenance or incorrect operation of the systems usually results from a combination of factors. First, maintenance budgets are often the first to be reduced or eliminated when money becomes tight. Second, contractors typically provide the building staff minimal or no training on how the systems are supposed to operate or be maintained. Finally, schools may lose institutional knowledge of the systems because of staff turnover and lack of communication. An environmental management system, which includes a hierarchy of responsibilities and protocols for training and transferring of duties, may help mitigate the loss of institutional knowledge.

Districts should create and execute a maintenance plan that addresses the following items:

- Educate the staff on the value of maintenance and how a properly functioning facility will help them educate their students.
- Establish a budget for maintenance.
- Hire qualified staff or contractors to perform tasks.
- Develop a preventive maintenance plan, including schedules for maintenance checks.
- Develop a predictive maintenance program to prevent problems from occurring.
- Use a work order system to track work orders, maintenance that has been performed, and the cost of each piece of equipment.
- Ensure that the maintenance staff has proper operation and maintenance manuals.
- Ensure the availability of recommended spare parts in the warehouse.
- Provide training to the maintenance staff.

High-performance schools are maintenance friendly. Building systems are easy to maintain, and the reduced operating costs from their energy-efficient design frees money that could be directed to support regular maintenance.

Commission the School

Commissioning is a systematic process of ensuring that all building systems perform interactively according to the contract documents, the design intent, and the district's operational needs. The commissioning process integrates the traditionally separate functions of design peer review; equipment startup; control system calibration; testing, adjusting, and balancing; equipment documentation; and facility staff training; it also includes the activities of documented functional testing and verification.

High-performance schools can be achieved only with some level of commissioning. No matter how carefully a school is designed, if the materials, equipment, and systems were not installed properly or are not operating as intended, the benefits of the high-performance design will not be achieved. Commissioning is a quality assurance program that is intended to show that the building has been constructed and performs as designed.

Commissioning is needed because many building systems do not operate as expected. A meta-analysis of findings from 85 studies of building commissioning (Mills et al. 2004) has revealed that buildings had an average of 32 deficiencies, the most common of which was HVAC malfunction. In many of the buildings, equipment that was specified in the plans was actually missing. Commissioning systematically uncovers such problems and monitors their solution.

Commissioning is occasionally confused with testing, adjusting, and balancing. Testing, adjusting, and balancing measure building air and water flows, but commissioning encompasses a much broader scope of work and typically involves four distinct phases: predesign, design, construction, and warranty. During the construction phase, commissioning calls for functional testing to determine how well the mechanical and electrical systems meet the operational goals established during the design process. Although commissioning can begin at the construction phase, districts receive the most cost-effective benefits when the process begins during the predesign phase, when the project team is assembled.

Commissioning can take place for either a single building system or the entire facility; however, the more comprehensive the commissioning, the greater the impact. Whichever level is chosen, a commissioning provider should be engaged during the design phase or earlier. It is therefore important that commissioning assignments—particularly those that state who will bear the cost of correcting conditions that do not meet specifications—are clearly spelled out in the beginning of the design process. For the best results, the provider should be an independent contractor or a member of the design team who is not directly involved in the design. The commissioning agent is responsible for implementing the commissioning plan, including the following tasks:

- Create a clear statement of the design intent of each building system. Write the commissioning specifications and incorporate them in the appropriate divisions of the construction documents.
- Carry out prefunctional and functional testing of all equipment and systems to be commissioned, using procedures designed in advance. Check installed equipment to ensure that all associated components and accessories are in place. Verify and document that systems are performing as expected and that all of the sensors and other system control devices are properly calibrated.
- Prepare comprehensive operation and maintenance manuals, and arrange for the training of the building operations staff.
- Ensure that all required documentation has been provided, such as a statement of the design intent and the operating protocols for all of the building systems. Give a final report with all of the commissioning documentation and recommendations to the district.
- Conduct ongoing monitoring for a specified time after the school is occupied to ensure that the equipment and systems continue to perform according to the design intent. Consider CO_2 monitoring systems in larger districts with well-equipped facilities management teams.

The Economics of High-Performance Schools

High-performance schools are cost effective for a number of reasons. For example, they can bring more money to the school by increasing average daily attendance; keep more money in the school by significantly reducing utility bills; and take advantage of currently available incentive programs (Kats et al. 2005).

Additional potential economic benefits flow from the avoided costs of workers' compensation claims and litigation. Discussed below are issues related to financing high-performance schools, including life-cycle costing, reduced operating expenses, increased funds, financial incentive and technical assistance programs, avoided costs, and reduced litigation risks.

Life-cycle Costing

School facilities are investments. State governments and local communities spend billions of dollars per year on building new facilities for current and future generations of students and on operating and maintaining existing facilities. Unfortunately, the institutional separation of operational and construction budgets can create schools that are economically, environmentally, and educationally poor investments.

Many high-performance measures can be incorporated into a school design without increasing costs, but additional investments can increase the health and efficiency of the school even further. However, conventional financing methodologies separate construction and operations budgets and sometimes omit future building costs in construction decisions. As a result, design measures that save money over the long term may be rejected because of higher initial costs. High-performance windows, for example, may cost more initially but may result in energy savings that pay for the extra costs in a few years and then continue to save the school money for years to come.

Life-cycle costing is a means of calculating and comparing different designs to identify the best investment over time. All building expenses that can be calculated are included in the analysis, including initial costs (design and construction); operating costs (energy, water, other utilities, and personnel);

and maintenance, repair, and replacement expenses. The values are adjusted for the time value of money to represent the true value of the investment. Predicted costs for alternative design approaches can then be compared, allowing the district to select the design that provides the lowest overall cost of ownership consistent with the desired quality level.

Life-cycle cost analysis, however, addresses only some of the benefits of high-performance design. Many benefits, such as improved health and test scores, are valuable but difficult to quantify monetarily. A more detailed description of life-cycle cost methods and techniques can be found at the website of the Center for High-performance Schools (http://www.chps.net) and on the center's Best Practices CD-ROM.

Reduced Operating Expenses

High-performance schools cost less to operate. School districts spend less for electricity, gas, water, maintenance, waste collection, and other ongoing operating costs, thereby enabling them to spend more money on salaries, books, teaching supplies, and other items with a more direct link to the true mission of schools: educating students.

How much savings can be expected? School districts can generally expect to save 30–40% on annual utility costs for new schools and 20–30% for renovated schools by applying high-performance design and sustainability concepts; these savings may even increase with more stringent energy measures. The potential for savings is greater in new schools because it is possible to steer clear of inefficiencies from the outset, thereby saving money year after year (fig. 23.6).

An integrated design is the key to savings of this magnitude. From the beginning of the design process, each of the building elements (windows, walls, building materials, air-conditioning, landscaping, etc.) is considered as a part of an integrated system of interacting components (fig. 23.7). Choices in one area often affect other areas; integrated design leverages these interactions to maximize the overall performance.

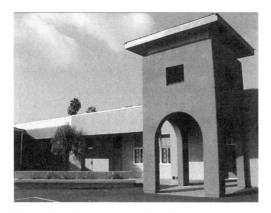

Figure 23.6. Saving money through energy measures. The San Diego Unified School District worked with San Diego Gas and Electric to find the most cost-effective and energy-efficient design solutions for Garfield Elementary School. The final design saves $100,000 annually. High-performance measures include external shading, highly insulated roofing, high-performance windows, T8 lighting, occupancy sensors, daylighting controls in selected spaces, skylights, and other measures. (Photo courtesy of San Diego Unified School District.)

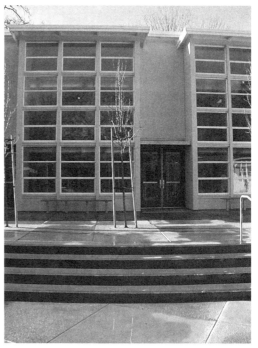

Figure 23.7. Great windows. These windows, viewed from the school courtyard, illuminate the large hallway and gathering space for middle school students. (Photo courtesy of Randy Karels.)

Avoidable Costs and Litigation Risk

The considerable costs of poor school IAQ are borne by students, staff, parents, and the community. In the school populations, the costs include poor health, reduced learning effectiveness, and increased frustration when IAQ problems become unmanageable. In particular, to the extent that overcrowded, poorly ventilated classrooms contribute to the spread of infectious diseases (e.g., colds, influenza) and poorly maintained carpets, dirty air ducts, and water-damaged materials contribute to asthma, allergy, and respiratory infections—some of which may have long-term health consequences—high-performance schools offer considerable potential for avoiding these associated costs, which are difficult to quantify. More easily counted are the strained budgets and staff resources expended by districts for facility repairs due to insufficient maintenance, community relations damage control, litigation, and workers' compensation claims. In addressing such problems, schools must use resources that would otherwise be available for educational and other programs.

References

American Society of Heating, Refrigeration, and Air-Conditioning Engineering. 2004. Ventilation for acceptable indoor air quality (Standards 62.1-2004). Available: http://www.ashrae.org.

Celano M, Geller R. 1993. Learning, school performance, and children with asthma: How much at risk? J Learn Disabil 26:23–32.

Daisey JM, Angell WJ. 1998. A survey and critical review of the literature on indoor air quality, ventilation, and health symptoms in schools. Berkeley: Environmental Energy Technologies Division, Lawrence Berkeley National Laboratory Report No. LBNL-41517. Available: http://www-library.lbl.gov/docs/LBNL/415/17/PDF/LBNL-41517.pdf [accessed 8 April 2005].

Daisey JM, Angell WJ, Apte MG. 2003. Indoor air quality, ventilation, and health symptoms in schools: An analysis of existing information. Indoor Air 13:53–64.

Heschong Mahone Group. 2003a. Daylighting in schools: Reanalysis report. Sacramento, CA: California Energy Commission (CEC Contract to New Buildings Institute No. P500-03-082-A-3). Available: http://www.newbuildings.org/downloads/FinalAttachments/A-3_Dayltg_Schools_2.2.5.pdf [accessed 15 January 2006].

Heschong Mahone Group. 2003b. Windows and classrooms: A study of student performance and the indoor environment. Available: http://www.new buildings.org/downloads/FinalAttachments/A-7_Windows_Classrooms_2.4.10.pdf [accessed 15 January 2006].

Illuminating Engineering Society of North America. 2000. Guide for educational facilities lighting. Document #IESNA RP-3-00. New York: Illuminating Engineering Society of North America.

Kats G, Perlman J, Jamadagni S. 2005. National Review of Green Schools: Costs, Benefits, and Implications for Massachusetts. Washington, DC: Capital E. Available: http://www.cap-e.com/ewebeditpro/items/O59F7707.pdf.

Kuller R, Lindsten C. 1992. Health and behavior of children in classrooms with and without windows. J Environ Psychol 12:305–317.

Lagus Applied Technologies. 1995. Air change rates in nonresidential buildings in California. Report P400-91-034BCN, prepared for the California Energy Commission. San Diego, CA: Lagus Applied Technologies.

Mannino DM, Homa DM, Akinbami LJ, Moorman JE, Gwynn C, Redd S. 2002. Surveillance for asthma, United States, 1980–1999. Mortal Morbid Weekly Rept Surveill Summ 51(SS-1) (March 29):1–13.

Mendell MJ, Heath GA. 2005. Do indoor pollutants and thermal conditions in schools influence student performance? A critical review of the literature. Indoor Air 15:27–52.

Mills E, Friedman H, Powell T, Bourassa N, Claridge D, Haasl T, Piette M. 2004. The cost effectiveness of commercial-buildings commissioning: A meta-analysis of energy and nonenergy impacts in existing buildings and new construction in the United States. LBNL-56637. Berkeley, CA: Lawrence Berkeley National Laboratory. Available: http://eetd.lbl.gov/emills/PUBS/PDF/Cx-Costs-Benefits.pdf [accessed 8 April 2005].

Nicklas M, Bailey G. 1996. Analysis of the performance of students in daylit schools. Raleigh, NC: Innovative Design. Available: http://www.innovativedesign.net/pdf/studentperformance.pdf [accessed 8 April 2005].

Niskar AS, Kieszad SM, Holmes A, Esteban E, Ruben C, Brody DJ. 1998. Prevalence of hearing loss among children 6 to 19 years of age. J Am Med Assoc 279(14):1071–1075.

Parcel G, Gilman S, Nader P, Bunce H. 1979. A comparison of absentee rates of elementary school children with asthma and nonasthmatic schoolmates. Pediatrics 64:878–881.

Piette MA, Nordman B, Greenberg S. 1994. Quantifying energy savings from commissioning: Preliminary results from the Pacific Northwest. In *Proceedings of the Second National Conference on Building Commissioning*. Berkeley, CA: Lawrence Berkeley National Laboratory.

Plympton P, Conway S, Epstein K. 2000. Daylighting in schools: Improving student performance and health at a price schools can afford. Presented at the American Solar Energy Society Conference, Madison, WI, June 16 [National Renewable Energy Laboratory, Golden, CO, NREL/CP-550-28049]. Available: http://www.deptplanetearth.com/pdfdocs/nrel_daylitschools.pdf [accessed 8 April 2005].

Rosen KG, Richardson G. 1999. Would removing indoor air particulates in children's environments reduce rate of absenteeism? A hypothesis. Sci Total Environ 234:87–93.

Rozelle R. 1968. Relationship between absenteeism and grades. Educ Psychol Meas 28:1151–1158.

Schneider M. 2002. Do school facilities affect academic outcomes? Washington, DC: National Clearinghouse for Educational Facilities. Available: http://www.edfacilities.org/pubs/outcomes.pdf.

Shendell DG, Winer AM, Weker R, Colome SD. 2004. Evidence of inadequate ventilation in portable classrooms: Results of a pilot study in Los Angeles County. Indoor Air 14:154–158.

U.S. Department of Energy. 2004. School operations and maintenance: Best practices for controlling energy costs. A guidebook for K–12 school system business officers and facilities managers. Prepared by Princeton Energy Resources International, HPowell Energy Associates, and Alliance to Save Energy. Washington, DC: Department of Energy. Available: http://www.energysmartschools.gov/attachments/SolutionCenter/SchoolEnergyGuidebookv2.pdf [accessed 8 April 2005].

Weitzman M. 1986. School absence rates as outcome measures in studies of children with chronic illness. J Chronic Dis 39:799–808.

24

David Mudarri

The Economics of Safe and Healthy Schools

■ *Summary*

- The operation of schools can be viewed in the same way as complex business operations that require smooth functioning, good staff, sound and healthy facilities, customer satisfaction, productive outcomes, and room for creativity and ingenuity.
- Each of these elements utilizes sound business practices to evaluate costs and benefits, assign resources, and then analyze the outcomes. ■

Suppose that a school system (or a single school) is considering a new educational program or a health intervention project or perhaps contemplating new construction. Perhaps school board members, PTA members, or interested citizens hear about the program and think it sounds like a good idea but have some doubts. To make an informed decision on whether the project is really worthwhile, they must have a systematic way to evaluate the issue in question. They hope that someone has done an economic analysis. If one has not been done, they may wish to request a breakdown of the estimated costs.

Alternatively, suppose that a school system is suffering financial constraints, and the school board or PTA members would like to turn to the marketplace for help. They contemplate selling snack foods, allowing restaurant chains to serve lunch to the students, or perhaps permitting other commercial interests to play a role in the school. They wish to balance the students' welfare with the need to provide revenue for the school, and they hope that someone can guide them through that process.

This chapter is designed to help with situations such as these and to help make the "business case" for safe and healthy schools. The first section deals with the economic evaluation of projects, policies, or proposals and provides a review of basic concepts and analytic techniques used to conduct economic evaluations. Most of the chapter is devoted to this subject. The second section introduces some basic concepts of economic behavior and the analysis of economic demand. This section is designed to help you assess the consequences of pricing and other strategies in programs in which goods and services are sold to students. This issue is less complex and is covered in less detail. The chapter concludes with three case studies (two real and one hypothetical) that help illustrate the principles described here.

Economic Analyses of Projects, Policies, or Proposals

Financial versus Economic Analysis

Economic analysis may seem similar to financial analysis, but it is broader. A financial analysis is limited to those aspects of a project for which there are direct budgetary implications (e.g., cost savings, revenue inflows, cost outflows). Such analysis is too limiting for most public programs that involve benefits that are not directly monetary (e.g., health, safety, environmental, and educational benefits). An economic analysis attempts to quantify these benefits and perhaps monetize them or, alternatively, develop a framework that incorporates consideration of these issues.

Types of Economic Analysis

Many types of economic analyses might be of interest to school personnel. Perhaps the most important—but sometimes difficult to understand—are those that either assess the economic value of benefits or evaluate the cost-effectiveness of various program options. This category includes cost-benefit analysis, cost-effectiveness analysis, and cost-utility analysis.

Cost–Benefit Analysis

In cost–benefit analysis, all or most of the costs and benefits are expressed in monetary units and then compared. If the benefits have a greater value than the costs, the project is deemed to be justified. In the real world, it is often difficult to evaluate all of the beneficial outcomes of a proposal in monetary terms. For example, what is the economic value of reducing school delinquency or improving student health? In addition, some benefits or costs may be only qualitatively included. Because of this, the cost-benefit analysis is an important factor in making decisions, but it is only one factor. Other political or community value considerations or the uncertainty of certain outcomes may outweigh the recommendations from such an analysis. Nevertheless, when a project or proposal has a range of various outcomes, cost-benefit analysis can be a powerful tool because the user can compare these outcomes on a consistent monetary basis.

Cost–effectiveness Analysis

Often a school system has already decided to fund a certain type of program and wishes only to determine the best approach. For example, perhaps the school already has a tobacco-use prevention program and is choosing among different proposals for implementing this program. The outcome measure for each proposal is the same—a quantified reduction in tobacco use. Which proposal is the most cost effective? To assess cost-effectiveness, one would estimate the tobacco reduction that could be achieved from each approach, as well as the cost of implementing each approach, and then calculate the ratio of the reduction in tobacco use to the cost. The proposal with the highest ratio would be the most cost effective (e.g., the lowest cost per cigarette avoided). Other types of projects would evaluate the cost per injury avoided or the cost per illness prevented. Unlike cost-benefit analysis, the monetary value of the outcome (e.g., reducing tobacco use, injuries, or illnesses in children) is not calculated, so these kinds of analysis are easier to do.

Cost–Utility Analysis

Cost–utility analysis is similar to cost-effectiveness, but it also evaluates the quality of the outcomes that might be derived from different program approaches. The most common use of cost–utility analysis is to determine the number of lives saved or spared from avoidable life-threatening illnesses. We all die eventually, and we have an expected life span, barring such illnesses. The quality of the years we have remaining depends on the degree to which such life-saving measures protect us from the debilitating aspects of an illness. Thus, a proposal that would preserve, on average, 20 years of life with no debilitating effects would be valued higher than a proposal that would preserve fewer years with a lower quality of life. How these are quantified and compared is subject to debate, although there are some accepted formulations referred to as "quality-of-life year" (QUALY) or disability-adjusted life year (DALY) measures. However, the weighting or scaling of any outcomes to reflect quality differences in other contexts might also be referred to as cost-utility analysis.

Direct versus Indirect Costs and Benefits

Costs and benefits may be monetary or nonmonetary, or they may be directly associated with a project or proposal. For example, consider a proposal to improve the indoor air quality for all schools in a district. Indoor air quality is important to the health and performance of children, as the school air may be overly polluted, contain allergens or irritants that overtly or subtly impact students, be too warm or too cold, or have uneven temperatures that affect student and teacher health, comfort, or performance (see chapter 10).

Direct impacts are those that affect the entity that is undertaking the proposal—in this case, the school district. Direct costs would be for labor and equipment to improve the school, and that may mean fixing the heating and cooling system, replacing some furnishings, improving maintenance and janitorial services, installing monitors, and other measures. Direct benefits might be (1) reduced cost of utilities (because of improved equipment efficiency); (2) fewer student and teacher absences; (3) an improved learning environment that could increase students' performance; (4) fewer complaints from parents, students, and staff, which weaken morale and take time and resources away from teaching and learning; and (5) possibly reduced litigation.

Indirect impacts are those that do not affect the entity. These may include fewer student illnesses and reduced medical expenditures for parents, less time that parents have to stay home to care for sick children and therefore miss work, and a greater attraction of young families into the school district. Often the indirect impacts will be of greater magnitude, but they may not be as persuasive in the final decisions. That is, it is doubtful that school systems would balance, dollar for dollar, a higher cost of equipment for the school with lower medical costs for parents. Such evaluations are dependent on the social and political context in which decisions are made and on how active and influential parents are in school decisions. In any case, both direct and indirect costs and benefits are important to consider. Analyses that skip over the indirect impacts could result in the wrong conclusions. Even if these indirect effects cannot be easily measured, they should at least be acknowledged and qualitatively discussed so they may be considered before a final decision is made.

Costs and Benefits over Time

Almost all projects will involve costs and benefits that accrue over time. With time, issues of inflation and the time value of money are involved, so a review of basic principles and techniques used for dealing with the time element of economic analysis is worthwhile.

Constant Dollars

The true cost of an item purchased is the value to the purchaser of the other things not purchased with the same money. With inflation, the cost of goods and services in general rise, so a dollar this year will buy fewer goods than the same dollar a few years ago. When comparing values of costs and benefits over time, it is important that the measuring device (in this case, dollars) remain stable in the sense of reflecting the true value of what is given up. Otherwise, the values in later years will be higher than in earlier years simply because of inflation, even if the true values have not changed. All economic comparisons over time, therefore, must be done in what is called "constant dollars" of a specified year. This is done by adjusting values in other years by an inflation index. Values are then reported in dollar values of a given year (e.g., 1997 dollars).

Discount Rates

When given a choice of receiving $1000 now or a year from now, most people would choose to receive it now rather than wait. This makes economic sense because, if you receive it now, you can put it into a savings account or otherwise invest it at some rate of return (e.g., 5%) so that you will have more money (e.g., $1050) a year from now. Looking at the same situation in reverse, you would need to discount next year's receipt of $1000 by some rate (e.g., 5%) to calculate its present value, which in this case would be only $952. This amount, if invested at the same rate of return, would be worth $1000 a year from now. In economic analysis, this is referred to as the time value of money, and the annual rate at which time values are compared is called the discount rate. In this example, the discount rate was 5%.

The choice of a discount rate is an important decision because it can greatly affect the outcome of an analysis where there are values over time. A high discount rate can seriously devalue benefits or costs that occur well into the future. For example, with a discount rate of 15%, the present value of a dollar 10 years from now is only $0.25 and only $0.06 in 20 years. Thus, when a discount rate is high, long term projects that accrue large benefits well into the future may be at a serious disadvantage in comparison with projects that offer more modest—but more immediate—benefits.

What is the appropriate discount rate to choose? There are two considerations in making this choice. When deciding whether to spend money now or later, a relevant consideration is the rate of return that the community is accustomed to receiving on financial investments having a risk equal to the risk or uncertainty of the current project—for example, the rate that would have to be paid to borrow money to finance the project. This might be 5–10%, depending on the circumstances. Because of the focus on current profits and the great uncertainties in the marketplace, corporations tend to use higher discount rates such as 10% or 15% or even higher. However, when considering projects with social outcomes that may accrue well into the future, perhaps spanning several generations of children, a low discount rate is more appropriate to avoid discounting future generations when making decisions. For projects that offer these types of societal benefits, a low social discount rate (e.g., 2–3%) is commonly used. In any case, it is always a good idea to calculate the economic implications of a project using more than one discount rate to see how sensitive the conclusions are to the discount rate that is chosen (see the "Sensitivity Analysis" section).

Techniques for Comparing Costs and Benefits over Time

To the uninitiated, the many different methods used to consider the time value of money in economic analyses can be confusing. However, they are all essentially the same, so understanding the basic principles is important.

Consider a renovation initiative for a school. Proposals include installing new heating, cooling, and ventilation equipment. The community has several diverse policies in place to save energy and reduce pollution and has participated in other initiatives to reduce our dependency on foreign oil. Therefore, there is a general desire to purchase

energy-efficient equipment. However, many people also argue that the energy-efficient equipment would cost too much. How would one go about evaluating which argument carries more weight? First, let's consider just the financial argument and then broaden it to include nonfinancial considerations.

The options are either to purchase more expensive equipment that is more energy efficient and thus costs less to operate or to buy less expensive, standard equipment that functions just as well except that it uses more energy and costs more to operate. This situation calls for evaluating two proposals with different cost streams over time. The expenses should be evaluated over the life cycle of the equipment. Let's assume the more efficient equipment costs $100,000 more to purchase and install initially but would reduce utility bills by an inflation-adjusted $10,000 per year for the first 10 years and approximately $7,000 for the next 10 years, after which the equipment would need to be replaced. Imagine that the school district would borrow the extra $100,000 to pay for the more expensive equipment.

End-of-time-period Analysis

One way to assess these choices would be to look at the situation after 20 years. For example, one might ask, if the school district used the utility bill savings each year to pay off the loan and continued to deposit the savings after the loan was repaid, what would the result be after 20 years? If the school district would be able to pay off the loan and have some savings left over, the energy-efficient equipment would be a financially superior option and vice versa. (A variation of this idea often used in business is payback period. The *payback period* is the number of years it takes for savings [or returns] to pay for the initial [or added] cost of a given alternative. Short payback periods are obviously preferred to longer ones. A payback period is a crude and inaccurate measure, and it is not useful when the time streams of costs and benefits of alternatives are not similar because it ignores benefits that lie in the distant future and ignores discounting.)

Rates of Return

An equivalent way of thinking about this problem is to compare rates of return. Do the energy savings represent a higher or lower rate of return than the interest the school district would have to pay if it borrowed the extra money to buy the energy-efficient equipment? If the rate of return is more than the actual borrowing rate, then the district should buy the energy-efficient equipment. (The internal rate of return [IRR] is a term often used in business to compare the future net earnings of a project with its initial cost. The IRR is the discount rate that makes the present value of future net earnings equal the cost of the project. A high IRR means the project is more profitable.)

Net Present Value

One could also compare the net present value of both options and choose the one with the higher net present value. The energy-efficient equipment costs $100,000 more initially, but if one computed the discounted present value of the annual energy savings for 20 years (discounted at the borrowing rate on the loan), would the discounted value be more or less than $100,000? If more, the energy-efficient equipment would be a better option financially. Sometimes present values are then translated into annual equivalent values, so that, rather than considering costs and benefits as if they were lump sums in the present, one considers them as a constant flow of costs and benefits each year.

In sum, one can compare either net values at the end of a time period, the rates of return, the present values, or the annual equivalent values. Most projects do not present such a simple set of alternatives as our example. Often the stream of benefits and costs is not uniform over the years. Thus, the calculations and comparisons are usually more complex, but they involve the same basic principles.

Most projects considered in business and in many public programs have a defined planning period in which costs and benefits are considered. However, what about programs that are likely to have lasting effects on society or the community for generations to come but have no defined planning period? Some analysts will choose a planning period for convenience. However, it is also appropriate to consider these effects as lasting in perpetuity and, using the chosen discount rate, convert the uneven flow of costs and benefits into constant annual equivalent flows, which are assumed to last forever.

How to Include Nonfinancial Costs and Benefits

The preceding life-cycle cost examples dealt with financial analysis of expenditure options—just the actual flows of money into and out of the school district. Suppose, however, that the lower utility bills were not sufficient to financially justify the project. In an economic analysis, other issues not involving actual money flows can also be assigned an economic value (monetized) and then incorporated into the evaluation. For example, since the community has other policies in place to reduce the use of fossil fuels (in order to decrease air pollution and lessen dependency on foreign oil), the value of energy-efficient equipment may go beyond just the savings in the utility bills. One might develop a community-based method of valuing those benefits and conduct the analysis accordingly. Alternatively, one might compute how valuable these extra benefits would have to be for the energy-efficient equipment to be worthwhile. The community could then decide whether the value of these extra benefits was worth the cost without ever really monetizing those benefits.

Valuing Health-related Benefits and Costs

Valuing Life-and-Death Issues

Essentially, two methods have been used to evaluate the negative impact of a premature death or, conversely, the benefit of preventing such a death. The first is to consider the death solely in market terms and to value it by the income that would have been earned had the person lived to life expectancy. This is often used because it is easy to calculate and purely market based, but it is fraught with social injustices. For example, it suggests that the life of a retired person, a low-income person, or a person with a disability (unable to work) has little worth and thus undervalues programs that save the lives of underprivileged, unemployed, or elderly people.

The other approach is to seek answers from the marketplace as to how people value the risk of death. For example, economists sometimes study different occupations and compare the wages in those that are very similar overall but different in the risk of death or injury. The difference in the wages is then taken as a measure of the compensation that people demand for the added risk. Thus, if there is a 1% difference in the risk of death and the income difference over the years for which the risk is calculated is $50,000, then the workers receive $5 million for each death incurred. These kinds of measures are called willingness-to-pay measures.

Finally, as mentioned earlier, the number of years of life saved is often used as a scaling factor to distinguish between saving the lives of people who have a long life ahead and of those who do not. Although it is often used and has much to justify it, it presents the problem of devaluing the lives of older people. Another complicating factor is that, as people age, they tend to value their remaining time more and more. These are complicated questions.

Valuing Health Outcomes

A similar issue involves the evaluation of health-based outcomes. For example, what is the value of preventing a single case of asthma? This is commonly determined by measuring the medical cost of asthma over the life of a person with the condition and then adding to that the cost of transportation, time lost from work, and other indirect costs. The problem is that this approach assumes that a person would not mind having asthma as long as someone paid for the medical and indirect costs. This is clearly an incomplete assumption since most people would prefer to be healthy in the first place. But how can the situation be assessed? Sometimes studies are undertaken through questionnaires and related techniques to ascertain the tradeoff that people would accept between having a disease and receiving compensation and not having the disease. The compensation they would accept becomes the willingness-to-pay measure.

Valuing Job Creation as a Benefit

A popular refrain of those who support some projects is that it creates jobs, so job creation becomes a big selling point. However, the question is not jobs per se, but *what* jobs? Making people sick from pollution or poor dietary habits can be said to create jobs in the health care industry, yet few would argue that this is a good social policy simply because it creates jobs. Indeed, when valuing the costs of pollution or poor dietary habits, one would probably measure the cost of health care, which includes the cost of paying health care workers, as a cost, not a benefit. Creating jobs can be a two-edged sword, so caution is in order to ensure that the jobs being created are divorced from the negative impacts of the proposal in question and also produce goods and services that are beneficial to society or the community.

Sensitivity Analysis

As one can see from this discussion, a degree of uncertainty is present with any estimate of economic costs and benefits. The uncertainty, which is often great, derives from choices the analyst makes in the process of conducting the evaluation. A sensitivity analysis would look at the choices that most affect the conclusions and then determine how the results would change if different choices were made. Often, a sensitivity analysis is used to provide a range of estimates or a best-case and a worst-case scenario. If the proposed project is deemed to be worthwhile even under the worst-case scenario or not worthwhile even under the best-case scenario, then the economic evaluation has a robust meaning. If it is worthwhile in the best-case but not the worst-case scenario, then the value of the project is less clear, and other factors not accounted for in the analysis will likely weigh more heavily in decisions about the project.

Institutional Issues

Capital versus Operating Budgets

One of the problems school systems and many other institutions face is that the capital budget that would pay for new schools and equipment is appropriated and administered separately from the operating budget. The previous examples using energy-efficient equipment suggests that one should consider paying for added capital costs for plant and equipment with the operational savings that may be associated with it. However, because the budgets are separate, those responsible for administering the capital budget tend to prefer less expensive equipment in order to stretch their resources as far as possible, irrespective of the overall long-term savings that might be achieved through reduced operating expenditures. This is a major barrier to the widespread use of life-cycle costing and often results in poorer-quality plant and equipment and thus increased operating costs.

Narrower versus Broader Perspectives

When only direct and immediate costs and benefits are considered in school decisions, education may be ill served. For example, school budgets are commonly very tight. Further, academic and facility-operating needs compete for funding within the same budget. As a result, school operating budgets tend to suffer because facilities are viewed as a necessary expense but not an investment in children's education. With maintenance budgets underfunded, facilities deteriorate over time. Indeed, conditions in many of the nation's schools are now characterized by appalling deficiencies. If decisions to reduce their maintenance budgets included a consideration of the impact of poor maintenance on the absentee rate of teachers and students, their illness rates, and their performance in schools, different budget decisions might arise. Indeed, initial indications are that academic outcomes and their precursors (e.g., attendance and good health) are significantly influenced by the quality of the school facilities, including indoor air, acoustics, and lighting. Thus, over long periods of time, considerations of capital and operating costs, investments in quality facilities, including energy-efficient and well-functioning equipment, and priority spending for maintenance may prove to be cost effective in terms of educational outcomes.

Beyond Educational Objectives

The principal mission of school districts is to educate the children of the community. However, schools are also institutions that reflect the community's values and either directly or indirectly instill them in the students. Schools are expected to provide an environment that does more than promote learning and foster healthy physical, mental, and emotional growth. At a minimum, they are expected to protect students from harmful situations, and they are frequently used as vehicles to deliver various health and social services, often in conjunction with other community institutions. Thus, many school systems have programs to steer children away from drugs and tobacco; reduce sexually transmitted diseases and teen pregnancies; reduce crime, violence, and bullying; improve nutrition; and promote socially acceptable skills. Thus, a host of school health and welfare programs with outcomes only indirectly related to education may be subject to economic evaluations.

Analysis of Programs to Sell Goods and Services to Students

Economic Demand Analysis

Increasingly, schools are being viewed as a marketplace in which the sale of economic goods (e.g., snacks) is providing a source of revenue. Minimizing the negative impact of these programs on children, while at the same time preserving the benefits of added revenue, may require some analysis of student economic behavior and the way students respond to various economic stimuli such as price or packaging. By altering price, packaging, and other incentives, schools may steer student behaviors in different directions. These changes will also impact the revenue from the sales. Finding the right balance will require some analysis of the economic demand for the goods or services being sold. Because food is the economic product that most commonly sold in schools and because dietary habits are critical to student health and school performance, it is used in this section as the context for assessing the potential for schools to influence students' economic choices.

Basic Determinants of Consumer Behavior

Economic demand analysis is simply the analysis of factors that affect consumer behavior, that is, the factors that enter into consumers' decisions to buy a product. The extent to which a factor influences student behavior, combined with the extent to which the school can influence or alter that factor, is a measure of how much influence the school system will have on the choices that students make. This analysis thus creates the context through which the school may alter the dietary habits of its students. The basic determinants of economic demand are tastes or preferences, income, relative prices, and incentives.

Tastes or Preferences

The first rule of marketing is to understand the customer. What drives students to seek out certain foods? This is the fundamental question that schools must first ask. An obvious answer is inherent personal tastes. But children are also influenced by their families, the culture around them, commercial advertising, and the personal tastes of others, as well as by what is considered "cool," their perception of nutritional needs, and many other factors—all intertwined and interrelated. In the context of changing behavior, the school must first consider which of these factors they can influence to improve nutritional choices. School personnel understand their students best, and because this is a relatively new subject area for schools, creativity and brainstorming may be required. However, school staff members may be surprised at some of the options they may have and be willing see how well they work.

Establishing a nutrition-conscious culture within the school system may be the first step. One obvious approach to this is basic education on nutritional needs and the consequences of poor dietary habits. How well do students understand the relationship between diet and consequences such as obesity, diabetes, heart disease, cancer, and other diseases? How well do they understand the nutritional value (or lack thereof) of various foods and how to choose the best among those that they like? Additional possibilities include the involvement of local leaders, including restaurant owners whose business the children frequent, effective advertising, and attractive packaging or presentation of nutritional foods. All of these activities are directed toward influencing students' tastes.

Income

One can think of income as acting as a constraint on purchases. The lower the income available to the purchaser, the fewer goods and services will be bought; there will be a tendency toward lower-priced items. This is true overall, but not necessarily within any goods category. For example, except for dire poverty, income is not likely to influence the quantity of food one eats, and although a low income is likely to discourage people from going to very high-priced restaurants or buying very pricey food items, these influences may not be relevant in the context of students' nutritional choices. However, it is true that lower-income families tend to have poorer nutritional eating habits that tend to higher fat, higher cholesterol, higher sugar, lower fiber content, and lower consumption of needed vitamins and minerals. The evidence suggests that this is not a question of not being able to afford

better nutrition, but the lack of perceived need to do so and the lack of understanding as to how to make nutritional choices within their budget constraints (Virginia Cooperative Extension Service 1993). To the extent that a family's habits influence children's habits in school, one consideration might be a program to educate families as well as students on nutritional needs, consequences of nutritional choices, nutritional values in foods, how to read labels, and how to make choices.

Relative Prices

The relative prices of foods and snacks sold in schools are probably the most easily manipulated by the school system and may have a significant effect on students' choices, particularly if used in combination with other programs to influence tastes. But why the term "relative prices" rather than just "prices"? Relative to what? When people make purchasing decisions, they generally compare the price of a product with that of potential substitutes. Thus, when buying a snack and choosing to consume an apple or a bag of chips, one would be influenced by how much each costs. If a school lowered the price of the apple and raised the price of the chips, one would expect more apples and fewer chips to be sold. The case is similar with drinks—choosing juice or chocolate milk instead of sodas, for example. In addition to the price of substitute products, the price of complementary products is also important. For example, students are more likely to purchase a hamburger and french fries rather than a hamburger and a dish of spaghetti and meatballs (although any combination is possible with some students). When items go together, a decline in the price of either one can increase the purchase of the other and vice versa, whereas a decrease or increase in the price of both will have a greater effect on each than the same change on just one of the items. Thus, knowledge of the substitutability or complementarity of foods should factor into the pricing decisions used to influence students' choices. Packaging complementary items that are nutritional and lowering the price on that package could be an effective strategy.

Incentives

Most incentives are like conditional price cuts. That is, "buy one and get the other half price" is equivalent to 25% off, but only if you buy two. Thus, the price incentive is conditional on the purchase of two instead of one. A variation on this theme is "buy the product at full price, and get a complementary product at a lower price or free." This is the same as packaging complementary products but offers another way of presenting it, which may have a different effect on sales. Another incentive offers coupons for nutritional foods that can accumulate to some value as they are collected. All these incentives can be used to alter the nutritional choices that students make.

Effects of Demand-altering Strategies on Revenues

When the price of a nutritional item falls, if sales of that item do not increase, then revenues for that item will fall. However, if sales increase, what happens to the revenues? Obviously, it depends on how much sales increase. If the percentage of increase in the quantity sold is equal to the percentage of decrease in price, revenues will remain the same. If the increase in the quantity sold is proportionally less than the decrease in price, revenues will fall and vice versa. Economists refer to this relationship as the "price elasticity" of demand.

Students select among the options available. As they choose to purchase one item, they are also opting not to purchase substitute items. In addition, they may decide to purchase complementary items. Thus the total revenues from food sales depend not only on the price elasticity of each product but also on the cross-elasticities of demand among products.

Similar concepts are applicable to any other measure designed to influence demand. To be able to predict the effect on revenue, one must have information about the responsiveness of the student body to these measures. Some of this information may be available from the literature, from other schools that have tried these approaches, or from marketing experts with access to unpublished information. If the information is not available, the school system may wish to systematically experiment and keep good records that can be analyzed in a scientific manner. Grants may also be available to help support such an effort. One of the case studies discussed below concerns a pricing and packaging strategy for vending machine snacks and demonstrates some of the principles involved in studying these issues.

Although the purchase decisions of students

combined with the relative prices will determine revenues, the cost to the school for each product under consideration is of equal concern. The combination of revenue change and cost change will determine the net revenue for each product available to the school. However, from a financial standpoint, it is the total revenues less total costs that matter. It may not be so bad to lose money on some nutritional items as a consequence of inducing their purchase, while making more money on other purchases that are being discouraged, to preserve a beneficial financial outcome.

Applying Basic Principles: Case Study Examples

This section briefly reviews how the basic principles of economic analysis have been or can be applied in real-world situations. The first example comes from a published cost-benefit study that assessed a proposed federal legislation to restrict smoking in all public buildings in the United States (Mudarri 1994). In this study, the health-related outcomes dealt with reducing life-threatening diseases and also included non–health-related outcomes. The second is a hypothetical situation in which a school asthma-intervention program is being proposed. The third study evaluated the effect of different pricing and packaging strategies on the sale of low-fat vending-machine snacks (French et al. 2001).

Costs and Benefits of Smoking Restrictions

This study is instructive because it estimates and values different kinds of outcomes (e.g., health, fire prevention, maintenance of buildings), deals with effects that cover very long time periods, incorporates a sensitivity analysis, and accounts for issues that could only be qualitatively evaluated. It is a cost-benefit analysis of proposed federal legislation that would restrict smoking in all buildings frequented by the public.

The objective of this analysis was to assess the costs and benefits that would occur each year from a federally mandated smoking-restriction policy. Future costs and benefits were discounted at a 3% rate to compute their present value and then converted to an equivalent annual rate. Current smoking prevalence and the prevalence of existing smoking policies were used as a baseline for measuring the effects of such a policy.

Smoking restrictions are designed to protect nonsmokers from exposure to secondhand smoke (environmental tobacco smoke). The main health effects assessed were the elevated risk of lung cancer and heart disease associated with exposure. Both of these diseases are life threatening and result in premature death to a portion of those exposed. This was evaluated using a willingness-to-pay measure of premature death derived independently from other analyses. Because only long-term exposure is associated with these diseases, time delays were estimated for the full realization of the health benefits, using the pattern of increasing lower risk over time that is known to occur after people stop smoking. Other results that were evaluated included estimated reductions in housekeeping and maintenance expenses in buildings where smoking is restricted and the reduced risk of smoking-related fires. These outcomes were considered to be realized at the inception of the smoking restriction. The major costs were implementation of the policy nationwide and in individual buildings plus the cost of providing smoking lounges in those buildings where smoking was an option.

Outcomes that were considered but not specifically evaluated were the expected increase in productivity by nonsmoking office workers and the potential reduction in productivity of smokers who could no longer smoke at their workstations. In addition, the study acknowledged that smokers would suffer some burden at having their need to smoke restricted, some would quit or cut back, and some people would fail to start smoking in the first place. These issues were quantitatively and qualitatively assessed but not included in the basic cost-benefit comparisons.

High and low estimates were derived principally from the uncertainty in making estimates of health outcomes. In addition, sensitivity analysis included considerations of how the estimates would change under alternate discount rates of 5% and 7%, alternate assumptions about changes in smoking prevalence, and alternate assumptions about the kinds of smoking restrictions that might take place over time in the absence of such a policy.

The study concluded that passage of the smoking restrictive legislation could achieve net benefits (i.e., benefits minus costs) of $39–$72 billion per year, excluding some potentially significant costs and benefits to smokers. Thus, the net costs to smokers would have to exceed $39 billion for the costs to surpass the benefits. Alternative discount rates and assumptions about future trends in the prevalence and the restriction of smoking that would occur in the absence of such legislation did not change the conclusion that the benefits of passing the legislation would exceed the costs by a substantial margin.

Costs and Benefits of a Hypothetical School Asthma-Intervention Program

The incidence of asthma in children has been rising rapidly over the last decade and has stimulated interest in developing asthma-management programs. (For more information on this subject, see chapter 28 on asthma.) School-based asthma-management programs might include the identification of children with asthma, assistance in determining their asthma triggers, access to medical treatment for asthma symptoms, including medications, and education and assistance in lifestyle changes (including changes in the school environment) to avoid exposure to those triggers. Costs and benefits would accrue to the school, to organizations that might be providing ancillary services, and to the families and their health insurance providers. Thus, both direct and indirect costs and benefits must be considered.

The advantage of managing children's asthma is that the use of medication, along with strategies to reduce exposure to asthma triggers, may reduce asthma episodes and their associated emergency room visits, hospitalizations, and absences from school. Even minor asthma episodes can disrupt a student's school activities.

From a school's perspective, the costs of implementing the program would essentially be personnel, administrative, and materials costs, all of which would depend on how the program is structured. Because children are exposed to asthma allergens at home as well as school and because exposure may require medical treatment, the program would probably have to include the training and education of parents, as well as children, plus the family physician or local clinic. Medical personnel from other community institutions or local physician volunteers may be available to train paraprofessionals, who in turn would train and educate the children and parents. School nurses would obviously be involved. In addition, removing allergens from the school environment (e.g., mold, animals, allergens embedded in upholstered furniture) could require the cooperation of teachers and other maintenance personnel. In other words, the most difficult part of estimating the cost of conducting such a program is formulating the structure of the project. Once that is done, estimating the costs could be fairly straightforward.

The impact of the program on outcomes such as visits to the nurse, absence from school, or trips to the emergency room could come either from programs administered elsewhere, in the general literature, from the educated judgments of local personnel, or a combination of these and other sources. Most often these sources would yield an estimate of the percentage of decline in these events. It would thus be necessary to establish the approximate number of the events associated with asthma in the student population to form a baseline to which the percentage of reductions could be applied. Thus, if there are 1,000 asthma-related visits to school nurses, 500 asthma-related absences from school, and 100 asthma-related emergency room trips by children in the school system, an estimated 50% reduction in the number of visits to the nurse and a 25% reduction in school absences and emergency room trips would translate to 500 fewer nurse visits, 125 fewer absences, and 25 fewer emergency room trips.

For a project such as this, it is probably sufficient to conduct a cost-effectiveness evaluation, that is, estimate the costs of administering the program along with the magnitude of the expected results. A judgment would then have to be made as to whether the outcomes expected would justify the cost. However, to the extent that other community services might be involved, including physician, emergency room, and hospitalization services, and to the extent that their cooperation, including their donation of resources, may be involved, some estimate of the value of these outcomes might also be helpful. For example, local health insurance agencies may find that their cooperation with the program would save them money. In that case, the cost of an average emergency room visit or hospitalization for an asthma patient would help support this argument to the agencies.

Pricing and Promotion Effects on Low-fat Vending-machine Snack Purchases

In this study, low-fat snacks were added to 55 vending machines in 12 secondary schools and 12 worksites. The prices were systematically altered in a scientific design using four pricing levels (equal price; reductions of 10%, 25%, and 50%). In addition, promotional conditions were systematically altered (no label, a low-fat label, and a low-fat label plus a promotional sign). The objective of the study was to observe how pricing and promotional strategies would alter food purchases and total revenues.

In general, one would expect that sales of low-fat snacks would increase with lower prices. But are the results significant enough to make the change worthwhile? Several previous studies described here had shown some dramatic effects, although not necessarily in school environments. For example, in one study, sales of low-fat vending-machine snacks increased by 80% when their prices were cut in half. In a worksite cafeteria, cutting salad bar prices in half increased sales threefold, and sales of fresh fruit and baby carrots in a school cafeteria increased two- to fourfold when prices were cut in half. Clearly, these pricing strategies greatly encouraged low-fat food sales. From the earlier discussion of the price elasticity of demand, it is clear that the revenues from the sales of the specific items whose prices were reduced rose in all of these cases. However, that result alone does not indicate how profits were affected.

The study at hand looked at the effect of price and promotion on sales as well as profits. The results show that price reductions of 10%, 25%, and 50% resulted in sales increases of 9%, 39%, and 93% respectively; thus, the substantial reductions in price of 25% and 50% had substantially higher increases in purchases of these foods. However, the very modest promotional strategies had a much smaller effect on sales. In addition, vending-machine profits were essentially the same under all conditions.

The fact that profits were the same does not necessarily imply a good outcome from a nutritional standpoint. Lowering the price of a product that someone purchases essentially leaves more money in that person's pocket—money that could be used to buy something else. This is what economists call the "income effect" of a price change. If students used that savings to buy a high-fat snack or bought twice as much of the low-fat snack, overall nutrition would not necessarily be enhanced. Thus, further research to ascertain the total impact on food choices would be valuable. Nevertheless, one way to lessen adverse outcomes and improve profits would be to raise the price of other foods slightly while lowering the price on the target foods. If other foods constituted the majority (e.g., 85%) of food sales, some very modest price increases could offset the price promotions on the target foods. Some experimentation with pricing strategies would be worth pursuing to find a balance that both promotes nutrition and protects the profitability of the program.

References

French SA, Jeffery RW, Story M, Breitlow KK, Baxter JS, Hannan P, et al. 2001. Pricing and promotion effects on low-fat vending snack purchases: The CHIPS Study. Am J Public Health 91(1):112–117.

Mudarri DH. 1994. The costs and benefits of smoking restrictions: An assessment of the Smoke-free Environment Act of 1993 (HR 3434). Washington, DC: Indoor Environments Division, U.S. Environmental Protection Agency.

Virginia Cooperative Extension Service. 1993. Applying cost benefit analysis to nutrition education programs: Focus on the Virginia Expanded Food and Nutrition Education Program. Publication No. 490_403. Available: http://www.ext.vt.edu/pubs/nutrition/490-403/490-403.html (accessed 15 January 2004).

25

Angelo J. Bellomo

Evaluating the School Environment

■ *Summary*

- Educators recognize that conditions in the learning environment can affect the health, safety, and well-being of teachers and students, directly impacting the ability of teachers to teach and students to learn.
- Regulatory standards and best management practices have been developed to control a number of health and safety factors in schools, including pesticide use, fire and safety risks, indoor air quality, traffic, pedestrian hazards, storage and handling of chemical cleaners and reagents, classroom acoustics, and emergency preparedness.
- Although identifying standards is a key step in improving school health and safety, inspections must routinely evaluate compliance with the applicable standards. Where schools have been inspected, a high rate of noncompliance has been observed.
- Improving conditions in U.S. schools will require implementation of a routine inspection and assessment program. The use of a standardized inspection template provides identification of compliance trends over time and the comparison of inspection data from different regions of the country. ■

Why Evaluate School Environments?

The Importance of School Conditions

A review of school infrastructure by the U.S. General Accounting Office (1995) found that more than half of the school buildings in the United States were in substandard condition and poorly maintained. A more recent survey found nearly 40% of Los Angeles schools in substantial noncompliance with applicable health and safety regulations (Los Angeles Unified School District 2005).

Teachers, architects, and environmental professionals recognize the relationship between conditions in the learning environment and the health and safety of school occupants. We know much less about the impact that school conditions have on academic performance, although this factor is frequently cited to justify increased funding for school repairs and modernization.

In view of current reforms in public education,

a better understanding of the relationship between school conditions and students' academic performance could engender major support for improving the quality of the learning environment. Although annual measures of academic performance are readily available for each of the nation's 50,000 schools, standardized assessment data on school conditions are clearly lacking. An important step in improving conditions in the learning environment is a routine inspection and evaluation program. Such inspections typically focus on identifying and mitigating risks to the health and safety of school occupants, but the data generated could also be used to examine the relationships between school conditions, students' health and safety, and academic performance.

This chapter presents an approach to routine inspections. A complementary source is the U.S. Environmental Protection Agency's Healthy School Environments Assessment Tool, or HealthySEAT. HealthySEAT, introduced in early 2006, is a free, downloadable software package designed to be customized and used by district-level staff to conduct voluntary self-assessments of their school (and other) facilities and to track and manage information on environmental conditions school by school. It can be found at www.epa.gov/schools/healthyseat. The Association for Supervision and Curriculum Development has also developed its own "Healthy School Report Card" Action Tool that helps administrators assess and address various aspects of student and staff health and well-being (Lohrmann et al. 2005).

Improving School Conditions through Inspection and Evaluation

The successful use of routine inspections to improve school health and safety involves a three-step process: (1) identifying school safety standards, (2) evaluating compliance with the applicable standards, and (3) implementing corrective action to achieve compliance with the standards. This approach provides school management with an effective orientation on school safety because it poses three key questions: What standards must be met to ensure the health and safety of students and staff? How well do we currently comply with these standards? What must be done to achieve full compliance with the standards? An inspection effort based on this approach optimizes the effective use of resources: The objective is to achieve compliance with the applicable standards, and all actions are directed toward this purpose.

A self-imposed or voluntary inspection program offers a number of benefits. First, hazardous conditions can often be identified and mitigated before they result in actual or perceived exposures of students and staff. Exposure to indoor air pollutants and other chemicals are common in the school environment and may particularly affect younger students or those with other susceptibilities such as asthma. Poor maintenance of building materials or improper precautions during building modernization may result in the uncontrolled release of lead paint debris or asbestos fibers. These incidents place school occupants at risk, often require the closure of rooms or entire buildings, and may disrupt classroom instruction for several days. Cleanup and abatement of a lead or asbestos release can be costly, and such incidents may expose the school district to substantial and continuing liability.

A second benefit is regulatory compliance. Schools are subject to a range of federal, state, and local health and safety regulations. Although regulatory inspections and enforcement within the school environment have historically been limited, this is likely to change with the current levels of public interest and investment in education. In addition, regulatory authorities generally support self-inspection efforts, and even if the agency identifies deficiencies, the fact that the school district conducts periodic inspections to detect and correct noncompliance may offer some defense.

Third, if health and safety risks are not promptly identified and corrected, they can often result in substantial public concern and associated media attention, both of which can redirect limited school resources from their primary mission of classroom instruction. A proactive self-inspection program demonstrates that school officials are committed to ensuring the safety of students and staff.

Finally, routine assessment of school conditions can produce the data necessary to justify funding for repairs or modernization or to assist in the prioritization of limited funding based on actual need.

Identifying School Health
and Safety Standards

The Nature and Scope
of School Safety Standards

Physical and operational conditions in a school can be evaluated in a number of ways, but each is dependent on a defined set of criteria or standards. Some standards are objective, whereas others are relatively subjective. For example, the requirement to maintain a fully charged fire extinguisher in a science laboratory is an objective standard, in that compliance with this requirement can be evaluated definitively, with little discretion on the part of the inspector. Other standards are more subjective and require greater judgment on the part of the inspector, such as the requirement that school staff be adequately trained in emergency procedures.

Generally, two types of safety standards are used in evaluating school conditions: regulatory standards and best management practices. Regulatory standards comprise federal, state, and local statutes and regulations and provide baseline requirements for a particular subject area. Best management practices are nonregulatory and are often developed as a supplement to regulation or in advance of the regulatory process. Together, regulatory standards and best management practices provide a useful set of criteria for assessing health and safety risks within the learning environment.

The process of defining a set of school safety standards must begin with a definition of the term "school safety." For many parents, school safety connotes the prevention of violence and other crimes on campus. For the health and safety inspector, the term often implies the management of potential chemical exposures resulting from the improper handling of laboratory reagents or art and craft supplies. The maintenance staff may see school safety more directly related to preventing the release of asbestos or lead during intrusive work on flooring, walls, ceilings, or other building components. For the emergency coordinator, the term may embody the efforts of school staff in preparing for and responding to emergencies.

A number of safety risks, ranging from asbestos and pesticide exposure to gun violence and acts of terrorism, have impacted schools in recent years. For this reason, it is important to define school safety broadly to cover the spectrum of health and safety risks within the learning environment.

Developing a School Safety
Standards Guidebook

The criteria for evaluating school conditions should be gathered from federal, state, and local laws and regulations dealing with school health and safety. Other appropriate but nonregulatory requirements, including school district policies, procedures, and best management practices, should also be identified. The resulting list of requirements should then be compiled into a school safety standards guidebook that specifies the requirements that schools should comply with to ensure the health and safety of students and staff. Additionally, the manual is a listing of the standards against which schools in the district will be inspected and evaluated.

Table 25.1 presents an excerpt from a sample health and safety standards guide. The manual should be organized as a listing of specific standards or requirements under each of several subject areas or categories. In preparing a standards guidebook, most school districts should consider including at least the safety-related categories given. As table 25.1 shows, each category may be further subdivided. This structure facilitates searching for specific safety requirements and examining them under a given category or type. The next column heading in the guide is a brief summary of the requirement, a feature that facilitates the use of the book by teachers, parents, and school staff.

Because the manual is also intended to guide the implementation of appropriate corrective action, the third column heading is Corrective Action for Identified Deficiency, which is a statement of necessary action to bring the facility into compliance with the given standard. The final column heading in the guidebook is Reference, where specific regulatory requirements may be found in the statutes or regulations or where the reader may find information about nonregulatory district policies or best management practices.

As schools conduct inspections and initiate efforts to improve the level of compliance, school personnel will gain experience in common problems and appropriate corrective measures. This information should be reviewed periodically to identify trends and assess the need for modifications to the standards and corrective actions listed in the

Table 25.1. Sample format: health and chemical safety standards guidebook

Type	Standard	Corrective action for identified	Reference
Lab safety	A chemical hygiene and safety plan shall be prepared and annually updated for all school science laboratories in compliance with District Bulletin 29.	Develop a written chemical hygiene and safety plan and ensure it is readily available to all employees. The plan should identify a coordinator and be revised at least annually.	8 California Code of Regulation (CCR) §5191; 29 CFR 1910.1450; Chemical Hygiene & Safety Plan
Hazard communication	A hazard communication program pursuant to District Bulletin 12 shall be implemented all district schools and administrative offices.	Implement a hazard communication program pursuant to District Bulletin 12 and applicable regulatory standards. To obtain a copy of the district's Hazard Communication Program Template, contact the Office of Health and Safety at (800) 555-5555.	8 CCR §5194; 29 CFR 1910.1200
	All containers of hazardous substances as defined in Code of Federal Regulations (CFR) Section 1910.1200 shall be labeled to identify the contents and appropriate hazard warnings.	Ensure that all hazardous substance containers within the facility are properly labeled, indicating identity of the contents and appropriate hazard warnings.	8 CCR §5194; 29 CFR 1910.1200
	A current Material Safety Data Sheet (MSDS) shall be maintained and readily available for each hazardous substance utilized at the facility.	Maintain current MSDSs for each hazardous substance used on-site. All MSDSs should be readily available to site personnel.	8 CCR §5194; 29 CFR 1910.1200
	Employees shall receive annual hazard communication training on chemicals used in their work areas.	Provide employees with annual hazard communication training on hazardous chemicals used in their respective work areas. Employees should be retrained when new hazards are introduced into the work place.	8 CCR §5194; 29 CFR 1910.1200

guidebook. Such action will ensure the continued appropriateness of the health and safety standards.

A useful supplement to the standards guidebook is an inspection checklist, which identifies key requirements to review during the inspection. The checklist should be derived from the guidebook but significantly scaled down for use in the field at the time of inspection. The checklist can also be useful to school personnel as a reminder of the scope of the inspection and the applicable safety requirements to be reviewed. An example of an inspection checklist that was developed for use by the Los Angeles Unified School District is shown in figure 25.1. The checklist is sectioned into the individual standards referenced in the guidebook, each of which includes several threshold criteria considered essential for a finding of compliance with the applicable standard.

The Inspection and Evaluation Process

The inspection and evaluation process involves three distinct phases: preinspection planning; inspection and evaluation; and postinspection documentation. The effectiveness of a school inspection program can be enhanced by carefully defining the work to be completed during each of these phases.

Phase 1: Preinspection Planning

In this phase, the inspector informs the appropriate school staff of the planned inspection and requests that relevant documentation be available for review at that time. This is done to facilitate the compliance assessment process and to ensure that appropriate personnel are available to participate in the inspection. Including staff members in the inspection process also serves to educate them about or remind them of applicable safety requirements.

The inspector also reviews the complaint and incident history for the school, previous inspection findings, and any outstanding deficiencies. In addition, the inspector should review worker injury data to determine whether the school has an elevated injury rate.

Phase 2: Inspection and Evaluation

The inspection should begin with a meeting between the inspector and the school principal and/or the facilities manager to explain the scope of the inspection and identify any health and safety issues requiring evaluation. The principal should be given copies of the standards guidebook and the inspection checklist and be advised that the purpose of the inspection is to assess compliance with the regulatory standards referenced in the guide.

The inspection should begin in the main office with a review of required regulatory postings and appropriate records. These records include accident and incident reports, the injury and illness prevention program, the asbestos management plan, and maintenance and repair logs. After the review of appropriate records, the inspection

should continue in all common areas of the school site, including the administrative offices, nurse's office, auditorium, library, playgrounds, and restrooms. The inspection should continue in 20–50% of all classrooms. At least one or two classrooms in each building should be inspected because the scope of conditions can vary in buildings of different ages and levels of repair. Certain classrooms, such as those used for shops, arts and ceramics, and science, will require greater attention. Finally, the inspection should include all specialty rooms and facilities such as boiler and HVAC rooms, chemical storage areas, and maintenance and refuse-holding facilities.

During the inspection, the inspector should carefully assess the extent of compliance with each of the requirements in the standards guidebook and the inspection checklist. The assessment should be based primarily on physical observations and interviews with the school administrator and appropriate plant maintenance personnel. The inspector may also receive input from teachers or other staff members during the course of the inspection.

The inspector may use various field instruments (see table 25.2) to assess conditions or evaluate compliance with specific physical or chemical parameters referenced in the guidebook. For ex-

Table 25.2. Equipment commonly used to evaluate conditions in the school environment

Equipment	Purpose
Sound level meter	Evaluate noise levels in classrooms and outdoor areas to assess acoustical quality. Assess occupational exposure to noise. Measurements expressed in decibels on the A-scale, dB(A).
Hygrometer	Measure relative humidity and temperature, typically in response to indoor air quality complaint.
Indoor Air Quality meter	Measure relative humidity, temperature, and carbon dioxide levels within room or building.
Light meter	Determine levels of indoor lighting in units of lumens or foot-candles.
Anemometer	Evaluate airflow in HVAC systems or exhaust hoods. Measurements expressed in cubic feet per minute, meters/second, or miles per hour.
XRF meter	Use X-ray fluorescence for determinations of the presence of lead-containing painted surfaces or lead-contaminated soils.
Multiple gas indicator	Assess the presence and concentration of carbon monoxide, hydrogen sulfide (in ppm), percentage of oxygen, or percentage of the lower explosive limit (for combustible gases).
Smoke tubes	Use smoke tubes that emit visible smoke in order to evaluate directional airflow in rooms and buildings; assess the effectiveness of exhaust hoods in science laboratories or other areas using volatile substances.
Drager tubes	Assess the presence and relative concentration of chemical vapors in rooms and buildings.
Emdex meter	Evaluate electromagnetic fields near power lines, transformers, and electrical panels.

OEHS
Office of Environmental Health & Safety
Facility Inspection Program
333 S. Beaudry Avenue, 20th Floor
Los Angeles, Ca 90017
Phone: (213) 241-3199
Fax: (213) 241-6816

SCHOOL SAFETY COMPLIANCE CHECKLIST
Los Angeles Unified School District

Date:
School:
Local District:

OEHS Inspector:
Inspection ID:

STANDARD	EVALUATION		
1. Accident Prevention	**Threshold Questions**	**YES**	**NO**
	Is there a written IIPP, which is current, complete, and readily available?	☐	☐
	Is the IIPP summary page posted in a conspicuous area?	☐	☐
	Is employee training provided on a regular basis and documented? *[Confer with school administration and review the available documentation.]*	☐	☐
	Is there a designated School Safety Committee that meets quarterly? *[Confer with school administration and review the available documentation.]*	☐	☐
	Does the Safety Committee perform and document semi-annual safety inspections?	☐	☐
	Is there evidence of follow up action to deficiencies noted during inspections? *[Review trouble call log.]*	☐	☐
	Does the school's Claims Rate compare favorably with the District wide average? *[Less than 120% of LAUSD average.]*	☐	☐
	Other Factors: *[mark factors requiring attention]* **Notes:**		
	☐ Accident Investigations ☐ Hazard Reporting	**Score:**	
	☐ New Employee Orientation ☐ Safety Inspections		
	☐ Enforcement/Discipline ☐ Personal Protective Equipment		
	☐ Safety Incentives ☐ OSHA Postings		
	☐ Accident Reporting ☐ Others		
2. Asbestos Management	**Threshold Questions**	**YES**	**NO**
	Is the Asbestos Management Plan kept in a designated location, readily available, and updated with the current 6-month and 3-year inspection results? *[Check that the update is consistent with AHERA regulations.]*	☐	☐
	Is there a procedure in place to have a review the Asbestos Management Plan prior to disturbing potential asbestos containing materials? *[Determine if Plant Manager has received 2-hour asbestos awareness training and if staff have been informed on the need to review the Asbestos Management Plan prior to disturbing any building material.]*	☐	☐
	Is all work on asbestos-containing materials performed by properly trained personnel? *[Evaluation should be based on staff interviews, field observations, and review of Contact Log.]*	☐	☐
	Other Factors: *[mark factors requiring attention]* **Notes:**		
	☐ VAT floors maintained ☐ Reporting of damaged ACBM	**Score:**	
	☐ Damage to ACBM ☐ Others		

OEHS School Safety Compliance Checklist
Revised 04/19/04

Page 1 of 5
OEHS File 2.5.6

Figure 25.1. Sample school safety compliance checklist, Los Angeles Unified School District.

STANDARD	EVALUATION	YES	NO
3. Fire/Life Safety	**Threshold Questions**		
	Are fire extinguishers checked monthly and serviced annually, clearly marked, and easily accessible?	☐	☐
	Are all exits and exit corridors free of obstructions?	☐	☐
	Are exits properly marked?	☐	☐
	Does each classroom equipped with security grilles have at least one with a releasable latch in compliance with District policy? *[Per Board of Education Report #15.]*	☐	☐
	Notes:		
	Score:		
	Other Factors: *[mark factors requiring attention]*		
	☐ Exit signs illuminated ☐ Exits unlocked & operable in single action		
	☐ Marked fire lane ☐ Occupant signs posted in assembly areas		
	☐ Fire extinguisher training ☐ Fire alarms tested weekly		
	☐ Posted emergency routes ☐ Flammable liquid storage		
	☐ Emergency lighting ☐ Others		
4. Campus Security	**Threshold Questions**	**YES**	**NO**
	Is the school perimeter secured with fencing in good condition & gates locked?	☐	☐
	Is there a visitor check in procedure in compliance with the Locked Campus Policy? *[Per Bulletin 33.]*	☐	☐
	Is there a written procedure for communicating classroom or play yard emergencies to the main office? *[Review written procedure and assess overall staff awareness of procedure.]*	☐	☐
	Is there adequate lighting for after school activities?	☐	☐
	Notes:		
	Score:		
	Other Factors: *[mark factors requiring attention]*		
	☐ Graffiti removed daily ☐ Discipline code		
	☐ Identification badges ☐ Secured food supply		
	☐ Crime reporting ☐ Exterior lighting		
	☐ Security signs ☐ Others		
5. Chemical Safety	**Threshold Questions**	**YES**	**NO**
	Is Hazard Communication training provided at time of initial assignment and when new hazards are introduced into the work place? *[Confer with school administration and review the available documentation.]*	☐	☐
	Is a chemical inventory kept in a designated location and readily available?	☐	☐
	Are MSDSs readily accessible for all chemicals listed on the inventory? *[MSDSs should be kept in a centralized location known to all staff members]*	☐	☐
	Are cleaners and other non-laboratory chemical products properly stored, secured, and disposed of?	☐	☐
	Notes:		
	Score:		
	Other Factors: *[mark factors requiring attention]*		
	☐ Personal Protective Equipment ☐ Gas cylinders secured		
	☐ Proper labeling & signs ☐ Emergency eyewash		
	☐ Grounding/Bonding ☐ Others		
	☐ Spill response kits		

STANDARD	EVALUATION		

6. Pest Management

	YES	NO
Threshold Questions		
Is the site free of evidence of a continuing pest infestation?	☐	☐
Is a copy of the District's IPM Handbook kept in a designated location and readily available?	☐	☐
Are the necessary annual and 72-hour notifications of pesticide use provided? *[Review available documentation.]*	☐	☐

Other Factors: *[mark factors requiring attention]*
☐ Record keeping ☐ Approved pesticides
☐ Fly fans or screen doors ☐ Refuse bins
☐ Staff trained ☐ Others
☐ Posted approved pesticide list

Notes:

Score:

7. Lead Management

	YES	NO
Threshold Questions		
Are buildings constructed prior to 1993 free of peeling or chalking paint?	☐	☐
Has a trouble call been placed for areas of peeling or chalking paint?	☐	☐
Are drinking fountains flushed daily and is a log maintained? *(Per Bulletin 55.)*	☐	☐

Other Factors: *[mark factors requiring attention]*
☐ Staff Awareness ☐ Others

Notes:

Score:

8. Restroom Facilities

	YES	NO
Threshold Questions		
Are all restrooms available for use; adequately stocked with toilet paper, soap, and paper towels; and maintained in sanitary condition? *[Evaluation should be based on visual inspection and review of Contact Log.]*	☐	☐
Are restroom inspections conducted regularly? *[At least twice daily.]*	☐	☐

Other Factors: *[mark factors requiring attention]*
☐ Adequate supervision ☐ Fixtures operating properly
☐ Restroom designation ☐ Adequate number of toilets/urinals
☐ Restroom ventilation ☐ Others

Notes:

Score:

9. Indoor Environment

	YES	NO
Threshold Questions		
Is the site free of evidence of potentially toxic or odorous emissions affecting the indoor environment? *[Evaluation should be based on staff interviews, field observations, and review of Contact Log.]*	☐	☐
Are classrooms and offices adequately lighted?	☐	☐
Are ventilation systems adequate & properly maintained? *[Evaluation should be based on visual observations and interview of Plant Manager.]*	☐	☐
Are classrooms free of excessive noise? *[Evaluation should be based on staff interviews, field observations, and review of Contact Log.]*	☐	☐

Other Factors: *[mark factors requiring attention]*
☐ Evidence of mold ☐ Continuing or multiple IAQ complaints
☐ Housekeeping ☐ Objectionable odor
☐ Thermal comfort ☐ Others
☐ Excessive dust

Notes:

Score:

STANDARD	EVALUATION	YES	NO
10. Maintenance & Repairs	**Threshold Questions**		
	Are facilities and equipment maintained in good repair?	☐	☐
	Have trouble calls been placed for necessary repairs?	☐	☐
	Are proper housekeeping practices followed in classrooms and on campus?	☐	☐
	Other Factors: *[mark factors requiring attention]*	**Notes:**	**Score:**
	☐ Furniture ☐ Approved TV mounts		
	☐ Landscaping ☐ Hopper rooms		
	☐ Unapproved vegetation ☐ Salvage disposal		
	☐ Broken windows ☐ Fall/Trip hazard		
	☐ Seismic bracing ☐ Secured electrical equipment		
	☐ Machine guarding ☐ Others		
	☐ Carpet condition		
11. Safe School Plan	**Threshold Questions**	**YES**	**NO**
	Is the "Safe School Plan" current and readily available?	☐	☐
	Are staff familiar with the SSP and their responsibilities?	☐	☐
	Does the "Safe School Plan" include procedures for: Violence Prevention, Emergency Preparedness, Crisis Intervention and Traffic & Pedestrian Safety? *[Consider use of Model Plan]*		☐ ☐
	Does the Safe School Plan comply with CEC Section 212?	☐	☐
	Other Factors: *[mark factors requiring attention]*	**Notes:**	**Score:**
	☐ Contact Information ☐ Prevention Programs		
	☐ School Planning Committee ☐ Crisis Intervention Training		
	☐ School Site Crisis Team ☐ Enforcement Programs		
	☐ Annual Safety Assessment ☐ Intervention Programs		
	☐ Crisis Intervention Handbook (1994) ☐ Others		
12. Emergency Preparedness	**Threshold Questions**	**YES**	**NO**
	Are emergency procedures current and readily available, and are staff familiar with their designated responsibilities?	☐	☐
	Is there an Emergency Response Plan that complies with regulatory requirements? *[Review "emergency preparedness" section of the Safe School Plan and compare "emergency response procedures" to the Model Emergency Response Plan for Schools.]*	☐	☐
	Are emergency supplies and equipment adequately stocked, properly maintained, and stored in designated locations? *[Review supplies and equipment in earthquake bin and designation locations. Refer to supply inventory listed in Reference Guides 801 and 802]*	☐	☐
	Is dedicated storage provided for emergency supplies?	☐	☐
	Other Factors: *[mark factors requiring attention]*	**Notes:**	**Score:**
	☐ Adequate water supply (1.5 gal./pp) ☐ Emergency drills		
	☐ Emergency training ☐ Annual emergency hazard assessment		
	☐ First-aid kits (1/400) ☐ Designated command post		
	☐ Office to room communication ☐ Toilet and Search and Rescue Supplies		
	☐ SEMS ☐ Others		

371

STANDARD	EVALUATION	YES	NO
13. Traffic & Pedestrian Safety	**Threshold Questions**		
	Have "Safe Routes" to school been designated? *[Safe Routes should be posted and distributed to parents.]*	☐	☐
	Are drop-off and pick-up points designated and supervised? *[Drop-off and pick-up points should be posted and distributed to parents.]*	☐	☐
	Are there recurring complaints, observed hazards, or a history of student injuries? *[Evaluation should be based on staff interviews, field observations, and review of Contact Log and School Police accident records.]*	☐	☐
	Notes:	**Score:**	
	Other Factors: *[mark factors requiring attention]*		
	☐ Annual meeting with traffic safety ☐ Crosswalks adequately marked		
	☐ Bi-annual with LAPD & School Police ☐ Traffic enforcement		
	☐ Accident reporting ☐ Others		
	☐ Adequate crossing guards		
14. Science Lab Safety	**Threshold Questions**		
	Is the Chemical Hygiene Plan kept in a designated location, readily available and are staff aware of their responsibilities?	☐	☐
	Has a Chemical Safety Coordinator been assigned by the Principal?	☐	☐
	Is a laboratory chemical inventory kept in a designated location and readily available?	☐	☐
	Are MSDSs readily accessible for all chemicals listed on the inventory? *[MSDSs should be kept in a centralized location known to all science staff.]*	☐	☐
	Is safety equipment adequate, available, and maintained in good condition?	☐	☐
	Are laboratory chemicals properly stored, secured and disposed of?	☐	☐
	Are all laboratory chemicals used at the school District-approved?	☐	☐
	Notes:	**Score:**	
	Other Factors: *[mark factors requiring attention]*		
	☐ Incompatible storage ☐ Fume hoods		
	☐ CSC training ☐ Outdated chemicals		
	☐ Eyewash/showers ☐ Over-accumulation of regents		
	☐ Personal Protective Equipment ☐ Others		
	☐ Fire extinguishers		
15. Off-Site Issues	**Threshold Questions**		
	Are off-site air emission sources affecting the school?	☐	☐
	Are off-site noise pollution sources affecting the school?	☐	☐
	Are there leaking transformers immediately adjacent to the school?	☐	☐
	Are industrial facilities adjacent or in close proximity to the school? *[Please note facility location, type of operations, and business name (if known)]*	☐	☐
	Are there multi-story buildings adjacent to the school?	☐	☐
	Notes:		
	Other Factors: *[mark factors requiring attention]*		
	☐ Abandoned vehicles ☐ Dead animals		
	☐ Sidewalk hazards (holes, cracking, etc.) ☐ Traffic/pedestrian hazards		
	☐ Truck/bus idling ☐ Fire hazards		
	☐ Rubbish ☐ Hazardous materials		
	☐ Rodent infestation ☐ Others		

372

ample, a classroom may be tentatively identified as having insufficient cooling or ventilation. Specific parameters for temperature, humidity, air flow, and the use of outside air may be spelled out but generally require measurement using a hygrometer, anemometer, or air meter (see table 25.2). Teachers and administrators often report excessive levels of classroom noise, which can be quickly assessed using a simple handheld meter to determine sound pressure levels in decibels; the resulting levels can then be compared to well-established standards for classroom noise and acoustics (see chapter 4). Other equipment commonly used during inspections includes a light meter to measure levels of classroom and hallway lighting; smoke tubes to evaluate air flow or the effectiveness of exhaust ventilation hoods; and an X-ray fluorescence (XRF) device to determine the presence of lead in painted surfaces.

The inspection and assessment process should be as comprehensive as possible, covering each of the standards listed in the guidebook. However, it is also important that the inspection process be viewed as a survey of school conditions and a general assessment of compliance with the applicable standards. The inspector may identify conditions or compliance issues that require consultation with legal counsel or a more detailed investigation by a trained expert. For example, the inspector may observe water damage on a classroom ceiling or wall. Although such a condition typically warrants the repair of defective equipment and the replacement of the affected ceiling or wall finishes, a more detailed assessment by a specialist (e.g., an industrial hygienist, a toxicologist, or various tradespeople in heating, air conditioning, and ventilation) will generally be required.

During the inspection, the inspector should record unsafe conditions and areas of noncompliance. In addition, the inspector may assign a compliance score of 1–10 for each of the standards listed in the guidebook or on the checklist. After the inspection, an exit interview should be conducted with the principal to review the findings and identify any items that require immediate attention. The principal will receive a corrective action notice (CAN) that details the necessary steps to bring the facility into compliance with applicable safety requirements (fig. 25.2) and a scorecard indicating the current level of fulfillment of each of the stan-

dards (fig. 25.3). These documents are discussed further in the next section.

Postinspection Documentation

The CAN (fig. 25.2) lists the corrective actions (column 3) necessary to bring the school into compliance with the respective standard (column 1). Standardized language for corrective actions may be taken directly from the inspection guidebook. This ensures consistency in the issuance of corrective actions and is appropriate in most cases. The standard language for any given corrective action may be modified by inserting a specific comment or location in column 4.

The CAN also includes a priority value of 1–4 for each of the actions and indicates the relative importance of taking the listed action (column 2). Peeling, lead-based paint in an area directly accessible to small children would likely receive a priority of 1, indicating the need for immediate correction. Alternatively, minor cracking in walkway pavement due to elevated tree roots may be assigned a priority value of 4, not requiring prompt action but indicating a condition that the inspector wished to bring to the attention of school management.

A due date should be established for each corrective action, and the CAN should be issued to school management within 10 days after the inspection. The principal should be asked to return a copy of the CAN within 30 days, indicating those items that have been corrected. Although this is a self-certification, it is generally an effective way to track compliance, especially if at least 5% of the self-certifications are independently reviewed by follow-up inspection. To track compliance efforts in response to inspections, a monthly exception report should be prepared to identify corrective action items still pending beyond the established due dates.

A compliance scorecard (fig. 25.3) is derived from the individual scores assigned to each of the standards on the inspection checklist. The individual scores may be converted to a percentage and assigned a value between 0 and 4 based on a scale considered appropriate by district management. In the example shown in figure 25.3, a value of 1–4 was assigned according to the following scale: 0–59% = 0; 60–69% = 1; 70–79% = 2; 80–89% =

Sample Corrective Action Notice

Inspection ID: **3362**

Inspection Date: 02/19/04

Facility Type: Senior High School
Enrollment: 1388

Local Area: 3
Inspector: Jim Smith

Principal: Ms. Mary Smith
Facility: Preston High School
Address: 3537 Fairfield Avenue
Los Angeles   CA   90027

Inspection Type:
Routine

Standard	Priority	Corrective Action	Location(s)	Due Date
Chemical Safety	1	Do not use chemicals that have not been approved.	Science Storage Room	ASAP
Fire/Life Safety	1	Repair, cover or provide guardrails to ensure safety for holes in floors, sidewalks, or other walking surfaces. If necessary, place a trouble call to Facilities Division.		ASAP
Fire/Life Safety	1	Utilize safety cans, flammable material cabinets or storage bunkers to store flammable materials.	Tool Room, Building A	ASAP
Accident Prevention	3	Ensure all employees are appropriately trained and made aware of the Injury and Illness Prevention Program.		03/26/04
Asbestos Management	3	Contact to H/S to conduct 6 month visual surveillance of each building known or suspected to contain Asbestos-Containing Material (ACM).		03/26/04

_____
Inspector

Jim Smith

Corrective Action Notice - Routine Inspection at Preston High School

Figure 25.2. Sample corrective action notice, Los Angeles Unified School District.

Sample Health & Safety Compliance Scorecard

Inspection Date: February 19, 2004
Facility Type: Senior High School
District: 1
OEHS Inspector: Jim Smith

Site Administrator: Ms. Mary Smith
Facility: Preston High School
Address: 3537 Fairfield Avenue
City: Los Angeles   **State:** CA   **Zip:** 90027

Standard	Compliance Scores (%)		
	Facility	**Local District 1**	**LAUSD**
Accident Prevention	60	73	61
Asbestos Management	60	76	75
Fire/Life Safety	30	63	57
Campus Security	60	78	75
Chemical Safety	50	68	64
Pest Management	80	74	73
Lead Management	60	71	70
Restroom Facilities	70	79	73
Indoor Environment	50	71	71
Maintenance and Repairs	50	70	66
Safe School Plan	80	83	75
Emergency Preparedness	50	69	70
Traffic and Pedestrian Safety	70	80	74
Science Lab Safety	50	55	55
SR	**1.00**	**1.78**	**1.50**
Overall Compliance Rating	**POOR**	**FAIR**	**FAIR**

Scoring Method: A compliance score of 1 to 10 is assigned to each of the 14 standards in the Compliance Checklist. If all threshold criteria are met for a standard, a minimum score of 7 is given. If all threshold criteria are not met for a standard, the maximum allowable score is 6. Each score is then converted to a percentage and assigned a value of 0-4 based on the following scale: 0% to 59% = 0; 60% to 69% = 1; 70% to 79% = 2; 80% to 89% = 3; 90% to 100% = 4. The "Scorecard Rating" (SR) is the average of the 14 values. An overall compliance rating of "Good", "Fair" or "Poor" is assigned to each facility based on the following SR values: 0.00-1.49 = Poor; 1.50-2.49 = Fair; 2.50-4.00 = Good.

N/R = Not Rated

Figure 25.3. Sample health and safety compliance scorecard, Los Angeles Unified School District.

3; 90–100% = 4. The scorecard rating is the average of the values assigned to each standard. An overall compliance rating of good, fair, or poor may then be assigned to each school, again based on a scale considered appropriate to district management. In figure 25.3, the overall ratings were derived from scorecard values using the following scale: 0.00–1.49 = poor; 1.50–2.49 = fair; 2.50–4.00 = good.

The use of a scorecard is effective in tracking improvements or other changes in compliance for a particular school or in comparing the results of different schools within a district. This information can provide an objective tool for the prioritization of schools for follow-up inspection, repairs, or modernization. For example, in the Los Angeles Unified School District, schools receiving a scorecard rating of Poor or a score of 50% or lower in any standard will be targeted for reinspection within 90 days to verify compliance.

Availability of Inspection Reports

Inspection reports and compliance scorecards should be made available to school staff, parents, and other members of the school community. Although access to the inspection findings can often generate significant interest and controversy, it provides a powerful tool for keeping school administrators and maintenance personnel properly focused on priority conditions and compliance issues. In addition, making inspection reports available is an effective way for school districts to demonstrate a clear commitment to the health and safety of students and school staff.

References

Lohrmann DK, Lewallen TC, Karwasinski P. 2005. Creating a healthy school using the healthy school report card: An ASCD action tool. Alexandria, VA: Association for Supervision and Curriculum Development.

Los Angeles Unified School District, Office of Environmental Health and Safety. 2005. School health and safety inspections and scorecard ratings. Available: http://www.lausd-oehs.org/fieldoperations_inspections.asp [accessed 26 March 2005].

U.S. General Accounting Office. 1995. School facilities: Condition of America's schools. GAO/HEHS-95-61. Washington, DC: Author.

26

Kathy Gips, Janice Nodvin, and I. Leslie Rubin

Children and Adults with Disabilities

■ *Summary*

- In the school environment, inclusiveness and individualization are primary goals in ensuring the full participation of students, staff, and visitors with disabilities.
- Planning and design must be multidisciplinary. The integration of people with disabilities includes awareness of legal standards and requirements, as well as consideration of inclusive language and attitudes.
- Four categories must be addressed to provide comfortable, effective surroundings for people with disabilities: mobility; dexterity; cognitive, emotional, and behavioral conditions; and sensory issues.
- Including the needs of people with disabilities when designing safe and healthy schools is a synergistic measure. Accessible design provides safety and usability for everyone. ■

Social policy relating to people with disabilities has progressed dramatically in recent years. In the past, people with disabilities were stigmatized and isolated; currently, the emphasis is on inclusiveness and integration. Throughout this book, various chapters emphasize that the needs of people with disabilities should be considered in creating safe and healthy school environments. Good lighting, for example, is essential for all students and staff, including those with visual impairments (chapter 3), and good acoustics are essential for everyone, including people with hearing impairments (chapter 4). In this chapter we focus on a wide range of attitudes and design features needed to achieve safe and healthy school environments for everyone, including those with disabilities (also see chapter 23).

Several themes run throughout this chapter. The first addresses inclusiveness, which requires that school facilities be inviting, friendly, and comfortably usable for everyone, including people with disabilities.

Second, considering the design needs of people with disabilities yields synergistic benefits for the greater society—the *curb cut principle*. Curb cuts that were originally intended for people in wheelchairs happen to benefit other people as well, such as older people who may have difficulty with steps that have no handrails, parents pushing strollers, people wheeling suitcases, and delivery staff with hand trucks.

A third theme is individualization. Educational planning for students with disabilities is not a "one-size-fits-all" process. Just as educational plans must be individualized, sometimes physical accommodations and adaptations must be planned around individual student and staff needs. That said, changes to the physical environment should anticipate a wide range of needs over time. For example, if hallway modifications are planned to accommodate students who use wheelchairs, planners should also consider that future students may have visual impairments or cognitive difficulties. Such needs should be included in the new design.

Tradeoffs represent a fourth theme. Certain environmental changes may work for some people but challenge others. For example, the bright lighting needed by people with some forms of low visual acuity may cause problems for those who need a dilated iris to see around a central opacity. Planning involves complex decision making and balancing of sometimes conflicting interests.

Finally, a multidisciplinary or, preferably, an interdisciplinary approach is presented. Expertise from many different specialties is important in creating healthy and safe school environments for students, staff, and others with disabilities. The interdisciplinary approach brings together input on the children, the educational processes, and the environment. It includes a medical approach, which is provided by primary care and specialty care pediatricians; and an educational approach involving regular classroom teachers, special education teachers, administrators, and roles for psychologists, speech therapists, occupational therapists, and physical therapists. In addition, in terms of designing school facilities, the interdisciplinary approach involves the expertise of architects. Participation of and input from students and staff with disabilities, their families, and advocates and other community members with disabilities are indispensable. Information on this approach, including details on specific developmental disabilities, has been comprehensively reviewed and is available elsewhere (Rubin and Crocker 2006).

Environmental changes are only part of the story of integration and inclusiveness. Arguably, the more important changes occur in attitudes. This chapter begins with a discussion of attitudes and language pertaining to disabilities, emphasizing the importance of "people-first" language and the outlooks it encourages. Next, we define disabilities and review the epidemiology of disabilities in schools, with information on the prevalence of various kinds of disabilities. The third section of the chapter is a review of legal requirements relevant to students, staff, parents, and others with disabilities. This section emphasizes the importance of addressing the needs of each person through an Individualized Education Program (IEP). Finally, design recommendations are offered for each part of the school to ensure that students and others with a wide range of disabilities can participate fully in all of the activities and services our schools provide.

Changing Views, Changing Language

Over the centuries, disabilities have been viewed through many lenses—from superstition and fear to science to compassion. Disabilities are more than biological facts; they exist in a social context and are the result of the way a person's abilities and needs interact with prevailing attitudes, environments, and opportunities.

Historically, in the United States, as in most other countries, people with disabilities lived in a society that had little understanding of or appreciation for those with physical, sensory, mental, and emotional disabilities. Some families and communities accepted people with disabilities. However, fear, shame, and confusion often led some people to hide or disown family members with disabilities. People with disabilities were often misdiagnosed, and few distinctions were made between people with cognitive disabilities, people with emotional disorders, people with cerebral palsy, and people with severe learning disabilities. Industrialization brought policies that segregated people with disabilities, including removing them from their families and placing them in large institutions. Some of these institutions offered education and training, whereas others were basically custodial. Over time, most of these institutions became overcrowded, and the people living in them were subjected to neglect and abuse.

Major changes began to emerge in the mid-twentieth century. The most important social changes occurred with the Civil Rights movement of the 1950s and 1960s. As various groups asserted their rights to fairness and nondiscrimination, the concept that people with disabilities had a right to an equal opportunity to participate in all aspects of society took hold and spread. Of note is the story of Rose Kennedy, mother of President John F. Kennedy, who, deeply affected by her own daughter's experience in institutional settings, championed a progressive approach to mental retardation. (The term "mental retardation," as it was then used, has since fallen into disfavor. The terms "developmental disabilities" [as a generic designation] or "cognitive disabilities" or "intellectual disabilities" [if specific to cognitive function] are currently preferred.) At the same time, society's realization of the deplorable conditions within large state institutions for people with disabilities resulted in the process of deinstitutionalization and the social concepts of "mainstreaming" and "normalization," in which people with intellectual and developmental disabilities are integrated into all aspects of society.

Before long, a landmark piece of legislation, the Education for All Handicapped Children Act of 1975 (Public Law 94-142), had enshrined a national commitment to Free Appropriate Public Education (FAPE) to all children with disabilities, regardless of the nature and degree of their handicaps.("Handicap" is the term that was used in the 1975 legislation, but that term has fallen into disfavor, and the term "disability" is currently preferred.) From then on, the momentum of the process was inexorable. The Special Olympics organization was created, acknowledging that people with intellectual and developmental disabilities are also eager to have a full range of activities and opportunities. The independent living movement, a national interest group that began in Berkeley, California, maintained that people with disabilities deserve the same civil rights, options, and control over choices in their lives as do people without disabilities, including "self-determination" or person-centered planning—the right to make one's own decisions rather than be subject to the decisions of professionals or agencies.

The evolution of attitudes has been paralleled by an evolution of language. Negative, degrading, or marginalizing terms have given way to terms that emphasize dignity and inclusiveness. For decades, people with disabilities were identified by their disability. In focusing on the specific disability, a person's strengths, abilities, skills, and resources were often ignored. For instance, the term "handicapped" is outdated, as mentioned above, and evokes negative images. The word derives from an old English bartering game, in which the loser was left with his "hand in his cap" and was thought to be at a *disadvantage*. Later, "disadvantage" was equated with having a disability label.

Table 26.1. People-first language vs. negative language

Negative language	Recommended language
Disabled	Person with a disability
Handicapped	Individual with a disability
Crippled	Child with a disability
Victim	
Spastic	
Patient (except in a hospital)	
Invalid	
Stricken	
Birth defect	Has had a disability since birth
Afflicted	Born with ____
Deformed	
Learning disabled	Has a learning disability
Brain damaged	Had a brain injury
Deaf	Hearing impairment
Deaf and dumb	Deaf/profoundly deaf (no hearing)
Deaf mute	Hard of hearing (some hearing)
	Nonverbal (limited speech)
Confined to a wheelchair	Person in a wheelchair
Restricted to a wheelchair	Uses a wheelchair
Wheelchair bound	Wheelchair user
Mental retardation	Intellectual disability
	Cognitive impairment

The preferred approach—known as people-first language—shows respect for the dignity of people with disabilities. People are recognized as individuals first and are then further characterized in terms of their specific disabilities. For example, "John, who has autism," and "My student, who has Down's syndrome," are preferable to "John is autistic" and "my Down's student." Further examples are shown in table 26.1.

Disabilities: Definitions and Epidemiology

Disability has multiple definitions, which can be confusing. Different definitions are used for specific reasons by various organizations and agencies, for example, by schools for educational planning or by pediatricians and psychologists for clinical reasons. State and federal agencies such as the Social Security Administration and the Veterans Administration may have specific terminology for administrative or situation-specific purposes (such as designated parking permits). Vocational rehabilitation agencies and insurance companies may define disability with other terms as well.

The legal definitions pertinent to schools are found in three federal laws: the Individuals with Disabilities Education Act (IDEA) of 1975 as amended (the revised name of the Education for All Handicapped Children Act), Section 504 of the Rehabilitation Act of 1973, also as amended, and the Americans with Disabilities Act (ADA) of 1990.

IDEA applies to children (not adults) and defines a child with a disability as one who has intellectual disabilities, a hearing impairment including deafness, a speech or language impairment, a visual impairment including blindness, a serious emotional disturbance, an orthopedic impairment, autism, a traumatic brain injury, "other health impairment," a specific learning disability, or multiple disabilities and who, by reason thereof, needs special education and related services.

Section 504 and the ADA apply to children and adults. For both of these laws, disability means a physical or mental impairment that substantially limits one or more of the major life activities; a record of such an impairment; or being regarded as having such an impairment.

Diagnostic terminology developed by the World Health Organization (WHO) is becoming widely accepted. WHO publishes the *International Classification of Functioning, Disability and Health* (ICF). The ICF focuses on health, functioning, and participation. Disability is viewed as the interaction among health conditions (diseases, disorders, injuries) that are features of the person and contextual factors such as social attitude, architecture, climate, terrain, and social structures. ICF combines a medical approach, which views disability as a feature of the person directly caused by disease, trauma, or other conditions, and a social approach, which views disability as a socially created problem that demands a political and social response. The synthesis of these two approaches leads to an understanding of individual difficulties in maximizing active participation in the community to the fullest extent of a person's abilities. This is most important in the school setting: recognizing that children may have difficulty participating actively, learning comfortably, and making progress and then responding with appropriate measures to help them overcome the barriers to achieving success through attain-

ment of their full potential. In this context, it is critical to appreciate the relationship between the environment and the individuals. This understanding applies to everyone but is particularly important for children and adults with disabilities.

It is also important to realize that most children with disabilities have more in common with average or typical children than they have differences. Many children with disabilities may differ from their peers in one or a few characteristics. A particular child may not see, hear, speak, learn, or walk as well as classmates but may be capable and even excel in another domain, such as social interactions, music, or computing. Although differences may be small, they can have a major impact on learning and socialization. Thus, it is the responsibility of the school to make sure that the impact of the disability is minimized through both the IEP process and environmental design.

Environmental Design

For design purposes, disability may be loosely divided into four categories: mobility; dexterity; cognitive, emotional, and behavioral conditions; and sensory. Each of these categories is greatly impacted by the built environment. Keep in mind, however, that the term "people with disabilities" includes millions of people with a broad range of abilities and limitations. What works for one person (or many people) does not necessarily work for everyone. Picture a 6-foot, 4-inch man with a bad back using a wheelchair-accessible public telephone. Two phones at different heights would be preferable.

Mobility

Impairments in mobility include cerebral palsy, spina bifida, other neurological conditions such as balance disorders, muscular dystrophy, paraplegia, multiple sclerosis, and other medical conditions such as heart disease and cancer, as well as having an amputated limb. People with mobility impairments may use manual wheelchairs, power wheelchairs, three-wheel scooters, forearm crutches, canes, walkers, braces, or no assistive device.

Mobility impairments may have diverse functional implications. A person who uses crutches (as do many others who do not use crutches) need stable, firm, nonslip walking surfaces. Most people with spinal cord injuries have an associated loss of sensation below their level of injury, so uninsulated hot water and drain pipes under the sink pose a burn hazard. Some kidney problems may require frequent fluid intake, so drinking fountains are essential—one for people who stand and one for those who use wheelchairs.

Dexterity

People with dexterity impairments may have difficulty grasping, twisting, pulling, pushing, or reaching. Lever hardware (rather than doorknobs), automatic controls, lowered-height reach range, and large pushbuttons that do not require much pressure are possible solutions.

Cognitive, Emotional, and Behavioral Disabilities

Cognitive, emotional, and behavioral disabilities constitute a broad category that includes specific learning disabilities, intellectual disabilities, autism spectrum conditions, attention deficit hyperactivity disorders, and a range of emotional and psychiatric diagnoses. This category of disability is characteristic of a large group of children in special education programs. In the last decade, attention deficit disorders have been increasingly identified as interfering with the education process, necessitating environmental modifications to reduce distractibility.

Currently, autism spectrum conditions have been the focus of diagnostic and remedial attention. These conditions require further consideration with regard to the ways in which noise, light, and crowding affect learning and behavior (see chapters 2, 3, and 4).

Sensory

Sensory disabilities include primarily vision and hearing impairment, but they also encompass speech and language impairments. People with visual impairment may have been blind from birth or have subsequently lost visual acuity; some may have selective visual disorders such as color blindness, depth perception difficulties, and problems adjusting from darkness to light.

People with hearing impairments may be deaf or hard of hearing from birth or have become deaf

Table 26.2. Extent of disability among noninstitutionalized children 5–15 years of age, United States, 2000

	Number	Proportion of total
Noninstitutionalized children 5–15 years of age	45,133,667	100.00
Children with no disability	42,518,748	94.2
Children with one disability	2,080,569	4.6
Sensory disability	238,498	0.5
Physical disability	161,401	0.4
Mental disability	1,604,363	3.6
Self-care disability	76,307	0.2
Children with two or more	534,350	1.2
Includes a self-care disability	342,711	0.8
Does not include a self-care disability	191,639	0.4

From U.S. Census Bureau (2000).

or hard of hearing after birth. Some may have auditory processing disorders.

Speech and language disorders range from sound substitutions to the inability to understand or use language or to use the oral-motor mechanism for functional speech. Some causes of speech and language disorders are hearing loss, neurological conditions, intellectual disabilities, and autism or physical conditions such as cleft lip or palate and vocal abuse and misuse. The various disabilities differ widely in prevalence (see table 26.2).

Legal Background

The Individuals with Disabilities Education Act is intended to guarantee that eligible children who require specialized services, including special education, receive a free appropriate public education designed to meet their unique educational needs. Special education instruction is to be provided in the least restrictive environment (LRE). Children with disabilities are to be educated with their typical peers in their neighborhood schools to the maximum extent possible. In addition, IDEA requires that children with disabilities have an equal opportunity to participate in extracurricular and nonacademic activities (i.e., children with disabilities will be everywhere in a school environment that children without disabilities will be).

ADA and Section 504 are broad civil rights laws

that apply to every aspect of American life: transportation; state, municipal, and county programs and services; private and public employment; businesses; nonprofit organizations; and, of course, public schools. Section 504 applies to entities that receive federal financial assistance (currently all or nearly all school districts). ADA applies regardless of whether an entity receives federal funds. Both laws cover anyone with a disability (children, parents, teachers, other staff, and the public), and both laws require that people with disabilities be in the most integrated setting appropriate. That is, children and adults with disabilities will be everywhere in a school environment that children and adults without disabilities will be.

The ADA and Section 504 contain specific design requirements, which differ for new construction, alterations, additions, and existing facilities (i.e., facilities that were in existence when the regulations went into effect). In July 2004 the U.S. Access Board released new design guidelines, the result of a decade-long review and update of the board's 1991 ADA Accessibility Guidelines. In the update, the board made its guidelines more consistent with model building codes (e.g., International Building Code) and with industry standards. The new Access Board 2004 guidelines have been adopted by the U.S. Department of Justice and will begin to apply to projects of various departments. Most federally funded construction projects beginning after May 8, 2006, must use the new guidelines (U.S. Access Board 2005). The federal government is working toward one design standard for all federal agencies, recipients of federal funds, and entities that have obligations under the ADA.

For existing facilities, rather than requiring full facility accessibility, Title II and Section 504 require school districts to operate each program so that, when viewed in its entirety, it is readily accessible to and usable by people with disabilities. Known as the program accessibility standard, this is one of the most important concepts in compliance planning. The concept of program accessibility is critical because it is a guideline in evaluating existing facilities and in formulating structural and nonstructural solutions to physical access problems in these facilities. For more information, see the chapter on program accessibility in *Compliance with the Americans with Disabilities Act: A Self-evaluation Guide for Public Elementary and Secondary Schools* (see the list of resources at the end of this chapter).

Private schools must comply with the ADA Standards for Accessible Design when undergoing new construction or alteration, provide reasonable accommodations for staff members with disabilities who need them, and make reasonable modifications for students with disabilities who need them. The ADA does not apply to schools owned or controlled by religious entities.

It is important to recall that the legal requirements in the ADA, Section 504, and state and local codes constitute minimum accessibility standards. Effective person-centered design goes beyond the legal requirements and invites both creativity and user participation. Individual abilities and limitations must also be considered. Students, teachers, or other staff with disabilities may need individual accommodations in order to function most effectively in the school environment.

Individual Needs: The Individual Education Program

Under IDEA, a student is required to have a comprehensive evaluation before special education and related services can be provided. The information gathered during the evaluation process is used by an interdisciplinary team to develop a plan that addresses the educational needs of a particular student—the Individualized Education Program (IEP). The IEP must include a statement of the child's present levels of educational performance, including how the disability affects the student's involvement and progress in the general curriculum, a statement of measurable annual goals, and benchmarks (short-term objectives). The IEP team, including the family, determines the placement and the special education, related services, and supplementary aids needed by each child with a disability.

IDEA requires that a child with a disability not be removed from the regular educational environment if the child's education can be achieved satisfactorily in regular classes with the use of supplementary aids and services. IDEA presumes that the first placement option considered for each student with a disability is the school and class the child would attend absent the disability. Before a child can be placed outside of the regular educational environment, the full range of supplementary aids and services that would facilitate the student's placement in the regular classroom setting must be considered. Following that, if a determination is made that a particular student cannot be educated satisfactorily in the regular educational environment even with the provision of appropriate supplementary aids and services, that student could then be placed in a setting other than the regular classroom. In all cases, placement decisions must be individually determined on the basis of the child's abilities and needs and not solely on factors such as category or significance of disability, availability of special education and related services, configuration of the service delivery system, availability of space, or administrative convenience. Rather, each student's IEP forms the basis for the placement decision.

Students with disabilities must be reevaluated if conditions warrant a reevaluation or the child's parents or teacher requests one; a reevaluation must take place at least once every 3 years.

Section 504 has similar (though less detailed and stringent) requirements concerning the needs of students with disabilities who do not need special education but nonetheless have a disability as defined under this law. Public schools must evaluate these children through an interdisciplinary team, which should identify the appropriate placement and the educational and related services needed. Again, the school district must place the student in a regular educational setting unless the team determines that, even with the use of supplementary aids and services, the child's education cannot be achieved satisfactorily in that setting.

Although private schools are not required to develop individual plans for students with disabilities, they do have an obligation to provide auxiliary aids and services, to make reasonable modifications, and to educate students with disabilities in the most integrated setting appropriate for those students (table 26.3).

Design Implications for Schools

Designing schools that meet the needs of people with disabilities is a process, not an event. It is not possible to present a checklist of design changes that, once completed, will ensure that a new school or adapted building is totally inclusive, safe, and healthy. This is an ongoing process of evaluating and adjusting the physical environment of the school buildings and grounds. There may be conflicts between the design needs of people with (and

without) disabilities. A teacher with limited mobility may require a warmer room temperature, which may be uncomfortable for more physically active students. A student with an emotional behavior disorder may feel distressed in a large teaching space where others are enjoying noisy interaction. Some of these issues can be addressed through design solutions that allow for choice and control. At other times, such as with room temperature, the solutions are more difficult.

As students grow and mature, their physical design needs often change. Some students may require additional space and facilities to manage their personal care. A child with an indwelling catheter may initially need privacy and space for an assistant to provide practical help and advice, but as the student becomes more independent and confident, may need an accessible restroom with good storage, waste disposal, and washing facilities. The following sections discuss various aspects of the physical environment as they pertain to students with disabilities, moving roughly from the outside to the inside of the school, including wayfinding, outdoor landscapes, getting to school, entrances, inside circulation, visual cues and lighting, changing floors, doorways, the auditory environment, auditoriums and other assembly areas, classrooms, support rooms, technician rooms, storage areas, cafeterias, the nurse's office, and restrooms. A final section addresses the challenges of emergency evaluation.

Wayfinding

Can students, parents, staff, and visitors orient themselves and find their way around the school buildings and grounds? Getting lost is stressful for everyone, and wayfinding is particularly important for people who have visual or cognitive impairments or limited stamina.

Wayfinding includes a broad set of design issues that affect the way in which people orient themselves and avoid getting lost. Students with certain forms of autism spectrum disorder can suffer increased levels of anxiety if the school building is difficult to understand, which can lead to stress and challenging behavior in the classroom. Some students may not be able to use the written word. For them, the use of colors, textures, and symbols within wayfinding systems becomes especially important. Recommendations for wayfinding design are shown in box 26.1.

Table 26.3. Disability statutes affecting public schools: a comparison of requirements

		Americans with Disabilities Act (Title II)	Section 504 of the Rehabilitation Act of 1973	Individuals with Disabilities Education Act
Who must comply?	Scope of coverage	All Programs and activities of state and local governments	All programs and activities of recipients of federal financial assistance	State and local education agencies funded under the Individuals with Disabilities Education Act
Who is protected?	Definition of disability	Noncategorical (covers people with a physical or mental impairment that substantially limits a major life activity, people who have a record of an impairment that substantially limits a major life activity, and people who are regarded as having such an impairment)	Noncategorical (covers people with a physical or mental impairment that substantially limits a major life activity, people who have a record of an impairment that substantially limits a major life activity, and people who are regarded as having such an impairment)	Categorical (covers specified disabilities only)
Oversight	Complaints	U.S. Department of Education, Office for Civil Rights	U.S. Department of Education, Office for Civil Rights	State Education Agency
Planning for compliance	Administrative requirements	Requires self-evaluation. Requires transition plan if structural modifications are needed if 50 or more employees.	Requires self-evaluation. Requires transition plan if structural modifications are needed.	Requires state plan submitted to Office of Special Education Programs
	Designation of responsible employee	Requires ADA coordinator if 50 or more employees	Requires Section 504 coordinator if 15 or more employees	Not required
	Grievance procedures	Required if 50 or more employees	Required if 15 or more employees	Procedural safeguards required
	Public notice	Requires ongoing notice of nondiscrimination on the basis of disability	Requires ongoing notice of nondiscrimination on the basis of disability	Requires notice to parents of child find activities
Employment	Reasonable accommodation	Required for qualified applicants or employees with disabilities, unless entity can demonstrate undue hardship	Required for qualified applicants or employees with disabilities, unless entity can demonstrate undue hardship	Not required
	Written job description	Advisable not specifically required	Advisable (not specifically required)	Not required
Facilities	Program accessibility	Requires services, programs, and activities in existing facilities to be readily accessible when viewed in their entirety	Requires services, programs, and activities in existing facilities to be readily accessible when viewed in their entirety	Not required

		Americans with Disabilities Act (Title II)	Section 504 of the Rehabilitation Act of 1973	Individuals with Disabilities Education Act
	Facilities accessibility	Requires compliance with ADA standards for accessible design or UFAS in new construction or alterations begun on or after 1/26/92; must comply with Access Board standards for federally funded construction started after May 8, 2006	Requires compliance with ANSI (R1971) in new construction or alterations begun on or after 6/3/77; compliance with UFAS or ADA Standards for Accessible Design if On or After 1/18/91; must comply with Access Board standards for federally funded construction started after May 8, 2006	Not required
	Maintenance of accessible features	required	Not required	Not required
Communication requirements	Auxiliary aids and services	Required for people with visual, hearing, and speech disabilities if necessary to provide effective communication	No requirement specified. Obligation exists to provide effective communication	Required only if written into the student's Individualized Education Program

UFAS = Uniform Federal Accessibility Standards.

Outdoor Landscapes

When climate, interest, and budget allow, include outdoor classrooms and sensory gardens in addition to the usual sports areas and playgrounds. At the very least, consider creating an outdoor gathering place or plaza that is outside the perimeter of the building or in an inner courtyard with seating areas, accessible paths, and plantings. At least part of the outdoor area should be in the sun during winter months and in the shade during the warmer months. Other suggestions are the following:

- Create a variety of spaces, including areas for large- and small-group discussions and activities, as well as quiet reflection.
- Do not use toxic plants, and arrange prickly or spiky plants so they can be easily identified or avoided.
- Maximize sensory experiences with scented plants, water, a variety of textured plants, wind chimes, and textured walls and seating.
- Make sure that paths are stable, firm, and slip resistant. Define the edges with materials of a different color and texture. Paths do not need to be paved.

- Consider providing an "animal relief area" for guide dogs and other assistive animals, separate from where humans will sit or gather.

Getting to School

To encourage integration without stigmatizing people with disabilities, the accessible route should be the same as that used by most people. External routes and level changes should minimize the effects of site gradients. Pedestrian slopes should be a maximum of 5% (1:20). Pedestrian paths of travel should connect site elements (e.g., public sidewalks, bus drop-off areas, parking lots, entrances, different buildings, playgrounds, ball fields) via the shortest routes possible. Because paths should be firm, slip resistant, smooth, and easy to maintain, materials to avoid in constructing them are bricks, cobblestones, rough-cut granite, and most pavers. Paths should also be at least 36 inches wide (48 inches or wider is preferable), with a cross slope no greater than 2% (1:50), have defined edges, and provide room for passing. Provide curb cuts wherever the path crosses a curb. Within 100 feet of entrances, there should be accessible passenger drop-off areas. In addition, students who are wait-

▪ *26.1. Recommendations for wayfinding*

- Entrance areas should be visible from driving and pedestrian routes and parking areas.
- Traffic and pedestrian patterns should be obvious.
- Pedestrian routes should contrast with driveways and parking areas in texture and visuals (light/dark).
- Provide visual and/or aural landmarks.
- Avoid visual clutter that might detract from or obscure entrances, pathways, places of arrival, and signs.
- Locate signs that direct people to entrances, to outdoor areas such as a sports field, and throughout their journey by providing information at junctures and long interior and exterior routes.
- Put signs with the international symbol of wheelchair accessibility at accessible entrances if any of the building entrances are not wheelchair accessible. Put signs at the inaccessible entrances indicating the direction of the accessible entrance. If all entrances are wheelchair accessible, the international symbol is not necessary at any entrance.
- If the building has more than one floor, is it obvious, when inside each entrance, where the elevator is? Is it obvious where the stairway is? If the gym, cafeteria, auditorium, or library are used by the public, is it obvious where they are and where the restrooms, water fountains, public phones, and other amenities are? If these items are not clearly visible, provide signs indicating their location and route.
- Directional and informational signs should have eggshell, matte, or some other nonglare finish. Characters and symbols should contrast with their background—either light characters on a dark background or dark characters on a light background—and be simple serif or sans serif type. Do not use all capitals in signs since they are difficult to read. Use sentence-style capitalization, or capitalize the first letter of each word. Add pictograms (such as the man/woman symbols at restrooms), which help people with cognitive disabilities, as well as those who do not know English.
- At permanent rooms and spaces such as classrooms, laboratories, libraries, restrooms, and auditoriums, signs should include the aforementioned, as well as Braille and raised characters. Mount permanent room signs on the wall, not the door, at 60" from the floor on the door latch side (not the hinged side).
- Signs, pedestrian paths, parking lots, and entrances should be well lit. ▪

ing for buses or for someone to pick them up should have indoor and outdoor waiting areas with places to sit, as well as room for wheelchair users. At outdoor waiting areas, canopies should protect people from sun, rain, and snow.

If a person has a mobility impairment and is not using a power wheelchair, distances can be daunting. For this reason, there should be accessible parking close to all entrances that students, the public, and staff might use, even if parking is not generally provided at those locations. Provide van-accessible spaces in addition to regular accessible spaces. (One in eight of these should be van accessible; the 2004 ADA Accessibility Guidelines recommend one in six.) These spaces need above-grade signs. The international symbol of wheelchair accessibility on the surface is good but not adequate since it may get covered up by snow. Provide side-walks along drives and clearly marked pedestrian walkways through parking lots and across vehicular drives. If the campus has several buildings and students travel between them, the pathways should be enclosed or covered where possible (fig. 26.1).

Entrances

Many people think of ramps when they think of access for people with disabilities, but if you can design or renovate a building to be accessible without ramps, do so. Not only are they sometimes unattractive, but they can also be dangerous and difficult to maneuver. If you install a ramp, provide stairs as well. People with certain mobility impairments who do not use wheelchairs find that stairs require less traveling and are easier to use. Where possible, fill and landscape the area at entrances

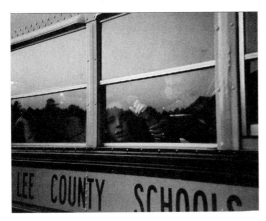

Figure 26.1. Transportation should be designed to include all children and is often a positive part of the child's school day. (Photo by Holly Markert.)

and provide a walkway (maximum 5% [1:20] slope) rather than a ramp. If you must construct a ramp because you are undertaking alterations or because of site constraints, use the least possible slope allowed by the site. An 8.33% (1:12) grade is the maximum steepness allowed, but this is not a goal. Many designers in cold climates either enclose or cover ramps or install heat coils in the surface to prevent buildup of snow and ice.

Automatic door-opening devices are wonderful for people with disabilities, parents with strollers, delivery people with hand trucks, and staff with rolling briefcases. Because building codes require that, for egress safety reasons, exterior doors not swing in, they usually swing out. However, this poses a slight hazard since an outward-swinging door can strike a child when in operation. Sliding doors are preferable, though more expensive. Outswinging doors should be set to open and close slowly, and generous, clear floor space should be provided so that people do not need to stand close to the doorway. Entrances should have level spaces that extend at least 60 inches on both sides of the doorway, which will offer stability for people entering and leaving the building.

Consider ways in which to avoid tripping hazards. Entrance mats are good at picking up dirt from shoes, wheelchairs, and other mobility devices, but they must be securely fastened. Doorways must provide at least 32 inches of clearance when open at 90°. If a building has double doors, at least one leaf of the doorway must provide 32 inches of clearance. Single doorways must provide

at least 18 inches (preferably 24 inches) of clear floor space on the latch-pull side of the door. This allows someone in a wheelchair or someone who uses canes or crutches to open the door without the door knocking into their mobility aid and pushing them backward.

These specifications are applicable to interior doors as well. In addition, thresholds at exterior doors should be less than 0.25 inch or beveled and no greater than 0.5 inch high (0.75 inch maximum for exterior sliding doors). Vestibules with two sets of doors must provide at least 48 inches from the edge of the door when open to the next doorway to allow maneuvering space. If the after-school-hours entrance is not the main public (accessible) entrance, be sure that all accessible amenities (parking, lighting, waiting area) are provided at the after-school-hours entrance as well. Steps should have consistent treads and risers with contrasting nosing, and handrails should be set at appropriate heights. Glass doors should include markings on the glass. If automatic door openers cannot be installed, exterior doors should require no more than 15 pounds of pressure for opening. Of course, the school may need to provide human assistance for people who are unable to operate doors themselves. Door hardware should be operable without tight grasping, pinching, or twisting.

Inside Circulation

Consider both the distances that students, staff, and visitors have to travel between activities and the complexity of the routes. Locate common spaces such as auditoriums, libraries, cafeterias, and gymnasiums in a central area surrounded by classrooms; common spaces should also be near an entrance so that students, staff, and visitors with limited mobility can reach them easily. Floor surfaces should be slip resistant, even when wet.

Thoughtful use of color and contrasting materials increases usability for people with cognitive disabilities and visual impairments. Examples include the following:

- stairway and ramp handrails that contrast with walls
- contrasting color at the edge of steps
- stairs that contrast with walls
- stair risers and treads that contrast with each other

- doorways that contrast with walls
- door hardware that contrasts with doors
- a unique color scheme for areas of the building or floors so that people have a quick sense of where they are (Color can be used to indicate both changes in directions in corridors and changes in floor levels.)
- landmark features such as seating, display areas, and artwork to help people orient themselves
- views to the outside and to other important parts of a building to help people find their way
- contrasting floor finishes and textures to define large open areas (Circulation can be difficult for students, especially those with visual and cognitive impairments.)
- no bold patterns such as stripes or checks on wall and floor coverings because these can be disorienting
- nonglare finishes on floor and wall coverings.

Visual Cues and Lighting

What students, staff, and visitors with visual impairments see may vary enormously. Some will see things clearly but within a very limited visual field, whereas others may have a loss of central vision. Some may have a loss of acuity, a blurring of vision, or a loss of color vision. Moreover, many of these conditions can occur together. Some people can see only shadows or cannot see at all. Because of these varying circumstances, people's needs sometimes conflict. For example, the use of higher than normal levels of lighting can help students whose visual acuity can be improved by the contraction of the iris, which produces a greater depth of field. However, for others, such as students who need a dilated iris to see around a central opacity, these higher light levels can cause problems.

Adequate contrast is needed between ceilings and walls since students with visual impairments often use the ceiling area to orient themselves and to identify the size of the space they are in.

Because of the inherent nature of visual impairments, people who are totally blind or have low vision occasionally walk into things. We can lessen these bruising incidents by making sure that travel paths are free from protruding objects. Most people with visual impairment who use a cane are trained to use both the touch technique and the diagonal

technique to detect objects. Generally, an adult who is using a cane will detect objects whose leading edges are no higher than 27 inches from the floor (this distance is lower for children).

The following safety measures can also be effective:

- Wing walls and alcoves can be used for elements such as water fountains, public telephones, and fire extinguishers.
- To ensure that a person's head does not hit overhanging objects, paths must provide at least 80 inches of vertical clearance. This is also an important consideration at open stairways and sloped walls.
- Overhanging objects that protrude more than 4 inches from a wall also should be at least 80 inches high.

Lighting is also important for students with hearing impairments. The teacher's face needs to be well lit to enable students to see facial expressions and the speaker's mouth and to read speech more easily (see chapter 3 for more details):

- Good levels of natural light should be created wherever possible.
- Lights should be positioned where they do not cause glare, reflection, confusing shadows, or pools of light and dark, which can be misleading.
- Uplighting, which is set above standing eye level, can be especially helpful in creating a glare-free environment.
- If possible, all lighting, whether natural or artificial, should be controllable and adjustable to suit the needs of individuals.
- Sudden changes in light levels should be avoided, as they can be disorienting.
- Some students and staff will need direct task lighting.

Changing Floors

How do people get from one floor to the other? Changes in level can be achieved in a number of ways, including the use of stairs, ramps, elevators, platform lifts, and stair lifts in certain situations.

- Full-sized, commercial elevators are preferred, but schools frequently use LULAs (limited-use, limited-access elevators) or wheelchair lifts because of budget or space constraints.

The latter should be used only in renovations, not in new construction.

- Stairglide wheelchair lifts are not recommended, but they may be the only solution in an older building if there is no space for a full-sized elevator, LULA, or vertical lift.
- One problem with LULAs and wheelchair lifts is that state elevator codes often require a key to operate them. In that case, provide signs at entrances and at the devices themselves, indicating where the key is kept (usually in the school office).
- Changes in level by ramp or stairs should be clearly indicated to avoid falls, stumbling, or loss of balance. This can be achieved through the use of color and tone, changes in texture, lighting, and signs.
- Step nosings should have contrasting colors. Mark the top and bottom steps with a contrasting stripe.
- Handrails that can be easily gripped should be provided on both sides of stairs and ramps.
- Rails should extend 12 inches beyond the top and bottom of stairs and ramps, unless the extension would protrude into a path of travel. The extra length gives people a place to rest and get their bearing and provides a tactile clue that a level change is ahead.

Doorways

Students and staff with disabilities should be given their own keys. Consider where the key will be for public after-hours use when the school office is closed. For students and staff with limited manual dexterity, keys may need to be redesigned or replaced with garage door opener–type controls or smart cards.

Clear door openings should be at least 32 inches wide. Thresholds should be flush. Fire doors should be held open by alarm-linked devices wherever possible.

Use door hardware that can be operated without tight grasping, pinching, or twisting, such as a lever, push bar, or loop type. Doors should be carefully weighted to open easily; hinged doors should be 5 pounds maximum. Automatic door-opening devices may be needed where doors are heavy or if people are unable to use any hardware.

Outline doorways with a contrasting border of color and finish. Doors should contrast with doorways and surrounding walls. Door hardware should contrast with the door. Visibility panels with safety glass should be provided at different levels to allow young students, students using wheelchairs, and standing students to see into a space.

The Auditory Environment

Acoustics have a profound influence on people with hearing disabilities, those with visual disabilities (who use sounds to help orient themselves), and those who find loud noises distressing (see also chapter 4).

- When determining where to locate a building, consider the proximity to noise sources such as roads and aircraft flight paths.
- When considering where to locate an addition or an activity, consider external noise sources such as delivery areas, bus stops, sports fields, and playgrounds, as well as inside noisy sources such as food preparation areas, the gym, HVAC systems, and music rooms.
- Open-plan areas can cause difficulties in controlling acoustics. Noise levels can be controlled by the use of buffer zones and physical barriers such as walls and windows.
- A TTY (also called Telecommunications Device for the Deaf or text telephone) is a terminal used for two-way text conversation over a telephone line. Install a TTY at public pay phones so that people who are deaf or cannot use the phone by voice can make outgoing calls. A TDD or TTY should also be available in the central office so that parents who are deaf can call the school and students who are deaf can call home.
- Phones used by students, parents, and visitors should also have volume control devices.
- Emergency warning systems should have visual, as well as audible, components. Install visual signals in classrooms, restrooms, corridors, and special-use areas, approximately one every 100 feet.

Auditoriums and Other Assembly Areas

Optimally, students who use wheelchairs and other mobility devices should have a range of seating options: front, back, middle. This is easier to accomplish in new construction than in renovations.

Wheelchair spaces should be dispersed and located next to seated companion spaces. Where there is a path of travel from the audience area to the stage, the path should be accessible (by vertical lift or ramp). Green rooms, dressing rooms, and other areas behind the stage should be on an accessible route and provide adequate clear space. Seating should contrast with floors and walls. Students and others may need to have seats reserved in the front rows. Both the stage and the seating area must be well lit. Where sign language interpreters may be present:

- provide direct lighting on the interpreter
- provide a dark, single-color background (which can be the wall) behind the interpreter
- reserve seats in the front rows so that students and others can see the presenters' faces, as well as the interpreter.

An assistive listening system (ALS) amplifies and delivers sounds (and not background noise) directly to the user. Auditorium and other large assembly areas should have permanently installed assistive listening systems. Portable systems can be used by students and teachers in classrooms or by parents with hearing disabilities who attend parent-teacher conferences or participate in parent night in the classroom. An ALS can be used alone or to augment sound amplification systems. When used with a sound amplification system, special equipment integrated into the system transmits the same signals to the ears of the person wearing an ALS receiver.

There are three general types of systems, named for the method of signal transmission: induction loop, frequency modulation (as in FM radio), and infrared. The choice of a specific system is individualized and should provide maximum benefit to the individual in the particular school setting with the available resources.

Electromagnetic (EM) fields can be a serious source of interference for hearing aids and assistive listening devices. Some interference comes from elements of the building environment, particularly from lighting and the electrical distribution system and equipment connected to it. In new construction, intrusive EM can be avoided by careful design and construction to isolate or shield areas where telephones and assistive listening devices will be used—offices, pay telephone banks, auditoriums, meeting rooms, and classrooms. Incoming electri-

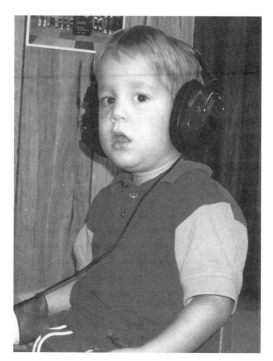

Figure 26.2. Assistive listening systems provide inclusive learning experiences to those students with hearing impairments. (Photo by Holly Markert.)

cal service, electrical rooms, and transformers should be isolated and shielded, and pipe entries grounded. Looped piping systems designed for multibuilding sites and campuses may require nonconductive isolators to prevent inadvertent current transmission (fig. 26.2).

Classrooms

Provide a variety of different-sized teaching spaces. Link large teaching spaces to smaller ones where assessment, support teaching, different kinds of therapy, and small-group study can take place. Provide space for equipment storage. Teaching spaces should be flexible and easily rearranged for different purposes and by various groups of students. Provide additional room within the teaching space for teaching assistants to work alongside students. Provide good lighting on the teacher's face to help students with vision and hearing impairments or with cognitive difficulties such as attention deficit disorder or autism spectrum disorder.

The average wheelchair's footprint is about 30 × 48 inches. Some students and teachers will stay in their wheelchairs. Others, however, may use a wheelchair only to get from class to class and then use crutches, another mobility device, or nothing within the classroom. Provide space where wheelchairs can be parked. Provide unobstructed routes at least 36 inches wide for people who use wheelchairs and other mobility devices.

Provide adjustable-height tables for working, computers, printers, and so on. Provide electric outlets for power wheelchairs and other equipment that may need to be recharged.

Consider where students who use wheelchairs are going to sit when other students are sitting on the floor. Students who use wheelchairs should be at eye level with their peers to encourage interaction. These students may need adaptive seating on the floor. Equipment that needs to be handled by students should have controls they can use without tight grasping, pinching, or twisting (fig. 26.3).

Select materials to provide sufficient acoustic absorption in a space. Curtains, acoustic ceilings, corkboard, and bulletin boards all increase the absorption in a space and reduce reverberation time. Choose floor coverings that muffle the sounds of equipment, footsteps, wheelchairs, and other mobility aids. The issue of floor coverings has been controversial in many schools. Although carpeting provides good sound absorption and is more comfortable to sit on than many other types of covering, carpeting can add to indoor air quality problems. Try using smaller, sectional, low-pile rugs or carpeting that can be easily (and frequently) cleaned. Provide rubber tips on chairs, tables, or other equipment that might be moved across the floor and create noise. Some schools have put tennis balls on the ends of chair legs. Some students may need a PA system or assistive listening device.

Differentiate a child's seat from other seats with contrasting colored tape on the back of the chair. Use a consistent color for the student's own areas such as storage cubby and coat hook. Use contrasting colors to differentiate between floor, walls, and ceilings. Contrasting molding at the intersection of floor and wall emphasizes the change in planes. Use contrasting colors on light switch plates and other controls.

Keep the location of furniture, equipment, and other objects in the room consistent, and keep the space uncluttered. Walking areas should be free of small items that are difficult to see. Keep doors and cabinets completely open or closed (not halfway). Differentiate areas of a room with different-colored and textured mats that contrast with the floor. Use placemats, colored paper, or tablecloths without patterns to define a student's work area. Provide adjustable reading stands that elevate books and writing materials. They bring the material closer and can reduce back and neck strain. Cover open shelves and other visually distracting areas. Solid-colored cloth is effective. Secure rugs and mats to the floor so that people do not trip on them.

Curtains and/or blinds on windows will control glare. Ideally, windows should be set back from the wall surface. If windows protrude, hang a dark mobile or strips of wide ribbon at windows that students are likely encounter. Replace fluorescent light bulbs that flicker, but avoid blue-spectrum bulbs. Use filters to reduce glare. Some students may need direct lighting. Gooseneck lights with incandescent bulbs and contrasting color controls work well, as do lamps with controls to adjust lighting levels. Student seating should not face direct lighting sources such as windows or lamps.

Support Rooms

Small-group rooms designed for flexible use are an invaluable resource for most schools. In some situations, it may be possible to use one room for a range of different functions. In others, a series of rooms may be needed. Support rooms could be used by

- staff members for one-on-one or small-group teaching, counseling, and therapy sessions
- speech and language therapists, occupational

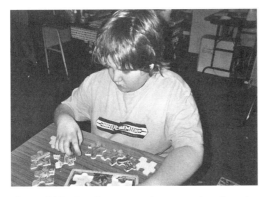

Figure 26.3. Simple games and toys may be adapted to suit the child's fine motor and coordination skills. (Photo by Holly Markert.)

therapists, educational psychologists, and physical therapists to store equipment and to work with students

- parents and guardians to meet with school staff and visiting therapists
- students who may be vulnerable or in need of additional support or who need to be removed from the classroom
- students who might develop social skills better in a smaller, less formal atmosphere than the classroom.

Technician Rooms

Technician rooms may be needed for adjustments, maintenance, and repair of equipment and aids if the number of students using assistive devices or technology is high.

Storage areas

Equipment and teaching resources for people with disabilities require adequate storage space. Extra space is needed throughout the school

- in entrance areas for storage of mobility aids, wheelchairs, and other equipment in teaching rooms, sports areas, and small-group roomsin rooms that technicians use to store equipment such as mobility aids and batteries.

Cafeterias

All students who choose to eat in the cafeteria should be provided with accessible spaces to enable them to eat in a dignified way with their peers. Extra circulation and seating space may be required to allow for students who use wheelchairs, walkers, canes, or crutches. Aisles should be at least 36 inches wide. Additional space may be required to provide parking space for wheelchairs.

Tray slides and serving counters should be designed with a maximum height of 34" to accommodate students in wheelchairs. Avoiding metal cutlery containers can help reduce noise levels, which will benefit students with hearing difficulties. Classroom recommendations are also appropriate for the cafeteria with respect to students with visual or cognitive difficulties.

The prevalence of severe food allergies in students has caused heated discussions about "peanut-free" buildings and/or cafeterias. Consider providing two separate eating areas; however, students with allergies should not be segregated.

Space and equipment may be needed for the preparation of special foods and storage of equipment. Space may be required for assistants to sit alongside students and help them eat.

Nurse's Office

The nurse's offices should have adequate room for

- students to move around freely and park their wheelchairs or other mobility devices
- students to be examined and treated, take medication, test glucose levels, or self-administer treatments in comfort and privacy
- assistants who may be needed to help the students maneuver themselves
- storage of medication, records, and information
- additional equipment such as hoists, changing tables, and showers
- students and staff who are not feeling well to rest in privacy.

Restrooms

Locate restrooms so that the distances people have to travel are not too great, and make sure that the routes are accessible. There should be an accessible restroom on each floor. People should not have to travel by elevator to reach a usable restroom.

The needs of students, staff, and visitors will vary. Consider providing changing tables for children with disabilities of all ages who need diapering. Some students might require the help of one or two assistants. Some might transfer laterally by themselves from a wheelchair to the toilet, requiring a low toilet seat, grab bars, and back supports. Others may require grab bars just for balance.

Most of us are familiar with wheelchair-accessible stalls, but fewer people are aware of "ambulatory" stalls, which are 36 inches wide with grab bars on both side walls. This stall is intended for someone who has difficulty walking, sitting from a standing position, or standing from a seated position. The parallel, horizontal grab bars are used simultaneously. The door should swing out and be hinged to self-close.

Schools should also consider providing single-user, wheelchair-accessible restrooms in addition to accessible stalls in multi-user rooms. Single-user rooms allow privacy and also provide room for assisting a person with a disability who needs help with toileting procedures such as catheterization or emptying colostomy bags and washing. In single-user restrooms or accessible stalls, consider installing alarm systems at different levels, including floor level, so that students can call for assistance.

Mobile hoists eliminate the need for human assistants to lift. They basically consist of a wheeled chassis—a boom that is raised to lift the user and lowered to position the user on the toilet. Some hoists attach to overhead tracking and can be used for independent transfers.

Provide visual emergency alarms. Auditory and visual alarms in the hallway will work for people who can hear, but not for people within rooms with closed doors (such as restrooms) who are deaf or severely hard of hearing.

Emergency Evacuation

The ADA requires areas of rescue assistance (or areas of refuge) in new buildings only. They are not required in buildings equipped with sprinkler systems that have built-in signals used to monitor the system's features. Areas of rescue assistance must meet specifications for fire resistance and ventilation. They may be incorporated into the design of fire stair landings or provided in other places. Areas of rescue assistance must have two-way communication devices so that users can place a call for evacuation assistance. Horizontal exits, which use fire barriers, separation, and other means to help contain the spread of fire on a floor, can substitute for areas of rescue assistance, provided they meet applicable building codes. Horizontal exits enable occupants to evacuate from one area of a building and go to another area or building on approximately the same level that provides safety from smoke and fire.

Many students with disabilities will be able to evacuate themselves, but some will need assistance. This should be discussed during each student's individual plan development. The same is true for staff with disabilities. Some may need a "buddy" to get out safely. Emergency evacuation chairs, which can be used to get people down stairs, are usually stored on the wall in stairways. People transfer from their wheelchair to the device, and an assistant rolls the device, which is on rubber tracks, down the

stairs. Portable wheelchair lifts are devices that attach under most standard wheelchairs and can be used indoors or outdoors. The user does not have to transfer from the wheelchair to the device, and an attendant can move a person in a wheelchair both up and down stairways.

Conclusion

Including the needs of people with disabilities when designing and creating healthy and safe schools will increase safety and usability for everyone. We all benefit from doorways that are easy to find, adjustable light levels, stable walking surfaces, and equipment that is easy to turn on and off. Universal design is a growing international trend. It is important that schools, which are so central to community life and in which children spend much of their time, be at the forefront of this movement toward more inclusive societies.

Resources

- ADA and Accessible IT Centers. Ten centers funded by the National Institute of Disability and Rehabilitation Research provide technical assistance, publications and training on the Americans with Disabilities Act, and accessible information technology in education. Telephone: 800-949-4232
  http://www.adata.org
- Adaptive Environments, Inc., Boston. This organization provides expertise in legally required accessibility plus promotion of best practices in human-centered or universal design. Resources include *Compliance with the Americans with Disabilities Act: A Self-evaluation Guide for Public Elementary and Secondary Schools,* a 277-page book published in 1995 jointly with the U.S. Department of Education, and "The ADA and Public Schools: Access for All," an 18-minute video. Telephone: 617-695-1225; E-mail: info@Adaptive Environments.org
  http://www.AdaptiveEnvironments.org
- Center for Inclusive Design and Environmental Access (IDEA Center), University of Buffalo School of Architecture and Planning. The center is dedicated to improving the design of

environments and products by making them more usable, safer, and more appealing to people with a wide range of abilities throughout their lives. Its web site includes information on schools.
http://www.ap.buffalo.edu/idea/
- Center for Universal Design, North Carolina State University. This national research, information, and technical assistance center evaluates, develops, and promotes universal design in housing, public and commercial facilities, and related products. Telephone: 800-647-6777. E-mail: cud@ncsu.edu
http://www.design.ncsu.edu:8120/cud
- Council for Exceptional Children. The council, which publishes *Research Connections in Special Education,* devoted its Fall 1999 issue (no. 5) to universal design.
http://ericec.org/osep/recon5/rc5cov.html
- Federal Resource Center for Special Education. The center supports a nationwide technical assistance network to respond to the needs of students with disabilities. Telephone: 202-884-8215
http://www.dssc.org/frc
- National Center on Accessing the General Curriculum (NCAC). The center's web site offers extensive materials on universal design.
http://www.cast.org/ncac/WhatisUDL372.cfm
- National Clearinghouse for Educational Facilities. The clearinghouse provides information on planning, designing, funding, building, improving, and maintaining schools, including articles on accessibility, acoustics, and indoor air quality. Telephone: 888-552-0624
http://www.edfacilities.org
- National Dissemination Center for Children with Disabilities. The center provides information on disabilities, IDEA, and related educational issues.
http://www.nichcy.org
- U.S. Access Board. The board provides publications and technical assistance on the ADA Accessibility Guidelines and the Uniform Federal Accessibility Guidelines. Telephone: 800-872-2253. E-mail: info@access-board.gov
http://www.access-board.gov
- U.S. Department of Education, Office of Civil Rights. This agency provides technical assistance, pamphlets, and complaint information on Section 504 of the Rehabilitation Act and

Title II of the ADA in education. Regional enforcement offices serve each state. Telephone: 800-421-3481 (voice); 877-521-2172 (TTY)
http://www.ed.gov/about/offices/list/ocr
- U.S. Department of Justice, Disability Rights Section. This agency maintains a website that provides extensive technical information on compliance with the ADA, including school recommendations.
http://www.usdoj.gov/crt/ada/liblist.htm

References

Barker P, Barrick J, Wilson R. 1995. *Building sight: A handbook of building and interior design solutions to include the needs of visually impaired people.* London: Royal National Institute for the Blind.

Brennan V, Peck F, Lolli D. 1992. *Suggestions for modifying the home and school environment: A handbook for parents and teachers of children with dual sensory impairments.* Watertown, MA: Perkins School for the Blind.

Calkins MP. 1988. *Design for dementia: Planning environments for the elderly and confused.* Owings Mills, MD: National Health Publishing.

Clarkson J, Keates S, Coleman R, Lebbon C, eds. 2003. *Inclusive design: Design for the whole population.* London: Springer-Verlag.

Greenman J. 1988. *Caring spaces, learning places: Children's environments that work.* Bellevue, WA: Exchange Press.

Population Reference Bureau. 2000. Analysis of data from the U.S. Census Bureau, Census 2000, Summary File 3 (Table PCT26).

Rubin IL, Crocker AC. 2006. *Medical care for children and adults with developmental disabilities,* 2nd ed. Baltimore, MD: Paul H. Brookes.

Sorensen RJ. 1979. *Design for accessibility.* Philadelphia: McGraw-Hill.

U.S. Access Board. 2005. Update of ADA and ABA Standards. Available: http://www.access-board.gov/ada-aba/standards-update.htm [accessed 12 April 2006].

U.S. Department of Education and Adaptive Environments, Inc. 1995. Self-evaluation guide for public elementary and secondary schools. Washington, DC: US Dept of Education.

Wilkoff W, Abed LW. 1994. *Practicing universal design: An interpretation of the ADA.* Philadelphia: Van Nostrand Reinhold.

World Health Organization. 2002. Toward a common language for functioning, disability, and health: The international classification of functioning, disability, and health (ICF). Geneva: WHO.

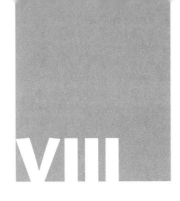

Health Services in Schools: Environmental Health Aspects

Julia Graham Lear

Health Services at School: Environmental Considerations

■ *Summary*

- The provision of health services at school—treating common ailments, caring for school ground injuries, and managing chronic diseases—is a daily occurrence in many U.S. schools.
- Professionals who deliver health care may need particular physical settings in which to practice.
- These professionals play a role in recognizing and controlling hazards and in achieving safe, healthy environments throughout the school. ■

School-based Health Care: The People and the Facilities

Health services are provided at schools across the nation and represent an opportunity not only to safeguard the health of students in general but also to promote environmental health. This chapter begins with an overview of school health services, describing the people, the facilities, and the clinical services, and then turns to aspects of school health services relevant to safe and healthy environments.

School Health Staff

Nurses represent the majority of health professionals in schools. While they have broad responsibilities, school nurses spend most of their time treating injuries and illnesses, both acute and chronic, rather than participating in population-focused activities such as disease and hazard surveillance. In 2000 there were an estimated 56,000 nurses in the nation's 92,000 public schools and about 5,000 more in the 25,000 private and parochial schools, according to the National Sample Survey of Registered Nurses (Spratley et al. 2002). Approximately one-third of these nurses were part-time employees, suggesting that fewer than 40% of schools have a full-time school nurse. The remaining schools were staffed with a nurse during some portion of the week or had no nurse at all. The nature of the school nurse's work is illustrated by the accounts in box 27.1.

Other health professionals who provide services at school include a diverse array of physical and mental health providers, including school psychologists, social workers, nurse practitioners, physicians, dentists, dental hygienists, nutritionists, physical therapists, and speech therapists. Guidance counselors, who offer primarily academic sup-

■ *27.1. School nurses' accounts of environmental health challenges*

I do a lot of work with students who have chronic conditions, but there is one that I am very involved with. Mary, I will call her, was admitted to General Springs Hospital last spring and was in the intensive care unit for several days due to uncontrolled asthma. As Somalian refugees, her family has had difficulty bridging language barriers and understanding how to manage Mary's disease. I was informed about her asthma diagnosis and have worked the 3 days a week I am at school to teach and reteach Mary about her medications and how she must take and interpret peak flow meter readings. I am in contact with the home health nurse and the doctor on a weekly basis, and I fax peak flow readings monthly to her doctor.

This year I have made home visits and continued patient education and treatment for Mary. When she was having trouble, twice this fall I have referred her to her doctor for emergency visits. I've learned that Mary was not letting her mother know she needed to go into the hospital. I know that what we do at school has helped Mary and prevented more inpatient hospitalizations.

*   *   *

One of our third-grade students brought gifts of necklaces back from Mexico and gave them to six of her friends. Most of the necklaces had mercury inside a blown glass chili pepper pendant that hung on a black cord. One morning I noticed that mercury was leaking out of one of the necklaces and getting on the hands of three girls. We later learned that several students had mercury stuck to the soles of their shoes. By the time I found out what was happening, the classroom and library were contaminated with mercury. I called the Seattle Poison Control Center, and the custodian called the school district's hazardous materials coordinator. The poison control center told us that a small amount of mercury was not alarming. Each child should wash the areas of skin that touched the mercury. The hazardous materials coordinator arrived within an hour. We were joined by the PTA president and a biologist, who brought along a machine that detects mercury. We scanned all the kids we identified as possibly contaminated. In the end, we confiscated three pairs of athletic shoes and one shirt, which were disposed of by the hazardous materials coordinator. I sent an e-mail to my school nurse colleagues, suggesting they be on the lookout for these necklaces. They are illegal in the United States, but travelers may bring them home as souvenirs or gifts. Teachers aren't trained to recognize these potentially poisonous gifts. We were all relieved to learn that the danger could be minimized with simple interventions.

(From school nurses in Seattle, Washington) ■

port, may also offer counseling on health matters and may therefore be regarded as health professionals. While some of these providers have few environmental requirements other than privacy and locked cabinets, others, such as dentists, physicians, or nurse practitioners, may need running water, special electrical outlets, or arrangements for daily disposal of infectious waste. The numbers of school-based health professionals are summarized in table 27.1.

In some schools, health centers provide medical care, mental health services, and, less commonly, dental care. In the 2000–2001 school year, there were approximately 1,500 such centers across the country (Center for Health and Health Care in Schools 2003).

Health aides, also referred to as paraprofessionals or unlicensed assistive personnel (UAPs), range from full-time staff members in the nurse's office or health suite to part-time staff (including school secretaries and teachers) who assume responsibility for medication management or other health-related duties in addition to their regular jobs. The term "unlicensed assistive personnel" refers to workers who are not licensed to perform nursing tasks but operate under the license and supervision of a reg-

Table 27.1. Health professionals at schools

Category	Number
School nurses	56,000 full-time and part-time
School psychologists	59,400 full-time and part-time
Social workers	39,600 full-time and part-time
Guidance counselors	81,000
School-based health center staff	1,500 centers staffed by a mix of nurse practitioners, clinical social workers, health aides, physicians, dentists, dental hygienists

From the Center for Health and Health Care in Schools (2003).

istered nurse. The UAPs have varying degrees of training or certification. Standards for UAP training are usually established by the state boards of nursing because the aides perform their functions as assistants to registered nurses. The number of school health aides who provide services across the United States is unknown but assumed to be substantial. These health staff all have facility and equipment requirements that relate to their responsibilities.

A Team Approach: Partnering for a Successful Health Office

Although school nurses or other health staff help identify and respond to environmental health issues within the school, other school personnel as well as community-based professionals are key partners in this work. Custodians, teachers, the principal, and parents are critical to supporting a well-designed and well-maintained health suite as well as implementing policies to protect student and staff health. (For some partners, especially parents and other volunteers, important confidentiality considerations arise, and these must be addressed.) For example, the custodian is critical to the proper disposal of infectious waste, and the health department can help respond to an infectious disease outbreak. Table 27.2 lists potential members of the health suite's support team and the roles they might play in achieving a healthy school environment.

School Health Facilities

The responsibilities of school health professionals differ considerably from those of teachers and ad-

Table 27.2. Partners to support a healthy health suite

Personnel	Function/perspective
School nurse or other school health professional	Provides first-aid and basic health services to students, documentation of student immunization status, provision of individual and group health education, care for children with disabilities, maintenance of children's school health records
Custodian	Has primary responsibility for cleaning the school, likely first responder in case of facility problems. A critical ally in anticipating problem areas and developing safe cleanup strategies.
Principal	Is in charge of the school. Without principal's support, improvements are impossible.
Parents	Have the greatest stake in the safety and well-being of their children. With sufficient education on the issues, they share the concerns of the school nurse and provide a higher level of political clout.
Science teachers	Are the most likely to have toxic materials stored in classroom. Need to partner with school nurse in checking for hazardous materials that require disposal
School district HQ members	Provide senior-level policy support
Facilities manager	Plays key role in ensuring adequate space for health suite in new buildings and maintaining and repairing health facilities in existing buildings. Critical in addressing air quality concerns, playground safety, sanitation, use of pesticides.
Community members	Provide support for school health functions, in partnership with health professionals
Health department	Can offer guidance in school response to disease outbreaks, provide information on school reporting requirements, and assist in immunization efforts
Waste management contractor	Provides information on state and local requirements for hazardous waste disposal

ministrators. Familiarity with their functions can assist school system leaders, space planners, and facility managers to anticipate the requirements for environmentally safe, well-functioning health facilities.

Tables 27.3 and 27.4 outline the primary functions of health staff and describe related facility needs. The central requirements for all health facilities are cleanliness, visual privacy, soundproofing, and accessibility for all students. Because adults do not always remember the privacy needs of students and their families, it bears repeating that, for school health professionals to do their job well, they must be provided with space that ensures both visual and auditory privacy. Locked cabinets for health records are also essential, as are private telephone lines that enable confidential conversation between the health office and students' families.

Table 27.5 describes the space guidelines for a school nurse's office, as suggested by the Council of Educational Facilities Planners International (Hawkins 1992). The council recommends that the nurse's office be located near the school administrative office, meet the federal requirements for accessibility, and accommodate educational displays that promote healthy behaviors and health-related events. Facility planners should keep in mind that mainstreaming children with special health care needs makes it particularly important that the health office, including exam rooms and bathroom facilities, be accessible to all students. (A more extensive discussion of this point is found in chapter 26.)

Clinical Services at School

Health services at schools are generally focused on children, although in some schools services are offered to teachers and staff members as well.

Clinical Services for Students

The profile of health services and health professionals may differ substantially from one school

Table 27.3. Environmental requirements for the school nurse's office

In-clinic school nurse functions	Facility requirements	Service requirements
General requirements	• Visual privacy and soundproofing • Accessibility • Easily cleaned surfaces (floors, walls, windows, countertops)	
Communication with family members, community physicians, and other community agencies about individual student and schoolwide health concerns	Private office with intercom to the administrative offices and electrical and cable connections for a telephone, computer, and modem access to the Internet	
Immunization records management	Locked student health records	
Medication and medical procedures management	• Locked medicine cabinet • Separate refrigerator for vaccines or medications requiring refrigeration	Regular testing of refrigerator temperature
Injury and illness management	• Locked supply cabinet for sterile supplies • Sick bay (a rest area with beds; physically separated from rest of office) • Exam room with sink with hot and cold water • Ice machine for icing injuries • Bathroom	Regular disposal of sharps and infectious waste
Referrals to community agencies	Separate telephone line that ensures confidential communication	
Health education and promotion	Space for educational displays and health promotion materials for students and family members	

Table 27.4. Environmental requirements for other school health professionals

School health professional	Functions	Facility requirements	Service requirements
School psychologist	• Evaluates students for placement in special education and monitors progress of students in this program • Counsels students and families. Also consults with and supports teachers and school administrators	• Office with visual privacy and soundproofing, • Locked cabinet for student files • Telephone • Secure Internet access	
School social worker	Links students and families with community agencies, provides individual and family counseling, may provide social services such as clothing and lunch money. Also consults with teachers	• Office with visual privacy and soundproofing • Locked cabinet for student files, • Telephone • Secure Internet access	
Guidance counselor	Assists students with course selection and scheduling. May also provide counseling to students.	• Office with visual privacy and soundproofing • Locked cabinet for student files, • Telephone • Secure Internet access	
Dentist and dental hygienist	Provides a range of preventive and restorative services, including dental exams, fluoride and dental cleaning, oral hygiene instruction, dental sealants, X-rays, and treatment and restorative services	• Soundproofing • Visual privacy • Depending on services to be provided, dental operatory with sink and dedicated electrical line for dental equipment • AC/fans if temperature-sensitive equipment is used • X-ray equipment	Regular disposal of sharps and infectious waste
School-based health center (employs two or more health staff)	Provides acute medical services as well as preventive care, assesses students for mental health problems, counsels students and parents, provides individual and group counseling. Less frequently, may offer dental services and nutritional support	• Soundproofing • Visual privacy • Space that facilitates infection control practices and universal precautions as required by state law or OSHA regulations • Telephone, secure Internet access • Exam rooms with sinks • Bathroom • Counseling office • Locked space for patient files, computer, drugs • Laboratory • Refrigerator	Regular disposal of sharps, infectious waste

district or school to another. With the exception of federally mandated health services for children with disabilities, state and local school boards and senior school system managers decide what health services will be provided and determine the number and types of health professionals to be employed. Individual principals may use discretionary funds or relationships with community providers to augment services provided by the school district.

Schools staffed with a full-time nurse and/or other health professionals will have access to a wide range of services. Particularly important are the provision of first aid, the management of medications for children experiencing acute and chronic

Table 27.5. Space guidelines for the school nurse's office in a high school

Portion of nurse's office	Square footage
School nurse office	150–175
Examination room	275–300
Waiting area	100–150
Rest area	100–150
Restroom	30–40

From the Council for Educational Facilities Planners International (1991).

health problems, and emergency medical services. (For an in-depth description of services required by students with asthma and allergies, see chapter 28.) Table 27.6 outlines the student screenings required by many school districts and the reported provision of those services by a nationally representative sample of elementary, middle, and senior high schools. Table 27.7 identifies the leading health services mandated by states and school districts. As chapter 26 points out, the health services required by students with disabilities go beyond those shown in table 27.7 and may be made available by community-based health providers.

Clinical Services for School Staff

Although some school health professionals have implemented health promotion programs for school employees, in most cases the health staff serves only students enrolled at the school. Several factors account for this arrangement, and limited staff support is likely the most important one.

Fewer than half of all schools have a full-time professional on-site. Even when there is a full-time health staffer, school health professionals are most commonly trained to treat the health problems of children. Taking care of adults may not be part of their skill set or something they enjoy. Even schools that support health promotion programs for their employees are not likely to provide them with health care services. Finally, in school districts that employ a health staff, the responsibilities of staff members may be governed by a contract between the school district and the teachers' union. Efforts to expand the responsibilities of school nurses could involve a renegotiation of that contract. All these factors limit health care provision to teachers and staff. (Occupational health care in schools is discussed in chapter 30.)

Protecting the Public's Health at School

School health services address environmental health in two major ways: primary prevention of environmental hazards and surveillance of both health effects and health hazards themselves. In addition, schools may provide some occupational health services.

Primary Prevention: Hazardous Waste Disposal

While school-based health care does not usually generate infectious or harmful materials, children

Table 27.6. Prevalence of health screening in schools

	School districts and various required services			Schools providing these services		
Type of screening	% Requiring screening	% Requiring parental notification	% Requiring teacher notification	% Of elementary schools	% Of middle/ junior high schools	% Of senior high schools
Hearing	88.4	98.5	85.5	90.1	63.9	50.3
Height/weight or BMI	38.4	81.1	33.1	52.6	37.8	31.8
Oral health	31.1	98.3	68.1	29.4	16.7	31.0
Scoliosis or posture	68.8	98.6	48.0	31.0	52.2	31.0
TB	17.1	93.7	59.8	5.9	7.0	5.8
Vision	90.4	98.5	84.8	92.1	68.3	53.4

From Brener et al. (2000).

Table 27.7. Percentage of states and school districts requiring school health services[a]

School health services	States (%)	School districts (%)
Administration of medications	64.0	93.7
First aid	48.0	91.1
CPR	42.0	81.5
Identification of or referral for physical, sexual, or emotional abuse	64.7	75.7
Crisis intervention for personal problems	20.4	64.8
Case management for students with chronic health conditions	32.6	60.8
Identification of or counseling for mental or emotional disorders	16.0	57.2
Identification or treatment of acute illness	28.0	50.0
Identification or treatment of chronic illness	32.6	46.5
Alcohol or other drug use treatment	8.2	46.2

From Brener et al. (2000).
[a]By type of service (top 10 services required).

inevitably bleed from playground injuries and vomit when sick, medical sharps (e.g., needles) have to be used, and some schools still have mercury thermometers and other sources of toxic substances. As a result, schools need to be prepared to address these hazards, safely dispose of medical sharps and potentially infectious waste, and eliminate mercury from the health office.

Disposing of Medical Sharps

Safe disposal of used needles and other medical sharps is essential to protect staff members who work in the health suite, those who clean it, and students who are treated there. All health suites should be supplied with puncture-proof containers to dispose of medical sharps, and these containers should be collected and replaced frequently. School systems should contact their local health department or solid waste management department to determine the disposal policies and procedures required in their community. They should also become familiar with federal requirements as outlined in the regulations of the Occupational Safety and Health Administration.

The Coalition for Safe Community Needle Disposal, a coalition of government agencies, waste as-

sociations, and private sector companies, is working with the U.S. Environmental Protection Agency (U.S. EPA) to assess and promote alternative methods for disposal of used medical sharps. The organization provides information on safe needle disposal through a help line at 1-800-643-1643. The web site of the U.S. EPA provides a listing of all state health and solid waste management departments at http://www.epa.gov/epaoswer/other/medical/. Additional information on this topic is available near the end of this chapter in the discussion of occupational health and safety in schools.

Disposing of Infectious Waste

A lengthier discussion of the role of school nurses and other health professionals in controlling infectious diseases appears later in the chapter. However, the safe disposal of infectious waste, a critical component of those activities, deserves attention here. As recommended by many state health departments, safe disposal of materials such as clothes or bandages soiled with blood or other body fluids is an essential part of a policy that implements universal precautions. All blood and body fluids should be treated as if they contain bloodborne infectious agents such as the human immunodeficiency virus (HIV) or hepatitis B virus.

The Virginia School Health Guidelines (Keen and Ford 1999) offer the following recommendations for disposing of potentially infectious materials:

- Contaminated supplies. All used or contaminated supplies, such as gloves, sanitary napkins, and bandages, except for needles and other sharp implements, should be placed in a plastic bag and sealed. The bag can be put in the regular garbage out of reach of children and animals.
- Used needles, syringes, and other sharps. These objects should be disposed of through arrangements with a local medical facility or health department. Until they can be transported, they should be stored immediately after use in a metal or other puncture-proof and leak-proof container.
- Bodily waste. Bodily waste such as urine, vomit, or feces should be disposed of in the toilet. Materials used to clean body fluids from the floor and other surfaces should be placed in a plastic bag, sealed, and discarded in the garbage.

All school districts and health professionals should contact their local board of health or sanitation department to learn of any local or state restrictions on the disposal of these potentially infectious materials.

Disposing of Mercury

Mercury is a hazardous chemical that can cause serious health problems, especially to children. Mercury exists in several chemical forms: elemental mercury (quicksilver), inorganic mercury, and organic mercury. Each form has different chemical properties and toxic effects. Children may be exposed to mercury through eating fish such as shark, tuna, and swordfish (because mercury that is released into the environment from the burning of fossil fuels and other industrial processes reaches waterways and concentrates in fish), dental amalgam (although only very low amounts of mercury are absorbed from this source), and thimerosal preservative in childhood immunizations (although current immunizations are generally free of thimerosal). Mercury exposures can occur in the school environment because certain equipment—blood pressure cuffs, thermometers, thermostat switches, and fluorescent light bulbs—may contain mercury. Some of this equipment can even be found in the health office. If this equipment breaks or is improperly disposed of, children may be exposed to mercury. In addition, mercury may be present in science laboratories, where it has traditionally been used in classroom experiments. School exposures generally involve elemental mercury, the familiar globules of silver liquid. This form of mercury vaporizes very readily and can easily be inhaled.

At high levels of exposure, inhaled mercury vapor can severely inflame the airways and lungs. Long-term exposure at lower levels primarily targets the nervous system. Early symptoms include insomnia, forgetfulness, loss of appetite, and mild tremors. More severe symptoms, after longer-term or higher exposures, include progressive tremors, emotional changes, and excessive sweating and salivation. Kidney damage may also occur. Fetuses and very young children are especially susceptible to mercury toxicity.

Very low or transient exposures to mercury are unlikely to cause symptoms. However, all exposures should be taken seriously. Federal and state governments have recommended a primary prevention approach, replacing mercury-containing equipment with mercury-free alternatives (University of Wisconsin 2003; U.S. EPA 2003). Fortunately, such alternatives are available. Until mercury is eliminated from schools, nurses and others should be prepared to manage mercury spills (see box 27.2). Mercury spill cleanup kits are commercially available, typically sold by vendors of laboratory safety supplies. The kits should be available in each room where mercury is present, and teachers and staff should be trained in their use.

Surveillance

Surveillance, in public health terms, may refer either to health conditions such as illnesses and injuries or to environmental hazards. Both kinds of surveillance may be part of a school health services program.

Disease Surveillance

Whether the perceived threat is an influenza outbreak or an anthrax attack, the school nurse is in a

---

■ 27.2. *Management of mercury spills in schools*

If mercury is spilled:

- Remove children from the area.
- Do not vacuum.
- Clean up the bead of mercury by rolling it onto a sheet of paper or sucking it up with an eyedropper.
- Place the mercury in an airtight container.
- Do not wash the mercury down the drain.
- Bag the paper and the eyedropper. Call environmental officials or the local health department for instructions on disposal.
- If a larger spill (exceeding 2 inches in diameter) occurs, leave the area, and contact the health department and fire authorities.
- If the spill is on a carpet, these recommendations do not apply. Consult a professional firm with expertise in mercury cleanup.

(Adapted from the Mercury in Schools Project of the University of Wisconsin Extension 2003). ■

position to provide early warning of emerging problems. Disease surveillance involves systematic collection of information about diseases. These data are then used by public health agencies to take actions to contain the spread of the disease. Disease incidence reporting also permits the monitoring of long-term trends and facilitates future planning for community-wide interventions. An electronic school health data system that enables nurses to record and retrieve information on student illnesses strengthens the capacity of health professionals to track incidents that were not immediately recognized as reportable illnesses. Unfortunately, most school systems continue to use paper documents to collect and report these data.

Each state maintains its own list of reportable diseases and may identify a subset of diseases that require health professionals to report the suspected illness by telephone to a designated local or state office. The state department of health should be contacted for information on which diseases are reportable, what information is required, who is responsible for reporting diseases, and to whom diseases are reported.

Infectious Disease Control

The emergence of new infectious diseases such as severe acute respiratory syndrome (SARS) and the reemergence of old infectious diseases such as tuberculosis have rekindled an awareness of the importance of protecting children from infectious disease and the role school nurses can play. The 2003 SARS epidemic demonstrated that, in an era when people travel easily and quickly between countries, the spread of diseases can be quick and deadly. Recent cases of measles in the United States are a reminder that certain diseases that have almost been eradicated in this country remain endemic in others. Failure to be vaccinated or a decision not to be vaccinated can have serious consequences for an individual and a community.

Vaccine-Preventable Diseases

Historically, a critical task for the school nurse has been documenting that children who are entering school have been immunized against vaccine-preventable diseases. Both states and school districts establish immunization requirements that students must meet before they can be admitted to kindergarten or first grade, middle or junior high school, and senior high school. Every state requires that entering kindergarteners be immunized against diphtheria, measles, and polio. Most school districts also require a tetanus immunization and a second measles-containing vaccine. Vaccines for other preventable diseases (e.g., chicken pox, hepatitis A and B, and *Haemophilus* influenza, type b) are required by some states and not by others. States typically require that health records reflect students' immunization status.

State laws have generally permitted students to be exempted from immunization requirements for medical, religious, and philosophical reasons. About 1 child in 20 entering first grade is currently unvaccinated for measles, according to estimates by the Centers for Disease Control and Prevention (CDC 2004), and even though two doses of measles-containing vaccine have been highly effective in preventing the spread of measles, there has been a 1% failure rate among recipients of two doses in recent outbreaks. It appears that most cases of measles are now imported; they are contracted by unvaccinated children or teenagers who travel to or arrive as adoptees from countries where measles is common and who then infect other children. In addition to documenting that children are properly immunized, school-based health professionals can play a critical role in educating families about the importance of immunization for children.

Non–Vaccine-Preventable Diseases

Control of non–vaccine preventable infectious diseases—those that spread through the intestinal tract and respiratory tract and through direct contact—is a challenge in schools, especially among younger children. Many schools do not have adequate hand-washing facilities; others do not maintain all of the sinks in working order. School-based health personnel can take the lead in promoting habits that reduce the likelihood of disease spread and in encouraging all staff members to make a well-maintained school a priority. Effective strategies to reduce the spread of infectious diseases include:

- promoting hand washing after using the bathroom and before preparing or eating food, which means making sure that bathrooms have an adequate supply of soap, running water, paper towels, and toilet paper
- teaching students and teachers to sneeze or

cough into their sleeve, keeping a supply of disposable tissues in the classroom and encouraging their use, and promoting hand washing after sneezing.

A major challenge to infection control is the degree to which parents and other caretakers work outside the home, making it difficult for a school nurse to send a sick child home. What is the nurse to do when parents send a sick child to school or a child becomes sick during the school day and there is no one available to take the child home? This dilemma has no easy solutions. Building parental understanding of the importance of controlling contagion, encouraging teachers to help parents develop emergency care plans, and giving

priority to sick-day planning with parents of children with a chronic disease are possible strategies. Nevertheless, this will remain an unresolved issue until a solution is developed that involves more than the individual parents of sick children.

Hazard Surveillance

As mentioned earlier, most schools do not have a full-time nurse on-site, and many have less than a half-time school nurse position. When present, school nurses tend to care for children's injuries or meet their acute or chronic health care needs. However, growing community concern about environmental hazards in school—mold problems, pesticides, hazards on the playground—have raised the visibility of these issues and increased the aware-

---

■ *27.3. The role of the school nurse in environmental health*

- Develop Individualized Health Plans (IHP), emergency plans, or 504 plans to address individual student sensitivity and health needs.
- Develop IHPs, emergency plans, or 504 plans for students with health impairment from toxin exposure.
- Develop a school committee to implement the EPA's Tools for Schools IAQ Management Program.
- Be aware of asbestos compliance activities (Asbestos Hazard Emergency Response Act, or AHERA) in your school and district.
- Promote the use of an Integrated Pest Management system for insect control in the school.
- Support environmental toxin exposure risk and management education programs for staff and children.
- Follow the EPA's hazardous waste management policies in your school and district.
- Participate in educational opportunities to learn and teach others about environmental toxins, their health impact, reduction, and exposure prevention.
- Participate in OSHA-required workplace safety teams to develop policies and practices that reduce hazard exposure.
- Be familiar with OSHA-required material safety data sheets, their content, and where to obtain them in your school.
- Become familiar with resources on promoting reduction of toxic exposures in children.
- Participate in community programs to protect children from environmental toxic exposure.
- Promote school and district policy development for management of potential hazards and activities in schools that advance safe environmental management.
- Support and enforce smoke-free school environments.
- Support students and staff who are interested in addressing environmental issues.
- Be aware of immediate care actions and first aid for anyone who has been exposed to chemical spills, toxin inhalation, or other toxin exposure.
- Assist in the development of school and district emergency response plans for chemical or toxin exposures.

(From the National Association of School Nurses 2004). ■

ness of a potential role for school health professionals.

While the school system's central administration is generally responsible for identifying and responding to environmental problems in the school building, a school nurse may be in a position to notice problems as they occur. The nurse is also in a position to recognize student or teacher health problems that may be reported and could be associated with environmental problems. In 2004, the National Association of School Nurses recognized the growing role of school nurses in environmental health at school by releasing an issue brief that both summarizes the challenges and describes the responsibilities associated with this expanding role (NASN 2004; see box 27.3). Federal and state environmental health offices, as well as private and nonprofit companies, have developed guides to assist school nurses with various aspects of these environmental health issues. For example, the EPA has issued an Indoor Air Quality Checklist for Health Officers and School Nurses (http://www.epa.gov/iaq/schools/tfs/healthof.html), and the University of Northern Iowa has released a National Program for Playground Safety Report Card (http://www.playgroundsafety.org/reportcard/index.htm).

Occupational Health for School Health Professionals and Students

The 1970 federal Occupational Safety and Health Act (OSHA) and similar laws adopted by some state governments mandate protections against unsafe procedures or exposure to health risks at the work site for private and some public school employees. The federal law applies to private employers, and some states have extended similar legal protection to public employees, including school employees. In any event, OSHA safety and health standards are widely adopted as best practice, if not mandatory rules. (Occupational health at school is more fully discussed in chapter 30.)

Three OSHA standards and their state equivalents are particularly important for health staff at school: protection against bloodborne pathogens, specific protections against needle sticks, and protection from the consequences of latex allergies. In those states in which federal and state OSHA protections are not mandated, school districts should be encouraged to adopt these standards as policy.

Bloodborne Pathogens

School nurses and other health staff such as health aides, physicians, and nurse practitioners are vulnerable to exposure to the HIV/AIDS, hepatitis B, and hepatitis C viruses through contact with children's blood, vomit, feces, and other bodily fluids. Each of these viruses may cause a serious or fatal disease. All school staff members should be instructed in the use of universal precautions, including the use of gloves, effective hand-washing techniques, and proper disposal of materials soiled with body fluids. Nurses may take the lead in ensuring that all school staff have received training and also have access to gloves and other materials necessary to handle potentially infectious fluids. Nurses or other health professionals should also have access to protective clothing and a mask or face shield if spattering of body fluids is anticipated (see box 27.4).

Needle Sticks

School health personnel are at risk for needle stick injuries. Nurses may immunize students, nurses and aides may assist a student in checking blood sugar or perform other minor lab work, and nurse practitioners and physicians may suture wounds. Safe storage of needles and other sharps in a puncture-resistant container is an essential component of a needle safety program. Practices such as recapping needles or leaving needles or sharps on surfaces rather than immediately disposing of them are associated with needle sticks. Other safety measures that can reduce the likelihood of needle sticks involve using needles that have been reengineered to provide greater protection to the user.

Latex Allergies

Gloves made from latex or natural rubber can protect health care workers from the transmission of many infectious diseases. However, frequent use of these gloves places health workers at risk for developing latex allergies ranging from mild to serious. Students with disabilities such as spina bifida or students with other disabilities who may require frequent bladder catheterization are also at increased risk of developing a latex allergy. Health care professionals may help students and their families identify nonlatex alternatives for necessary equipment and medical devices.

Mild reactions to latex include skin redness,

▦ *27.4. Bloodborne pathogen rules for schools*

The Occupational Safety and Health Administration has issued standards for employers (including schools) to reduce risks for workers exposed to blood or other body fluids. The application of these standards to public schools varies by state; OSHA standards apply to all private schools. The OSHA standards requires employers of workers at risk for occupational exposure to body fluids do the following:

- Determine which employees are potentially at risk for occupational exposure.
- Write and annually update an exposure control plan.
- Provide personal protective equipment (e.g., gloves).
- Provide initial and annual training for staff.
- Offer hepatitis B vaccine to employees identified as at risk for occupational exposure.
- Provide postexposure management of employees who have exposure incidents.
- Maintain records of training and exposure incidents.

(From OSHA 2001). ▦

---

rash, hives, or itching. More severe reactions include an array of respiratory symptoms such as runny nose, sneezing, itchy eyes, scratchy throat, and respiratory difficulty. Severe anaphylactic reactions are possible. To prevent triggering a latex allergy, the National Institute for Occupational Health and Safety (NIOSH) recommends switching from latex to nonlatex gloves. If latex gloves must be used, then NIOSH suggests choosing reduced-protein, powder-free latex gloves, avoiding oil-based hand creams or lotions (which can cause glove deterioration), washing hands with mild soap, drying thoroughly after using gloves, and frequently cleaning areas and equipment contaminated with latex-containing dust (NIOSH 1999). Both staff and students with latex allergies should learn to recognize the symptoms of this allergy and consider taking precautions that include carrying an adrenaline kit to treat severe allergic reactions, wearing a medic-alert bracelet, and carrying a pair of latex-free gloves in the event of a medical emergency (Spina Bifida and Hydrocephalus Association of Canada 2004).

Other precautions include:

- using nonlatex gloves for activities that are not likely to involve contact with infectious materials
- using powder-free latex gloves with reduced protein content when barrier protection is essential to protect against infectious materials

- taking actions to reduce the chance of reactions to latex: not using oil-based hand creams or lotions (which can cause glove deterioration) when wearing latex gloves; washing hands with a mild soap and drying thoroughly after removing latex gloves; frequently cleaning areas and equipment contaminated with latex-containing dust (NIOSH 2000).

Safe Working Conditions for Students with Outside Jobs

Every 6 minutes, on average, a student sustains an on-the-job injury that necessitates a trip to an emergency department. Low-income youth are more likely than more affluent youth to work in hazardous industries such as manufacturing, construction, and agriculture (Castillo et al. 1999; Runyan and Zakocs 2000). These teens are especially in need of health and safety training and knowledge about their employment rights. School nurses and physicians who provide physical exams and sign work permits for students can help protect young workers by knowing the federal and state rules associated with youth employment and helping students understand the importance of a safe working environment.

NIOSH has developed a special web site on young worker safety and health that provides information on specific workplace hazards (http://www.cdc.gov/niosh/topics/youth/), and the Mas-

■ *27.5. Sample questions on the health and safety of a child's workplace*

Floors and walkways

- Are exits marked and walkways kept clear?
- Do you know where to get buckets and mops to clean up spills?
- Are stairways clear?
- Do stairways have handrails?

Ladders

- Do ladders appear to be in good condition?
- Do ladders have safety feet?
- Are nonmetal ladders used when there is a chance of electrical shock?

Housekeeping

- Are toilet facilities kept clean and ventilated?
- Do toilet facilities have sinks with hot and cold water and disposable paper towels?

(From Massachusetts Department of Education) ■

sachusetts Department of Education has created the Work-based Learning Plan Toolkit (http://www .doe.mass.edu/stc/wbl_resource/toolkit), which includes a two-page checklist to help teachers, parents, and students assess the safety of student work sites. Sample questions from the checklist appear in box 27.5.

Conclusion

The school health suite has both its own environmental requirements and an opportunity to partner with school staff, students, and parents to create a healthy environment in the larger school setting. The challenge for school health professionals is how to respond to new, schoolwide environmental obligations in light of fiscal and staffing constraints over which they have little control.

The most important barrier to an enlarged role for school health professionals is the limited time available to the many nurses and other health staff who serve part-time in several schools. An addi-

tional constraint is the limited training many of them have received concerning environmental health problems. Successfully carrying out duties such as disease and hazard surveillance in the absence of such training is challenging. The absence of computerized data management hinders surveillance functions. At the school district level, lack of clarity as to who defines the environmental health responsibilities of the health staff, who articulates the policies and procedures related to the health suite, and what environmental training is available to health staff creates additional obstacles to action.

Despite these challenges, school health professionals remain the most promising candidates for coordinating building-based efforts to protect and develop a healthy school environment. They treat the consequences of unsafe playgrounds, can track the spread of infectious disease from classroom to classroom, take note of increased complaints about air quality and poor building maintenance, and follow procedures used to control pests in the school cafeteria. No one else in the building has as many opportunities to understand the scope and depth of environmental health issues at school.

With most school districts allocating limited resources to health personnel, school nurses or other school-based health professionals may be unable fully to implement the agenda outlined in this chapter. Given this resource-to-challenge dilemma, school health professionals might consider focusing their environmental health work on a few priorities. Because the daily work of a school nurse involves contact with sick students and staff, the priority environmental health assignment for the nurse's office may be disease surveillance. Training the nurse and equipping the office for that responsibility would not only achieve an important public health goal but also lay a foundation for identifying and reporting other hazards within the school. Regardless of the priorities that a school district selects, the challenge for each school district is to ensure that the school health staff are given the support and the resources to do their job effectively.

Resources

School-based Health Care: The People

- Brener ND, Burstein GR, DuShaw ML, Vernon ME, Wheeler L, Robinson J. 2001. Health services: Results from the school health policies and programs study 2000. J Sch Health 71(7):294–300.

- Kort M. 1984. The delivery of primary health care in American public schools. J Sch Health 54(11):453–457.
- Schwab N, Gelfman MHB, eds. 2001. *Legal issues in school health services: A resource for school administrators, school attorneys, school nurses.* North Branch, MN: Sunrise River Press.

School-based Health Care: Facilities

- Butin D. 2000. School health centers. Washington, DC: National Clearinghouse for Educational Facilities. Available: http://www.edfacilities.org/pubs/healthctr3.html
- Maryland State Department of Education. 2002. School health services: A facility planning and design guide for school systems. Baltimore: Maryland State Department of Education. To order: Division of Business Services, School Facilities Branch, 200 W. Baltimore Street, Baltimore, MD 21201. Telephone: 410-767-0098.
- National Clearinghouse for Educational Facilities. Health Services Facilities. http://www.edfacilities.org/rl/health_centers.cfm

Clinical Health Services

- Brener ND, Burstein GR, DuShaw ML, Vernon ME, Wheeler L, Robinson J. 2001. Health services: Results from the school health policies and programs study 2000. J Sch Health 71(7):294–300.
- Goodman IF, Sheetz AH, eds. 1995. The comprehensive school health manual. Boston: School Health Unit, Bureau of Family and Community Health, Massachusetts Department of Public Health. Order through Massachusetts Statehouse Bookstore, telephone 617-727-2834.
  http://www.mass.gov/dph/fch/schoolhealth/cshm.htm
- Texas Department of State. 2002. The Texas guide to school health programs. Health Services, Office of Family Health, Adolescent, and School Health Division. Available: http://www.dshs.state.tx.us/schoolhealth/pgramguide.shtm

Protecting the Public's Health at School: Primary Prevention

- Minnesota Department of Health. 1996. Disposal of infectious/hazardous waste. In Minnesota School Health Guide.
  http://www.health.state.mn.us/divs/fh/mch/schoolhealth/guide/chapter4.html#disposal
- University of Wisconsin Extension, Solid and Hazardous Waste Education Center. 2003. Mercury in schools: What can schools and teachers do to reduce the presence of mercury in schools?
  http://www.mercuryinschools.uwex.edu/schools

Protecting the Public's Health at School: Surveillance

- National Association of School Nurses. 2001. Position statement: Infectious diseases. Scarborough, ME: National Association of School Nurses.
  http://www.nasn.org/positions/2001psinfectious.htm

Occupational Health and Safety for Health Professionals and Students

- National Association of School Nurses. 2000. Position statements: Natural rubber latex allergy. Scarborough, ME: National Association of School Nurses.
  http://www.nasn.org/positions/2000pslatex.htm
- National Association of School Nurses. 2003. Position statement: Regulations on bloodborne pathogens in the school setting. Scarborough, ME: National Association of School Nurses.
  http://www.nasn.org/positions/2003psbloodborne.htm
- National Institute for Occupational Safety and Health. 1997. Preventing allergic reactions to natural rubber latex in the workplace. DHHS publication no. 97-135.
  http://www.cdc.gov/niosh/latexalt.html
- National Institute for Occupational Safety and Health. 2000. What every worker should know: How to protect yourself from needles-

tick injuries. DHHS publication no. 2000-135.
http://www.cdc.gov/niosh/2000-135.html

- Occupational Safety and Health Administration. 2001. Occupational exposure to bloodborne pathogens: Needlestick and other sharps injuries, final rule. Fed Reg 66:5317–5325.
- Virginia Department of Health, Office of Family Health, School Health Program. 1999. Virginia school health guidelines. Appendix C: Universal precautions and infectious diseases. http://www.vahealth.org/schoolhealth/onlinepubs.htm#vshguidelines

References

Brener ND, Burstein GR, DuShaw ML, Vernon ME, Wheeler L, Robinson J. 2000. The School Health Policies and Programs Study (SHPPS): Health services. J Sch Health 71(8):294–304.

Castillo DN, Davis L, Wegman DH. 1999. Young workers. Occup Med 14(3):519–536.

Center for Health and Health Care in Schools. 2003. 2002 state survey of school-based health center initiatives. Washington, DC: George Washington University Medical Center. Available: http://www.healthinschools.org/survey2002 [accessed 26 March 2005].

Centers for Disease Control and Prevention. 2004. National Immunization Program. Coverage estimates for school entry vaccinations, 2003–2004 school year. Available: http://www2.cdc.gov/nip/schoolsurv/nationalAvg.asp [accessed 26 March 2005].

Hawkins HL. 1992. Guide for school facility appraisal. Scottsdale, AZ: Council of Educational Facility Planners International.

Keen TP, Ford N, eds. 1999. Virginia school health guidelines, 2d ed. Richmond: Virginia Department of Health, Division of Child and Adolescent Health. Available: http://www.vahealth.org/schoolhealth/onlinepubs.htm#vshguidelines [accessed 16 January 2006].

Massachusetts Department of Education, Office for School to Career Transition. n.d. The Massachusetts Work-based Learning Plan Toolkit. Health and safety checklist. http://www.doe.mass.edu/stc/wbl_resource/toolkit/ [accessed 26 March 2005].

National Association of School Nurses. 2004. Issue brief: Environmental concerns in the school setting. Castle Rock, CO: NASN. Available: http://www.nasn.org/briefs/2004briefenvironmental.htm [accessed 26 March 2005].

National Institute for Occupational Safety and Health. 1999. Latex allergy: A prevention guide. DHHS (NIOSH) Publication No. 98-113. Available: http://www.cdc.gov/niosh/98-113.html [accessed 26 March 2005].

Occupational Safety and Health Administration, U.S. Department of Labor. Occupational safety and health standards: Bloodborne pathogens. 29 CFR 1910.1030. 1991, amended 1992, 1996, 2001.

Runyan CW, Zakocs RC. 2000. Epidemiology and prevention of injuries among adolescent workers in the United States. Annu Rev Public Health 21:247–269.

Spina Bifida and Hydrocephalus Association of Canada. 2004. Latex allergies: Questions and answers. Winnipeg: SBHAC. Available: http://www.sbhac.ca/index.php?page=latex [accessed 26 March 2005].

Spratley E, Johnson A, Sochalski J, Fritz M, Spencer W. 2000. The registered nurse population: Findings from the National Sample Survey of Registered Nurses. U.S. DHHS, Health Resources and Service Administration, Bureau of Health Professions, Division of Nursing. Available: http://bhpr.hrsa.gov/healthworkforce/reports/rnsurvey/ [accessed 26 March 2005].

University of Wisconsin Extension. 2003. Mercury in schools. Available: http://www.mercuryinschools.uwex.edu/home.htm [accessed 26 March 2005].

U.S. Environmental Protection Agency. 2003. Safe mercury management. Available: http://www.epa.gov/epaoswer/hazwaste/mercury/school.htm [accessed 26 March 2005].

W. Gerald Teague

Care of Asthmatic and Allergic Students

■ *Summary*

- Asthma is the most prevalent chronic illness that affects children in school.
- A close partnership, built on open communication and preparedness, is necessary among school personnel, parents, and health professionals in order to optimize outcomes for children with asthma in the school environment.
- School personnel should be able to recognize the signs and symptoms of an asthma attack, assess its severity, and initiate treatment.
- Children with asthma must have ready access to a reliever (rescue) medication that is inhaled to relieve symptoms.
- School professionals also have a role in prevention. ■

Asthma is the most prevalent chronic illness that affects children in school. The symptoms of asthma, such as wheezing and coughing, tend to wax and wane, but the underlying problem, inflammation of the airways, tends to persist. Even mild cases of asthma can be fatal, so proper diagnosis, treatment, and prevention are essential. School pro-

fessionals also have a role in prevention by modifying factors that exacerbate asthma.

By recognizing the symptoms of asthma, school personnel may be able to detect a child's asthma even before parents and physicians are aware of it. Although there is no known cure for asthma, the daily use of anti-inflammatory medications ("controllers") can prevent attacks in most cases. School personnel should be able to recognize the signs and symptoms of an asthma attack and initiate treatment. Children with asthma must have ready access to a reliever ("rescue") medication that is inhaled to relieve symptoms. During an asthma attack, students should be allowed to use their rescue inhaler immediately and be escorted to the clinic if necessary for further evaluation, treatment, contact with the legal guardian, and emergency transport, if required. This chapter presents more details about each of these issues.

Asthma is the most common chronic disorder of childhood, affecting 4–11% of children (Mellinger-Birdsong et al. 2000). Nearly 5 million people in the United States younger than 18 years of age have asthma (National Center for Environmental Health 2005). Between 1980 and 1994, the prevalence of asthma increased 75% overall and

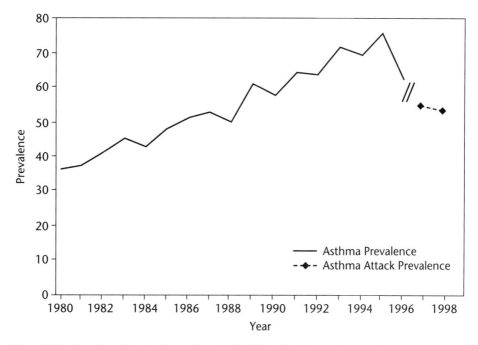

Figure 28.1. Prevalence (per 1,000 population) of childhood asthma in the United States, National Health Interview Survey, 1980–1998. This survey was redesigned in 1997, resulting in a discontinuity in the trend. (Data from CDC 2000.)

74% among children 5–14 years of age (Mannino et al. 2002; National Center for Environmental Health 2005; see fig. 28.1).

The sharpest rise in asthma was seen in preschool children under the age of 6 years. Asthma is among the top three causes for admission to the hospital during childhood, and even in its mild form, asthma can be fatal. The number of children dying from asthma increased almost threefold, from 93 in 1979 to 266 in 1996. Exacerbations of asthma are responsible for a significant number of lost days of school and work the world over. Asthma may interfere with participation in sports

and has a profound impact on the quality of life both for the child and family. In the United States alone, the direct and indirect costs associated with asthma in children and adolescents are an estimated $3.2 billion annually.

Asthma has a major impact on the classroom. According to the Centers for Disease Control and Prevention (2002), asthma accounts for 14 million lost days of school missed annually in the United States (National Center for Environmental Health 2005). The total number of school absences due to asthma more than doubled from 1980 to 1990 (see table 28.1; Mannino et al. 2002). Relatively little is

Table 28.1. Impact of asthma on school attendance and physical activity among children 5–17 years of age with self-reported asthma

	1980–1982	1985–1987	1990–1992	1994–1996
School absences per year (millions)	6.6	11.4	14.6	14.0
School absence days per child with asthma per year	4.9	4.4	4.7	3.7
Percentage with > 1 absence days in the previous 2 weeks	8.0%	8.1%	7.7%	5.4%
Percentage with activity limitation caused by asthma	27.2%	20.3%	27.6%	23.6%

From the National Health Interview Survey, 1980–1996. Table abstracted from Mannino et al. (2002).

known about the effects of asthma on individual school performance. However, apart from children's increased absences and missed assignments, asthmatic symptoms are likely to interfere with students' ability to concentrate in the classroom. Similarly, medications that are known to treat asthma, including short-acting rescue inhalers such as albuterol, may have side effects that decrease attentiveness.

What Is Asthma?

Asthma is a chronic disorder that primarily affects the airways, the network of branching tubes that funnel air into the lungs. The defining features of asthma are

- recurrent episodes of coughing, wheezing, chest tightness, and shortness of breath, usually in response to one or more triggers
- inflammation of the airways that persists in the absence of symptoms
- narrowing of the airways, as demonstrated by obstruction to air flow (measures of obstruction include a reduced peak expiratory flow rate and/or a reduced forced expired volume in 1 second [FEV_1])
- "twitchiness" of the airways, manifested by sudden narrowing in response to various triggers, including exposure to allergens, irritants, or viral infections.

Two features differentiate asthma from other lung diseases: persistent inflammation of the airways and narrowing of the airways, or bronchospasm (Busse and Lemanske 2001). A third feature that makes it different from other lung diseases is its episodic nature; symptoms tend to appear suddenly and then diminish over time.

Even when asthma symptoms such as wheezing and coughing are minimal, inflammation of the airways tends to persist (Busse and Lemanske 2001). This inflammation is due to certain kinds of cells called eosinophils, mast cells, and T lymphocytes, which congregate in the airways and cause inflammation. When activated, these inflammatory cells produce powerful irritants that narrow the airways; thus, children with persistent asthma must be treated daily with anti-inflammatory medications, termed controllers, to prevent asthma attacks.

■ *28.1. Asthma case study 1*

JR is a 16-year-old male who has had moderate, persistent asthma since he was 4 years old. JR is allergic to dust mites and ragweed and typically has asthma attacks from October through February, especially in association with upper respiratory tract infections. He has been admitted to the hospital three times with asthma but has not required admission in the past 3 years since starting daily treatment with a combination of fluticasone, a steroid inhaler, and montelukast, a tablet medication that blocks leukotrienes (toxic substances produced as part of allergic inflammation). Before starting these medications, JR would typically miss 10–20 days of school per year because of asthma symptoms. Now that his asthma is better controlled with maintenance preventive therapy, he misses fewer than 2 days of school per year. During the winter months, JR usually needs to use albuterol, an inhaled medication with immediate effects, at least once or twice per day to control coughing and wheezing. He is able to participate in sports at school but has to use an albuterol inhaler 20 minutes before vigorous activities to prevent chest tightness and shortness of breath. ■

Approximately two-thirds or more of children with asthma have allergies. When children are allergic, their immune system reacts to substances in the environment (allergens) by producing antibodies. Some children with allergies suffer chronic irritation of the skin (eczema) or lining of the nose (rhinitis). Allergies may also cause asthma attacks when the inhaled allergen triggers certain cells in the airways to release irritant chemicals. The most important common allergens that cause serious asthma attacks are dust mites, cockroaches, furred and feathered animals, and molds. Many of these allergens are found in the school environment (Almqvist et al. 1999; Lonnkvist et al 1999; Tortolero et al. 2002), and avoiding them is an important step in preventing asthma attacks.

School professionals can help to prevent asthma exacerbations by addressing asthma triggers in the school setting: minimizing allergens in the classroom, avoiding the use of aerosolized irritants, and limiting vigorous outdoor activity in the late afternoon on days when the ground ozone level is predicted to reach unhealthy levels.

How Do You Know When a Child Has Asthma?

The most important symptom of asthma in a child is a persistent dry cough. Many children cough briefly when they have a common cold; however, a cough that persists for several days in the absence of a stuffy nose is typical of asthma. In fact, up to one-fourth of children with asthma have no symptoms other than a cough. Other symptoms of asthma include wheezing, frequent clearing of the throat, and a tight or even painful sensation in the chest. Children rarely cough so hard that they produce sputum, a thick, sticky substance made in the airways. Because many children with asthma have nasal allergies, at school they present with frequent nasal stuffiness and allergic shiners—dark-appearing eye sockets that often give the child a raccoonlike appearance.

The more severe the asthma, the more frequent and severe are the symptoms (National Institutes of Health 2002). Children with mild, persistent asthma, the most common severity level, have symptoms two to five times per week. Children with moderate, persistent asthma have daily symptoms and use a rescue medication daily. Children with severe asthma have near-continuous symptoms that may significantly threaten their school performance. School personnel can be extremely helpful in the recognition and treatment of asthma by being aware of these symptom patterns, especially when they occur in students with frequent absences. Nighttime asthma attacks are especially disruptive of school performance, as they interrupt sleep.

School personnel should contact the student's legal guardian whenever they are concerned that poor asthma control is having an adverse effect on classroom performance. Proper medication can usually minimize or prevent this problem.

How to Assess the Severity of an Asthma Attack

School personnel should be familiar enough with asthma to be able to assess the severity of an asthma attack. This helps them respond appropriately, including identifying children in need of immediate medical attention.

Mild

A mild asthma attack usually features a persistent dry cough, sometimes accompanied by wheezing. The affected child may have a stuffy nose and other signs of an upper respiratory infection, an important cause of asthma attacks. The student may appear distracted but is breathing comfortably and fully aware of the surroundings. Asthma attacks at this stage can usually be averted with the use of a rescue inhaler, but the symptoms may return 4–8 hours later unless the child receives a second type of medication, a controller, to limit the inflammatory reaction in the airways.

Moderate

A moderate asthma attack usually progresses over 1–2 days or may be preceded by weeks of uncontrolled cough. The student appears to be breathing rapidly and is clearly uncomfortable but can still respond directly to questions. There is audible wheezing, and the child may be able to walk short distances but with some difficulty. If the attack progresses, breathing becomes more difficult, and the child begins to use the neck muscles. Asthma attacks that have progressed to this level should be treated immediately with a rescue medication (albuterol) in preparation for contacting the child's legal guardian and arranging transport to a medical care facility.

Severe

In a severe asthma attack, the student is visibly distressed, breathing rapidly, anxious, sitting upright, and often unable to answer questions with more than a single-word response. Wheezing may actually go away as the child gets tired. As the amount of oxygen in the blood drops, the child then has a dark gray to bluish appearance. In the advanced stages of a severe asthma attack, the child becomes progressively unresponsive and may lose consciousness. An asthma attack of this severity is a medical emergency. School personnel should administer oxygen if it is available, give albuterol up to 3 times over 60 minutes, and summon emergency rescue personnel.

Treatment of Asthma at School

School personnel can play two key functions in managing a child's asthma: (1) recognizing asthma and intervening appropriately with students who are undiagnosed or undertreated, and (2) maintaining optimal environmental conditions to prevent attacks. Teachers should be encouraged to become familiar with the pattern of asthma in individual students and, through communication with their legal guardians, understand the appropriate treatments to be used at school. In an effort to avoid being noticed by their classmates, children with asthma often suppress their symptoms and avoid treatment in the classroom. School personnel can identify such students by noticing those with a persistent cough. On the playground, students with asthma often have limited capacity to participate in vigorous activities and may take a long time to recover from them.

Indoor air quality issues are described in detail in chapter 10, and toxins in the school setting are described in chapter 15, so they are not covered in this chapter. It is important to recognize that, in addition to common inhaled allergens such as dust mite, mold, and cockroach (Tortolero et al. 2002), school environments can also contain high levels of volatile organic compounds, especially formaldehyde, a known airway irritant. Perhaps the most important building-related problems impacting indoor air quality in schools are inadequate outdoor air ventilation and water damage, which result in secondary mold growth (Daisey and Angell 1998).

Medications to treat asthma are divided into two main categories: relievers (also termed rescue medications) and controllers (see box 28.2; National Institutes of Health 2002). Relievers are used when needed to treat attacks, whereas controllers are used on a routine basis to minimize inflammation and prevent attacks. School personnel should be familiar with reliever medications, as they have immediate effects and are medications a

---

▇ *28.2. Medications to treat asthma*

Rescue or Reliever Medications
Purpose: to immediately reverse the symptoms of asthma
Onset of action: within a few minutes of use
Common side effects: jitteriness, muscle tremor, anxiety, rapid heartbeat
Categories and specific drugs:

- short-acting beta-agonists: albuterol (Proventil, Ventolin, Accuneb), pirbuterol (Maxair), levalbuterol (Xopenex)
- anticholinergics: ipratropium bromide (Atrovent)
- combinations: albuterol/ipratropium bromide (Combivent, Duoneb)

Controller Medications
Purpose: to prevent or control asthma exacerbations
Onset of action: days to weeks
Common side effects: none short term, but long-term side effects possible
Chemical and brand names:

- inhaled corticosteroids: budesonide (Pulmicort), fluticasone (Flovent), beclomethasone (Qvar), flunisolide (Aerobid), triamcinolone (Azmacort)
- leukotriene antagonists: montelukast (Singulair), zafirlukast (Accolate)
- long-acting beta-agonists: salmeterol (Serevent), formoterol (Foradil)
- mast-cell stabilizers: cromolyn (Intal), nedocromil (Tilade)
- methylxanthines: theophylline (Theodur, Theochron, Uniphyl)
- combinations: fluticasone/salmeterol (Advair), budesonide/formoterol (Symbicort) ▇

---

child with asthma is most likely to need at school. Because the airways open in response to relievers, they are often called bronchodilators. The most frequently used reliever medication is albuterol. Albuterol can be administered in two ways: with an inhaler, which is a convenient pocket-sized device that delivers a puff of medicine from a pressurized canister, or with a nebulizer, a larger, electrically powered device that forms a mist that the child can breathe with a face mask or mouthpiece. Most students with asthma carry an albuterol inhaler, but school policies often do not allow them to use their rescue medications at school. Such policies should be revised to permit immediate access to rescue medication for asthmatic students for self-administration or for administration by a school nurse or teacher, as most appropriate to the circumstances.

Controller medications are anti-inflammatory drugs taken once or twice daily either as inhalers or pills, typically before and after school. Accordingly, students usually do not use controller medications while at school. Students with severe asthma may need to take inhaled steroids or oral steroids late in the afternoon, often around 3:00 P.M., and should be permitted to do so.

The Athlete with Asthma

Any vigorous activity can trigger coughs and wheezes in a child with asthma. In fact, some children have a specific type of asthma triggered only by exercise, a condition called "exercise-induced bronchospasm" (EIB). (Bronchospasm refers to the narrowing of the airways; this term is preferable to "exercise-induced asthma," as exercise induces a narrowing of the airways rather than the full syndrome referred to as asthma.) Children with EIB typically have significant limits in their capacity for exercise. Sports that involve sprinting or bursts of activity such as basketball and soccer are most likely to trigger asthmatic symptoms, especially on dry, cool days. In a child with EIB, the shortness of breath and cough may actually worsen in the first minute or so after the child stops the activity. A coach may mistakenly attribute this symptom pattern to poor physical fitness and inappropriately exhort the child to resume exercise.

A student with known EIB should use an albuterol inhaler at least 20 minutes before any vigorous physical activity. Alternatively, students may use a drug known as formoterol instead of albuterol. The advantage of formoterol is that it has a much longer duration of effect than albuterol. Salmeterol also has a role in preventing EIB, but it must be used at least 1–2 hours before the vigorous activity, as it has a delayed onset of action. Montelukast, a controller medication that prevents an entire class of inflammatory chemicals known as leukotrienes, is also an excellent treatment for preventing EIB in children, but it should be used in advance and only in association with albuterol.

Exercise is an excellent treatment per se for children with asthma, as it improves the clearance of secretions from the airways and improves overall fitness. However, children with asthma often avoid exercise and sports because of undertreated EIB. With proper treatment, children with asthma can participate safely and benefit greatly from sports. Coaches should never exhort a student with known EIB to exercise when the child is having difficulty.

How to Handle Air Pollution Episodes

Air pollution refers to a wide range of contaminants in the air. This topic is discussed in detail in chapter 12, but because air pollution can have direct effects on children with asthma, it is also reviewed here. The two most important pollutants known to threaten health are ozone and particles. "Smog," a word derived from the combination of "smoke" and "fog," does not have a precise definition but includes both ozone and particles. Scientific studies have shown that breathing polluted air is harmful. Initially, temporary changes in lung function can occur without causing any symptoms. When symptoms do appear, they include cough, chest tightness or congestion, wheezing, inability to breathe deeply, and fatigue. Changes in heart rhythm and blood pressure have been linked to breathing particles. Everyone is susceptible to the effects of smog if exposure is high enough. However, children with asthma tend to be particularly vulnerable. Studies in many cities have shown that episodes of wheezing increase when air pollution levels rise (Teague and Bayer 2001; Tolbert et al. 2000) and decrease when the air is cleaner (Friedman et al. 2001).

The U.S. Environmental Protection Agency (EPA) rates air quality on a 0–500 scale known as the Air Quality Index (AQI). Medical research has clarified the health risk associated with each level, and health warnings are set accordingly. As the AQI increases, the risk of symptoms increases. The EPA conveys this information using a color-coded scale: Green represents 1–50; yellow, 51–100; orange, 101–150; and so on through red, purple, and maroon. Some people are more sensitive, experiencing symptoms at AQI levels below 100, while others are less sensitive. At AQI above 150–200, most people are affected. Current air quality information

■ *28.3. Asthma case study 2*

KB was a 12-year-old African-American male with lifelong severe asthma. He had been under the care of asthma specialists for most of his life. Despite treatment with oral and inhaled corticosteroids, he had experienced multiple admissions to the hospital for asthma. Approximately 2 days before his death, KB was seen by his pulmonary specialist for increased asthma symptoms and given a burst of oral corticosteroids. He improved, and on the morning of his death, he walked to a neighborhood bus stop to attend school. When the school bus arrived, KB experienced sudden shortness of breath. He collapsed and could not be revived. The cause of his death was determined to be an acute asthmatic exacerbation. A bill was recently passed by the Georgia legislature bearing KB's name to mandate that children have access to asthma rescue medication while at school. ■

■ *28.4. Asthma case study 3*

JW is a 16-year-old female who started having shortness of breath and chest tightness at school. She first noticed the symptoms during third-period band practice, when it became increasingly difficult to play the French horn. The symptoms increased in severity, leading to a hospital admission to evaluate her chest pain. JW had a normal cardiac evaluation and was referred to a psychiatrist for treatment of depression. She had pulmonary function tests in the hospital that showed a small decrease in the amount of air exhaled in 1 second, or the FEV_1. JW saw a pulmonary specialist, who recommended that she maintain a symptom diary at home and school and use a portable device to measure peak expiratory flow rate whenever she felt short of breath. The monitor records showed that every time JW attended classes in a temporary modular building at school, within 1–2 hours she would experience chest discomfort and a decrease in peak expiratory flow rate. On weekends and during holidays, she had no symptoms and had normal peak expiratory flow rates. Air-sampling studies of the modular school building showed high levels of formaldehyde, a known volatile organic compound and airway irritant. JW was treated with inhaled budesonide, a steroid, and salmeterol, a long-acting bronchodilator, and avoided the modular building. Her symptoms immediately improved, and within one year she was symptom free with normal pulmonary function. ■

and forecasts for the next day are available via roadside advisory signs, television, radio, and the Internet.

School personnel should monitor the air quality for their region and take appropriate action when the AQI is predicted to reach unhealthy levels (orange or higher). Typically, unhealthy ozone levels are the most common air pollution event and occur in large urban areas between May and September. On days when the ground ozone reaches unhealthy levels, the levels tend to peak in the late afternoon to early evening hours. On such days, school personnel should excuse students with asthma from vigorous outdoor activities scheduled for the late afternoon (Teague et al. 2002). On days when the ground ozone level is expected to reach unhealthy levels for everyone, outdoor activities should be moved indoors or rescheduled.

Coordinated School Health Programs to Address Asthma

The Centers for Disease Control and Prevention (CDC 2002) has published a strategy based on six

key elements to address asthma within a coordinated school health program. These elements are abstracted in box 28.5 and provide an implementation plan. A complementary publication published by the National Institutes of Health's National Asthma Education and Prevention Project, *Managing Asthma: A Guide to Schools*, provides specific action steps for school staff members (NAEPP 2002). Although this guide and other government publications (NAEPP 1997a, 1997b) focus on integrated school health responses to asthma, it is vital not to overlook the needs of individual students.

■ *28.5. Coordinated school health plan for asthma*

1. Establishment management and support systems:

- Designate a person to coordinate asthma activities at the district and school levels
- Use school health records to identify and track students with asthma
- Focus on students with poorly managed asthma

2. Provide appropriate school health services for students with asthma:

- Obtain written asthma action plan for all students with asthma
- Ensure that students have immediate access to medications prescribed by a physician and approved by parents
- Use standard emergency protocols for students in respiratory distress

3. Provide asthma education for students and school staff:

- Educate students with asthma and the school staff on asthma basics and management

4. Provide a safe and healthy school environment to reduce asthma triggers:

- Prohibit tobacco use at all times.
- Reduce indoor allergens and irritants
- Use integrated pest-management techniques

5. Provide safe physical education opportunities:

- Provide modified activities as indicated by a student's action plan
- Ensure that students have access to rescue medications before and during activities

6. Coordinate school, family, and community efforts to better manage asthma symptoms and reduce absences among students with asthma

(From CDC 2002). ■

In particular, such programs should focus on students with poorly managed asthma as demonstrated by frequent school absences, health care provider office visits, hospitalizations, and requests for rescue medication from the school clinic.

The School Clinic

The school clinic should be an area in the school that is easily accessible to students, faculty, and staff and where routine health problems can be addressed. Typically parents will provide health information about their children at the start of the school year, and this information should be accessible to the teachers and the school health staff. Not all schools have a full-time nurse, although schools within a district may share a nurse on a rotating schedule. As a result, other school personnel may assume responsibility for asthma prevention and treatment activities. Although policies may vary, students may generally store their inhaler in the school clinic. If that is the case, then the students and teachers must have easy access to the medication whenever such treatment is warranted according to information provided by the parent or health-care provider.

References

Almqvist C, Larsson PH, Egmar AC, Hedren M, Malmberg P, Wickman M. 1999. School as a risk environment for children allergic to cats and a site for transfer of cat allergen to homes. J Allergy Clin Immunol 103:1012–1017.

Busse WW, Lemanske RF. 2001. Advances in immunology: Asthma. N Engl J Med 344:350–362.

Centers for Disease Control and Prevention. 2000. Measuring childhood asthma prevalence before and after the 1997 redesign of the National Health Interview Survey, United States. Mortal Morbid Weekly Rept 49(40):908–911.

Centers for Disease Control and Prevention. 2002. Strategies for addressing asthma within a coordinated school health program. Atlanta, GA: Centers for Disease Control and Prevention, National Center for Chronic Disease Prevention and Health Promotion. Available: http://www.cdc.gov/HealthyYouth/asthma/index.htm [accessed 7 March 2005].

Daisey JM, Angell WJ. 1998. A survey and critical review of the literature on indoor air quality, ventilation, and health symptoms in schools. LBNL-41517. Berkeley, CA: Lawrence Berkeley National Laboratory.

Friedman MS, Powell KE, Hutwagner L, Graham LM, Teague WG. 2001. Impact of changes in transportation and commuting behaviors during the 1996 Summer Olympic Games in Atlanta on air quality and childhood asthma. J Am Med Assoc 285:897–905.

Lonnkvist K, Hallden G, Dahlen SE, Enander I, van Hage-Hamsten M, Kumlin M, et al. 1999. Markers of inflammation and bronchial reactivity in children with asthma, exposed to animal dander in school dust. Pediatr Allergy Immunol 10:45–52.

Mannino DM, Homa DM, Akinbami LJ, Moorman JE, Gwynn C, Redd SC. 2002. Surveillance for asthma, United States, 1980–1999. In CDC Surveillance Summaries (March 29). Mortal Morbid Weekly Rept 51(SS-1):1–13.

Mellinger-Birdsong AK, Powell KE, Iatridis T. 2000. Georgia asthma report. Publication no. DPH00.65H. Atlanta: Georgia Department of Human Resources.

National Asthma Education and Prevention Program. 1997a. How asthma friendly is your school? Bethesda, MD: National Asthma Education and Prevention Program, National Heart, Lung, and Blood Institute. Available: http://www.nhlbi.nih.gov/health/public/lung/asthma/friendhi.htm [accessed 7 March 2005].

National Asthma Education and Prevention Program. 1997b. Resolution on asthma management at school. Bethesda, MD: National Asthma Education and Prevention Program, National Heart, Lung, and Blood Institute. Available: http://www.nhlbi.nih.gov/health/public/lung/asthma/resolut.htm [accessed 7 March 2005].

National Asthma Education and Prevention Program. 2002. Managing asthma: A guide for schools. Bethesda, MD: National Heart, Lung, and Blood Institute.

National Center for Environmental Health, Air and Respiratory Health Branch. 2005. Asthma's impact on children and adolescents. Atlanta, GA: Centers for Disease Control and Prevention. Available: http://www.cdc.gov/asthma/children.htm [accessed 7 March 2005].

National Institutes of Health. 2002. Clinical practice guidelines: Expert panel report 2: Guidelines for the diagnosis and management of asthma. NIH Publication 97-4051. Rockville, MD: Author

Teague WG, Bayer CW. 2001. Outdoor air pollution: Asthma and other concerns. Pediatr Clin North Am 48(5):1167–1184.

Teague WG, Chang M, Gottschalk M, Tolbert P, Redd S, Frumkin H, et al. 2002. Smog and physical activity advisory. Technical Advisory Subcommittee of the Clean Air Campaign and Southeast Pediatric Environmental Health Specialty Unit. Available: www.cleanaircampaign.com/index.php/cac/content/download/250/1289/file/cac_health_advisory_guidelines.pdf [accessed 14 January 2006].

Tolbert PE, Mulholland JA, MacIntosh DL, Xu F, Daniels D, Devine OJ, et al. 2000. Air quality and pediatric emergency room visits for asthma in Atlanta, Georgia, USA. Am J Epidemiol 151:798–810.

Tortolero SR, Bartholomew LK, Tyrrell S, Abramson SL, Sockrider MM, Markham CM, et al. 2002. Environmental allergens and irritants in schools: A focus on asthma. J Sch Health 72:33–38.

29

Harry Keyserling

Infectious Disease in Schools: Prevention and Control

■ *Summary*

- School environments provide ideal conditions for transmission of infectious diseases, but information on the frequency of infections in school children is limited.
- Major infectious agents contribute to brain infections, hepatitis, respiratory infections, diarrheal diseases, sexually transmitted diseases, and skin infections.
- Because infectious diseases are transmitted primarily by direct contact with hands, a stringent hand-washing program can be effective in reducing transmission.
- The most effective prevention strategies must also encompass regular environmental cleaning, comprehensive animal policies, immunizations, isolation of infected people, and mass prophylaxis in some cases. ■

Early school health programs were initiated in the 1800s. The primary goal of these efforts was to contain the spread of communicable diseases in the school setting. During the last century, tremendous progress has been made in sanitation and nutrition, as well as in the development and use of antibiotics and immunizations. Administrators and teachers can help prevent the spread of infectious diseases in schools by increasing their knowledge of the principles of disease transmission, learning how to recognize infectious disease emergencies, and working with health departments and community physicians to respond to local epidemics.

Incidence and Impact of Selected Infections in Childhood

Schools provide an environment that fosters the transmission of common infections. Large numbers of students are in close contact for long periods of time, and young children are susceptible to numerous infectious agents. In addition, hand hygiene facilities may be limited, classroom pets are sometimes handled improperly, and parents often allow infected children to attend school.

Limited information is available on the frequency of infections in school-aged children. The school nurse or a designated person should have written guidelines for reporting illnesses to the health department (American Academy of Pediatrics 2003). Local health departments, in turn, document information on selected infections required by law to be reported (notifiable diseases); these

421

data are collated and reported by the U.S. Centers for Disease Control and Prevention (CDC). Although each state health department establishes and distributes this list of reportable diseases to licensed physicians, reporting of other diseases to the state is entirely voluntary. This passive surveillance system tends to underestimate common diseases but is more accurate for rare diseases.

The most recent national estimates for common infections, based on a parental questionnaire survey, were reported by CDC's National Center for Health Statistics. The data used in the report were collected in the 1988 National Health Interview Survey on Child Health, which included children from birth through 17 years of age (Hardy 1991). Information was collected on infections during the preceding year. Approximately 122,000 people in 50,000 households were interviewed. Thirty-eight percent of children had at least one of the nine infectious diseases on the questionnaire:

- repeated ear infections
- repeated tonsillitis or enlarged adenoids
- pneumonia
- frequent diarrhea or colitis
- bladder or urinary tract infections
- mononucleosis
- hepatitis

■ *29.1. Steps of an outbreak investigation*

- An increase in disease activity is reported to public health authorities.
- The public health authorities determine whether an investigation is necessary.
- A case definition is established (e.g., vomiting and diarrhea in a classroom that occurred over a 3-day period).
- Cases are identified and counted (using diagnostic tests if available).
- Using statistical and epidemiologic methods, patterns in the occurrence of the disease are described.
- Factors that increase or decrease the risk of disease are analyzed.
- Prevention and control measures are initiated.
- Results of the investigation are communicated to parents and school officials. ■

- meningitis
- rheumatic fever.

Eleven percent reported two or more infections. Most of the infections were reported more frequently among white non-Hispanic children than black non-Hispanic or Hispanic children. Girls were more than five times as likely to have urinary tract infections compared with boys. Among teenagers 13–17 years of age, repeated tonsillitis was the most common disorder, reported in 5%.

Repeated ear infection was the most common disease in all children up to 17 years of age, with an annual incidence of 9 per 100 children, followed by repeated tonsillitis (4.7/100 children), pneumonia (1.7/100 children), urinary tract infection (1.5/100 children), frequent diarrhea or colitis (1.4/100 children), and mononucleosis (0.5/100 children). Hepatitis, meningitis, and rheumatic fever were rarely reported. Among children 12–17 years of age, mononucleosis occurred in 1.1 per 100 children.

The average annual number of lost school days per child was 2.8 for ear infections, 4.7 for tonsillitis, 5.5 for pneumonia, 2.0 for urinary tract infection, 2.0 for diarrhea or colitis, and 6.5 for mononucleosis. Hospitalizations for infections were rare. Approximately one-quarter of children with pneumonia were hospitalized. Less than 7% of children with repeated tonsillitis or ear infections were hospitalized.

Viral respiratory infections were not covered in the 1988 Health Interview Survey. These infections are common, occurring six to eight times per year in children younger than 2 years of age. Annual influenza epidemics affect 30–60% of school-aged children. Influenza cases are often first noted in schools before spreading to the general population.

Specific questions related to infectious disease in the school-age population have not been included in national surveys since 1991. Based on the latest national surveys, which were revised in 1997, in 2001 about one-quarter of school-aged children (5–17 years of age) had missed no school in the past year because of illness or injury (Bloom et al. 2003). Six percent of children missed 11 or more days of school because of illness or injury. Low-income families were more than twice as likely to have absences of 11 days or more (10% vs. 4%). In households headed by single mothers, children were twice as likely to have been absent for 11 or more days, compared with families with two parents.

Types of Infectious Agents

Viruses, bacteria, fungi, parasites, and infestations compose the major types of infections. Viruses are the smallest microorganisms that cannot survive independently and require an appropriate host for replication. Examples of viral infections include influenza, polio, hepatitis A, herpes simplex, rabies, and human immunodeficiency virus (HIV). Bacteria are microorganisms that can reproduce independently from a host organism. Examples of bacterial infections include *Streptococcus pyogenes* (the cause of strep throat), tuberculosis, and meningococcus (a cause of bacterial meningitis). Fungi are larger organisms that often cause superficial skin infections such as ringworm. Parasites are even larger organisms. Examples of parasitic infections include malaria and pinworms. Infestations occur when tiny animals burrow into the skin. Scabies and lice fall into this category.

Routes of Transmission

Normal childhood activities result in the transmission of infectious agents on a daily basis. Our noses and throats, gastrointestinal tracts, and skin contain billions of bacteria. Infectious agents can be transmitted in a school setting through four major mechanisms:

- through the air
- by direct contact such as shaking hands or salivary exchange during kissing
- through vectors such as mosquitoes or ticks
- by contact with objects such as tissues, toothbrushes, or combs that have been contaminated with infectious material.

What Happens When a Child Is Exposed to an Infectious Agent?

When a child is exposed to microorganisms, the concentration of infectious particles must be greater than a certain threshold for the infection to be successfully transmitted. Often the child becomes colonized with the agent, but symptoms do not develop. The colonization can occasionally last for months; during this time, the child may transmit the disease regardless of whether symptoms develop. For example, someone shakes hands with a person and acquires staphylococcal bacteria. The bacteria start growing on the recipient's skin, but no symptoms occur. The bacteria remain on the person's skin for many months; during that period the person may transmit the bacteria to others. Most of us have staphylococcal bacteria on our skin. Some of the bacteria are more likely to cause infections than other types. Most of the time, the bacteria do not cause problems. If the person has a skin abrasion or cut, the bacteria can then establish a portal of entry, and a local wound infection may occur.

Some infections may be mild and not cause any symptoms. For example, when influenza circulates through a community, a few people are infected yet do not develop any symptoms, but are able to transmit the virus to others.

The *incubation period* is the interval between becoming infected and developing symptoms. Some infections, such as influenza, have short incubation periods (1–5 days). Others have intermediate incubation periods, such as chickenpox (7–21 days), hepatitis A (15–50 days), and infectious mononucleosis (30–50 days). Some infections have prolonged incubation periods, such as rabies (up to 6 years) and human immunodeficiency virus (HIV), the infection that leads to AIDS (up to 15 years).

Unfortunately, for many infections, the highest risk of transmission occurs shortly before any symptoms develop. Mild illness is common in children attending daycare, preschool, and elementary school. Many children are infectious but do not have any symptoms. Most children do not need to miss school when experiencing a mild respiratory illness. However, if symptoms interfere with the child's ability to participate in classroom activities or require extensive attention by classroom teachers, the child should be sent home until symptoms resolve. Closing schools during influenza epidemics has not been shown to limit the spread of the disease in the community. For some infections, isolation of individuals is recommended until appropriate medications are administered or until the body's immune system controls the infection. Table 29.1 offers additional recommendations about exclusion from school for infectious illnesses.

Table 29.1. Common infectious illnesses[a]

Disease, illness, organism	How is it spread?	When is child most contagious?	Return to school[b]
Chicken pox[c] (varicella)	Airborne or direct contact with droplets from nose or mouth and skin lesions of infected individuals	From 2 days before rash until all lesions are dry and crusted	When all lesions have crusted (usually 7–8 days)
Cold sore (herpes simplex)	Direct contact with infected oral lesions or secretions	While lesions are present	After lesions are scabbed over
Common cold (upper respiratory infection)	Contact with droplets from nose, eyes, or mouth (virus can live in environment 24 hours)	Variable (from day before symptoms appear until symptoms resolve)	No exclusion, unless fever is present or child is too ill to attend
Conjunctivitis (pinkeye) (may be viral, bacterial, or allergic)	Contact with secretions from eyes or with contaminated surfaces	Variable (allergic conjunctivitis is not contagious)	When cleared by physician or after 24 hours of treatment *if* bacterial
Croup	Contact with droplets from nose, eyes, or mouth	Variable (usually from day before symptoms appear and for 3 days of illness)	When breathing comfortably, cough has improved, and no fever for 24 hours
Ear infection (otitis media)	Not contagious	Not contagious	No exclusion unless child is too sick to attend
Fever 100.4° or higher; no specific reason known or identified	Unknown until illness is identified; safe to assume it may be spread by contact with any secretions	Unknown; assume child is contagious while fever is present	After 24 hours without fever and child is behaving normally
Fifth disease[c] (parvovirus): "slapped cheek" appearance and a lacy rash	Contact with droplets from nose, eyes, or mouth	During the week before the rash develops	No need to restrict once rash has appeared
Gastroenteritis, bacterial (*E. coli, Salmonella, Shigella, Campylobacter, Yersinia*)	Contact with stool from infected person; ingestion of contaminated food, beverages, or water (especially raw eggs or improperly cooked meats)	When diarrhea is present	When diarrhea is resolved. *E. coli* and *Shigella* require two negative stool cultures
Gastroenteritis, viral (adenovirus, rotavirus, norovirus)	Contact with stool, saliva, or vomit from infected person either directly or from contaminated surfaces	From 2 days before illness until vomiting and diarrhea improve	When no fever or vomiting for 24 hours and fewer than 5 stools/day
German measles[c] (rubella)	Contact with droplets from nose, eyes, or mouth of infected person; may be transmitted to fetus across the placenta	From 5 days before until 7 days after rash appears	Typically 7 days after rash appears
Giardia (a parasite that causes diarrhea)	Contact with infected stool or consumption of contaminated water or food	When diarrhea is present	When stools are formed or fewer than 5/day
Hand, foot-and-mouth disease (Coxsackie virus)	Contact with stool; oral or respiratory secretions	May be contagious for several weeks after infection	When no fever for 24 hours and child is behaving normally
Head lice (pediculosis)	Close contact with infested individuals; sharing combs, brushes, hats, or bedding	When there are live insects on the head	After treatment, if crawling lice are gone. Nits need to be removed; however, nits alone should not be a reason for exclusion.

Disease, illness, organism	How is it spread?	When is child most contagious?	Return to school[b]
Hepatitis A	Eating contaminated food or water; close contact with infected individuals; contact with infected stool	From 2 weeks before the illness until 1 week after jaundice (yellow skin) has begun	After 1 week from the onset of jaundice
Hepatitis B[c]	From contaminated needles, blood, bloody secretions, ear piercing, tattooing, sexual activity	Virus can be spread at any time with the listed contact	When cleared by physician
Impetigo (staphylococcus or streptococcus skin infection)	Person-to-person skin contact (especially nasal discharge or hands)	Until active lesions are gone or after 24 hours on antibiotics	After at least 24 hours of topical or oral antibiotics
Influenza	Contact with droplets from nose, eyes, or mouth of infected person	Variable (from the day before, until after the first 5 days of illness)	After 24 hours without fever and when other symptoms are improving
Measles (rubeola)	Airborne or direct contact with droplets from nose, eyes, or mouth of infected person	From 4 days before the rash begins until 4 days after the rash appears	At least 5 days after the appearance of the rash
Meningitis, bacterial	Contact with droplets from nose, eyes, or mouth of infected person	Unknown (probably from several days before symptoms appear until at least 24 hours of antibiotic treatment)	After at least 24 hours of antibiotic treatment, including antibiotics to eliminate carrier state
Meningitis, viral (enterovirus)	Contact with droplets from nose, eyes, mouth, or stool of infected person	From the day before the illness until fever has subsided	After 24 hours without fever and child is behaving normally
Mononucleosis (mono) Epstein-Barr virus	Close personal contact with droplets from nose, eyes, or mouth of infected person	Probably several days before the illness until the fever has subsided	After 24 hours without fever unless child is too sick to attend
Mumps	Contact with droplets from nose, eyes, or mouth of infected person	Peak infectious time begins 2 days before swelling but may range from 7 days before to 9 days after	Typically 9 days after parotid gland begins to swell
Pinworms	Pinworms cause rectal itching. Microscopic eggs found on hands of infected children may contaminate surfaces. Infections spread through ingestion of eggs.	Eggs may survive up to 2 weeks after treatment and after rectal itching stops. Reinfection is common.	No exclusion, but treatment should be given to reduce spread
Pneumonia (viral or bacterial)	Contact with droplets from nose, eyes, and mouth of infected person. Some viruses can live on surfaces up to 24 hours.	Variable (from the day before symptoms appear through the first 3 days of the illness)	No exclusion needed unless child has fever or is too ill to attend
Ringworm (tinea capitis, corporis, pedis), fungal infection of scalp, body, or feet	Direct skin contact with infected people or animals or with surfaces contaminated with fungus; scalp lesions from contact with barber clippers or shared brushes	From onset of lesions until treatment begins	No exclusion, but treatment should be given to reduce spread

(continued)

Table 29.1. (*Continued*)

Disease, illness, organism	How is it spread?	When is child most contagious?	Return to school[b]
Scabies (mites that burrow under the skin, causing severe itching)	Skin contact with infested individuals; contact with bedding or clothes of infested person	From up to 8 weeks before skin rash appears until it has been treated	The day after adequate treatment begins
Sinusitis	Not contagious	Not contagious	No exclusion unless child is too sick to attend
Strep throat/scarlet fever	Contact with droplets from nose and mouth	From onset of symptoms until 24 hours after treatment begins	After at least 24 hours of antibiotic treatment and no fever for 24 hours
Tuberculosis	Airborne or contact with droplets from nose and mouth of infected person. Children usually contract TB from close contact with an infected adult.	Children with TB usually are not infectious to others	Only when health department gives permission

[a]Adapted from Common Infectious Illnesses poster, 2000 edition, comp. by the Georgia Department of Human Resources Division of Public Health and Children's Healthcare of Atlanta.
[b]Exceptions to the exclusion/return-to-school guidelines listed on this chart may be made by local personnel on a case-by-case basis.
[c]These diseases may be of particular concern to staff members who are pregnant or trying to become pregnant. Follow-up with obstetric health-care provider is recommended after known or suspected exposure.

A major principle of isolation is the physical separation of an infected person from the general population. Close contact is required for transmission, with the exception of a few infections such as chicken pox, measles, and tuberculosis, where the infectious agents can remain suspended in the air for hours. Respiratory infections can be limited by teaching children appropriate respiratory etiquette practices. For patients who are coughing or sneezing, the use of handkerchiefs and tissues can limit the spread of disease. In a hospital setting, facial masks for certain infections are recommended.

As normal children develop, they are better able to respond to infections because of a more mature immune system, having received appropriate immunizations and been exposed to many infectious agents. Children with chronic medical problems such as diabetes, kidney and liver disease, or sickle cell disease are predisposed to have more severe infections. Children who are receiving chemotherapy for cancer or who have had transplants are similarly vulnerable. It is important for teachers and administrators to be aware of any medical conditions that predispose school children to severe infections. Some schools have policies recommending that parents of high-risk children be immediately informed of any infections noted in classmates.

■ *29.2. Respiratory hygiene and cough etiquette*

- Cover the nose and mouth when coughing or sneezing.
- Use tissues to contain respiratory secretions.
- Dispose of tissues in the nearest wastebasket after use.
- Wash hands after contact with respiratory secretions.
- Wash hands after contact with contaminated materials or objects.
- Do not allow children to share handkerchiefs or tissues.
- Tissues should be readily available to all students and staff in all classrooms. ■

Infections in School-age Children

Infectious Disease Emergencies

Any febrile illness in a child with a poorly functioning immune system should have a prompt medical evaluation. This includes children with sickle cell disease, children with an abnormal immune system, children receiving chemotherapy, children on immunosuppressive therapy after transplants, or children receiving immunosuppressive therapy for diseases such as rheumatoid arthritis or inflammatory bowel disease.

Any child who has a cough and significant difficulty breathing should have a medical evaluation. Symptoms of a brain infection, such as headache, stiff neck, seizures, or change in mental status, should be evaluated promptly. Symptoms of a bone or joint infection, such as difficulty and pain on movement of an extremity, should be evaluated. Fever associated with a rapidly progressive skin rash may represent a serious systemic bacterial infection that needs immediate diagnosis and antibiotic therapy.

Brain Infections

Meningitis (inflammation of the spinal cord) may be caused by viruses, bacteria, or fungi. During the summer months, enteroviruses often cause community outbreaks. These infections have no specific therapy and do not result in significant brain damage. After the introduction of vaccines against *Haemophilus influenzae* and *Streptococcus pneumoniae,* bacterial meningitis was dramatically reduced. The major cause of bacterial meningitis in the United States is now *Neisseria meningitides.* A vaccine is available that prevents some cases of meningococcal disease. In rare cases, meningoencephalitis (infection of brain and spinal cord) results from West Nile virus, which is transmitted by mosquitoes.

Hepatitis

Several viruses cause liver infections (hepatitis). Hepatitis B and C are serious because they can cause chronic infections that may lead to long-term medical problems such as cirrhosis and liver cancer. Immunization against hepatitis B is required before school entry in the United States, with the first dose being administered in the newborn period. Unfortunately, no vaccine for hepatitis C is available currently.

Hepatitis A virus is transmitted from contaminated food or infected stools. Infections associated with diapered children in daycare centers may be decreased by appropriate disinfection of changing tables. An effective vaccine is currently recommended for all children at one year of age and for international travelers.

Respiratory Infections

Viral respiratory infections are common. Young children, particularly those in daycare settings, may have as many as 10 infections in the first year of life. Agents include respiratory syncytial virus, metapneumovirus, adenovirus, parainfluenza virus, and influenza. The first encounters with respiratory viruses usually occur in the first three years of life and can cause runny nose, sneezing, coughing, wheezing, sore throat, and pneumonia. Vaccines against influenza are available for children older than 6 months of age and must be administered every year for maximum protection against the disease. Influenza season in the United States usually occurs between November and March.

Viruses or bacteria frequently cause ear infections (otitis media), sinusitis, and bronchitis, particularly in children younger than three years. In the last few years, national initiatives have promoted the judicious use of antibiotics and a decrease in the use of antibiotic therapy for these common ailments.

Some cases of pharyngitis and tonsillitis are caused by bacteria known as group A streptococcus. Children may complain of sore throat, swollen glands, and abdominal pain. Numerous diagnostic tests are available, and a course of antibiotics is recommended to prevent transmission and complications of these diseases.

Eye infections (conjunctivitis) may be caused by bacteria or viruses. Some types of viral conjunctivitis (adenovirus) are highly contagious. Children or staff members with this type of conjunctivitis need to stay out of school until the eye inflammation has resolved.

Diarrheal Diseases

Vomiting and loose stools are often caused by infectious agents. Many different viruses, bacteria, and parasites can cause acute gastroenteritis. Children with symptomatic gastroenteritis should be excluded from school until their symptoms have resolved. The main goal of therapy for gastroenteritis is to provide supplemental fluids to prevent dehydration. Antibiotics are rarely necessary and potentially prolong the disease process.

Sexually Transmitted Diseases

A number of infections can be transmitted through sexual contact (oral, genital, and anal). Bacterial infections include syphilis, gonorrhea, chlamydia, and chancroid; viral infections include herpes, HIV, hepatitis B, and human papilloma virus (HPV). Trichomonas is a parasitic infection. Sexually transmitted diseases (STDs) may not cause any symptoms or may include vaginal or penile discharge, pain on urination, skin ulcers, or warts. HPV causes warts and cervical cancer. Vaccines are currently under development for HIV and HPV. Untreated genital infections may lead to infertility and other medical complications. Accurate diagnosis is important for appropriate therapy and counseling, and partner evaluation is essential to limit the spread of infections.

Other than vaccination for hepatitis B, the primary methods for prevention of STDs include abstinence, barrier methods such as condoms, and limiting the number of sexual partners.

Skin Infections

Herpes simplex is a common viral infection that causes recurrent fever blisters. About 1% of the population is shedding virus from oral secretions at any random time. Infections can be spread by kissing or contact sports such as wrestling. All children should be advised to avoid contact with oral secretions of other students and not to share cups or bottles. Excluding symptomatic children with herpes from routine school activities is not justified, but it is reasonable to exclude students with obvious mouth or skin lesions from wrestling or rugby. Careful cleaning of wrestling mats routinely after use with a 1:64 dilution of household bleach (1 cup of bleach diluted in 1 gallon of water) is recommended, with a contact time of a minimum of 30 seconds. The bleach solution may be wiped off or allowed to air dry.

Impetigo is a local skin infection caused by bacteria. Redness and drainage of pus in one or more areas of the skin may occur. Antibiotics are useful in treating such skin infections. The risk of transmission of impetigo is dramatically decreased after 1 day of antibiotics.

Ringworm (tinea corporis) is a fungal infection that may involve the face, trunk, or limbs. It is usually red, circular, and scaly. Itching is common. Local medication applied to the affected areas is usually successful. When ringworm occurs on the scalp (tinea capitis), more aggressive therapy is necessary. Until they have been treated, students with ringworm should not share combs, hair brushes, hats, or hair ornaments. Other types of fungal skin infections include jock itch (tinea cruris), which occurs in the groin and upper thighs, and athlete's foot (tinea pedis), which occurs on the foot or between the toes. The fungi are acquired by contact with skin scales from an affected person or contact with fungi in damp areas such as swimming pools, locker rooms, and shower rooms. The risk of ringworm in schools can be decreased by not sharing towels, appropriately laundering towels, and disinfecting shower areas. Students with tinea pedis should be excluded from swimming pools and from walking barefoot on locker room and shower floors until treatment has been started.

Scabies is a red rash caused by mites in the upper layers of the skin. A major feature is severe itching, particularly at night. Within the household, scabies is transmitted in clothing and bedding. In schools, direct skin contact is the major route of transmission. Several medications are available to treat scabies.

Lice usually occur on the head but may also occur on the body or pubic area. The most common symptom of head lice is itching; however, many children are asymptomatic. Lice or eggs (nits) may be found in the hair, often behind the ears or near the neck. Lice infestations in children attending schools or daycare are common. Transmission is by direct contact with the hair of an affected person or contact with objects such as combs, hair brushes, and hats. Children with scabies or head lice should be excluded from school until treatment is initiated.

Prevention of Infections

Environmental Control

Appropriate architectural design of the physical plant in schools and daycare centers can decrease the risk of infections (Donowitz 1996). Areas for different activities such as diaper changing, play, and food preparation should be separated. Appropriate sinks, soap, and towels should be available in all restroom facilities. Sinks should be easily accessible near diaper-changing areas.

Environmental surfaces should be nonporous and easily cleaned by disinfectants. Toys should be cleaned and disinfected daily, and toys that are contaminated by saliva or feces should be cleaned immediately. Individual bedding should not be shared and should be washed at least weekly. Other surfaces that require special cleaning attention include wrestling mats, sleeping mats, blankets, and therapy equipment. The handling of blood contamination of surfaces is discussed in box 29.3.

Regularly scheduled environmental cleaning, including vacuuming, sweeping, dusting, and washing, is important to kill infectious agents that may be present on surfaces in the building. The U.S. Environmental Protection Agency registers products as detergents or disinfecting agents for cleaning the environment. Because many agents can be toxic, it is important in daycare and school settings to use appropriate chemicals that achieve disinfection but do not pose toxic risks to students or staff. Standard household cleaning products are usually adequate. Additional information about cleaning can be found in chapter 14.

■ *29.3. Handling blood exposures (nose bleeds, lacerations, and bites)*

- Use gloves when having direct contact with blood.
- Control bleeding by applying pressure with gauze pads.
- Disinfect blood spills with bleach or alcohol.
- Dispose of contaminated materials in plastic trash bags.
- Wash hands after removing gloves.
- If students or teachers have direct blood exposure to skin, eyes, or mouth, wash blood off immediately with soap and water, and contact local medical resources.
- Intact skin does not require physician evaluation or other measures beyond cleaning the area with soap and water and informing the child's parent.
- If a student or teacher is bitten, clean the bite wound with soap and water immediately and seek medical advice. ■

Because carpets are extremely difficult to maintain, the use of carpets and rugs should be limited to administrative areas rather than classrooms.

Pet and Animal Policies

Animals are a significant reservoir of infectious agents. Schools that are considering the use of pets or other animals must carefully weigh the potential risks and benefits. Students should wash their hands thoroughly after any contact with an animal. Additional information about this topic is presented in chapter 7.

Immunizations

All states mandate certain immunizations for school entry. The U.S. Public Health Service, the American Academy of Pediatrics, and the American Academy of Family Physicians recommend that certain vaccines be given to all children (see box 29.4). Waivers from the school immunization requirements vary from state to state and are based on medical conditions and religious and philosophical convictions. High levels of immunization coverage in the United States have dramatically decreased the incidence of vaccine-preventable diseases.

Mass Prophylaxis

In certain situations such as exposure to meningococcal disease or tuberculosis, antibiotics may be administered to classrooms or entire schools. Decisions to undertake such measures are made by the health department and school officials.

Infection Control

The primary means of infectious disease transmission is through direct contact with infected hands. An active hand-washing program should help reduce disease transmission.

A study in 1997 demonstrated that when elementary school children in Michigan washed their hands four times a day, the risk of school absenteeism decreased significantly (Master et al. 1997). Six classrooms of 143 students 5–12 years of age were in the hand-washing group, and eight classrooms of 162 students were the control group (children washed their hands without any special encouragement or monitoring). Students in the hand-washing group washed their hands when they arrived at school, before lunch, after lunch, and before going home. Information collected during the flu season in 1996 showed the hand-washing group

---

▦ *29.4. Recommended childhood vaccinations*

- hepatitis B: three doses before 18 months of age
- diphtheria/tetanus/pertussis (whooping cough): five doses before 6 years of age, and a booster dose for adolescents
- *Haemophilus influenzae* type b (Hib): two to three doses before 15 months of age
- poliovirus: four doses before 6 years of age
- measles, mumps, rubella (MMR): two doses before 6 years of age
- varicella (chickenpox): one dose before 18 months of age
- pneumococcal: four doses before 15 months of age
- influenza: annual vaccine beginning after 6 months of age
- hepatitis A: two doses between one and two years of age
- meningococcal: one dose for adolescents

(Based on recommendations of the Centers for Disease Control and Prevention 2004) ▦

▦ *29.5. Hand-washing guidelines*

When to wash your hands:

- before, during, and after you prepare food
- before you eat
- after you use the bathroom
- after handling animals or animal waste
- when your hands are dirty
- more frequently when someone in your home is sick.

How to wash your hands:

- First, wet your hands and apply liquid or clean bar soap. Place the bar soap on a rack, and allow it to drain.
- Next, rub your hands together vigorously and scrub all surfaces.
- Continue for 10–15 seconds, or about the length of time it takes to sing "Happy Birthday" twice. It is the soap combined with the scrubbing action that helps dislodge and remove germs.
- Rinse well and dry your hands. ▦

---

lost 116.5 school days compared with 175 school days for the control group. Absenteeism due to infectious diseases (respiratory and gastrointestinal illness) was reduced 25% in the hand-washing group compared with the control group. Another study conducted in kindergarten and first-grade classes from a suburban school in Chicago had similar results (Kimel 1996). During the 2-month study period, absenteeism was significantly higher in the students who were in the control group.

An Associated Press report of a large county-wide experiment in 20 West Virginia elementary schools supported hand-washing programs. After teachers encouraged students to wash their hands four times a day, absenteeism fell by 1%.

Several resources are available to support hand-washing programs in schools (Rodriguez 2002). The Minnesota Health Department has a curriculum to support hand washing (http://www.health.state.mn.us/handhygiene/toolkit/curricula/index.html). Another resource is available from the CDC at http://www.cdc.gov/ncidod/op/handwashing.htm.

Conclusion

School environments have many conditions amenable to the transmission of infections. Infectious diseases are a common cause of absence from school. Simple prevention strategies can reduce the transmission of infections from person to person. Hand washing, immunization strategies, and isolation of infected people are reviewed in this chapter as examples of strategies with a high likelihood of success at reducing transmission.

Resources

- Association for Professionals in Infection Control and Epidemiology
  www.apic.org
- Centers for Disease Control and Prevention
  www.cdc.gov
- Infectious Disease Society of America
  www.idsociety.org

- Pediatric Infectious Disease Society
  www.pids.org
- Society for Health Care Epidemiology of
  America
  www.shea-online.org
- World Health Organization
  www.who.int

References

American Academy of Pediatrics Committee on Infectious Diseases. 2003. Red book: 2003 report of the Committee on Infectious Diseases, 26th ed. Elk Grove Village, IL: American Academy of Pediatrics.

American Academy of Pediatrics Committee on School Health. 2004. *School health: Policy and practice,* 6th ed. Elk Grove Village, IL: American Academy of Pediatrics.

Bloom B, Cohen RA, Vickerie JL, Wondimu EA. 2003. Summary health statistics for U.S. children: National Health Interview Survey, 2001. National Center for Health Statistics. Vital Health Stat 10(216):1–54.

Donowitz LG, ed. 1996. *Infection control in the child care center and preschool,* 3d ed. Baltimore, MD: Williams and Wilkins.

Hardy AM. 1991. Incidence and impact of selected infectious diseases in childhood. National Center for Health Statistics. Vital Health Stat 10(180): 1–22.

Kimel LS. 1996. Handwashing education can decrease illness absenteeism. J Sch Nurs 12(2):14–16, 18.

Master D, Hess Longe SH, Dickson H. 1997. Scheduled hand washing in an elementary school population. Fam Med 29(5):336–339.

Rodriguez S. 2002. The importance of school-based hand-washing programs. J Sch Nurs (October; Suppl.):19–22.

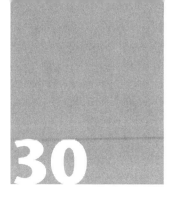

Darryl Alexander

Occupational Health and Safety for Faculty and Staff

■ *Summary*

- Schools are not only educational institutions; they are also workplaces for teachers, administrators, and staff.
- Numerous work-related hazards are found in schools, including chemical hazards, indoor air problems, stress, ergonomic hazards, and infectious diseases.
- An occupational health approach to these problems, including recognition, elimination, and control of hazards, personal protective equipment when appropriate, administrative controls, and training can help protect the health and safety of school employees. ■

Many activities and processes in schools have implications for the health and well-being of staff members as well as children. The chapters of this book focus primarily on creating safe and healthy school environments for children, but it is also critically important to address the occupational health and safety concerns of the adults who spend their working lives in schools.

Some occupational health and safety concerns relate to exposures that both children and staff

share. For example, as chapters 10 and 11 point out, indoor air quality and mold problems affect both students and staff members, although the pattern of responses may differ in adults and children. The prevalence of asthma appears to be greater in education employees than the general working population; whether this is due to school exposure or other factors is not known (National Institute for Occupational Safety and Health 2003). Other occupational health issues, such as some ergonomic concerns, are more specific to teachers and other employees. These often go unrecognized as work related and are addressed as individual concerns.

The overall impact of school work on staff health and well-being is not fully understood, but a comprehensive occupational health and safety approach to identifying, preventing, and eliminating hazardous exposures will go a long way to protecting and promoting the health of teachers and other school personnel. This chapter describes a range of occupational health concerns, some that potentially affect all staff members and some that are specific to certain job categories. It also offers recommendations for a model occupational health program in a school setting.

Occupational Hazards Shared by All School Employees

Stress

Occupational stress may have a significant effect on health and well-being. It may result from work organization and management, from the physical environment, or from both. Stress, in turn, can contribute to teacher burnout (Farber 1991).

Organizational issues that lead to stress, according to the Karasek model, include a combination of high job demand and low decision control (Karasek 1979). People with high job demands perceive excessive task requirements or workload, time pressure, and conflicting demands. They describe themselves as "working very hard," "working very fast," and "not having enough time to get the job done." These conditions are common among teachers, especially when budget cutbacks lead to high class loads and little time to plan or prepare. People with low workplace control say that they lack influence at work and are unable or unauthorized to make decisions or impact their job, conditions that may apply when hierarchical management structures are in place, curricula are inflexible, and class schedules are rigid. However, high job demands are not necessarily bad; when combined with high control, demanding jobs can be highly stimulating and motivating. A third dimension of the workplace, social support, can mitigate some of the effects of stress.

Physical environments with environmental problems may also be a source of stress. Poor air quality, noisy conditions, leaking roofs, classrooms and kitchens that are too hot or too cold, and moldy conditions are commonly cited by school employees as stressful. Inspiring students in these conditions creates added stress; even if students do not suffer symptoms, they may be inattentive and distracted.

Few studies have been conducted on the impact of stress on teachers. One longitudinal study of new teachers found that depressive symptoms, self-esteem, job satisfaction, and motivation to teach were all related to stressful conditions at work; support from supervisors, colleagues, and nonwork sources improved symptoms levels and self-esteem (Schonfeld 1996, 2001). A Canadian study of elementary school teachers found high and constant job demands with little time for physical or mental relaxation; teachers reported that they loved their work and were dedicated to the children but also felt that job burnout was a real risk and that they would not likely reach retirement (Messing et al. 1997). A series of studies among primary and high school teachers in England found that high job demands (as measured by questionnaire items such as "The pace of work in my job is very intense") and low job control (as measured by questions such as "I have freedom to decide what I do in my job") were associated with high blood pressure, elevated cortisol levels, and other signs of stress, not only during the workday but in the evenings as well (Steptoe 2000; Steptoe and Cropley 2000; Steptoe et al. 1999, 2000). Again, social support helped modulate the stress response. There is some evidence that stress may be even more prevalent and troubling among certain categories of teachers, such as those who teach children with disabilities (Jennett et al. 2003).

Improved research is needed to characterize the impact of stress and poor environmental conditions on teachers and teaching. Indications are, though, that poor environmental quality combined with nonsupportive, high-demand, low-control working conditions may contribute significantly to poor health outcomes for teachers and classroom staff.

Moreover, job stress may affect other school staff members who also confront the combination of high demands and low control. Custodial staff, food service workers, and secretaries in many schools are confronting staff cutbacks that result in increasing workloads. The effects may include increased risk of anxiety, depression, and cardiovascular disease (Belkic et al. 2004).

Asbestos

Nearly two decades after the passage of the Asbestos Hazard Emergency Response Act (AHERA) of 1987, asbestos exposure remains a problem in some older schools (see chapter 10). Custodial maintenance workers are often required to remove and replace broken vinyl asbestos floor tile, remove asbestos-containing lagging on leaking pipes, and patch and repair blown-on asbestos on gym and auditorium ceilings. Other school employees are passively exposed to friable asbestos whenever asbestos-containing building material (ACBM) is disturbed.

Little research has been conducted to determine the extent of the impact of this exposure on school staff, but the few existing studies deserve attention and response. In Wisconsin, statewide surveillance for mesothelioma, a cancer uniquely associated with asbestos exposure, found 22 patients between 1959 and 1989 whose asbestos exposure had likely occurred in schools (Anderson et al. 1991). Twelve were school teachers, and 10 were school maintenance employees. In 9 of the 12 school teacher cases, the only potential source of asbestos exposure identified was at school. The investigators also found two school clusters of cases among the 12 teachers investigated. In four of the ten maintenance employees, the disease was attributed to asbestos exposure at school. Another report described four cases of mesothelioma in teachers; again, the teachers' only apparent exposure to asbestos was in the schools in which they taught, although none had personally handled it (Lilienfeld 1991).

Two other studies provide further evidence of asbestos exposure among school custodial and maintenance workers. One (Oliver et al. 1991) reported that 21% of custodial study participants with no known asbestos exposure outside of school had developed pleural plaques, a marker of asbestos exposure, and 18% had restrictive changes on pulmonary function testing. The other study (Levin and Selikoff 1991) documented chest X-ray abnormalities consistent with asbestos scarring in 28% of a large cohort of New York City Board of Education custodians with no known asbestos exposure outside of school. The prevalence of this finding increased with length of employment; 53% of custodians who had begun employment 35 or more years earlier were affected.

Asbestos exposures in schools, whether to spray-on insulation, ceiling tiles, or pipe insulation, remains an occupational hazard years after it was installed.

Occupational Hazards of Teachers and Teachers' Aides

Teaching has traditionally been considered a relatively safe job, and work-related symptoms, illnesses, and injuries among classroom staff are rarely recognized in school settings. There are probably several reasons for this. The "industry of education" does not utilize hazardous processes, in contrast to, say, manufacturing. Toxic chemicals and hazardous operations are not used to make a final "product," and classroom staff do not typically engage in tasks that would lead to injuries. This perception is typically shared by administrators who focus on pedagogy and improved student performance and who are not trained to recognize potential exposures and related illnesses and injuries. Furthermore, school employees themselves have not been trained to recognize hazards and to report work-related injuries and illnesses.

However, research has demonstrated patterns of illnesses and injuries associated with teaching. These include violence, voice disorders, infectious diseases, bladder problems, and ergonomic issues.

Violence

Much has been written about violence at schools (see chapter 19). While much of the focus is on the traumatic effects of violence on children, teachers and other staff are also affected. According to the Bureau of Justice (Duhart 2001), teachers and other staff have some of the highest rates of workplace assaults in the country; junior high and special education teachers have rates that rival those of mental health care workers. Similarly, a national study of workers' compensation claims for work-related assaults found that teachers account for a large proportion of claims for assaults (Hashemi and Webster 1996). Of 28,692 such claims filed between 1993 and 1996, schools accounted for nearly 12%, a larger proportion than any other industry. Three-quarters of the school claims were from women.

In addition to the direct effects of violent acts, violence can have lasting impacts on teachers' mental health (Levenson et al. 2000). This may be a significant contributor to workplace stress, and in severe cases, it may result in posttraumatic stress disorder.

Voice Disorders

Teachers and teacher assistants (paraprofessionals) suffer a higher rate of voice disorders than other working people. Smith et al. (1997) compared the frequency and effects of voice symptoms in teachers to a group of people employed in other occupations. Teachers were more likely to report having voice problems and symptoms than nonteachers, and more than one in five teachers had missed workdays due to voice problems, compared to none of the nonteachers. A related study (Smith et al. 1998) found that more than 38% of teachers complained that teaching had an adverse impact on their voice and that 39% of these had cut back on teaching activities as a result. Female teachers reported more acute and chronic voice problems than males. These research results suggest that teaching is a high-risk occupation for voice disorders and that this may have significant work-related economic effects.

Several factors may contribute to voice disorders in teachers, including poor indoor air quality, the presence of irritants and other air contaminants, and low humidity. In addition, the noise created by heating, ventilating, and air-conditioning (HVAC) systems, poor acoustic design in classrooms, and crowded classrooms may also contribute to teachers' straining their voices to be heard (American National Standards Institute and Acoustical Society of America 2002).

Infectious Disease

Schools are some of the most densely populated institutions in our society, and in some cases, budget cuts and the resulting crowding have increased density even above traditional high levels. School enrollment is expected to increase to historic numbers at least until 2009, and most school districts do not anticipate any relief in crowding.

Crowding and inadequate ventilation may combine to play an important part in the transmission of many communicable diseases in schools. Crowding is a risk factor for respiratory infections in both children (Cardoso et al. 2004) and adults (Jaakkola and Heinonen 1995; see chapter 2). Moreover, people in buildings with reduced air supply may have an increased risk of exposure to infectious droplet nuclei transmitted by building occupants (Brundage et al. 1988; Myatt et al. 2004; see also chapter 10). In particular, rhinovirus, a frequent cause of the common cold, may be transmitted over large distances. Other studies have shown that relative humidity may have an influence on rates of respiratory infections in building occupants. The survival or infectivity of infectious disease agents appears to decrease in environments

with a humidity range of 40–70%, and people in buildings with mid-range humidity levels have demonstrated lower rates of respiratory infections (Arundel et al. 1986). These research results suggest that classrooms with crowded conditions and suboptimal air quality may increase teachers' risk of respiratory infections (see also chapter 29).

As early as 1923, a study in New York schools found that students in fan-ventilated rooms suffered 70% more respiratory illnesses than students in window-ventilated classrooms (New York State Commission on Ventilation 1923). Although there is little evidence available on teachers, one study has found a high rate of acute respiratory infections among teachers compared with the general working population (Whelan et al. 2002).

Of special concern are some communicable diseases that are more dangerous to adults than to children. A case in point is fifth disease. Fifth disease, or erythema infectiosum, is a viral infection caused by parvovirus 19. In children it results in a mild illness with low-grade fever, headache, and stuffy nose, followed by a typical bright red rash that begins on the face (a "slapped face" appearance) and spreads to the abdomen, arms, and legs. This illness resolves quickly and completely. However, in adults who have never been infected, "fifth" can have a significant health impact, including a rheumatoid arthritis-like syndrome (Keeler 1992; Naides 1993). In addition, acute infection with parvovirus 19 during pregnancy is associated with miscarriage and fetal hydrops (or accumulation of fluid in tissues; Al-Khan et al. 2003). There is some evidence that school and day-care personnel are at increased risk of fifth disease. For example, a CDC study of day-care personnel during an outbreak of fifth disease showed that nearly 20% of susceptible personnel were newly infected (Gillespie et al. 1990). Anecdotal reports of miscarriage among teachers in schools with outbreaks of fifth disease raise the question of whether the risk of miscarriages is elevated among teachers because of the danger of fifth disease.

Teachers can be exposed to students with other viral infections, including rhinovirus, influenza, varicella, and cytomegalovirus, and with streptococcal and staphylococcal bacterial infections. Pertussis or whooping cough has been of recent concern for several reasons: The disease has increased in incidence in recent years (Zanardi et al. 2002), many children are not being immunized (Lyons et al. 2004), immunity among immunized children wanes 5–15 years after their last immunization (Everett et al. 2004), outbreaks in schools have been documented (Brennan et al. 2000), and a vaccine has only recently been licensed for adults.

School employees who are immunocompromised—those with diabetes, cancer, and other diseases and/or those on immune-suppressing medications—may be especially vulnerable to infection. Many teachers continue teaching in this condition during treatment for diseases such as breast cancer.

Staff exposure to communicable infection merits more attention. At a minimum, teachers and other school employees should be advised to keep their immunizations current according to the CDC Advisory Committee on Immunization Practice (ACIP). In addition, administrators should revisit policies that penalize teachers and classroom personnel who stay home when they contract an infectious disease.

Bladder Infections and Problems

One of the penalties of rigid classroom schedules is that teachers may be unable to use the restroom as needed. In a survey of nearly 800 teachers in Iowa, four in five reported needing to urinate at times other than breaks, and half reported drinking less while at work to reduce their need to go to the bathroom (Nygard and Linder 1997). In this study 15.8% of respondents reported a urinary tract infection during the preceding year, 13.4% reported urge incontinence at least weekly, and 17.6% reported stress incontinence at least weekly, leading 19% to wear pads while working. Teachers who drank less at work were more likely to have had a urinary tract infection during the previous year than women who drank the volume they desired at work (21.2% vs. 9.9%). Many anecdotal reports corroborate this study. A kindergarten teacher reported that she literally had to take her class with her to the restroom every day because she had no one to cover her classes. A teacher in a large urban school reported that she had twenty minutes every day for lunch and personal needs; with the restroom located at least five minutes away from her classroom, she had to decide each day whether to go to the restroom or eat lunch. Teachers and teaching assistants are probably at risk for bladder problems and infections when they lack adequate opportunities to go to the restroom.

Ergonomics

Teaching is not often considered physically demanding work. However, as described in more detail in chapter 6, work can take a toll on joints and muscles for some classroom and related staff. Crowded schools often leave many teachers without dedicated classrooms; many are forced to move from room to room with books and equipment. Special education teachers and paraprofessionals sometimes function as health-care workers as they handle students with physical disabilities who may need repositioning in a wheelchair, lifting from chair to floor, or diapers changed. Special education teachers and paraprofessionals may perform repetitive motions as they use manipulative toys and games with their students, placing them at risk of conditions such as carpal tunnel syndrome. Librarians may also have to lift boxes of books, placing them at risk of back injuries. Teachers and other classroom staff appear to be at risk of back pain as they spend the day bending, squatting, and kneeling to assist students; the problem is especially troublesome for primary and elementary school teachers who sit in "kiddy" chairs or find themselves sitting on the floor. In addition, standing for long periods of time may increase teachers' risk of plantar fasciitis, a painful inflammation of connective tissue of the foot (fig. 30.1).

New technology and computers in classrooms offer important educational benefits, but they may also come with ergonomic risks for teachers and other school staff. One survey of 218 elementary school teachers in Oregon found that each day they spent an average of 1–2 hours on the computer at school and an additional 2–3 hours on the computer at home (Williams 2001). Eighty percent reported that they experienced discomfort during computer use at home and school. The most common discomfort was in the necks, shoulders, lower back, wrists, and eyes. These results corresponded closely to results in office workers. As computer use in schools increases, associated ergonomic problems may become more common.

Vocational and Career/Technical Education

Vocational educators and career/technical educators confront a number of hazards in their work, many of which are often unrecognized. Examples include cosmetology shops, where nail polishes

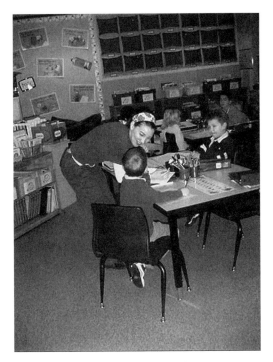

Figure 30.1. When teachers work with young students, they often bend over to interact at the child's level, an uncomfortable and potentially dangerous position. (Photo by Diane Tien.)

■ *30.1. A custodial worker*

John R., a longtime custodian in a New Jersey school district, recalls that he and his co-workers had to replace their shoes several times each year because the floor stripper they used literally ate holes through the soles. Not only did their shoes get destroyed, but John and some of his fellow custodians also had irritated skin, headaches, and other symptoms they now associate with the solvents in the stripper. After several years, the school district finally replaced the floor stripper with one with less-toxic ingredients. Larry M., another custodian in a Texas school district, says that he and his coworkers hate the propane-powered floor buffers they use; they constantly get nauseous from the fumes. Despite their complaints, the school district has not changed the equipment. ■

and removers, hair dyes and rinses, and hair straighteners are used, often without adequate ventilation. Building trade shops, auto body shops, and printing operations in schools are in effect industrial settings, except that the equipment is often older and the local ventilation is more likely not to function.

Occupational Hazards of Other School Staff

Custodial and Maintenance Workers

The work-related hazards and associated injuries and illnesses for custodians may be more obvious but are overlooked in many schools. Deferred maintenance and tight budgets translate into fewer custodial employees, no new equipment, and shortcuts in operations and maintenance.

School custodians sustain a wide range of potentially hazardous exposures, including quaternary ammonia, phenols, disinfectants, corrosives,

pesticides, solvents, dust, mold, and other bioaerosols. These exposures may increase the risk of work-related asthma, dermatitis, and nervous system symptoms. When training is scant or nonexistent, custodians may mix incompatible chemicals with tragic effect. To this day, some custodians still mix bleach with ammonia; some have died from the released chlorine gas, while others have suffered severe lung damage.

Musculoskeletal injuries and back strain are common among custodial and maintenance workers. Lifting furniture and books and handling heavy, often antiquated, equipment contribute to these problems. Falls, slips, and trips are common and may result in injuries. Women in these jobs are especially at risk because most equipment—from vacuums, mops, and buckets to floor buffers—is designed for men.

Food Service Workers

Food service work is performed primarily by women, yet it requires frequent and heavy lifting and transferring of food, dishes, and commercial utensils. The work also requires standing for long hours on hard surfaces. As a result, these workers have high rates of musculoskeletal injuries, affect-

---

▧ *30.2. A food service worker*

On a typical day, Mary L. prepares breakfast and lunch for more than 3000 students in her school and two neighboring schools. She may bake muffins, which requires lifting large trays in and out of the oven. If chili is on the menu that day, she stirs hundreds of pounds of it and ladles it into shipping containers. The kitchen is hot, the grill exhaust does not work, and the floor is always wet because the dishwasher leaks. The task she hates most is hauling the frozen food into the walk-in freezer; it's cold, and lifting those heavy boxes onto high shelves is difficult. She goes home totally exhausted after standing on her feet for nearly all of her eight hours. She has to lie down to recover so that she can prepare food for her own family. Her back, shoulders, and feet have hurt for fifteen years, and her doctor has told her that she has two bad discs in her back. She cannot find any shoes that help. Despite the aches, pains, occasional burns, and cuts, she loves her job and she loves the students. ▧

---

omatic hydrocarbons (PAHs), even if there is local exhaust ventilation (Vainiotalo and Matveinen 1993). The health consequences of exposure to these concentrations of airborne impurities in a commercial kitchen have not yet been documented.

Secretaries and Clerical Staff

School secretaries and clericals confront the new age of technology with mixed emotions. They welcome the computers. However, the computers often do not come with modern workstations. Instead they frequently sit on old desks without keyboard trays. Also with the computers come expectations of far higher workloads, including record keeping and word processing. Unfortunately, staff members are often excluded from the selection of software and inadequately trained for using new software (fig. 30.2).

School secretaries fit the classic stress model of high demand and low control. They need to meet the demands of administrators and teachers, act as crisis managers during incidents such as student medical emergencies, monitor students with behavioral problems, and deal with angry parents.

---

ing the back, shoulders, and upper and lower extremities (Huang et al., 1988). Heavy lifting, awkward postures, and the repetitive use of the hands and arms are associated with these disorders (Bernard 1997).

Food service workers face additional hazards. School kitchens are frequently hot and poorly ventilated, and the heat and humidity can reach extreme levels in the warmer months. Even acclimated workers may complain of heat stress symptoms. Food service workers typically are responsible for cleaning their ovens, grills, and fryers. The work often involves using heavy-duty degreasers and corrosive oven cleaners in spaces with no ventilation. Machine guarding is often missing from slicers and other cutting equipment, increasing the risk of serious cuts or even amputation. Finally, food service workers are frequently exposed to cooking fumes. Kitchens that use ordinary frying methods, such as grilling meats and deep-frying foods, may have high air levels of fat aerosols including acroleins, formaldehyde, and polycyclic ar-

---

▧ *30.3. A secretary*

Elaine P., a school secretary, can identify many stressful aspects of her job. She has to juggle competing demands from the principal, teachers, and other staff members, deal with irate parents, and manage misbehaving students sent to the office, alongside her routine responsibilities of keeping records and supporting the administration. Elaine never really gets a break, and she has been followed to the bathroom by a principal who needed something completed right away. She has a headache most afternoons, perhaps from the copy machines near her desk in a small, unventilated alcove. She has also started to develop muscle strains and sprains from cradling the phone while she types on the computer keyboard on her desk. She inherited her chair when she started working for the district 17 years ago. ▧

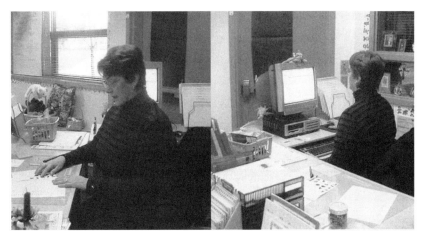

Figure 30.2. Comfort may be improved if the writing surface and the computer keyboard are at different heights. (Photo by Diane Tien.)

School secretaries often find themselves in the position of working "informal" overtime with no compensation to catch up with paperwork at the end of the day. These conditions can increase the risk of stress and stress-related conditions.

Bus Drivers and Garage Mechanics

There are no data available on the occupational health of school bus drivers or school garage mechanics. However, studies of urban bus drivers and garage mechanics help identify potential hazards for these workers. Both school bus drivers and mechanics are potentially exposed to diesel fumes, a mixture of particulates and gases that increases the risk of cancer, cardiovascular and respiratory disease, and other diseases (U.S. Environmental Protection Agency 2002; Kagawa 2002). The highest exposure to diesel fumes occurs in yards in the morning, when buses are often idle for long periods of time before the morning runs. Other exposures occur during the repair of engines, on the streets and highways, and while idling at schools.

School bus drivers share the same exposure to musculoskeletal hazards as their urban bus driver counterparts. The most common hazards described for them include whole-body vibration, sedentary positions, twisting the neck and shoulders, and forceful movements to operate controls (Krause et al. 1997). The primary complaints related to these exposures include lower back pain and injury (herniated discs), sciatica, neck and shoulder pain, and hand problems.

■ *30.4. A bus driver*

Evelyn T. is leaving her bus driver job after 22 years because her asthma is becoming difficult to manage, and she and her physician believe that this difficulty may be job related. Every morning she arrives at the bus yard, where she is exposed to the diesel exhaust of more than 50 buses idling for over an hour. Idling the bus during the winter months so that students do not have to ride on a cold bus exposes her to yet more exhaust. Her inhaler gives only temporary relief. Although she can cope with the other hazards of her job, she has been attacked twice by special education students, resulting on one occasion in an injury that required two lost days of work, and her back pain is manageable but worrisome. However, the asthma will make her leave the job a few years before she had planned. ■

Occupational Health and Safety Programs for Schools

Very few school systems have occupational health and safety programs. There are a few barriers to overcome before meaningful and effective programs can be put in place, some of which are attitudinal. First, schools must be recognized as workplaces as well as institutions of learning. Currently, the Occupational Safety and Health Act applies to public employees in only 26 states and jurisdictions—the federally certified "state plan" states that have opted to cover their public employees and to implement OSHA standards in public workplaces, including schools. Without this protection, public school employees may have no enforceable rights to safe and healthy workplaces. State policy that recognizes the occupational health needs of public employees would do much to ensure their protection.

School systems must also understand that they lose more by ignoring work-related problems than by trying to resolve them. Passing on the costs of work-related illness or injury to health insurance plans ultimately taxes the system's budget. Paying substitutes or losing skilled workers also constitutes a cost to the school system.

School systems should implement health and safety programs under the direction of staff members who are knowledgeable about occupational safety and health strategies and can assess hazards and make recommendations for controls. Industrial hygiene and safety management techniques can be readily applied to schools. The standard approach is based on a hierarchy of controls, including environmental changes (through engineering controls), personal protective equipment, and administrative procedures.

The most effective method for controlling hazardous exposures is the use of environmental changes. For example, substitution of a hazardous cleaning material with a safe one would eliminate the danger from the environment. Similarly, engineering controls separate workers from hazardous exposures by means of a physical or mechanical barrier. An efficient, well-maintained HVAC system that provides sufficient filtered air is an example of an engineering approach to indoor air quality. Other engineering controls would include acoustical barriers to reduce noise levels and local exhaust ventilation in technical career shops, kitchens, and bus garages.

The second tier in the hierarchy of controls is personal protective equipment (PPE) such as gloves, safety glasses, earplugs, and hardhats. This approach is less effective and desirable than environmental change because it permits the continued presence of hazards in the environment, it is more prone to failure, and workers often dislike using PPE. However, PPE is appropriate when environmental changes cannot be accomplished. In schools, science teachers should be provided with the appropriate PPE for the types of chemicals they use.

The third tier in the hierarchy of controls is administrative controls. One example is rotating workers through exposures, thus removing them for periods of time to reduce their cumulative exposure. This is the least effective way to protect them because there may be substantial uncontrolled exposures during the times of exposure. However, this method may have some merit in school settings. For example, if a hot kitchen cannot be effectively cooled, food service workers should be given ample breaks (and water) to prevent heat stress.

In addition to designating knowledgeable staff to oversee the occupational safety and health program, schools can take several steps toward effective program development. These include partnerships, policies, data collection, and training.

Two kinds of partnerships are important: those within the school system and those with external partners. Within the school system, a process that includes all stakeholders—administrators, teachers, staff, health-care professionals, parents—can be effective. Some school systems have joint labor-management health and safety committees that fulfill this role. External partnerships with qualified occupational health clinics are also very useful; these facilities can provide assistance with data collection, clinical evaluations, training, and other functions. In many parts of the country, academic medical centers offer this resource.

Policies can be adopted by a board of education to help promote safe and healthy workplaces. For example, a board might adopt relevant OSHA standards for record keeping, hazard communication, protection from bloodborne pathogens, and other issues.

Data collection is essential to effective occupational safety and health management to help identify problems, target resources effectively, and monitor the success of interventions. A standard public health approach is surveillance for on-the-job injuries and suspected work-related illnesses. This requires establishing an effective reporting system, with defined criteria for reporting, that all school staff are trained and encouraged to use. An annual assessment or analysis of occupational illnesses and injuries should be conducted, and reports made to key staff.

Finally, employees should receive training on the identification and prevention of work-related illnesses and injuries. This instruction should be tailored to the job and any associated hazards. Employees who are trained should acquire knowledge of job hazards and control strategies, attitudes that include alertness to hazards and an orientation toward safety, and behaviors such as reporting hazards.

These steps are fairly universal approaches to establishing occupational health and safety programs. In addition to these generic tactics, certain unique components would be very appropriate in schools that confront specific challenges. Examples include infectious diseases, asthma, ergonomics, and violence.

Infectious Diseases

School districts should establish infectious disease policies for employees, including providing information and immunizations. Schools should strongly consider offering teachers and staff standard immunizations as recommended by the Advisory Committee on Immunization Practice at no cost since they are routinely exposed to communicable diseases. Information is especially vital to women of child-bearing age and employees with compromised immune function. As new immunizations such as the acellular pertussis vaccine become licensed for adults, these should be offered to staff.

Asthma

An asthma monitoring and management program for both staff and students would be beneficial (see chapter 28). Asthma is prevalent in children, and as mentioned earlier, school employees show an excess occurrence as well. Schools should monitor asthmatics to ascertain whether their conditions are exacerbated by conditions in schools and try to accommodate those staff members as well as assisting them with control strategies.

Ergonomics

As chapter 6 points out, ergonomics programs for staff members can help reduce chronic back pain and other musculoskeletal disorders. The school employees most at risk include food service workers, custodians and maintenance personnel, bus drivers, school secretaries, and those special education paraprofessionals or aides who physically lift and handle students with disabilities. Components of an ergonomics program include assessment of risk factors (e.g., awkward posture, repetitive motion, heavy lifting, keying, unequal loading, whole body vibration) in each job category. Approaches to eliminating ergonomic hazards can be designed and implemented with the assistance of the school employees, who can help evaluate new equipment and software for ergonomic "friendliness." Bus drivers might evaluate the seats and controls of new buses; custodians might evaluate buffers, vacuums, buckets, and waste collection systems, special education assistants and health aides could test new lifts for transferring children to and from wheelchairs and changing tables, and clerical staff could help choose the optimal workstations for their needs.

School violence prevention programs have become more prevalent since the tragic Columbine High School shooting incident. In attempting to reduce violence among students, these programs should focus both on student welfare and on the impact of assaults (or even threats of violence) on staff. The United Federation of Teachers in New York City has established a program that collects data on assaults on teachers, paraprofessionals, nurses, and school secretaries (the union's members) and reports these data to the New York City Board of Education. It also provides assistance to assault victims. An experienced team assists the victim in finding medical care, filing workers' compensation claims and/or criminal charges if appropriate, and reintegrating into the school (counseling and support) when the teacher is ready to return. This program is a model for other locations.

References

Al-Khan A, Caligiuri A, Apuzzio J. 2003. Parvovirus B-19 infection during pregnancy. Infect Dis Obstet Gynecol 11(3):175–179.

American National Standards Institute and Acoustical Society of America. 2002. Acoustical performance criteria, design requirements, and guidelines for schools. S 12.60-2002. Melville, NY: Author.

Anderson H, Hanrahan L, Schirmer J, Higgins D, Sarow P. 1991. Mesothelioma among employees with likely contact with in-place asbestos containing material. Madison: Wisconsin Division of Health.

Arundel AV, Sterling EM, Ginn JH, Sterling TD. 1986. Indirect health effects of relative humidity in indoor environments. Environ Health Perspect 65: 351–361.

Belkic K, Landsbergis PA, Schnall PL, Baker D. 2004. Is job strain a major source of cardiovascular disease? Scand J Work Environ Health 30(2):85–128.

Bernard BP, ed. 1997. Musculoskeletal disorders and workplace factors: A critical review of epidemiologic evidence for work-related musculoskeletal disorders of the neck, upper extremity, and low back. Cincinnati, OH: National Institute of Occupational Safety and Health.

Brennan M, Strebel P, George H, Yih WK, et al. 2000. Evidence for transmission of pertussis in schools, Massachusetts, 1996: Epidemiologic data supported by pulsed-field gel electrophoresis studies. J Infect Dis 181:210–215.

Brundage JF, Scott RM, Lednar WM, Smith DW, Miller RN. 1988. Building-associated risk of febrile acute respiratory diseases in army trainees. J Am Med Assoc 259:2108–2112.

Cardoso MR, Cousens SN, de Goes Siqueira LF. 2004. Crowding: Risk factor or protective factor for lower respiratory disease in young children? BMC Public Health 4(1):19.

Duhart DT. 2001. National Crime Victimization Survey: Violence in the workplace, 1993–1999. NCJ 190076. Washington, DC: U.S. Department of Justice, Bureau of Justice Statistics, Office of Justice Programs. Available: http://www.ojp.usdoj.gov/bjs/pub/pdf/vw99.pdf.

Everett S, Jacobson M, Halldorson S, Savoini D, Supalla B, Goodykoontz S. 2004. School-associated pertussis outbreak: Yavapai County, Arizona, September 2002–February 2003. Mortal Morbid Weekly Rept 53(10):216–219.

Farber BA. 1991. *Crisis in education: Stress and burnout in the American teacher.* San Francisco, CA: Jossey-Bass.

Gillespie SM, Cartter MI., Asch S, Rokos JB, Gary GW, Tsou CJ, et al. 1990. Occupational risk of human parvovirus B19 infection for school and day-care personnel during an outbreak of erythema infectiosum. J Am Med Assoc 263(15):2096–2097.

Hashemi L, Webster BS. 1996. Non-fatal workplace violence workers' compensation claims. J Occup Environ Med 40(6):561–567.

Huang J, Ono Y, Shibata E. 1988. Occupational exposure: Musculo-skeletal disorders in lunch centre workers. Ergonomics 31(1):65–75.

Jaakkola JJ, Heinonen OP. 1995. Shared office space and the risk of the common cold. Eur J Epidemiol 11:213–216.

Jennett HK, Harris SL, Mesibov GB. 2003. Commitment to philosophy, teacher efficacy, and burnout among teachers of children with autism. J Autism Developmental Disord 33:583–593.

Kagawa J. 2002. Health effects of diesel exhaust emissions: A mixture of air pollutants of worldwide concern. Toxicology 181–182:349–353.

Karasek RA. 1979. Job demands, job decision latitude, and mental strain: Implications for job redesign. Admin Sci Q 24:285–307.

Keeler ML. 1992. Human parvovirus B-19: Not just a pediatric problem. J Emerg Med 10(1):39–44.

Krause N, Ragland DR, Greiner BA. 1997. Physical workplace and ergonomic factors associated with the prevalence of back and neck pain in urban transit workers. Spine 22:2117–2126.

Levenson RL, Jr., Memoli M, Flannery RB, Jr. 2000. Coping with psychological aftermath of school violence: The teacher and the assaulted staff action program. Int J Emerg Mental Health 2(2):105–112.

Levin SM, Selikoff IJ. 1991. Radiological abnormalities and asbestos exposure among custodians of the New York City Board of Education. Ann NY Acad Sci 643:530–539.

Lilienfeld DE. 1991. Asbestos associated pleural mesothelioma in school teachers: A discussion of four cases. Ann NY Acad Sci 643:454–486.

Lyons B, Stanwyck C, McCauley M. 2004. Vaccination coverage among children entering school, United States, 2003–2004 school year. Mortal Morbid Weekly Rept 53:1041–1043.

Messing K, Seifert AM, Escalona E. 1997. The 120-s minute: Using analysis of work activity to prevent psychological distress among elementary school teachers. J Occup Health Psychol 2:45–62.

Myatt TA, Johnston SL, Zuo Z, Wand M, Kebadze T, Rudnick S, et al. 2004. Detection of airborne rhinovirus and its relation to outdoor air supply office environments. Am J Respir Crit Care Med 169: 1187–1190.

Naides SJ. 1993. Parvovirus B19 infection. Rheum Dis Clin North Am 19(2):457–475.

National Institute for Occupational Safety and Health, Division of Respiratory Disease Studies. 2003. Work-related lung disease surveillance report 2002. Atlanta: Centers for Disease Control and Prevention.

National Toxicology Program. 2002. *Report on Carcinogens,* 10th ed. Research Triangle Park, NC: Author.

New York State Commission on Ventilation. 1923. The prevalence of respiratory diseases among children in schoolrooms ventilated by various methods. In *Ventilation: Report of the New York State Commission on Ventilation.* New York: Dutton.

Nygard I, Linder M. 1997. Thirst at work: An occupational hazard? Int Urogynecol J 8:340–343.

Oliver LC, Sprince NL, Green R. 1991. Asbestos-related abnormalities in school maintenance personnel. Ann NY Acad Sci 643:521–529.

Schonfeld IS. 1996. Relation of negative affectivity to self-reports of job stressors and psychological outcomes. J Occup Health Psychol 1(4):397–412.

Schonfeld IS. 2001. Stress in 1st-year women teachers: The context of social support and coping. Genet Soc Gen Psychol Monogr 127(2):133–168.

Smith E, Gray SD, Dove H, Kirchner L, Heras H. 1997. Frequency and effects of teachers' voice problems. J Voice 11(1):81–87.

Smith E, Kirchner HL, Taylor M, Hoffman H, Lemke JH. 1998. Voice problems among teachers: Differences by gender and teaching characteristics. J Voice 12(3):328–334.

Steptoe, A. 2000. Stress, social support, and cardiovascular activity over the working day. Int J Psychophysiol 37(3):299–308.

Steptoe A, Cropley M. 2000. Persistent high job demands and reactivity to mental stress predict future ambulatory blood pressure. J Hypertension 18(5):581–586.

Steptoe A, Cropley M, Griffith J, Kirschbaum C. 2000. Job strain and anger expression predict early morning elevations in salivary cortisol. Psychosom Med 62(2):286–292.

Steptoe A, Cropley M, Joekes K. 1999. Job strain, blood pressure, and responsivity to uncontrollable stress. J Hypertension 17:193–200.

U.S. Environmental Protection Agency. 2002. Health assessment document for diesel exhaust. EPA/600/8-90/057F. Washington, DC: Author.

Vainiotalo S, Matveinen K. 1993. Cooking fumes as a hygienic problem in the food and catering industries. Am Ind Hygiene Assoc J 54(7):376–382.

Whelan EA, Lawson CC, Grajewski B, Petersen MR, Pinkerton LE, Ward EM, et al. 2002. Prevalence of respiratory symptoms among female flight attendants and teachers. Med Lav 93:396–397.

Williams IM. 2001. Elementary school teachers' working comfort while using computers in school and home. Presentation. International Ergonomics Association (IEA). Available: http://education.umn.edu/kls/ecee/pdfs/ElementarySchoolTeachersinger.pdf.

Zanardi L, Pascual FB, Bisgard K, Murphy T, Wharton M. 2002. Pertussis: United States, 1997–2000. Mortal Morbid Weekly Rept 51(04):73–76.

Index